SALEM HEALTH

COMPLEMENTARY
& ALTERNATIVE
MEDICINE

SALEM HEALTH

COMPLEMENTARY
& Alternative Medicine

Volume 2

Editors

Richard P. Capriccioso, M.D.
University of Phoenix

Paul Moglia, Ph.D.
South Nassau Communities Hospital

SALEM PRESS
A Division of EBSCO Publishing
Ipswich, Massachusetts   Hackensack, New Jersey

Note to Readers

The material presented in *Salem Health: Complementary and Alternative Medicine* is intended for broad informational and educational purposes. Readers who suspect that they or someone they know has any disorder, disease, or condition described in this set should contact a physician without delay. This set should not be used as a substitute for professional medical diagnosis. Readers who are undergoing or about to undergo any treatment or procedure described in this set should refer to their physicians and other health care providers for guidance concerning preparation and possible effects. This set is not to be considered definitive on the covered topics, and readers should remember that the field of health care is characterized by a diversity of medical opinions and constant expansion in knowledge and understanding.

Library of Congress Cataloging-in-Publication Data

Complementary & alternative medicine / editors, Richard P. Capriccioso, Paul Moglia.
   p. ; cm. — (Salem health)
Complementary and alternative medicine
Includes bibliographical references and indexes.
   ISBN 978-1-58765-870-9 (set : alk. paper) — ISBN 978-1-58765-871-6 (vol. 1) — ISBN 978-1-58765-872-3 (vol. 2) — ISBN 978-1-58765-873-0 (vol. 3) — ISBN 978-1-58765-874-7 (vol. 4)
   I. Capriccioso, Richard P. II. Moglia, Paul. III. Title: Complementary and alternative medicine. IV. Series: Salem health (Ipswich, Mass.)
   [DNLM: 1. Complementary Therapies–Encyclopedias–English. WB 13]
   LCclassification not assigned
   615.503–dc23

2011051023

Contents

Contents

Complete List of Contents

Volume 1

Volume 2

Volume 3

Complete List of Contents

Volume 4

Complete List of Contents

SALEM HEALTH

COMPLEMENTARY
& Alternative Medicine

D

Damiana

CATEGORY: Herbs and supplements

RELATED TERM: *Turnera diffusa*

DEFINITION: Natural plant product used to treat specific health conditions.

PRINCIPAL PROPOSED USE: Increase male sexual capacity

OTHER PROPOSED USES: Asthma, depression, difficulty achieving orgasm in women, digestive problems, impotence in men, menstrual disorders, respiratory diseases

OVERVIEW

The herb damiana has been used in Mexico for some time as a male aphrodisiac. Classic herbal literature of the nineteenth century describes it as a tonic, or general body strengthener.

THERAPEUTIC DOSAGES

The proper dosage of damiana is 2 to 4 grams taken two to three times daily, or as directed on the label.

THERAPEUTIC USES

Damiana continues to be a popular aphrodisiac for males. However, if it does work, the effect appears to be rather mild. No scientific trials have been reported.

Damiana is also sometimes said to be helpful for treating asthma and other respiratory diseases, depression, digestive problems, menstrual disorders, and various forms of sexual dysfunction, such as impotence in men and inability to achieve orgasm in women. However, there is no real evidence that it works for any of these conditions.

Like the herb uva ursi, damiana contains arbutin, although at a concentration about ten times lower. Arbutin is a urinary antiseptic, but the levels present in damiana are probably too small to make this herb a useful treatment for bladder infections.

SAFETY ISSUES

Damiana appears to be safe at the recommended dosages. It appears on the U.S. Food and Drug Administration's Generally Recognized as Safe (GRAS) list and is widely used as a food flavoring. The only common side effect of damiana is occasional mild gastrointestinal distress. However, because damiana contains low levels of cyanide-like compounds, excessive doses may be dangerous. Safety in young children, pregnant or nursing women, or those with severe liver or kidney disease is not established.

EBSCO CAM Review Board

FURTHER READING

Duke, J. A. *CRC Handbook of Medicinal Herbs.* Boca Raton, Fla.: CRC Press, 1985.

Newall, C., L. A. Anderson, and J. D. Phillipson. *Herbal Medicines: A Guide for Health-Care Professionals.* London: Pharmaceutical Press, 1996.

Willard, T. *The Wild Rose Scientific Herbal.* Calgary, Alta.: Wild Rose College of Natural Healing, 1991.

See also: Asthma; Herbal medicine; Sexual dysfunction in men; Uva ursi.

Dance movement therapy

CATEGORY: Therapies and techniques

RELATED TERMS: Dance, dance therapy, bodily movement therapy, movement therapy

DEFINITION: A body-based technique to enhance emotional and physical well-being.

PRINCIPAL PROPOSED USES: Depression, eating disorders, physical therapy, psychotic disorders, schizophrenia

OTHER PROPOSED USES: Autism, head injuries, learning and mental disabilities

OVERVIEW

One of the creative arts therapies, dance movement therapy is defined by the American Dance Therapy Association (ADTA) as "the psychotherapeutic use of movement as a process that furthers the emotional, cognitive, social and physical integration of the individual." Many practitioners consider Marian Chace to be the pioneer of dance movement therapy.

Chace began teaching dance in Washington, D.C., after retiring from the Denishawn Dance Company in 1930. She had noticed that some of her students were more interested in the emotions that they felt while dancing than in learning the techniques of modern dance. Intrigued, Chace learned that they valued the catharsis of feelings they experienced while dancing. Some of these students were concurrently undergoing traditional psychotherapy with psychiatrists, who noticed that their patients felt more refreshed and unburdened after their lessons with Chace. The psychiatrists began to send other patients to Chase's classes, and they noted the positive change that dance appeared to inspire.

Chace was then invited to volunteer with those considered too disturbed to participate in therapy. The nonverbal approach of dance elicited improvement, and by the 1950s, Chace's methods were subjected to serious study.

MECHANISM OF ACTION

The principle behind dance movement therapy is that dance is the most fundamental of all the arts, requiring no external materials. It is a communication of the psyche, expressed through self-directed movement. Dance movement therapists assume that the body, mind, and spirit are interconnected, allowing for direct access to feelings, cognition, and behavior. Bodily movement simultaneously provides the means of both intervention and assessment in this mode of therapy. Participants are encouraged to choose their own music and to begin moving to it in their own ways.

The dance movement therapist begins by empathically mirroring the participant's actions, and then extends and expands them into a nonverbal statement of emotion that can release the participant from any fixed muscular patterns. Next, participants are gently coaxed into a circle and led into movement extensions with verbal narration. Once the group is a more cohesive unit, the therapist notes the styles of the participants and leads into the development of a global psychological theme for the session, with questions to shed light on individual conflicts. The session ends with communal movement from all participants to provide closure.

Early Thoughts on Dance as Therapy

Before developing dance movement therapy in the 1940s, Marian Chace reflected on how she came to understand the significance of nonverbal communication in therapeutics.

Out of observing the non-verbal communication of individuals taking their first classes, I began to understand and meet the needs for which they were asking help. Instead of feeling frustration when they lagged behind the more adequate pupils, I tried to empathize with them as people.

Obviously, my teaching was undergoing change. Unconsciously, my centering for all pupils became a support of them as people as well as dancers. While the students at the school found satisfaction in various ways, I think of the whole period of the 1930s for me as one of intense absorption in learning about non-verbal communication.

Source: Marian Chace, quoted in *Marian Chace: Her Papers*, edited by Harris Chaiklin, 1975. 15-16.

USES AND APPLICATIONS

Chace believed that dance served as a medium for communication for the most disturbed psychiatric patients, such as schizophrenics. However, today dance movement therapists work with groups and individuals of all ages who have widely differing problems. They may work in private practice, wellness clinics, rehabilitation centers, nursing homes, and schools. The focus on positive body movement may help clients with eating disorders and body issues. The nonverbal conflict revelations and resolutions may help dysfunctional families develop communication skills, and those who have been through trauma such as abuse or violence may find a new mode of constructive coping. The physical therapy uses of dance movement therapy are self-evident, and it is often used with the frail and elderly.

Disease prevention and health promotion, a new area of specialization in dance movement therapy, is beginning to be used in programs for people with chronic medical conditions such as cardiovascular disease, chronic pain, and hypertension. Research on the effectiveness of dance movement therapy has investigated certain settings, such as prisons and homeless shelters, and specific populations, such as the mentally disabled, suicidal persons, the visually and hearing impaired, and autistic persons.

SCIENTIFIC EVIDENCE

A 1993 study suggested that dance movement therapy improved balance, rhythmic discrimination, mood, social interaction, and energy level in older persons with neurological damage. A 2010 study evaluated the influence of dance movement therapy on the perception of well-being in women with chronic fatigue syndrome. Seven persons attended a four-month program and were tested both before and after the program. Their perceptions of physical well-being improved by an average of 25.8 percent, and their perceptions of psychological well-being improved by 22.7 percent.

A 2008 dance movement therapy intervention group of persons with dementia improved in a task of visual-spatial ability and planning, whereas the control group either remained unchanged or deteriorated slightly. Dance movement therapy appears to be effective in treating cognition and self-care abilities in dementia.

A 2006 study assessed mildly depressed adolescents after twelve weeks of dance movement therapy. All self-report measurements of distress decreased significantly after the twelve weeks. In addition, both serotonin and dopamine levels increased in that group. Thus, dance movement therapy may help to decrease depression both by relieving perceptions of distress and by lowering neurotransmitter levels.

CHOOSING A PRACTITIONER

Chace helped to organize the ADTA in 1966 and served as its first president. The ADTA has a code of ethics and standards for professional clinical practice, education, and training. Course work for dance movement therapy includes classes on theory and practice, observation and analysis, human development, psychopathology, cultural diversity, research, and group therapy. The ADTA maintains a registry of dance movement therapists who meet these stringent standards.

Persons certified (as Dance Therapist Registered, or DTR) have master's degrees and seven hundred hours of supervised clinical internship. The certification Academy of Dance Therapists Registered (ADTR) is then awarded with the completion of 3,640 hours of supervised clinical internship. Persons interested in dance movement therapy can find qualified practitioners through the ADTA Web site (http://www.adta.org).

SAFETY ISSUES

There are no known safety issues with dance movement therapy.

Eugenia M. Valentine, Ph.D.

FURTHER READING

American Dance Therapy Association. http://www.adta.org.

Levy, Fran J., ed. *Dance Movement Therapy: A Healing Art.* 2d rev. ed. Reston, Va.: National Dance Association, 2005. The definitive book on the history and development of dance therapy, from its beginnings with Marian Chace to its expansion.

Sadler, Blair L., Annette Ridenour, and Donald M. Berwick. *Transforming the Healthcare Experience Through the Arts.* San Diego, Calif.: Aesthetics, 2009.

See also: Art therapy; Exercise-based therapies; Manipulative and body-based practices; Massage therapy; Mind/body medicine; Music therapy; Progressive muscle relaxation; Tai Chi; Walking, mind/body; Yoga.

Dandelion

CATEGORY: Herbs and supplements
RELATED TERM: *Taraxacum officinale*
DEFINITION: Natural plant product used to treat specific health conditions.
PRINCIPAL PROPOSED USES: None
OTHER PROPOSED USES: Constipation, detoxification, fluid retention, liver support, nutritional supplement

OVERVIEW

The common dandelion, enemy of suburban lawns, is an unusually nutritious food. Its leaves contain substantial levels of vitamins A, C, D, and B complex and of iron, magnesium, zinc, potassium, manganese, copper, choline, calcium, boron, and silicon.

Worldwide, the root of the dandelion has been used for the treatment of a variety of liver and gallbladder problems. Other historical uses of the root and leaves include the treatment of breast diseases, water retention, digestive problems, joint pain, fever, and skin diseases.

The most active constituents in dandelion appear to be eudesmanolide and germacranolide, substances

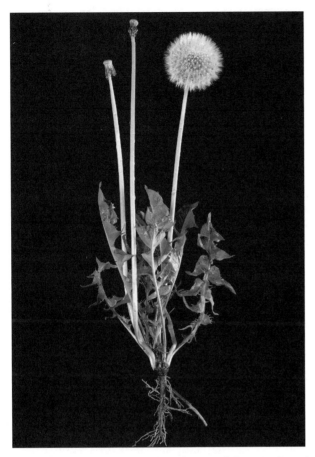

Dandelion roots and leaves have been used for a variety of ailments. (©Igor1509/Dreamstime.com)

unique to this herb. Other ingredients include taraxol, taraxerol, and taraxasterol, along with stigmasterol, beta-sitosterol, caffeic acid, and p-hydroxyphenyl-acetic acid.

THERAPEUTIC DOSAGES

A typical dosage of dandelion root is 2 to 8 grams, three times daily (of dried root); 250 milligrams, three to four times daily of a 5:1 extract; or 5 to 10 milliliters, three times daily of a 1:5 tincture in 45 percent alcohol. The leaves may be eaten in salad or cooked.

THERAPEUTIC USES

Dandelion leaves are widely recommended as a food supplement for pregnant women because of the many nutrients they contain. The scientific basis for any other potential use of dandelion is scanty.

Dandelion leaves have been found to produce a mild diuretic effect, which has led to its proposed use for people who experience mild fluid retention, such as may occur with premenstrual syndrome (PMS). However, no double-blind, placebo-controlled studies have been reported on the effectiveness of dandelion for this purpose.

In the folk medicine of many countries, dandelion root is regarded as a liver tonic, a substance believed to support the liver in an unspecified way. This led to its use for many illnesses traditionally believed to be caused by a "sluggish" or "congested" liver, including constipation, headaches, eye problems, gout, skin problems, fatigue, and boils. Building on this traditional thinking, some modern naturopathic physicians believe that dandelion can help detoxify or clean out the liver and gallbladder. This concept has led to the additional suggestion that dandelion can reduce the side effects of medications processed by the liver and can relieve symptoms of diseases in which impaired liver function plays a role. However, while preliminary studies do suggest that dandelion root stimulates the flow of bile, there is no meaningful scientific evidence that this observed effect leads to any of the foregoing benefits.

Dandelion root is also used like other bitter herbs to improve appetite and treat minor digestive disorders. When dried and roasted, it is sometimes used as a coffee substitute. Finally, dandelion root is sometimes recommended for mild constipation.

SAFETY ISSUES

Dandelion root and leaves are believed to be quite safe, with no side effects or likely risks other than rare allergic reactions. Dandelion is on the GRAS (Generally Recognized as Safe) list of the U.S. Food and Drug Administration and has been approved for use as a food flavoring by the Council of Europe.

However, based on dandelion root's effect on bile secretion, Germany's Commission E has recommended that it not be used by persons with obstruction of the bile ducts or other serious diseases of the gallbladder, and that it be used only under physician supervision by those with gallstones.

Some references state that dandelion root can cause hyperacidity and thereby increase ulcer pain, but this concern has been disputed. Because the leaves contain so much potassium, they probably resupply any potassium lost due to dandelion's mild diuretic effect, although this has not been proven. Persons with known allergies to related plants, such as chamomile and yarrow, should use dandelion with caution.

There are no known drug interactions with dandelion. However, based on what is known about the effects of dandelion root, there might be some risk when combining it with pharmaceutical diuretics or drugs that reduce blood sugar levels. In addition, persons taking the medication lithium should use herbal diuretics such as dandelion leaf only under the supervision of a physician.

Safety in young children, pregnant or nursing women, or those with severe liver or kidney disease has not been established. Also, persons taking diuretic drugs, lithium, insulin, or oral medications that reduce blood sugar levels should use dandelion only under a doctor's supervision.

EBSCO CAM Review Board

FURTHER READING

Leung, A. Y., and S. Foster. *Encyclopedia of Common Natural Ingredients Used in Food, Drugs, and Cosmetics.* 2d ed. New York: Wiley; 1996.

McGuffin, M., ed. *American Herbal Products Association's Botanical Safety Handbook.* Boca Raton, Fla.: CRC Press, 1997.

Murray, M. T. *The Healing Power of Herbs: The Enlightened Person's Guide to the Wonders of Medicinal Plants.* 2d ed. Rocklin, Calif.: Prima, 1995.

Pyevich, D., and M. P. Bogenschutz. "Herbal Diuretics and Lithium Toxicity." *American Journal of Psychiatry* 158 (2001): 1329.

See also: Constipation; Detoxification; Diuretics, loop; Lithium; Liver disease; Premenstrual syndrome (PMS).

Dawkins, Richard

CATEGORY: Biography
IDENTIFICATION: British scientist, professor, and major public critic of alternative medicine
BORN: March 26, 1941; Nairobi, Kenya

OVERVIEW

Richard Dawkins, a British scientist, professor, popular science writer, and filmmaker, is probably best known for his revolutionary ideas about genes, the

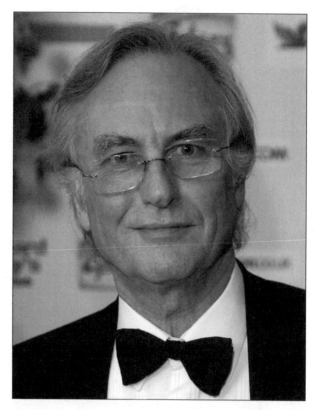

Richard Dawkins. (Getty Images)

basic genetic material of all living things. His books include *The Selfish Gene* (1976) and *The Extended Phenotype* (1983). In these works, Dawkins asserts that these molecular building blocks (genes) not only influence the organism in which they are housed but also impact the world around the organism (that is, as an "extended phenotype"). A large proportion of his writings has focused on defining and redefining this concept.

Dawkins also is critical of religion and related philosophies and practices, arguing that they are inconsistent with scientific evidence. Dawkins is a self-proclaimed atheist and humanist, and based on his collection of work, he relies heavily on logic and the systematic scientific method to critique various "unproven" philosophies and methods. He has also been a vocal critic of traditional types of medicine, including complementary and alternative medicine (CAM), and has defined them as a "set of practices which cannot be tested, [which] refuse to be tested, or [which] consistently fails tests."

Dawkins has written and spoken on this topic for many years, and he continues to be an adversary of many believers in such practices. He wrote the foreword to John Diamond's posthumous book *Snake Oil and Other Preoccupations* (2001), which focuses solely on debunking alternative medicine. In his foreword, Dawkins writes that alternative medicine is harmful, particularly because it serves to distract diseased and ill persons from seeking more successful conventional methods that have been proven effective using scientific means. "There is no alternative medicine," he writes, and "there is only medicine that works and medicine that doesn't work." In addition, he has often cited that the placebo effect is largely responsible for the apparent successes of alternative techniques. That is, any given unproven, alternative medicinal treatment may cause an ailing person to feel better (or actually improve the person's overall health somewhat), despite its having no physiological benefits to the person. To extrapolate from this logic, he is essentially arguing that a person could be given inexpensive sugar pills (or any other placebo), along with the promise of healing, to achieve the same effect as that gained from expensive, ineffective alternative treatments.

In his documentary film *The Enemies of Reason* (2007), Dawkins discusses the many differences between the scientific method and what he terms "superstition." In particular, he discusses many types of CAM, arguing that these methods should be rigorously evaluated by the scientific method before being accepted as useful to the medical community. He also focuses on a discussion of homeopathy, or the use of ultra-diluted substances to treat various ailments. To summarize, Dawkins indicates the placebo effect may also be largely responsible for claimed successes in this line of therapy. In the film, he and others argue that practicing homeopaths use various excuses to avoid testing the validity of their methods, claiming they cannot afford large randomized clinical trials, or that their treatments are individualized to patients, and, therefore, are inappropriate for inclusion in such standardized testing. These issues are largely at the core of the disagreement between proponents and opponents of alternative medicine.

Dawkins also is concerned about the overpopulation of planet Earth. He has been openly critical of religions and cultures that forbid or condemn modern-day contraceptives, and he has been skeptical of "traditional" or "natural" forms of birth control that are relatively ineffective, compared with more modern approaches.

Dawkins was awarded a doctor of science degree by the University of Oxford in 1980. He also has honorary doctorate degrees in science from several other universities around the world. He was elected Fellow of the Royal Society of Literature in 1997 and of the Royal Society in 2001. He is also a member of the Oxford University Scientific Society. In addition to these honors, he has received prestigious awards and other marks of distinction for his contributions to science. Dawkins was a professor at the University of Oxford from 1995 to 2008.

Brandy Weidow, M.S.

FURTHER READING

Dawkins, Richard. *Unweaving the Rainbow: Science, Delusion, and Appetite for Wonder.* New York: Mariner Books, 2000. Dawkins discusses his views on the relationship between science and the arts. This discussion at times crosses over to the shortcomings of what he claims is pseudoscience, including complementary and alternative medicine.

Diamond, John. *Snake Oil and Other Preoccupations.* New York: Vintage Books, 2001. This book aims to debunk practices that fall under the general category of alternative medicine. Dawkins wrote the foreword of this book.

Schrage, Michael. "Revolutionary Evolutionist." *Wired*, July, 1995. Also available at http://www.wired.com/wired/archive/3.07/dawkins_pr.html. The author reviews some of Dawkins's contributions to science and popular culture.

See also: Barrett, Stephen; Clinical trials; History of alternative medicine; Popular practitioners; Pseudoscience; Sampson, Wallace; Scientific method; Spirituality; Traditional healing.

Deer velvet

CATEGORY: Herbs and supplements
RELATED TERMS: Deer antler, velvet antler
DEFINITION: Natural animal product used to treat specific health conditions.
PRINCIPAL PROPOSED USE: Male sexual dysfunction
OTHER PROPOSED USES: Adaptogen, cancer prevention, drug addiction support, immune support, liver protection, osteoarthritis, osteoporosis treat-

ment, pain control, rheumatoid arthritis, sports performance and bodybuilding enhancement

OVERVIEW

Deer velvet is the common name of a product made from the still-growing antlers of deer, during a stage when they are covered in soft velvety hair. New Zealand is a major exporter of deer velvet, shipping tens of millions of U.S. dollars worth to Asia and the United States each year.

According to Asian tradition, deer velvet has tonic properties, meaning that it tends to enhance energy and vitality. More recently, it has been called an adaptogen. This term, invented by early Soviet scientists, refers to a hypothetical treatment that can be described as follows: An adaptogen should help the body adapt to stresses of various kinds, whether heat, cold, exertion, trauma, sleep deprivation, toxic exposure, radiation, infection, or psychological stress. Furthermore, an adaptogen should cause no side effects, should be effective in treating a variety of illnesses, and should help return an organism toward balance regardless of the cause of illness.

The only indisputable example of an adaptogen is a healthful lifestyle. By eating right, exercising regularly, and generally living a life of balance and moderation, a person will increase physical fitness and the ability to resist illnesses of all types. The herb ginseng is widely said to have adaptogenic properties. However, there is no reliable evidence that any herb or supplement actually has adaptogenic properties, and the term is not accepted by conventional medicine.

THERAPEUTIC DOSAGES

A typical dosage of deer antler is 1 gram daily, taken all at once or divided throughout the day.

THERAPEUTIC USES

In the 1960s, an injectable form of deer velvet was used by Japanese physicians to treat male sexual dysfunction. Deer velvet first gained popularity in the United States beginning in the late 1990s. Numerous books and Web sites claim that deer velvet can enhance sexual performance by increasing levels of male hormones. However, these claims are based on extremely preliminary research. Only double-blind, placebo-controlled studies can actually prove a treatment effective, and the one study of this type reported for deer antler failed to find evidence of benefit.

In this study, thirty-two healthy men age forty-five to sixty were given either deer velvet (1 gram [g] daily) or placebo for twelve weeks. The results showed no significant change in sexual function or male hormone levels in the treated group, compared with the placebo group. Also, a six-month, double-blind, placebo-controlled study of 168 people with rheumatoid arthritis failed to find that elk velvet antler enhanced the effectiveness of conventional treatment for rheumatoid arthritis.

Deer antler contains cartilage. On this basis, and based on one study in dogs, cartilage has been promoted as a treatment for osteoarthritis; however, cartilage is not a proven treatment for this condition. Numerous other proposed benefits of deer velvet are based on test-tube studies or other forms of evidence that are too preliminary to rely upon. These claimed benefits include cancer prevention, drug addiction support, immune support, liver protection, osteoporosis treatment, pain control, and sports performance and bodybuilding enhancement.

SAFETY ISSUES

Other than occasional allergic reactions, deer velvet does not appear to cause many obvious, immediate side effects. However, there are concerns based on contamination with the tranquilizers and anesthetics used during the process of removing the horn from the deer. One of the substances used, xylazine, is carcinogenic, and studies have found that low but potentially dangerous levels of xylazine are contained in deer antler products.

Another set of risks derives from the proposed effects of deer velvet: raising male hormone levels. If deer velvet does increase male hormones as it is advertised to do, this could lead to a range of potential problems; however, as noted, there is no real evidence that deer velvet actually does raise such hormones. Finally, safety of deer velvet use in young children, pregnant or nursing women, and people with severe liver or kidney disease has not been established.

EBSCO CAM Review Board

FURTHER READING

Allen, M., et al. "A Randomized Clinical Trial of Elk Velvet Antler in Rheumatoid Arthritis." *Biological Research for Nursing* 9 (2008): 254-261.

Conaglen, H. M., J. M. Suttie, and J. V. Conaglen. "Effect of Deer Velvet on Sexual Function in Men and

Their Partners." *Archives of Sexual Behavior* 32 (2003): 271-278.

See also: Sexual dysfunction in men; Sports and fitness support: Enhancing performance; Stress.

Depression, mild to moderate

CATEGORY: Condition

DEFINITION: Treatment of mild to moderate emotional illness.

PRINCIPAL PROPOSED NATURAL TREATMENTS: Repetitive transcranial magnetic stimulation, St. John's wort

OTHER PROPOSED NATURAL TREATMENTS: Acetyl-L-carnitine, acupuncture, Ayurveda, beta-carotene, chromium, damiana, dehydroepiandrosterone, exercise, fish oil, 5-hydroxytryptophan, folate, ginkgo, hatha yoga, inositol, lavender, massage, multivitamins, nicotinamide adenine dinucleotide, phenylalanine, phosphatidylserine, pregnenolone, S-adenosylmethionine, saffron (*Crocus sativus*), traditional Chinese herbal medicine, tyrosine, vitamin B_6, vitamin B_{12}, zinc

INTRODUCTION

Depression is a common emotional illness that varies widely in its intensity. Many of the natural treatments described in this section have been evaluated in people with major depression of mild to moderate intensity. This apparently contradictory language indicates a level of clinical depression that is significantly more intense than simply feeling "blue," but it is not as disabling as major depression of severe intensity, which usually requires hospitalization.

Typical symptoms of major depression of mild to moderate severity include depressed mood, lack of energy, sleep problems, anxiety, appetite disturbance, difficulty concentrating, and poor stress tolerance. Irritability can also be a sign of depression.

More severe depression includes markedly depressed mood complicated by symptoms such as slowed speech, slowed (or agitated) responses, markedly impaired memory and concentration, excessive (or diminished) sleep, significant weight loss (or weight gain), intense feelings of worthlessness and guilt, recurrent thoughts of suicide, and lack of interest in pleasurable activities. This form of clinical depression is a dangerous and excruciating illness. The emotional structure of the brain has frozen into a pattern of misery that cannot be altered by willpower, a change of scenery, or the most earnest efforts of friends.

One of the earliest successful treatments for major depression was shock therapy. This technique is in some ways analogous to rebooting a computer, and in cases of major depression, its effects were revolutionary. For the first time, a reliable way was available to help people with severe major depression.

However, shock treatment was overused at first and became unpopular as a result of this overuse; ethical concerns over this type of treatment also arose. The accidental discovery of antidepressant drugs provided a route with fewer interventions. The original antidepressants, known as monoamine oxidase inhibitors (MAOIs), could be used with major depression as successfully as shock treatment. However, MAOIs can cause serious and even fatal side effects.

Subsequently, antidepressants with progressively fewer side effects came on the market, but most of them still caused significant fatigue. Because fatigue is one of the most characteristic symptoms of mild to moderate depression, such medications were seldom found useful for anything other than severe depression. With the appearance of the selective serotonin reuptake inhibitor (SSRI) class of antidepressants, however, there was a practical option for depression that was less than catastrophic. In no time, enormous numbers of people began taking Prozac and similar drugs for mild to moderate depression and for the related, but more mild, condition known as dysthymia.

The big advantage of the SSRIs is that they usually do not cause severe fatigue. Many people find them to be entirely free of side effects. However, side effects are not uncommon and include sexual disturbances (such as impotence in men and, in women, the loss of the ability to experience an orgasm), insomnia, and nervousness. The antidepressant drug Wellbutrin is an option for people who have sexual side effects from SSRIs.

PRINCIPAL PROPOSED NATURAL TREATMENTS

Alternative medicine offers numerous options for treating depression, but only one has strong scientific evidence behind it: the herb St. John's wort.

St. John's wort. Numerous double-blind, placebo-controlled studies have examined the effectiveness of

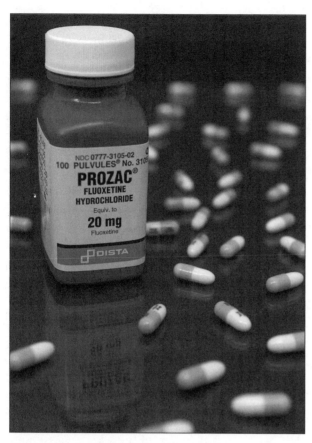

Prozac is used to treat mild to moderate depression. (Bloomberg via Getty Images)

St. John's wort for the treatment of mild to moderate major depression, and most have found the herb more effective than placebo. In addition, several studies have found that St. John's wort is at least as effective as standard antidepressants, including fluoxetine (Prozac), sertraline (Zoloft), citalopram (Celexa), and paroxetine (Paxil).

A 2008 detailed review of twenty-nine randomized, placebo-controlled trials found that St. John's wort was consistently more effective than placebo and just as effective as standard antidepressants. The total number of persons in these trials runs into the several thousands and compares favorably to the evidence base for approved drugs. St. John's wort has also shown some promise for severe major depression, but the evidence is quite limited. St. John's wort alone should never be relied on for the treatment of severe depression.

Much has been made of two double-blind, placebo-controlled trials performed in the United States that failed to find St. John's wort more effective than placebo for mild to moderate depression. However, two studies cannot overturn a body of positive research. Approximately 35 percent of double-blind studies involving pharmaceutical antidepressants have also failed to find the active agent significantly more effective than placebo. As if to illustrate this, in the more recent of the two trials in which St. John's wort failed to prove effective, the drug Zoloft also failed to prove effective. The reason for these negative outcomes is not that Zoloft (or any other drug) does not work. Rather, statistical effects can easily hide the benefits of a drug, especially in a condition like depression in which there is a high placebo effect and no truly precise method for measuring symptoms.

St. John's wort seldom causes immediate side effects. However, it interacts adversely with many critical medications and may present other safety issues.

OTHER PROPOSED NATURAL TREATMENTS

There are many other herbs and supplements that may be helpful in depression, although the evidence for them is not as strong as that for St. John's wort.

Folate. In the body, the vitamin folate works in tandem with the supplement S-adenosylmethionine. Observational studies have suggested that depressed people have reduced folate levels, and some evidence hints that folate supplements may help alleviate depression. In addition, people with particularly low folate levels may respond poorly to antidepressants.

Based on these findings, a study examined the effects of combining folate with antidepressant treatment. This ten-week, double-blind, placebo-controlled trial of 127 people with severe major depression found that folate supplements at a dose of 500 micrograms daily significantly improved the effectiveness of Prozac in female participants. Improvement in male participants was not significant, but blood tests conducted during the study suggest that higher intake of folate might be necessary for men.

S-adenosylmethionine. The supplement S-adenosylmethionine (SAMe) has been widely marketed for the treatment of depression, but the evidence to indicate that it works remains incomplete. Several double-blind, placebo-controlled studies have found SAMe effective in relieving depression; however, most of these studies were small and poorly reported. In addition, many used injected SAMe rather than the oral supplement. Furthermore, the most recent and best-designed of these, a double-blind, placebo-controlled study of 133 depressed people, actually failed to find intravenous SAMe more effective than placebo.

In addition to placebo-controlled studies, several trials have compared SAMe with antidepressant drugs in the tricyclic family. Again, many of these studies were poorly reported and designed, or they used injected SAMe rather than the oral supplement. Of the studies using oral SAMe, the best was a six-week double-blind trial of 281 people with mild depression. The results showed that SAMe was about as effective as the drug imipramine. However, the lack of a placebo group in this trial makes the results less than fully reliable.

Other small studies have also compared the benefits of oral or intravenous SAMe to those of tricyclic antidepressants and have found generally equivalent results, although, again, poor reporting and inadequacies of study design (such as too limited a treatment interval) mar the meaningfulness of the outcomes.

Ginkgo biloba. The herb *Ginkgo biloba* is used mainly for age-related mental decline such as that from Alzheimer's disease. However, during the studies on impaired mental function, researchers frequently observed improvements in mood and relief from symptoms of depression. This incidental discovery led scientists to investigate whether ginkgo might be useful as an antidepressant treatment.

One double-blind study, published in 1990, evaluated this effect in sixty people who had depressive symptoms and signs of dementia. The results showed significant improvements among participants given ginkgo extract instead of placebo.

Another study followed forty depressed people older than age fifty years who had not responded successfully to antidepressant treatment. Those who were given ginkgo showed an average drop of 50 percent in scores on the Hamilton Depression scale, whereas the placebo group showed only a 10 percent improvement.

In 1994, research was reported that may shed light on the mechanism by which ginkgo may reduce depression. This study examined levels of serotonin receptors in rats of various ages. When older rats were given ginkgo, the level of serotonin-binding sites increased. However, the same effect was not observed in younger rats. The researchers theorized that ginkgo may block an age-related loss of serotonin receptors. Reduced receptors for serotonin may mean that the body needs more serotonin to produce a normal effect. Thus, ginkgo might improve the brain's ability to respond to serotonin (in older people). However, this is still highly speculative.

Phenylalanine. Phenylalanine is a naturally occurring amino acid that is consumed in daily diets. There is some evidence that phenylalanine supplements may help reduce symptoms of depression.

Phenylalanine occurs in right-hand and left-hand forms, known as D-phenylalanine and L-phenylalanine, respectively. Some studies have evaluated the D form and others have evaluated a mixture of the D and L forms. Both formulations may provide some measure of relief for symptoms of depression. The mixed form (DLPA) is the one most commonly available in stores.

A 1978 study compared the effectiveness of D-phenylalanine with the antidepressant drug imipramine (taken in daily doses of 100 mg) and found them to be equally effective. A total of sixty people were randomly assigned to either one group or the other and followed for thirty days. D-phenylalanine worked more rapidly, producing significant improvement in only fifteen days.

Another double-blind study followed twenty-seven people, one-half of whom received DL-phenylalanine and the other half imipramine in higher doses of 150 to 200 mg daily. When the participants were reevaluated in thirty days, the two groups had improved by the same amount.

It seems that no properly designed studies comparing phenylalanine to placebo have been conducted. Until these studies are performed, phenylalanine cannot be considered a proven treatment for depression, but it is certainly promising.

5-hydroxytryptophan. When the body manufactures serotonin, it first makes 5-hydroxytryptophan (5-HTP). The theory behind taking 5-HTP as a supplement is that providing the one-step-removed raw ingredient might raise serotonin levels.

There have been several preliminary studies of 5-HTP. The best of these trials was a six-week study of sixty-three people given either 5-HTP (100 mg three times daily) or an antidepressant in the Prozac family (50 mg three times daily). The results showed equal benefit between the supplement and the drug. Actually, 5-HTP worked a little better, but from a mathematical perspective, the difference was not statistically significant. 5-HTP caused fewer and less severe side effects than the drugs in the Prozac family. The only real complaint was occasional mild digestive distress.

Fish oil. It has been suggested that fish oil or the related substance ethyl-EPA (eicosapentaenoic acid) may be helpful for people with depression. For example, a four-week, double-blind, placebo-controlled trial evaluated the potential benefits of fish oil in twenty persons with depression. All but one of the participants were also taking standard antidepressants and had been for a minimum of three months. By week three of the trial, the level of depression had improved to a significantly greater extent in the fish oil group than in placebo group. In addition, a double-blind, placebo-controlled study of seventy people with depression who did not respond well to drug treatment found that the addition of ethyl-EPA (a modified form of a primary ingredient of fish oil) improved the response. Similarly, a double-blind study that evaluated the antidepressant effect of EPA plus fluoxetine found the combination to be more effective than fluoxetine or EPA alone after four weeks of treatment.

In another study, forty people who had committed repeated acts of self-harm were given either fish oil or placebo for twelve weeks. The results indicated that fish oil supplementation markedly reduced measures of suicidal ideation and well-being. However, the best and most recent studies have failed to find benefit.

A meta-analysis (formal statistical review of evidence) published in 2007 failed to find convincing evidence of benefit. The largest (seventy-seven participants) study in this review failed to find fish oil more effective than placebo for treatment of depression. Two subsequent studies enrolling almost three hundred people also failed to find benefit. A third placebo-controlled study found no benefit for fish oil in improving "mental well-being" among 320 older adults without a diagnosis of depression.

Exercise. Exercise may be helpful for depression. In a review published in the journal *Sports Medicine*, researchers analyzed the published research on this subject and concluded that exercise does help. In seven of eight studies reviewed, various forms of exercise proved beneficial for depression. Aerobic exercise, weight training, dancing, and racquetball all produced improvements in mood compared to no exercise.

However, the findings of the one negative study reported in this review cast doubt on the other studies. In this trial, some participants exercised while others took a course at a school and did not exercise. The results: Equal benefits were seen in both groups. This suggests that it may not be the exercise itself that is helping, but rather the general effects of participation in an organized activity.

Another feature of the positive studies also tends to cast doubt on the value of exercise per se in depression. One might think that if it were exercise itself improving mood, the more effectively the participants exercised, the greater the effect. However, no correlation was seen between how much participants increased their physical fitness and how significantly their depression improved.

Repetitive transcranial magnetic stimulation. Repetitive transcranial magnetic stimulation (rTMS) involves the application of low-frequency magnetic pulses to the brain. A growing body of evidence suggests, on balance, that rTMS may be helpful for depression.

In a well-designed trial, for example, seventy people with major depression were given rTMS or sham rTMS in a double-blind setting for two weeks. The results showed that participants who had received actual treatment experienced significantly greater improvement than those receiving sham treatment.

In another trial involving ninety-two older persons whose depression had been linked to poor blood flow to the brain (vascular depression), actual rTMS was significantly more effective than a sham rTMS. Benefits were more notable in younger persons.

In a particularly persuasive piece of evidence, researchers pooled the results of thirty double-blind trials involving 1,164 depressed persons and determined that real rTMS is significantly more effective than sham rTMS.

Two separate studies suggest that rTMS may be an effective additional treatment for the 20 to 30 percent of depressed people for whom conventional drug therapy is not successful. Another group of researchers pooled the results of twenty-four studies involving 1,092 persons and found rTMS to be more effective than sham for treatment-resistant depression. ECT (electroconvulsive therapy, or shock treatment) is often used for people who fall in this category, but rTMS may be an equally effective and less traumatic alternative.

Other herbs and supplements. Like ginkgo, the supplement phosphatidylserine is used mainly for mental decline in the elderly, but it may also offer antidepressant benefits. Limited evidence hints that acetyl-L-carnitine may also offer benefits for the elderly and, potentially, for younger people.

Diets low in vitamin B_6 or vitamin B_{12} have been associated with symptoms of depression. While there is little direct evidence that taking these supplements can help depression, deficiencies of vitamin B_6 are common and vitamin B_{12} deficiencies occur more often with advancing age, so it may be a good idea to take these vitamins on general principles. Nonetheless, a randomized trial involving 299 men older than age seventy-five years found that a daily supplement containing a combination of vitamins B_6, B_{12}, and folate was no better than placebo at preventing depression in a two-year period.

Other micronutrients are also commonly deficient in the elderly. A small study among nursing home residents found that low levels of the mineral selenium was associated with depression. Moreover, eight weeks of mineral supplementation tended to improve the mood of the most seriously depressed persons with low selenium levels.

In a small, double-blind, placebo-controlled study, tincture of lavender enhanced the antidepressant effectiveness of the drug imipramine. Also, the hormone dehydroepiandrosterone has shown some promise for depression.

When depression is characterized by rapid mood changes, excessive sleeping and eating, a sense of leaden paralysis, and extreme sensitivity to negative life events, the condition is called atypical depression. A small (fifteen participants), double-blind, placebo-controlled study found that chromium picolinate might be helpful for this form of depression; however, a much larger study failed to find convincing benefits. One study found weak evidence that zinc supplements may enhance the effectiveness of standard antidepressants.

According to five preliminary double-blind studies, the use of the herb saffron (*Crocus sativus*) at 30 mg daily is more effective than placebo and just as effective as standard treatment for major depression. However, all these studies were small and were performed by a single research group in Iran. Larger studies and independent confirmation will be necessary to determine whether saffron truly is effective for depression. Two studies of somewhat questionable validity reported benefit with an herbal combination used in traditional Chinese herbal medicine (Free and Easy Wanderer Plus).

Beta-carotene, damiana, nicotinamide adenine dinucleotide, pregnenolone, and tyrosine are also sometimes recommended for depression, but there is no meaningful evidence that they work. Also, a double-blind study of forty-two people with severe depression found no improvement with the supplement inositol. Similarly, the use of multivitamin mixtures has failed to prove more effective than placebo.

Alternative therapies. Ayurveda, hatha yoga, massage, and relaxation therapies have all been studied for their effectiveness against depression, but results have been largely unconvincing. Studies on acupuncture as a treatment for depression have shown mixed results. In a review of twenty trials involving two thousand persons with major depression, researchers concluded that real acupuncture's effectiveness was comparable to that of antidepressants but was no more effective than sham acupuncture for this population. Other studies have not found this benefit, though. There is some suggestion that combining acupuncture with fluoxetine (Prozac) may hasten the effect of the antidepressants and allow for a lower dose.

HERBS AND SUPPLEMENTS TO USE ONLY WITH CAUTION

Various herbs and supplements may interact adversely with drugs used to treat depression.

EBSCO CAM Review Board

FURTHER READING

Akhondzadeh Basti, A., et al. "Comparison of Petal of *Crocus sativus* L. and Fluoxetine in the Treatment of Depressed Outpatients." *Progress in Neuro-Psychopharmacology and Biological Psychiatry* 31 (2007): 439-442.

America, A., and L. S. Milling. "The Efficacy of Vitamins for Reducing or Preventing Depression Symptoms in Healthy Individuals: Natural Remedy or Placebo?" *Journal of Behavioral Medicine* 31 (2008): 157-167.

Bretlau, L. G., et al. "Repetitive Transcranial Magnetic Stimulation (rTMS) in Combination with Escitalopram in Patients with Treatment-resistant Major Depression." *Pharmacopsychiatry* 41 (2008): 41-47.

Butler, L. D., et al. "Meditation with Yoga, Group

Therapy with Hypnosis, and Psychoeducation for Long-Term Depressed Mood." *Journal of Clinical Psychology* 64 (2008): 806-820.

Coelho, H. F., K. Boddy, and E. Ernst. "Massage Therapy for the Treatment of Depression." *International Journal of Clinical Practice* 62 (2008): 325-333.

Duan, D. M., et al. "Efficacy Evaluation for Depression with Somatic Symptoms Treated by Electroacupuncture Combined with Fluoxetine." *Journal of Traditional Chinese Medicine* 29 (2009): 167.

Ford, A. H., et al. "Vitamins B$_{12}$, B$_6$, and Folic Acid for Onset of Depressive Symptoms in Older Men." *Journal of Clinical Psychiatry* 69 (2008): 1203-1209.

Grenyer, B. F., et al. "Fish Oil Supplementation in the Treatment of Major Depression." *Progress in Neuro-Psychopharmacology and Biological Psychiatry* 31 (2007): 1393-1396.

Hallahan, B., et al. "Omega-3 Fatty Acid Supplementation in Patients with Recurrent Self-Harm." *British Journal of Psychiatry* 190 (2007): 118-122.

Jorm, A. F., A. J. Morgan, and S. E. Hetrick. "Relaxation for Depression." *Cochrane Database of Systematic Reviews* (2008): CD007142. Available through *EBSCO DynaMed Systematic Literature Surveillance* at http://www.ebscohost.com/dynamed.

Linde, K., M. M. Berner, and L. Kriston. "St. John's Wort for Major Depression." *Cochrane Database of Systematic Reviews* (2008): CD000448. Available through *EBSCO DynaMed Systematic Literature Surveillance* at http://www.ebscohost.com/dynamed.

Zhang, W. J., X. B. Yang, and B. L. Zhong. "Combination of Acupuncture and Fluoxetine for Depression." *Journal of Alternative and Complementary Medicine* 15 (2009): 837

Zhang, Z. J., et al. "The Effectiveness and Safety of Acupuncture Therapy in Depressive Disorders." *Journal of Affective Disorders* 124 (2010): 9-21.

See also: Bipolar disorder; Fish oil; 5-hydroxytryptophan; Folate; Ginkgo; Mental health; Phenylalanine; St. John's wort.

Detoxification

CATEGORY: Therapies and techniques
RELATED TERMS: Colonic irrigation, fasting, high colonics, liver-flushing

DEFINITION: The removal from the body of toxins, such as certain chemicals added to food and the mercury in silver dental fillings.

OVERVIEW

The concept of detoxification plays a major role in many schools of alternative medicine, including Ayurveda, naturopathy, and chiropractic. In this context, the term refers to a belief that toxins accumulated in the body are a major cause of disease and that health can be promoted by removing these toxins through various means.

The toxins referred to in this theory are said to have several major sources and include the following: chemicals added to processed foods, such as preservatives; chemicals that enter the food chain through the use of pesticides, artificial fertilizers, and drugs given to food animals; toxins produced in the intestines from improper digestion; toxins produced in the bloodstream from stress; pharmaceutical medications, nearly all of which are regarded as essentially toxic by proponents of detoxification; toxins present in the general environment, such as automobile exhaust, cigarette smoke, the aluminum in antiperspirants, and the formaldehyde released by new carpet; toxins in water; and toxins introduced through the use of mercury in silver dental fillings.

These toxins are said to cause a wide variety of chronic illnesses, from multiple sclerosis and migraine headaches to cancer and rheumatoid arthritis. Alternative practitioners use various methods with the intention of removing the toxins. One such recommendation has made it into conventional wisdom: drinking at least two quarts (or one-half gallon) of water per day. Other detoxification methods include fasting (on juice, water, fruit, or brown rice), using "cleansing" herbs and supplements (such as olive oil and lemon juice to flush the liver, dandelion root to purge the gallbladder, or psyllium seed to cleanse the colon), taking high colonics, receiving intravenous vitamin C, and removing mercury fillings.

The removal of toxins is often said to cause a temporary flare-up of illness. This reaction is generally interpreted as a positive sign, but also as a call for careful medical management to avoid causing harm on the way to healing.

SCIENTIFIC EVIDENCE

In general, there is little to no scientific support for

detoxification methods. Aside from specific toxicities such as lead or arsenic, medical researchers have observed no general phenomenon of toxification. For this reason, it is difficult to scientifically validate whether detoxification actually works.

Most detoxification approaches essentially remain unexamined, rather than proved or disproved, and rely on reasonable concepts but no hard evidence for their justification. Mercury-filling removal is a typical example. Many alternative practitioners believe that the mercury in silver dental fillings is a cause of numerous health problems and should be removed to prevent or treat disease. However, although it is a matter of indisputable fact that mercury can be toxic, scientific evaluation generally indicates that mercury levels in people with mercury fillings are far below those necessary to cause toxic symptoms. Opponents of the use of mercury respond that some people are sensitive to mercury in very low amounts, and that those people will therefore benefit from filling removal even if they are not experiencing actual toxicity. This could certainly be true. However, despite numerous unreliable anecdotes, there is no meaningful evidence that removing mercury fillings can treat or prevent any disease.

Much the same can be said about the other popular detoxification methods. However, in the case of one form of detoxification, colon cleansing, the theory behind the technique is definitely wrong. According to this nineteenth-century theory, known as colon health or colon hygiene, years of bad diet cause the colon to become caked with layer upon layer of accumulated toxins. This accumulation is said to resemble sedimentary rock. High colonics, which are essentially enemas that reach far into the large intestine, are said to release the accumulated buildup and thereby restore health.

However, physicians have performed colon examinations to search for colon cancer in millions of persons, and their findings do not support the theory. Most of the persons given these examinations are middle-aged or older, and not many have devoted their lives to healthy diets and clean colons. According to the colonic hygiene theory, colon examinations on such persons should turn up concrete-like deposits. However, all that shows up during a typical colonoscopy is fresh, pink flesh. Proponents of colonics do not seem to have assimilated this information, and they continue to recount theories about the colon that were shown to be untrue decades ago.

SAFETY ISSUES

The safety of detoxification methods varies widely. While drinking one quart of water a day is undoubtedly benign and mercury-filling removal is unlikely to be harmful, other methods might be risky. High colonics have occasionally resulted in serious internal injury, and intravenous therapies, being highly invasive, must be handled with a certain degree of sophistication to avoid causing harm. Considering that detoxification has not been proven useful, one should try the more moderate of its various methods if one wants to try detoxification at all.

EBSCO CAM Review Board

FURTHER READING

Cohen, M. "'Detox': Science or Sales Pitch?" *Australian Family Physician* 36 (2007): 1009-1010.

Crinnion, W. J. "The CDC Fourth National Report on Human Exposure to Environmental Chemicals: What It Tells Us About Our Toxic Burden and How It Assists Environmental Medicine Physicians." *Alternative Medicine Review* 15 (2010): 101-109.

Dodes, J. E. "The Amalgam Controversy." *Journal of the American Dental Association* 132 (2001): 348-356.

Ernst, E. "Colonic Irrigation: Therapeutic Claims by Professional Organisations." *International Journal of Clinical Practice* 64 (2010): 429-431.

Genius, S. J., et al. "Human Detoxification of Perfluorinated Compounds." *Public Health* 124 (2010): 367-375.

See also: Ayurveda; Cavity prevention; Chelation therapy; Naturopathy.

Devil's claw

RELATED TERM: *Harpagophytum procumbens*
CATEGORY: Herbs and supplements
DEFINITION: Natural plant product used to treat specific health conditions.
PRINCIPAL PROPOSED USES: Back pain, gout, loss of appetite, mild stomach upset, muscle pain, osteoarthritis, rheumatoid arthritis

OVERVIEW

Devil's claw is a native herb of South Africa, so named because of its rather peculiar appearance. Its large tuberous roots are used medicinally, after being chopped up and dried in the sun for three days. Native South Africans used the herb to reduce pain and fever and to stimulate digestion. Colonists brought devil's claw home to Europe, where it became a popular treatment for arthritis.

THERAPEUTIC DOSAGES

A typical dosage of devil's claw is 750 milligrams three times daily of a preparation standardized to contain 3 percent iridoid glycosides.

THERAPEUTIC USES

In modern Europe, devil's claw has been used to treat all types of joint pain, including osteoarthritis, rheumatoid arthritis, and gout. Devil's claw also is used for soft-tissue (muscle-related or tendon-related) pain. Like other bitter herbs, devil's claw is said to improve appetite and relieve mild stomach upset.

SCIENTIFIC EVIDENCE

The evidence for devil's claw is fairly preliminary, with the largest and most well-designed studies showing marginal benefits at best. Most studies have evaluated the herb for treatment of arthritis.

A double-blind study compared devil's claw to the European drug diacerhein. Diacerhein is a member of a drug category not recognized in the United States: the so-called slow-acting drugs for osteoarthritis (SADOAs). Unlike anti-inflammatory drugs such as ibuprofen, SADOAs do not provide immediate relief, but rather act over a period of weeks to gradually reduce arthritis pain. The supplements glucosamine and chondroitin have been proposed as natural SADOAs.

In this trial, 122 persons with osteoarthritis of the hip or knee (or both) were given either devil's claw or diacerhein for four months. The results showed that devil's claw was as effective as diacerhein, as measured by pain levels, mobility, and need for pain-relief medications (such as acetaminophen or ibuprofen). While this might seem impressive, diacerhein itself is only slightly effective, and in such cases, comparative studies must use a placebo group to achieve reliable results.

Another double-blind study followed eighty-nine persons with rheumatoid arthritis for two months. The group given devil's claw showed a significant decrease in pain intensity and improved mobility. A third double-blind study of fifty people with various

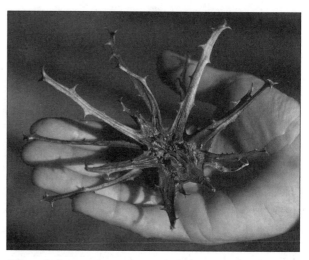

The tuberous roots of devil's claw are used medicinally. (Martin Harvey/Getty Images)

types of arthritis found that ten days of treatment with devil's claw provided significant pain relief. A fourth study compared devil's claw against Vioxx, an anti-inflammatory drug no longer on the market. While it was widely reported that devil's claw was as effective as the drug, the study was too small to produce statistically meaningful results.

Other studies have evaluated devil's claw for treatment of muscular tension and discomfort. One of these studies was a four-week, double-blind, placebo-controlled trial that evaluated sixty-three persons with muscular tension or pain in the back, shoulder, and neck. The results showed significant pain reduction in the treatment group, compared with the placebo group. However, a double-blind study of 197 persons with back pain found devil's claw marginally effective at best. Similarly unimpressive results were seen in an earlier double-blind study of 118 people with back pain.

It remains unclear how devil's claw might work. Some studies have found an anti-inflammatory effect, but others have not. Apparently, the herb does not produce the same changes in prostaglandins as standard anti-inflammatory drugs.

SAFETY ISSUES

Devil's claw appears to be safe, at least for short-term use. In one study, no evidence of toxicity emerged at doses many times higher than recommended. In a review of twenty-eight clinical trials, researchers found no instances where adverse effects were more common than those associated with a placebo. Minor adverse effects, most gastrointestinal in nature, occurred in roughly 3 percent of patients.

Devil's claw is not recommended for people with ulcers. Also, a six-month open study of 630 people with arthritis showed no side effects other than occasional mild gastrointestinal distress. According to one case report, devil's claw might increase the potential for bleeding in persons taking warfarin (Coumadin).

Safety in young children, pregnant or nursing women, or those with severe liver or kidney disease has not been established. Persons taking blood-thinning medications such as warfarin or heparin should note that devil's claw might enhance the effect of these drugs, possibly producing a risk of bleeding.

EBSCO CAM Review Board

FURTHER READING

Chrubasik, S., et al. "A Randomized Double-Blind Pilot Study Comparing Doloteffin and Vioxx in the Treatment of Low Back Pain." *Rheumatology* 42 (2003): 141-148.

Leblan, D., P. Chantre, and B. Fournie. "*Harpagophytum procumbens* in the Treatment of Knee and Hip Osteoarthritis: Four-Month Results of a Prospective, Multicenter, Double-Blind Trial Versus Diacerhein." *Joint, Bone, Spine* 67 (2000): 462-467.

Schulz, V., R. Hansel, and V. E. Tyler, eds. *Rational Phytotherapy: A Physicians' Guide to Herbal Medicine.* 3d ed. New York: Springer, 1998.

Vlachojannis, J., B. D. Roufogalis, and S. Chrubasik. "Systematic Review on the Safety of *Harpagophytum* Preparations for Osteoarthritic and Low Back Pain." *Phytotherapy Research* 22 (2008): 149-152.

See also: Gastrointestinal health; Osteoarthritis; Pain management; Rheumatoid arthritis.

Diabetes

CATEGORY: Condition

RELATED TERMS: Diabetes mellitus, diabetes prevention

DEFINITION: Treatment of the condition that causes blood sugar to reach toxic levels and to damage tissues and major organs.

PRINCIPAL PROPOSED NATURAL TREATMENTS

- *Blood sugar control:* Aloe, chromium (alone or with biotin), ginseng
- *To correct nutritional deficiencies:* Calcium, magnesium, manganese, taurine, vitamin B_{12}, vitamin C, zinc

OTHER PROPOSED NATURAL TREATMENTS

- *Blood sugar control:* Arginine, Ayurvedic combination herbal therapies, berberine (goldenseal), black tea, biotin, bitter melon, caiapo, carnitine, cayenne, cinnamon, cod protein, coenzyme Q_{10}, *Coccinia indica*, dehydroepiandrosterone, fenugreek, garlic, genistein, glucomannan, green tea, guggul, gymnema, holy basil, lipoic acid, magnesium, medium-chain triglycerides, melatonin, milk thistle, niacinamide, nopal cactus, oligomeric proanthocyanidins, onion, ooolong tea, pterocarpus, qigong, *Salacia oblonga, Salvia hispanica*, salt bush, traditional Chinese herbal medicine, vanadium, vitamin E, zinc

HERBS AND SUPPLEMENTS TO USE ONLY WITH CAUTION: Conjugated linoleic acid, *Ginkgo biloba*, rosemary, selenium

INTRODUCTION

Diabetes has two forms. In the type that develops early in childhood (type 1), the insulin-secreting cells of the pancreas are destroyed (probably by a viral infection) and blood levels of insulin drop nearly to zero. However, in type 2 diabetes (usually developing in adults), insulin remains plentiful, but the body does not respond normally to it. (This is only an approximate description of the difference between the two types.) In both forms of diabetes, blood sugar reaches toxic levels, causing injury to many organs and tissues.

Conventional treatment for type 1 diabetes includes insulin injections and careful dietary monitoring. Type 2 diabetes may respond to lifestyle changes alone, such as increasing exercise, losing weight, and improving diet. Various oral medications are also often effective for type 2 diabetes, although insulin injections may be necessary in some cases.

PRINCIPAL PROPOSED NATURAL TREATMENTS

Several alternative methods may be helpful when used under medical supervision as an addition to standard treatment. They may help stabilize, reduce, or eliminate medication requirements or may correct nutritional deficiencies associated with diabetes.

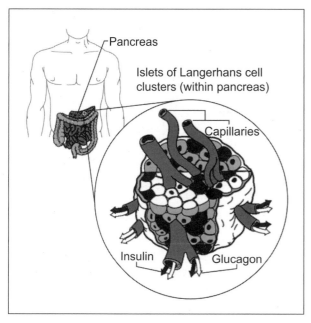

Location of the pancreas, with a section showing the specialized cells (islets of Langerhans) that produce the sugar-metabolizing hormones.

However, because diabetes is a dangerous disease with many potential complications, alternative treatment for diabetes should not be attempted as a substitute for conventional medical care. Other natural treatments may be helpful for preventing and treating complications of diabetes, including peripheral neuropathy, cardiac autonomic neuropathy, retinopathy, and cataracts.

Treatments for improving blood sugar control. The following treatments might be able to improve blood sugar control in type 1 or type 2 diabetes, or both. However, for none of these is the evidence strong. The mere fact of joining a study tends to improve blood sugar control in people with diabetes, even before any treatment is begun. Presumably, the experience of being enrolled in a trial causes participants to watch their diet more closely. This indicates that for diabetes, as for all conditions, the use of a double-blind, placebo-controlled method is essential. Only if the proposed treatment proves more effective than placebo can it be considered to work in its own right.

For those persons in which a natural treatment for diabetes works, it is essential to reduce their medications to avoid hypoglycemia. For this reason, medical supervision is necessary.

Chromium. Chromium is an essential trace mineral that plays a significant role in sugar metabolism. Some evidence suggests that chromium supplementation may help bring blood sugar levels under control in type 2 diabetes, but it is far from definitive.

A four-month study reported in 1997 followed 180 Chinese men and women with type 2 diabetes, comparing the effects of 1,000 micrograms (mcg) chromium, 200 mcg chromium, and placebo. The results showed that HbA1c (glycated hemoglobin) values (a measure of long-term blood sugar control) improved significantly after twp months in the group receiving 1,000 mcg, and in both chromium groups after four months. Fasting glucose (a measure of short-term blood sugar control) was also lower in the group taking the higher dose of chromium.

A double-blind, placebo-controlled trial of seventy-eight people with type 2 diabetes compared two forms of chromium (brewer's yeast and chromium chloride) with placebo. This rather complex crossover study consisted of four eight-week intervals of treatment in random order. The results in the sixty-seven participants who completed the study showed that both forms of chromium significantly improved blood sugar control. Positive results were also seen in other small, double-blind, placebo-controlled studies of people with type 2 diabetes. However, several other studies have failed to find chromium helpful for improving blood sugar control in type 2 diabetes. These contradictory findings suggest that the benefit, if it exists, is small.

A combination of chromium and biotin might be more effective. Following positive results in a small pilot trial, researchers conducted a double-blind study of 447 people with poorly controlled type 2 diabetes. One-half of the participants were given placebo and the rest were given a combination of 600 milligrams (mg) of chromium (as chromium picolinate) and 2 mg of biotin daily. All participants continued to receive standard oral medications for diabetes. During the ninety-day study period, participants who were given the chromium-biotin combination showed significantly better glucose regulation than participants who were given placebo. The relative benefit was clear in levels of fasting glucose and in levels of HgA1c (glycated hemoglobin).

One placebo-controlled study of thirty women with gestational diabetes (diabetes during pregnancy) found that supplementation with chromium (at a dosage of 4 or 8 mcg chromium picolinate for each kilogram of body weight) significantly improved blood sugar control. Chromium has also shown some promise for helping diabetes caused by corticosteroid treatment.

Ginseng. In double-blind studies performed by a single research group, the use of American ginseng (*Panax quinquefolius*) appeared to improve blood sugar control. In some studies, the same researchers subsequently reported possible benefit with Korean red ginseng, a specially prepared form of *P. ginseng.*

A different research group found benefits with ordinary *P. ginseng.* However, in other studies, ordinary *P. ginseng* seemed to worsen blood sugar control rather than improve it. (Another research group found potential benefit.) It seems possible that certain ginsenosides (found in high concentrations in some American ginseng products) may lower blood sugar, while others (found in high concentration in some *P. ginseng* products) may raise it. It has been suggested that because the actions of these various ginseng constituents are not well defined, ginseng should not be used to treat diabetes until more is known.

Aloe. The succulent aloe plant has been valued since prehistoric times as a topical treatment for burns, wound infections, and other skin problems. Today, evidence suggests that oral aloe might be useful for type 2 diabetes.

Evidence from two human trials suggests that aloe gel (the gel of the aloe vera plant, and not the leaf skin, which constitutes the drug aloe) can improve blood sugar control. A single-blind, placebo-controlled trial evaluated the potential benefits of aloe in either seventy-two or forty people with diabetes. (The study report appears to contradict itself). The results showed significantly greater improvements in blood sugar levels among those given aloe over the two-week treatment period.

Another single-blind, placebo-controlled trial evaluated the benefits of aloe in people who had failed to respond to the oral diabetes drug glibenclamide. Of the thirty-six people who completed the study, those taking glibenclamide and aloe showed definite improvements in blood sugar levels over forty-two days compared with those taking glibenclamide and placebo. While these are promising results, large studies that are double-blind rather than single-blind will be needed to establish aloe as an effective treatment for improving blood sugar control.

Cinnamon. Cinnamon has been widely advertised as an effective treatment for type 2 diabetes and for high cholesterol. The primary basis for this claim is a single study performed in Pakistan. In this forty-day study, sixty people with type 2 diabetes were given cinnamon at a dose of 1, 3, or 6 grams (g) daily. The results reportedly indicated that the use of cinnamon improved blood sugar levels by 18 to 29 percent, total cholesterol by 12 to 26 percent, LDL (bad) cholesterol by 7 to 27 percent, and triglycerides by 23 to 30 percent. These results were said to be statistically significant compared to the beginning of the study and to the placebo group.

However, this study has some odd features. The most important feature is that the study found no significant difference in benefit among the various doses of cinnamon. This is called lack of a "dose-related effect," and it generally casts doubt on the results of a study.

In an attempt to replicate these results, a group of Dutch researchers performed a carefully designed six-week, double-blind, placebo-controlled study of twenty-five people with type 2 diabetes. All participants were given 1.5 g of cinnamon daily. The results failed to show any detectable effect on blood sugar, insulin sensitivity, or cholesterol profile. Furthermore, a double-blind study performed in Thailand enrolling sixty people, again using 1.5 g of cinnamon daily, also failed to find benefit. However, a double-blind study of seventy-nine people that used 3 g instead of 1.5 g daily did find that cinnamon improved blood sugar levels. In addition, a small study evaluated cinnamon for improving blood sugar control in women with polycystic ovary disease, and it too found evidence of benefit. Regarding type 1 diabetes, a study of seventy-two adolescents failed to find benefit with cinnamon taken at a dose of 1 g daily.

A meta-analysis (formal statistical review) of all published evidence concluded that cinnamon has no effect on blood sugar levels in people with diabetes. The evidence regarding cinnamon as a treatment for diabetes is highly inconsistent, suggesting that if cinnamon is indeed effective, its benefits are minimal at most.

Other treatments studied for their effect on blood sugar control. The food spice fenugreek might also help control blood sugar, but the supporting evidence is weak. In a two-month double-blind study of twenty-five people with type 2 diabetes, the use of fenugreek (1 g daily of a standardized extract) significantly improved some measures of blood sugar control and insulin response compared with placebo. Triglyceride levels decreased and HDL (good) cholesterol levels increased, presumably because of the enhanced insulin sensitivity. Similar benefits have been seen in animal studies and open human trials. However, it is possible that the effects of fenugreek come from its dietary fiber content.

A few preliminary studies suggest that the Ayurvedic (Indian) herb gymnema may help improve blood sugar control. It might be helpful for mild cases of type 2 diabetes when taken alone or with standard treatment (under a doctor's supervision in either case).

Studies in rats with and without diabetes suggest that high doses of the mineral vanadium may have an insulin-like effect, reducing blood sugar levels. Based on these findings, preliminary studies involving humans have been conducted, with some promising results. However, of 151 studies reviewed, none was of sufficient quality to judge if vanadium is beneficial in type 2 diabetes. The researchers did find that vanadium was often associated with gastrointestinal side effects. Furthermore, there may be some cause for concern given the high doses of vanadium used in some of these studies.

The following herbs are proposed for helping to control blood sugar, but the supporting evidence regarding their potential benefit is, in all cases, at best preliminary; for some, there are as many negative results as positive: agaricus, blazei, berberine (goldenseal), black tea, caiapo, cod protein, cayenne, *Coccinia indica* (also known as *C. cordifolia*), garlic, green tea, guggul, holy basil (*Ocimum sanctum*), maitake, milk thistle, nopal cactus (*Opuntia stredptacantha*), onion, oolong tea, oligomeric proanthocyanidins, *Salacia oblonga*, *Salvia hispanica* (a grain), and salt bush. Additionally, the supplements arginine, carnitine, coenzyme Q_{10} (CoQ_{10}), dehydroepiandrosterone (DHEA), glucomannan, lipoic acid, melatonin with zinc, and vitamin E might also help control blood sugar levels to a slight degree.

One placebo-controlled study found hints that the use of medium-chain triglycerides by people with type 2 diabetes might improve insulin sensitivity and aid weight loss. The herb bitter melon (*Momordica charantia*) is widely advertised as effective for diabetes, but the scientific basis for this claim is limited to animal studies, uncontrolled human trials, and other unreliable forms of evidence. The one properly designed (that is, double-blind, placebo-controlled) study of bitter melon failed to find benefit. Conjugated linoleic acid (CLA) has shown promise in preliminary trials. However, other studies have found that CLA might worsen blood sugar control.

One study found that insulin metabolism in 278 young, overweight persons improved on a calorie-restricted diet rich in fish oil from seafood or supplements compared with those on a diet low in fish oil. Though preliminary, the results suggest that fish oil may help delay the onset of diabetes in susceptible persons. In another study of fifty people with type 2 diabetes, 2 g per day of purified omega-3-fatty acids (fish oil) was able to significantly lower triglycerides levels. However, it had no effect on blood sugar control.

Other herbs traditionally used for diabetes that might possibly offer some benefit include *Anemarrhena asphodeloides*, *Azadirachta indica* (neem), *Catharanthus roseus*, *Cucurbita ficifolia*, *Cucumis sativus*, *Cuminum cyminum* (cumin), *Euphorbia prostrata*, *Guaiacum coulteri*, *Guazuma ulmifolia*, *Lepechinia caulescens*, *Medicago sativa* (alfalfa), *Musa sapientum* L. (banana), *Phaseolus vulgaris*, *Psacalium peltatum*, *Rhizophora mangle*, *Spinacea oleracea*, *Tournefortia hirsutissima*, and *Turnera diffusa*.

Combination herbal therapies used in Ayurvedic medicine have also shown some promise for improving blood sugar control. One study attempted to test the effectiveness of whole-person Ayurvedic treatment involving exercise, Ayurvedic diet, meditation, and Ayurvedic herbal treatment. However, minimal benefits were seen.

A double-blind study of more than two hundred people evaluated the effectiveness of a combination herbal formula used in traditional Chinese herbal medicine (Coptis formula). This study evaluated Coptis formula with and without the drug glibenclamide. The results hint that Coptis formula may enhance the effectiveness of the drug but that it is not powerful enough to treat diabetes on its own. Another randomized trial, this one lacking a control group, found no added benefit for Tai Chi in the treatment of blood glucose and cholesterol levels among fifty-three people with type 2 diabetes during a six-month period.

One study claimed to find evidence that creatine supplements can reduce levels of blood sugar. However, because dextrose (a form of sugar) was used as the "placebo" in this trial, the results are somewhat questionable. In another study, the herb *Tinospora crispa* did not work, and it showed the potential to cause liver injury.

One study found hints that the supplement DHEA might improve insulin sensitivity. However, a subsequent and more rigorous study failed to find benefits. Relatively weak evidence hints that genistein (an isoflavone extracted from soy) might help control blood sugar.

It has been suggested that if a child has just developed diabetes, the supplement niacinamide (a form of niacin, also called vitamin B$_3$) might slightly prolong what is called the honeymoon period. This is the interval during which the pancreas can still make some insulin and the body's need for insulin injections is low. However, the benefits (if any) appear to be minor. A cocktail of niacinamide plus antioxidant vitamins and minerals has also been tried, but the results were disappointing. Niacinamide has also been tried for preventing diabetes in high-risk children. According to most studies, fructo-oligosaccharides (also known as prebiotics) do not improve blood sugar control in people with type 2 diabetes.

Massage therapy has shown some promise for enhancing blood sugar control in children with diabetes. A review of nine clinical trials found insufficient evidence to support the traditional Chinese practice of qigong as beneficial for treatment of type 2 diabetes.

TREATING NUTRITIONAL DEFICIENCIES

Both diabetes and the medications used to treat it can cause people to fall short of various nutrients. Making up for these deficiencies (through either diet or the use of supplements) may or may not help with diabetes specifically, but it should make a person healthier overall. One double-blind study, for example, found that people with type 2 diabetes who took a multivitamin-multimineral supplement were less likely to develop an infectious illness than those who took placebo.

People with diabetes are often deficient in magnesium, and inconsistent evidence hints that magnesium supplementation may enhance blood sugar control. People with either type 1 or type 2 diabetes may also be deficient in the mineral zinc. Vitamin C levels have been found to be low in many people on insulin, even though these persons were consuming seemingly adequate amounts of the vitamin in their diets. Deficiencies of taurine and manganese have also been reported. The drug metformin can cause vitamin B$_{12}$ deficiency. Taking extra calcium may prevent this.

PREVENTION

Niacinamide. Evidence from a large study conducted in New Zealand suggests that the supplement niacinamide might reduce the risk of diabetes in children at high risk. In this study, more than twenty thousand children were screened for diabetes risk by measuring certain antibodies in the blood (ICA antibodies, believed to indicate risk of developing diabetes). It turned out that 185 of these children had detectable levels. About 170 of these children were then given niacinamide for seven years (not all parents agreed to give their children niacinamide or to have them stay in the study for that long). About ten thousand other children were not screened, but they were followed to see if they developed diabetes.

The results were positive. In the group in which children were screened and given niacinamide if they were positive for ICA antibodies, the incidence of diabetes was reduced by almost 60 percent. These findings suggest that niacinamide is an effective treatment for preventing diabetes. (The study also indicates that tests for ICA antibodies can very accurately identify children at risk for diabetes.)

An even larger study that attempted to replicate these results in Europe (the European Nicotinamide Diabetes Intervention Trial) failed to find benefit. This study screened 40,000 children at high risk and selected 552. The results were negative. The rate of diabetes onset was not statistically different in the group given niacinamide compared with those given placebo. Another study also failed to find benefit.

Dietary changes. The related terms "glycemic index" and "glycemic load" indicate the tendency of certain foods to stimulate insulin release. It has been suggested that foods that rank high on these scales, such as white flour and sweets, might tend to exhaust the pancreas and therefore lead to type 2 diabetes. For this reason, low-carbohydrate and low-glycemic-index diets have been promoted for the prevention of type 2 diabetes. However, the results from studies on this question have been contradictory and far from definitive.

There is no question, however, that people who are obese have a far greater tendency to develop type 2 diabetes than those who are relatively slim; therefore, weight loss (especially when accompanied by increase in exercise) is clearly an effective step for prevention. One review suggests that a weight decrease of 7 to 10 percent is enough to provide significant benefit.

Other natural treatments. Studies investigating the preventive effects of antioxidant supplements have generally been disappointing. In an extremely large double-blind study, the use of vitamin E at a dose of 600 international units every other day failed to reduce the risk of type 2 diabetes in women. Another large study, which enrolled male smokers, failed to find benefit with beta-carotene, vitamin E, or the two taken together. Another large study of female health professionals who were more than forty years old with or at high risk for cardiovascular disease found that long-term supplementation (an average of just more than nine years) with vitamin C, vitamin E, or beta-carotene did not significantly reduce the risk of developing diabetes compared with placebo. In a smaller (but still sizable) trial involving a subgroup of these same women, supplementation with vitamins B_6 and B_{12} and folic acid also did not reduce risk of type 2 diabetes.

Several observational studies suggest that vitamin D may also help prevent diabetes. However, studies of this type are far less reliable than double-blind trials. One observational study failed to find that high consumption of lycopene reduced risk of developing type 2 diabetes.

SUPPLEMENTS TO USE ONLY WITH CAUTION

In a double-blind, placebo-controlled study of sixty overweight men, the use of conjugated linoleic acid (CLA) unexpectedly worsened blood sugar control. These findings surprised researchers, who were looking for potential diabetes-related benefits with this supplement. Other studies corroborate this as a potential risk for people with type 2 diabetes and for overweight people without diabetes. Another study, however, failed to find this effect. Nonetheless, people with type 2 diabetes or who are at risk for it should not use CLA except under physician supervision.

Unexpected results also occurred in a study of vitamin E. For various theoretical reasons, researchers expected that the use of vitamin E (either alpha tocopherol or mixed tocopherols) by people with diabetes would reduce blood pressure; instead, the reverse occurred. People with diabetes should probably

monitor their blood pressure if they take high-dose vitamin E supplements.

There are equivocal indications that the herb ginkgo might alter insulin release or insulin sensitivity in people with diabetes. The effect, if it exists, appears to be rather complex; the herb may cause some increase in insulin output and, yet, might actually lower insulin levels overall through its effects on the liver and perhaps on oral medications used for diabetes. Until this situation is clarified, people with diabetes should use ginkgo only under the supervision of a physician.

Despite hopes to the contrary, it does not appear that selenium supplements can help prevent type 2 diabetes, but rather might increase the risk of developing the disease. Contrary to earlier concerns, vitamin B_3 (niacin) and fish oil appear to be safe for people with diabetes. A few early case reports and animal studies had raised concerns that glucosamine might be harmful for persons with diabetes, but subsequent studies have tended to allay these worries.

Finally, if any herb or supplement does in fact successfully decrease blood sugar levels, this could lead to dangerous hypoglycemia. A doctor's supervision is strongly suggested

EBSCO CAM Review Board

FURTHER READING

Ahuja, K. D., et al. "Effects of Chili Consumption on Postprandial Glucose, Insulin, and Energy Metabolism. *American Journal of Clinical Nutrition* 84 (2006): 63-69.

Altschuler, J. A., et al. "The Effect of Cinnamon on A1C Among Adolescents with Type 1 Diabetes." *Diabetes Care* 30 (2007): 813-816.

Basu, R., et al. "Two Years of Treatment with Dehydroepiandrosterone Does Not Improve Insulin Secretion, Insulin Action, or Postprandial Glucose Turnover in Elderly Men or Women." *Diabetes* 56 (2007): 753-766.

Boshtam, M., et al. "Long Term Effects of Oral Vitamin E Supplement in Type II Diabetic Patients." *International Journal for Vitamin and Nutrition Research* 75 (2006): 341-346.

Bryans, J. A., P. A. Judd, and P. R. Ellis. "The Effect of Consuming Instant Black Tea on Postprandial Plasma Glucose and Insulin Concentrations in Healthy Humans." *Journal of the American College of Nutrition* 26 (2007): 471-477.

Elder, C., et al. "Randomized Trial of a Whole-System Ayurvedic Protocol for Type 2 Diabetes." *Alternative Therapies in Health and Medicine* 12 (2006): 24-30.

Lee, M. S., et al. "Qigong for Type 2 Diabetes Care." *Complementary Therapies in Medicine* 17 (2009): 236-242.

Li, Y., T. H. Huang, and J. Yamahara. "Salacia Root, a Unique Ayurvedic Medicine, Meets Multiple Targets in Diabetes and Obesity." *Life Sciences* 82 (2008): 1045-1049.

Mackenzie, T., L. Leary, and W. B. Brooks. "The Effect of an Extract of Green and Black Tea on Glucose Control in Adults with Type 2 Diabetes Mellitus." *Metabolism* 56 (2007): 1340-1344.

Pi-Sunyer, F. X. "How Effective Are Lifestyle Changes in the Prevention of Type 2 Diabetes Mellitus?" *Nutrition Reviews* 65 (2007): 101-110.

Ramel, A., et al. "Beneficial Effects of Long-Chain N-3 Fatty Acids Included in an Energy-Restricted Diet on Insulin Resistance in Overweight and Obese European Young Adults." *Diabetologia* 51 (2008): 1261-1268.

Shidfar, F., et al. "Effects of Omega-3 Fatty Acid Supplements on Serum Lipids, Apolipoproteins, and Malondialdehyde in Type 2 Diabetes Patients." *Eastern Mediterranean Health Journal* 14 (2008): 305-313.

Song, Y., et al. "Effects of Vitamins C and E and Beta-Carotene on the Risk of Type 2 Diabetes in Women at High Risk of Cardiovascular Disease." *American Journal of Clinical Nutrition* 90 (2009): 429-437.

Ward, N. C., et al. "The Effect of Vitamin E on Blood Pressure in Individuals with Type 2 Diabetes." *Journal of Hypertension* 25 (2007): 227-234.

See also: Aloe; Chromium; Cinnamon; Diabetes, complications of; Ginseng; Insulin.

Diabetes, complications of

CATEGORY: Condition

RELATED TERMS: Autonomic neuropathy, cardiac autonomic neuropathy, cataracts, diabetic neuropathy, diabetic retinopathy, peripheral neuropathy

DEFINITION: Treatment of the condition that causes toxic blood sugar levels and organ and tissue damage.

PRINCIPAL PROPOSED NATURAL TREATMENTS

- *Peripheral neuropathy:* Acetyl-L-carnitine, evening primrose oil (gamma-linolenic acid), lipoic acid, vitamin B
- *Cardiac autonomic neuropathy:* Lipoic acid

OTHER PROPOSED NATURAL TREATMENTS

- *Cardiac autonomic neuropathy:* Vitamin E
- *Cataracts:* Bilberry
- *Foot ulcers:* Tinospora cordifolia
- *Immunity and infections:* Multivitamin-multimineral supplements
- *Lower leg swelling (microangiopathy):* Oxerutins
- *Peripheral neuropathy:* Fish oil, magnet therapy, selenium, vitamin E
- *Retinopathy:* Bilberry, oligomeric proanthocyanidins

INTRODUCTION

Diabetes is an illness that damages many organs in the body, including the heart and blood vessels, nerves, kidneys, and eyes. Most of this damage is believed to be caused by the toxic effects of abnormally high blood sugar, although other factors may play a role too.

Tight control of blood sugar greatly reduces all complications of diabetes. Some of the natural treatments described here also may help.

PRINCIPAL PROPOSED NATURAL TREATMENTS

Several dietary and herbal supplements may help prevent or treat some of the common complications of diabetes. However, because diabetes is a dangerous disease, alternative treatment should not be attempted as a substitute for conventional medical care.

Natural treatments helpful in general for improving cholesterol and triglyceride profiles may be useful to people with diabetes. Contrary to some early concerns, both fish oil and niacin (treatments used for improving triglyceride and cholesterol levels, respectively) appear to be safe for people with diabetes.

High levels of blood sugar can damage the nerves leading to the extremities, causing pain and numbness. This condition is called diabetic peripheral neuropathy. Nerve damage may also develop in the heart, a condition named cardiac autonomic neuropathy. Following is a discussion of three natural supplements–acetyl-L-carnitine, lipoic acid, and gamma-linolenic acid–that have shown promise for the treatment of diabetic nerve damage.

Acetyl-L-carnitine. The supplement acetyl-L-carnitine

(ALC) has shown promise for diabetic peripheral neuropathy. Two fifty-two-week, double-blind, placebo-controlled studies involving 1,257 people with diabetic peripheral neuropathy evaluated the potential benefits of ALC taken at 500 milligrams (mg) or 1,000 mg daily. The results showed that the use of ALC, especially at the higher dose, improved sensory perception and decreased pain levels. In addition, the supplement appeared to promote nerve fiber regeneration. ALC has also shown some promise for cardiac autonomic neuropathy.

Lipoic acid. Lipoic acid is widely advocated for the treatment of diabetic neuropathy. However, while there is meaningful evidence for benefits with intravenous lipoic acid, there is only minimal evidence to indicate that oral lipoic acid can help.

A double-blind, placebo-controlled study that enrolled 503 people with diabetic peripheral neuropathy found that intravenous lipoic acid helped reduce symptoms in a three-week period. However, when researchers substituted oral lipoic acid for intravenous lipoic acid, benefits ceased.

Benefits were seen with oral lipoic acid in a study published in 2006. In this double-blind, placebo-controlled trial, 181 people with diabetic peripheral neuropathy were given either placebo or one of three doses of lipoic acid: 600, 1,200, or 1,800 mg daily. During the five-week study period, benefits were seen in all three lipoic acid groups compared with the placebo group. However, while this outcome may sound promising, one feature of the results tends to reduce the faith one can put in them: the absence of a dose-related effect. Ordinarily, when a treatment is effective, higher doses produce relatively better results. When such a spectrum of outcomes is not observed, one wonders if something went wrong in the study.

Other than this one study, the positive evidence for oral lipoic acid in diabetic peripheral neuropathy is limited to open studies of minimal to no validity and to double-blind trials too small to be relied upon.

Lipoic acid has also been advocated for cardiac autonomic neuropathy, and one study did find benefits: The DEKAN (Deutsche Kardiale Autonome Neuropathie) study followed seventy-three people with cardiac autonomic neuropathy for four months. Treatment with 800 mg of oral lipoic acid daily showed significant improvement compared with placebo, and no important side effects. Preliminary evidence hints that lipoic acid may be more effective for neuropathy if it is combined with gamma-linolenic acid.

Gamma-linolenic acid. Gamma-linolenic acid (GLA) is an essential fatty acid in the omega-6 category. The most common sources of GLA are evening primrose oil, borage oil, and black currant oil.

Many studies in animals have shown that evening primrose oil can protect nerves from diabetes-induced injury. Human trials have also found benefits. A double-blind study followed 111 people with diabetes for one year. The results showed an improvement in subjective symptoms of peripheral neuropathy, such as pain and numbness, and objective signs of nerve injury. People with good blood sugar control improved the most. A much smaller double-blind study also reported positive results.

OTHER PROPOSED NATURAL TREATMENTS

A four-month, double-blind, placebo-controlled trial found that vitamin E at a dose of 600 mg daily might improve symptoms of cardiac autonomic neuropathy. Vitamin E and selenium have also shown promise for diabetic peripheral neuropathy. Intriguing evidence from a small study suggests that vitamin E may also help protect people with diabetes from developing damage to their eyes and kidneys. However, a large, long-term study failed to find vitamin E effective for preventing kidney damage. (Vitamin E also did not help prevent coronary artery disease.) In a review of thirteen randomized trials, researchers found inadequate evidence for the effectiveness of B vitamins for peripheral neuropathies (diabetic or otherwise).

The supplement inositol has been tried as a treatment for diabetic neuropathy, but the results have been mixed. In preliminary studies, fish oil has shown some promise for diabetic neuropathy, but human trials have not been performed.

Diabetes can cause swelling of the ankles and feet by damaging small blood vessels (microangiopathy). A preliminary, double-blind, placebo-controlled trial suggests that oxerutins might be helpful for this condition.

Weak evidence suggests that the herb bilberry may help prevent eye damage (cataracts and retinopathy) caused by diabetes. Pycnogenol, a source of oligomeric proanthocyanidins (OPCs), has also shown promise for diabetic retinopathy.

It has been suggested that vitamin C may also help prevent cataracts in diabetes, based on its relationship to sorbitol. Sorbitol, a sugar-like substance that tends to accumulate in the cells of people with diabetes, may play a role in the development of diabetic cataracts. Vitamin C appears to help reduce sorbitol buildup, but the evidence that vitamin C provides significant benefits by this route is indirect and far from conclusive. Another study suggests that vitamin C might be helpful for reducing blood pressure in people with diabetes. The herb *Tinospora cordifolia* and honey (applied topically) have shown some promise for speeding healing of diabetic foot ulcers.

Magnetic insoles, a form of magnet therapy, have shown some promise for the treatment of diabetic peripheral neuropathy. A four-month, double-blind, placebo-controlled, crossover study of nineteen people with peripheral neuropathy found a significant reduction in symptoms in those using the insoles compared with those using placebo insoles. This study enrolled people with peripheral neuropathy of various causes; however, reduction in the symptoms of burning, numbness, and tingling was especially marked in those cases of neuropathy associated with diabetes.

Another type of magnetic therapy, involving low-frequency, repetitive magnetic pulses generated by an electric current, was no better than a placebo at relieving painful peripheral neuropathy among sixty-one people who had long-term diabetes. In another study, however, high-frequency magnetic fields applied repetitively to the brain were more effective than placebo in reducing pain and improving quality of life among twenty-eight subjects with peripheral neuropathy.

One small, double-blind, placebo-controlled study suggests that regular use of multivitamin-multimineral supplements may reduce the incidence of infectious illness in people with diabetes. Another study failed to find that general nutritional supplementation accelerated healing of diabetic foot ulcers.

EBSCO CAM Review Board

FURTHER READING

Ang, C. D., et al. "Vitamin B for Treating Peripheral Neuropathy." *Cochrane Database of Systematic Reviews* (2008): CD004573. Available through *EBSCO DynaMed Systematic Literature Surveillance* at http://www.ebscohost.com/dynamed.

Barringer, T. A., et al. "Effect of a Multivitamin and Mineral Supplement on Infection and Quality of Life." *Annals of Internal Medicine* 138 (2003): 365-371.

Eneroth, M., et al. "Nutritional Supplementation for Diabetic Foot Ulcers." *Journal of Wound Care* 13 (2004): 230-234.

Manzella, D., et al. "Chronic Administration of Pharmacologic Doses of Vitamin E Improves the Cardiac Autonomic Nervous System in Patients with Type 2 Diabetes." *American Journal of Clinical Nutrition* 73 (2001): 1052-1057.

Montori, V. M., et al. "Fish Oil Supplementation in Type 2 Diabetes." *Diabetes Care* 23 (2000): 1407-1415.

Purandare, H., and A. Supe. "Immunomodulatory Role of *Tinospora cordifolia* as an Adjuvant in Surgical Treatment of Diabetic Foot Ulcers." *Indian Journal of Medical Sciences* 61 (2007): 347-355.

Shukrimi, A., et al. "A Comparative Study Between Honey and Povidone Iodine as Dressing Solution for Wagner Type II Diabetic Foot Ulcers." *Medical Journal of Malaysia* 63 (2008): 44-46.

Wrobel, M. P., et al. "Impact of Low Frequency Pulsed Magnetic Fields on Pain Intensity, Quality of Life, and Sleep Disturbances in Patients with Painful Diabetic Polyneuropathy." *Diabetes and Metabolism* 34 (2008): 349-354.

See also: Carnitine; Cataracts; Diabetes; Fish oil; Gamma-linolenic acid; Lipoic acid; Vitamin B.

Diabetes: Homeopathic remedies

CATEGORY: Homeopathy
RELATED TERMS: Diabetes insipidous, diabetes mellitus, juvenile diabetes
DEFINITION: Homeopathic treatment for diabetes

OVERVIEW

Diabetes is a chronic disease that affects the body's ability to use sugar. Type 1, or insulin-dependent, diabetes is characterized by an inability of the pancreas to produce insulin, and type 2, or non-insulin-dependent, diabetes is characterized by an inability of insulin to exert its normal physiological effects.

In type 1 diabetes, sometimes called juvenile diabetes, the body cannot make insulin, which helps the body turn the sugar obtained from the food into a source of energy. Type 1 occurs more frequently in children and young adults but accounts for only 5 to 10 percent of the total diabetes cases in the United States. Type 2 diabetes, also called adult-onset diabetes, is marked by defective insulin production and the development of tissue resistance to insulin.

Symptoms and Effects

Symptoms of diabetes can include excessive urination, thirst, weight loss, and a lack of energy. However, diabetes is often present without symptoms and may exist for many years without a person noticing it. Certain organs are more vulnerable to the damaging effects of chronically high blood sugar levels. These organs are the eyes, the kidneys, the nerves, and the large blood vessels, such as in the heart.

Homeopathic Remedies

Conventional methods of treatment for diabetes include diet, exercise, moderation in alcohol use and smoking, and monitoring blood glucose. A health treatment classified as other than standard Western medical practice is referred to as complementary and alternative medicine (CAM). CAM encompasses a variety of disciplines and includes treatments such as diet and exercise, mental conditioning, and lifestyle changes. Examples of CAM therapies are acupuncture, guided imagery, chiropractic treatment, yoga, hypnosis, biofeedback, aromatherapy, relaxation, herbal remedies, and massage. CAM therapies for diabetes include the following:

Ginseng. Studies have shown that North American ginseng may improve blood sugar control and levels of glycosylated hemoglobin, a form of hemoglobin in the blood used to monitor blood glucose levels over time.

Chromium. Chromium is an essential trace mineral that has an important role in carbohydrate and fat metabolism and helps body cells properly respond to insulin. Studies regarding the effectiveness of chromium supplementation on diabetes management have not been conclusive. A 2008 study compared the diabetes medication sulfonylurea taken with 1,000 micrograms of chromium with sulfonylurea taken with a placebo. Results from the study showed that people taking the chromium had significant improvements in insulin sensitivity. Another study concluded that there was no significant difference in glycosylated hemoglobin, body mass index, blood pressure, or insulin requirements across the three groups.

Evaluating Diabetes-Treatment Claims

The Federal Trade Commission recommends checking all over-the-counter products with a health care provider before purchase. Fraudulent marketers peddle products that sound like cures for diabetes, but these products do not, and cannot, work as promised. Here are some tips on how to spot scams.

A promise that a product can cure diabetes is a tip-off to a rip-off. There is no pill, patch, tea, herb, or other "miracle" treatment one can buy on the Web that can make diabetes disappear.

Advertisements that promise too much generally deliver nothing. One should not buy any product that claims it can do it all, such as stabilize blood sugar, end the need for insulin, regenerate the pancreas, reduce bad cholesterol, and cause easy weight loss.

A product that claims to be a "scientific breakthrough" may be a bust. Researchers around the world are racing to find better treatments for diabetes, so genuine scientific discoveries make front-page news. If the first news about a supposed scientific breakthrough is through an advertisement on the Web, be suspicious of that claim.

Magnesium. Magnesium is a mineral found naturally in foods such as green leafy vegetables, nuts, seeds, and whole grains, and in nutritional supplements. Magnesium is needed for more than three hundred biochemical reactions in the body. It helps regulate blood sugar levels and is needed for normal muscle and nerve function, heart rhythm, immune function, and blood pressure, and for bone health. Some studies suggest that low magnesium levels may worsen blood glucose control in type 2 diabetes. Research also has shown that magnesium supplementation may improve insulin sensitivity and lower fasting glucose levels.

Cinnamon. Studies of the use of cinnamon in managing diabetes are inconclusive. Some research demonstrates that cinnamon significantly reduces fasting blood-glucose levels. However, the American Diabetes Association suggests that there is no significant difference in glycosylated hemoglobin or lipid profiles related to the use of cinnamon.

Zinc. The mineral zinc plays an important role in the production and storage of insulin. Food sources of zinc include fresh oysters, ginger root, lamb, pecans, split peas, egg yolk, rye, beef liver, lima beans, almonds, walnuts, sardines, chicken, and buckwheat. Some research shows that persons with type 2 diabetes have suboptimal zinc status because of decreased absorption and increased excretion of zinc.

Aloe vera gel. Although aloe vera gel is better known as a home remedy for minor burns and other skin conditions, recent animal studies suggest that aloe vera gel may help people with diabetes. A Japanese study evaluated the effect of aloe vera gel on blood sugar and found that compounds from the gel reduced blood glucose and glycosylated hemoglobin levels.

Plant foods. Most plant foods are rich in fiber, which is beneficial for helping control blood sugar levels. The following plant foods have been found to help people with type 2 diabetes: brewer's yeast, buckwheat, broccoli, okra, peas, fenugreek seeds, and sage. There are no clinical trials with promising results for many of the other herbs being proposed for diabetes, such as garlic, ginger, ginseng, hawthorn, and nettle. Persons with diabetes who are considering taking any of these herbal substances should first consult a doctor.

FURTHER CONSIDERATIONS

Although many alternative therapies are considered to be natural, one should take caution when using them. The following recommendations will ensure safe usage of alternative treatments: Discuss any drugs, including herbal products, with a doctor before taking them; report any side effects, such as nausea, vomiting, rapid heartbeat, anxiety, insomnia, diarrhea, or skin rashes, to one's health care provider and stop taking the herbal product immediately; avoid preparations made with more than one herb; look for scientific-based sources of information; purchase only those brands that list the herb's common and scientific names, the name and address of the manufacturer, a batch and lot number, expiration date, dosage guidelines, and potential side effects.

Sandra C. Hayes, D.Ph.

FURTHER READING

"Alternative Treatments for Diabetes." Available at http://diabetes.webmd.com/guide/alternative-medicine.

Khan, A., et al. "Cinnamon Improves Glucose and Lipids of People with Type 2 Diabetes." *Diabetes Care* 26, no. 12 (2003): 3215-3218.

Kleefstra, N., et al. "Chromium Treatment Has No Effect in Patients with Poorly Controlled, Insulin-Treated Type 2 Diabetes in an Obese Western Population." *Diabetes Care* 29, no. 3 (2006): 521-525.

Martin, J., et al. "Cromium Picolinate Supplementation Attenuates Body Weight Gain and Increases Insulin Sensitivity in Subjects with Type 2 Diabetes." *Diabetes Care* 29, no. 8 (2006): 1826-1832.

See also: Cholesterol, high; Diabetes; Diabetes, complications of; Diet-based therapies; Exercise; Obesity and excess weight; Pancreatitis.

Diarrhea

CATEGORY: Condition
RELATED TERMS: Loose bowel movements, loose stools
DEFINITION: Treatment of acute and chronic loose bowel movements.
PRINCIPAL PROPOSED NATURAL TREATMENT: Probiotics
OTHER PROPOSED NATURAL TREATMENTS: Acupuncture, bilberry, carob, chamomile, colostrum, *Eleutherococcus*, fiber, fructo-oligosaccharides, folate, food allergen identification and avoidance, goldenseal, green banana, lactase, marshmallow, pectin, red raspberry, sangre de drago, slippery elm, tormentil root (*Potentilla tormentilla*), Witch hazel, wood creosote, zinc
SUPPLEMENTS TO AVOID: Magnesium, vitamin C

INTRODUCTION

Diarrhea can occur for many reasons. Food poisoning and infections are the most common causes of acute (short-lived) diarrhea. Chronic diarrhea may be caused by ongoing illnesses of the digestive tract, such as inflammatory bowel disease and irritable bowel syndrome.

Conventional treatment for diarrhea involves addressing the cause, if possible, and, in some cases, treating symptoms with medications that slow down the action of the digestive tract.

PRINCIPAL PROPOSED NATURAL TREATMENTS

Supplements called probiotics have shown considerable promise for safely preventing or treating various kinds of diarrhea. The following section summarizes much of the evidence regarding this treatment.

Probiotics. Certain bacteria and fungi play a helpful role in the body. For this reason, they are known collectively as probiotics ("prolife"). Some of the most common include the yeast *Saccharomyces boulardii* and the bacteria *Lactobacillus acidophilus*, *L. bulgaricus*, *L. reuteri* (often studied in the proprietary form *Lactobacillus* GG), *L. plantarum*, *L. casei*, *B. bifidus*, *S. salivarius*, and *Streptococcus thermophilus*.

The digestive tract is like a rainforest ecosystem, with billions of bacteria and yeasts. Some of these internal inhabitants are more helpful to the body than others. Probiotics not only help digestive tract function but also reduce the presence of less healthful organisms by competing with them for the limited available space. For this reason, the use of probiotics can help prevent infectious diarrhea.

Antibiotics being taken to treat an infection can disturb the balance of the inner ecosystem by killing friendly bacteria. When this occurs, harmful bacteria and yeasts can move in and flourish, which can lead to diarrhea. Probiotic therapy may help prevent this problem. Probiotics also appear to be helpful for preventing or treating forms of diarrhea with different causes.

Travelers' diarrhea. According to some studies, it appears that the regular use of various probiotics can help prevent travelers' diarrhea, an illness caused by eating contaminated food, usually in developing countries. One double-blind, placebo-controlled study followed 820 people traveling to southern Turkey and found that the use of a probiotic called *Lactobacillus* GG significantly protected against intestinal infection.

An even larger double-blind, placebo-controlled study found benefits from using the yeast product *S. boulardii*. This trial enrolled three thousand Austrians traveling to a variety of countries. The greatest benefits were seen in travelers who visited North Africa and Turkey. The researchers noted that the benefit depended on consistent use of the product, and that a dosage of 1,000 milligrams (mg) daily was more effective than 250 mg daily.

Substances called prebiotics are thought to enhance the growth of probiotics. On this basis, prebiotics called fructo-oligosaccharides (FOS) have been suggested for preventing travelers' diarrhea. However, in a 244-participant double-blind study, FOS at a dose of 10 grams (g) daily offered only minimal benefits.

Areas of Interest to Researchers on Probiotics

- What is going on at the molecular level with the "good" bacteria themselves and how they may interact with the body (such as the gut and its bacteria) to prevent and treat diseases

- Issues of quality. For example, what happens when probiotic bacteria are treated or are added to foods? Is their ability to survive, grow, and have a therapeutic effect altered?

- The best ways to administer probiotics for therapeutic purposes, and the best doses and schedules

- Probiotics' potential to help with the problem of antibiotic-resistant bacteria in the gut

- Whether probiotics can prevent unfriendly, harmful bacteria from getting through the skin or mucous membranes and traveling through the body (which can happen with burns, shock, trauma, or suppressed immunity)

Infectious diarrhea. Children frequently develop diarrhea caused by infectious viruses. Probiotics may help prevent or treat this condition and may also be useful for viral diarrhea in adults. A review of the literature published in 2001 found thirteen double-blind, placebo-controlled trials on the use of probiotics for acute infectious diarrhea in infants and children. Ten of these trials involved treatment, and three involved prevention. Benefits have been seen in subsequent studies too, including one that involved almost one thousand infants. Overall, the evidence strongly suggests that the use of probiotics can significantly reduce the severity and duration of diarrhea and perhaps help prevent it.

One double-blind, placebo-controlled trial of 269 children (age one month to three years) with acute diarrhea found that those treated with *Lactobacillus* GG recovered more quickly than those given placebo. The best results were seen among children with rotavirus infection. (Rotavirus can cause severe diarrhea in children.) In another double-blind, placebo-controlled study, *Lactobacillus* GG helped prevent diarrhea in 204 undernourished children. In addition to

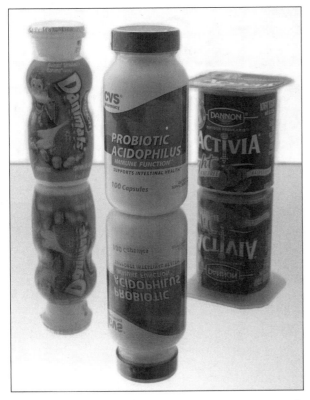

Probiotics have shown promise in preventing or treating diarrhea. (Washington Post/Getty Images)

Lactobacillus GG, the probiotics *Bifidobacterium bifidum, S. thermophilus, L. casei, L. reuteri, S. boulardii,* and *Escherichia coli Nissle* (a safe strain of *E. coli*) have also shown promise for preventing or treating diarrhea in infants and children. However, probiotic therapy is probably not helpful for acute, severe, dehydrating diarrhea. (Diarrhea in young children can be serious. If it persists for more than a couple of days or is extremely severe, the child's physician should be consulted.) In addition, a large (211-participant) double-blind, placebo-controlled study found that adults with infectious diarrhea can also benefit from probiotic treatment.

Antibiotic-related diarrhea. The results of most double-blind and open trials suggest that probiotics, especially *S. boulardii* and *Lactobacillus* GG, may help prevent or treat antibiotic-related diarrhea (including the most severe form, *Clostridium difficile (diarrhea).* One study found *L. rhamnosus* effective in children, and another study found that *L. casei* was effective in hospitalized patients.

It is sometimes said that it is useless to begin probiotic treatment until after the antibiotics are finished. However, evidence appears to indicate that it is better to begin treatment with probiotics at the initial use of antibiotics and then to continue probiotic treatment for a week or two afterward. Diarrhea that occurs in the context of antibiotics may be dangerous, so one should consult a doctor if this is the case.

Inflammatory bowel disease. Crohn's disease and ulcerative colitis fall into the family of conditions known as inflammatory bowel disease. Chronic diarrhea is a common feature of these conditions.

A double-blind trial of 116 people with ulcerative colitis compared a special probiotic treatment using *E. coli* to a relatively low dose of the standard drug mesalazine. The results suggest that this probiotic treatment might be as effective as low-dose mesalazine for controlling symptoms and maintaining remission.

Another study found *S. boulardii* helpful for treating diarrhea resulting from Crohn's disease. However, two studies failed to find benefit with *Lactobacillus* probiotics.

Other forms of diarrhea. Preliminary evidence suggests that probiotics may be helpful for reducing diarrhea and other gastrointestinal side effects caused by cancer treatment (radiation or chemotherapy). Another study found that *S. boulardii* can increase the effectiveness of standard treatment for amoebic infections. Small double-blind studies suggest *S. boulardii* might be helpful for treating chronic diarrhea in people with human immunodeficiency virus (HIV) infection and hospitalized persons who are being tube-fed.

Premature infants weighing less than 2,500 grams (5.5 pounds) are at risk for a life-threatening intestinal condition called necrotizing enterocolitis (NEC). In a study that pooled the results of nine randomized, placebo-controlled trials involving 1,425 infants, probiotic supplementation significantly reduced the occurrence of NEC and death associated with it. Also, a subsequent study found similar benefits in very low birth weight infants weighing less than 1,500 grams (3.3 pounds).

Irritable bowel syndrome. People with irritable bowel syndrome (IBS) experience cramping digestive pain, alternating diarrhea and constipation, and other symptoms. In some people, diarrhea predominates. Although the cause of IBS is not known, one possibility is a disturbance in healthy intestinal bacteria. Based on this theory, probiotics have been tried as a treatment for IBS with diarrhea, but the results have been inconsistent. One study tested the potential effectiveness of a traditional Chinese herbal remedy for diarrhea-predominant IBS, but failed to find benefit.

OTHER PROPOSED NATURAL TREATMENTS

A large (255-participant), double-blind, placebo-controlled study found that the use of a product containing apple pectin and chamomile significantly improved symptoms of acute diarrhea in children aged six months to six years. A small double-blind study found that an extract of tormentil root (*Potentilla tormentilla*) reduced the severity and duration of rotavirus infection in children. Another study of the same herb found that it was approximately as effective as the drug loperamide for the treatment of nonspecific diarrhea in adults. The herbal extract was particularly effective for reducing symptoms of abdominal cramping.

A preliminary double-blind study found that an extract of the Amazonian herb sangre de drago might be helpful for diarrhea associated with HIV infection. The supplement medium-chain triglycerides also has shown promise for this purpose.

Wheat germ might enhance the effects of standard treatments for giardiasis. Also, a double-blind clinical trial of forty-one infants with diarrhea found that carob powder (at a dose of 1 g per kilogram of body weight daily) significantly speeded resolution of diarrhea compared with placebo.

The herb *Eleutherococcus* might be useful in the treatment of antibiotic-associated diarrhea. Brewer's yeast, a bitter-tasting product recovered from the beer-making process, might also be helpful. The herb goldenseal contains berberine, a substance with antimicrobial properties. One study suggests that berberine can help in diarrhea caused by the *E. coli* bacterium. However, it is not clear that goldenseal itself would have the same effect. The herbs barberry and Oregon grape also contain berberine.

Allergy to milk and other foods may trigger diarrhea. Milk can also cause diarrhea in a completely different way–through lactose intolerance. This condition is the inability to digest milk sugar, and it occurs in many adults. The use of the enzyme lactase should help.

Weak (and in some cases inconsistent) evidence partially supports the use of the following as treatments for various forms of diarrhea: colostrum, a special extract of egg yolk, fiber, folate, and green banana. Zinc has been shown to be beneficial for acute diarrhea in children, the most convincing evidence coming from studies done in developing countries. This suggests that zinc is most useful for this condition in the presence of a nutritional deficiency.

Other herbs that are suggested for diarrhea but have no meaningful supporting evidence include agrimony, bilberry, blackberry leaf, marshmallow, oak bark, red raspberry, slippery elm, and witch hazel. The supplement glutamine has been advocated for chronic diarrhea, but again, there is no meaningful supporting evidence.

Wood creosote is the principal ingredient in seirogan, a widely used traditional herbal treatment for diarrhea. It has undergone a certain amount of safety testing and appears to be relatively safe for short-term use. Efficacy, however, is unclear. Acupuncture has been studied for its beneficial effects on diarrhea, but there is no compelling evidence for its effectiveness.

SUPPLEMENTS TO AVOID

Excessive intake of vitamin C or magnesium can cause diarrhea.

EBSCO CAM Review Board

FURTHER READING

Alfaleh, K., and D. Bassler. "Probiotics for Prevention of Necrotizing Enterocolitis in Preterm Infants." *Cochrane Database of Systematic Reviews* (2008): CD005496. Available through *EBSCO DynaMed Systematic Literature Surveillance* at http://www.ebscohost.com/dynamed.

Beausoleil, M., et al. "Effect of a Fermented Milk Combining *Lactobacillus acidophilus* Cl1285 and *Lactobacillus casei* in the Prevention of Antibiotic-Associated Diarrhea." *Canadian Journal of Gastroenterology* 21 (2007): 732-736.

Briand, V., et al. "Absence of Efficacy of Nonviable *Lactobacillus acidophilus* for the Prevention of Travelers' Diarrhea." *Clinical Infectious Diseases* 43 (2006): 1170-1175.

Gao, X. W., et al. "Dose-Response Efficacy of a Proprietary Probiotic Formula of *Lactobacillus acidophilus* CL1285 and *Lactobacillus casei* LBC80R for Antibiotic-Associated Diarrhea and *Clostridium difficile*-Associated Diarrhea Prophylaxis in Adult Patients." *American Journal of Gastroenterology* 105 (2010): 1636-1641.

Guandalini, S. "Probiotics for Children with Diarrhea: An Update." *Journal of Clinical Gastroenterology* 42, suppl. 2 (2008): S53-S57.

Henker, J., et al. "Placebo Versus Probiotic *Escherichia coli Nissle* 1917 for Treating Diarrhea of Greater than Four Days Duration in Infants and Toddlers." *Pediatric Infectious Disease Journal* 27 (2008): 494-499.

Hickson M, et al. "Use of Probiotic *Lactobacillus* Preparation to Prevent Diarrhoea Associated with Antibiotics." *British Medical Journal* 335 (2007): 80.

Lazzerini, M., and L. Ronfani. "Oral Zinc for Treating Diarrhoea in Children." *Cochrane Database of Systematic Reviews* (2008): CD005436. Available through *EBSCO DynaMed Systematic Literature Surveillance* at http://www.ebscohost.com/dynamed.

Leung, W. K., et al. "Treatment of Diarrhea-Predominant Irritable Bowel Syndrome with Traditional Chinese Herbal Medicine." *American Journal of Gastroenterology* 101 (2006): 1574-1580.

Lin, H. C., et al. "Oral Probiotics Prevent Necrotizing Enterocolitis in Very Low Birth Weight Preterm Infants." *Pediatrics* 122 (2008): 693-700.

Mao, M., et al. "Effect of a Lactose-Free Milk Formula Supplemented with Bifidobacteria and Streptococci on the Recovery from Acute Diarrhoea." *Asia Pacific Journal of Clinical Nutrition* 17 (2008): 30-34.

Patro, B., D. Golicki, and H. Szajewska. "Meta-analysis: Zinc Supplementation for Acute Gastroenteritis in Children." *Alimentary Pharmacology and Therapeutics* 28 (2008): 713-723.

Zaman, S., et al. "B 221, a Medical Food Containing Antisecretory Factor Reduces Child Diarrhoea." *Acta Paediatrica* 96 (2007): 1655-1659.

See also: Crohn's disease; Gas, intestinal; Irritable bowel syndrome (IBS); Lactose intolerance; Nondairy milk; Probiotics.

Diarrhea in children: Homeopathic remedies

CATEGORY: Homeopathy

DEFINITION: The use of highly diluted remedies to treat loose bowel movements, both acute and chronic, in children.

STUDIED HOMEOPATHIC REMEDIES: *Arsenicum; Chamomilla;* classical homeopathic remedy; *Podophyllum*

INTRODUCTION

Diarrhea, or loose bowel movements, can occur for many reasons. Food poisoning and infections are the most common causes of acute diarrhea. Chronic diarrhea, such as inflammatory bowel disease and irritable bowel syndrome, may be caused by ongoing illnesses of the digestive tract.

Appropriate treatment involves addressing the cause of the diarrhea, if possible. In many cases, however, all that can be done is to treat the symptoms.

Prolonged or severe diarrhea can be dangerous, especially in small children and the elderly. The greatest health risk is severe dehydration. This can often be corrected through the use of special oral solutions, but in some cases intravenous fluids may be required.

SCIENTIFIC EVALUATIONS OF HOMEOPATHIC REMEDIES

Two trials investigating the treatment of childhood diarrhea with homeopathic remedies were performed in Nicaragua and a third one was performed in Nepal, all by a single research group. Overall, the results suggest benefit with homeopathic treatment determined by classical homeopathic evaluation.

The first study followed eighty-one Nicaraguan children aged six months to five years, each of whom had acute diarrhea. Each child had a classical homeopathic evaluation and then was assigned an individual remedy in the potency 30c (centesimals) or placebo. The results showed statistically significant improvement in the treated group compared with the placebo group. (Both groups were also treated with standard oral fluid solutions to counteract dehydration.) Positive results were also reported in a similar study of 126 Nepalese children.

However, a trial of much the same design but including only thirty-three children failed to find meaningful evidence of benefit. For statistical reasons, studies with fewer participants are relatively likely to miss actual benefits; therefore, this study does not tend to invalidate the other two studies.

Another study by the same researchers enrolled 292 Honduran children with acute diarrhea and tested a fixed combination containing five popular homeopathic remedies. The combination remedy failed to prove more effective than placebo.

TRADITIONAL HOMEOPATHIC TREATMENTS

Classical homeopathy offers many possible homeopathic treatments for diarrhea. These therapies are chosen based on various specific details of the person seeking treatment.

When a child has diarrhea that is characterized by profuse, foul-smelling stools that are watery, gushing, and painless, and the child has a great thirst for large quantities of cold water, then his or her condition may fit the symptom picture for the homeopathic remedy *Podophyllum*. The child might also be fidgety and restless. However, when a child is generally hot, desires cold drinks, and has colicky, slimy, foul-smelling diarrhea with green stools that look like green grass, his or her condition might fit the symptom picture for the homeopathic remedy *Chamomilla*.

When a child is restless, anxious, and fearful; feels much worse around midnight; and has painful diarrhea with burning sensations, he or she may fit the symptom picture for homeopathic *Arsenicum*. Other characteristic symptoms include a red, sore anus; discomfort that is relieved by hot applications; and the complaint of feeling chilly, especially on the arms and legs.

EBSCO CAM Review Board

FURTHER READING

Jacobs, J., B. L. Guthrie, et al. "Homeopathic Combination Remedy in the Treatment of Acute Childhood Diarrhea in Honduras." *Journal of Alternative and Complementary Medicine* 12 (2006): 723-732.

Jacobs, J., L. M. Jimenez, S. Malthouse, et al. "Homeopathic Treatment of Acute Childhood Diarrhea: Results from a Clinical Trial in Nepal." *Journal of Alternative and Complementary Medicine* 6 (2000): 131-139.

Jacobs, J., L. M. Jimenez, S. S. Gloyd, et al. "Homeopathic Treatment of Acute Childhood Diarrhea: A Randomized Clinical Trial in Nicaragua." *British Homeopathic Journal* 82 (1993): 83-86.

Pappano, D., et al. "Why Pediatric Health Care Providers Are Not Using Homeopathic Antidiarrheal Agents." *Journal of Alternative and Complementary Medicine* 13 (2007): 1071-1076.

See also: Diarrhea.

Dietary Supplement Health and Education Act

CATEGORY: Organizations and legislation
DEFINITION: Established federal regulations for the manufacture, marketing, and use of dietary supplements in the United States.
Date: Signed on October 25, 1994

HISTORY OF THE ACT

The Dietary Supplement Health and Education Act (DSHEA) was created in response to the growing popularity of dietary supplements in the United States. The act amended the Food, Drug, and Cosmetic Act of 1938. In response to the federal government's priority of citizen health, members of Congress proposed DSHEA after studies revealed that 50 to 70 percent of adults use dietary supplements. Congress also recognized that the dietary supplement industry is a major contributor to the U.S. economy and that its regulation made sense both for consumers and for the industry.

Research has demonstrated that dietary supplements may contribute to health maintenance and to the prevention of chronic diseases such as heart disease, birth defects and disorders, and cancer. Research also has shown that there are rarely any safety issues with the use of supplements.

Lobbyists for the industry and other consumer groups strongly supported DSHEA. Consequently, U.S. president Bill Clinton signed DSHEA into law on October 25, 1994.

RULES AND REGULATIONS

DSHEA marked the first time that dietary supplements were defined by law. A dietary supplement is a product other than tobacco that is intended to supplement a person's diet. According to DSHEA, a supplement must contain either a vitamin, mineral, herb, or other botanical, amino acid, concentrate, metabolite, or extract (or a combination of these ingredients). The dietary supplement must be listed as such and cannot be labeled as the only component of a meal or diet, nor can it be a food additive. The DSHEA also stipulates the forms in which these supplements may be sold: capsule, powder, soft gel, gel cap, tablet, or liquid.

To enforce safety standards, the U.S. Food and Drug Administration (FDA) has regulatory power over

Dietary Supplement Health and Education Act of 1994

Following is an excerpt from section 2 of the Dietary Supplement Health and Education Act of 1994, in which the U.S. Congress finds that:

(1) improving the health status of United States citizens ranks at the top of the national priorities of the Federal Government;

(2) the importance of nutrition and the benefits of dietary supplements to health promotion and disease prevention have been documented increasingly in scientific studies;

(3) (A) there is a link between the ingestion of certain nutrients or dietary supplements and the prevention of chronic diseases such as cancer, heart disease, and osteoporosis; and (B) clinical research has shown that several chronic diseases can be prevented simply with a healthful diet, such as a diet that is low in fat, saturated fat, cholesterol, and sodium, with a high proportion of plant-based foods;

(4) healthful diets may mitigate the need for expensive medical procedures, such as coronary bypass surgery or angioplasty;

(5) preventive health measures, including education, good nutrition, and appropriate use of safe nutritional supplements, will limit the incidence of chronic diseases and reduce long-term health care expenditures;

(6) (A) promotion of good health and healthy lifestyles improves and extends lives while reducing health care expenditures; and (B) reduction in health care expenditures is of paramount importance to the future of the country and the economic well-being of the country;

(7) there is a growing need for emphasis on the dissemination of information linking nutrition and long-term good health;

(8) consumers should be empowered to make choices about preventive health care programs based on data from scientific studies of health benefits related to particular dietary supplements; ...

(13) although the Federal Government should take swift action against products that are unsafe or adulterated, the Federal Government should not take any actions to impose unreasonable regulatory barriers limiting or slowing the flow of safe products and accurate information to consumers;

(14) dietary supplements are safe within a broad range of intake, and safety problems with the supplements are relatively rare; and

(15) (A) legislative action that protects the right of access of consumers to safe dietary supplements is necessary in order to promote wellness; and (B) a rational Federal framework must be established to supersede the current ad hoc, patchwork regulatory policy on dietary supplements.

---

dietary supplements as food, rather than as medication. Under the DSHEA, the FDA is responsible for determining if a supplement is unsafe, that is, if insufficient information exists regarding the risk for a significant illness or injury. The FDA, however, does not test or evaluate a given product. The manufacturer must submit safety information a minimum of seventy-five days before marketing a new dietary ingredient and must notify the FDA within thirty days of marketing the product.

Under the Nutrition Labeling and Education Act of 1990, companies were not required to obtain authorization from the FDA before labeling a product a dietary supplement. The DSHEA, however, changed this when it created the Commission on Dietary Supplement Labels to evaluate the best means for providing current, accurate, and scientifically valid information to consumers.

According to DSHEA, the product must first claim a benefit related to a nutrient deficiency, must include information on the prevalence of the disease or condition the product addresses, and must include information on the product's mechanism of action. Also, the label must specifically state that the product is not intended to diagnose, treat, cure, or prevent any disease. The supplement label also must list the name and the per-serving quantity of each ingredient. Unlike prescription medications, supplement labels do not include reference or recommended daily intake (RDI) or daily recommended value (DRV).

DSHEA also regulates the marketing of dietary supplements. Written works, such as book chapters or

Dietary Supplement Safety

The word "dietary" may lead people to believe that supplements are as safe as foods. While this is often the case, many supplements have health effects, and side effects, similar to those of medications. However, because dietary supplements are not strictly regulated (as are drugs), consumers should be well informed about purchasing and using these products.

Dietary supplements are consumable products that contain one or more substances, usually natural, that are formulated to achieve a specific health effect. Three main groups of dietary supplements are nutritional, botanical, and miscellaneous.

- *Nutritional supplements.* These provide nutrients that are naturally present in food and have well-established health-related functions. These nutrients are isolated from foods and often provided at much higher concentrations. Examples include amino acids, fatty acids, and high-dose vitamins and minerals.

- *Botanical supplements.* These are herbal products containing concentrates or extracts from plants such as *Ginkgo biloba*, saw palmetto, and St. John's wort.

- *Miscellaneous supplements.* These include a variety of nonherbal substances from many sources that are not normally found in the human diet but are purported to have beneficial health effects. Examples include shark cartilage, DHEA (a steroid hormone precursor), and chondroitin.

The U.S. Food and Drug Administration (FDA) ensures that medicines, but not dietary supplements, are reasonably safe and effective. Government regulators consider dietary supplements to be more like food than medicine. Therefore, supplement makers are not held to the same strict approval standards as the drug industry. One reason for this is that dietary supplement manufacturers often cannot afford to do the level of research necessary to meet these FDA standards for safety and effectiveness. Drug companies spend billions of dollars on such research each year.

In 1994, the U.S. Congress passed the Dietary Supplement Health and Education Act (DSHEA). This act states that a dietary supplement may be sold without scientific evidence of effectiveness, as long as no specific health-benefit claims are made in its advertising or labeling. The manufacturer can only provide information about the intended use or potential benefits of the product. For example, a ginkgo label may not use the phrase "effective treatment for Alzheimer's dementia," but it can use the phrase "may be useful for boosting memory in the elderly."

DSHEA also allows lower safety standards for dietary supplements. Manufacturers need only show that their product is "reasonably expected to be safe," but DSHEA does not specify what evidence is required to make this safety assertion. In addition, once a product is on the market, it is up to the government to show that it is unsafe and that it should be withdrawn. Such a withdrawal is called a postmarket recall. These recalls do occur with drugs as well, but many consumer-advocacy groups claim that the public is at greater risk with dietary supplements because they do not undergo the stringent premarket scrutiny that drugs do. For example, the substance ephedra was banned from the market in the United States after a number of deaths, strokes, and heart attacks were attributed to its use.

Still, others argue that comparable vigilance is not necessary for these "natural" products, which are often gentler and less toxic than highly concentrated, chemically based drugs. While this may be true, "natural" does not necessarily mean "safe." Plants, after all, produce some of the most powerful poisons on earth. Additionally, it is known that vitamins and minerals in mega-doses cause toxicity. Furthermore, people taking prescription drugs may also take dietary supplements. Even if a supplement is considered safe, it can still interfere with the function of other medicines a person is taking.

Another issue closely related to safety and effectiveness is the concentration and purity of the product. When you purchase an FDA-approved drug, you know exactly what you are getting, down to the last milligram.

This is not always true of dietary supplements. Herbs, in particular, often contain many different constituents in addition to the active ingredient. Studies have shown that some supplements contain no active ingredients, while others contain much higher concentrations than the label indicates. It also is not uncommon for supplements to contain substances that are not listed on the label, some of which may be biologically active. Currently, U.S. government regulation does not ensure that what is on the label of a dietary supplement is actually in the bottle or package.

Richard Glickman-Simon, M.D.;
reviewed by Brian Randall, M.D.

scientific journal articles, may only be used in marketing a supplement if they contain data that is correct, balanced, and not misleading. This supporting literature may not endorse a specific brand or manufacturer and may not be displayed adjacent to the supplement that is for sale.

IMPLICATIONS AND CONTROVERSIES

The enactment of DSHEA allowed the dietary supplement industry to grow substantially. In 1994, the year DSHEA was enacted, total sales for the industry averaged $4 billion. In 2007, sales were estimated to be approximately $21 billion. Most transactions now occur on the Internet, through Web sites, which are not regulated by DSHEA.

DSHEA increased the FDA's ability to establish and enforce new labeling and potency standards. The FDA can take criminal action against violating companies and can ban supplements from the market. One case in which the FDA removed a product from the market was that of the well-publicized weight loss supplement ephedra, which was banned after several reports of adverse side effects in persons who had taken the supplement.

DSHEA brought greater attention and oversight to a previously unregulated industry. Still, critics of DSHEA call for even greater reform. Years after Congress proposed that the act's passage would reduce major illness and economic burden, the United States has seen neither result.

Even with DSHEA in place, dietary supplements are assumed to be safe unless proven otherwise. Manufacturers, rather than the FDA, determine the quality specifications of their product. Unlike prescription medications, dietary supplements do not come with package inserts describing potential negative interactions or side effects. Thus, consumers are left without a clear way of determining if a supplement is safe.

Although DSHEA has had a substantial impact on the dietary supplement industry, collaborative work among the U.S. government, consumers, and medical researchers and providers is still needed to further improve the industry. This quality control will ensure that consumers make the best-informed medical decisions.

Janet Ober Berman, M.S., CGC

FURTHER READING

Dietary Supplement Health and Education Act of 1994. Available at http://ods.od.nih.gov/about/dshea_wording.aspx. The online version of the act.

Dietary Supplements Labels Database. http://dietarysupplements.nlm.nih.gov. A service of the National Library of Medicine.

Office of Dietary Supplements (ODS). http://ods.od.nih.gov. The Web site of the agency that was formed through the enactment of the law. ODS is part of the National Institutes of Health.

Saldanha, Leila G. "The Dietary Supplement Marketplace: Constantly Evolving." *Nutrition Today* 42, no. 2 (2007): 52-54. An editorial detailing the financial implications of the act and the effects that the act may have on the growing supplements industry.

Seamson, Matthew J., and Kevin A. Clauson. "Ephedra: Yesterday, DSHEA, and Tomorrow: A Ten Year Perspective on the Dietary Supplement Health and Education Act of 1994." *Journal of Herbal Pharmacotherapy* 5, no. 3 (2005): 67-86. Detailed history and outline of the act's key points and its application to the case of ephedra and other dietary supplements.

See also: Codex Alimentarius Commission; Food and Drug Administration; Herbal medicine; Office of Dietary Supplements; Regulation of CAM; Supplements: Introduction; Vitamins and minerals.

Diet-based therapies

CATEGORY: Therapies and techniques
RELATED TERM: Nutritional therapies
DEFINITION: Complementary and alternative therapies using special diets to improve health, increase longevity, and prevent and treat specific health conditions and diseases.
PRINCIPAL PROPOSED USES: Asthma, diabetes, heart disease, high cholesterol, obesity
OTHER PROPOSED USES: General health, longevity, quality of life

OVERVIEW

Diet-based therapy uses specialized dietary regimens to promote wellness and to prevent and treat specific diseases, including cancer, cardiovascular disorders, and diabetes. Some low-fat vegetarian diets can help reverse arterial blockages that cause coronary artery disease and may help prevent or slow the progression of prostate and other cancers. Persons who follow a specific type of diet have reported cancer remission. It usually takes months or years for benefits to be observed. Diet therapies are more likely to be effective if practiced as a preventive measure against disease or if started early after the onset of disease.

Some diet-based movements, such as breatharianism, claim that food and even water are not necessary for living. Believers claim that human life can be sustained by a vital force whose energy comes from sunlight and by the nutrients of fresh air. Another diet therapy based on religious beliefs is fruitarianism, which involves a diet based solely on the intake of fruits, nuts, and seeds. This diet therapy is practiced by people who call themselves fruitarians and who believe that fruits are the original diet of humankind, a diet that stems from the time of Adam and Eve. Some followers of this practice will eat only fallen fruits.

Regardless of philosophical or religious beliefs, however, humans need a balanced diet to be healthy. People with chronic diseases and some types of cancer can enhance their quality of life by improving the quality of their daily meals, shifting or replacing eating habits, and being more aware about calorie intake.

MECHANISM OF ACTION

Some studies show that several diets based on fruits can improve lipid profiles and glucose tolerances and can stop the weight-gain tendency in some people. The intake of nuts, olive oil, and fish can reduce bad cholesterol. Reducing saturated fats in daily meals can reduce triglycerides in the blood. Potassium from fruits can also reduce muscle pains. It is well known that a diet low in salt (sodium) can help to reduce blood pressure.

USES AND APPLICATIONS

Diets have been used to treat hypertension. One of the most important science based-diets designed to control blood pressure is the Dietary Approaches to Stop Hypertension (DASH) diet, which is promoted by the National Heart, Lung, and Blood Institute, part of the National Institutes of Health (NIH).

The DASH diet is a plan that is low in saturated fats, cholesterol, and total fat. It emphasizes the intake of fruits, vegetables, fat-free or low-fat milk and milk products, whole grain products, fish, poultry, and nuts. The diet is low in lean red meat, sweets, added

sugars and sugar-containing beverages. It is rich in potassium, magnesium, calcium, protein, and fiber.

Type 2 diabetes is another chronic disease that can be partially controlled by diet. The ideal diabetic meal consists of a combination of foods, such as bread, products that are high in fat, dairy items that provide protein, and starchy vegetables. Most of the protein in a diabetic diet comes from chicken, fish, lean beef, or dairy. Servings and portions in diabetic diets depend on a person's level of physical activity.

Cardiovascular diseases can also be prevented and controlled by diet. Histological studies show that vascular injury accumulates from adolescence, making it extremely important to monitor one's lifestyle and diet from childhood to prevent a heart condition in the future. Any diet designed to control or prevent cardiovascular disease most be low in saturated fats (less than 7 percent of the daily diet) and low in cholesterol (less than 300 milligrams per day for healthy adults and less than 200 milligrams per day for adults with high levels of low-density lipoprotein, or bad, cholesterol).

The American Cancer Society recommends that people with cancer not undertake a dietary program as an exclusive or primary means of treatment. A macrobiotic diet is one of the most common diets followed by persons with cancer. It is based on whole cereal grains, especially brown rice, and is low in processed foods. Another diet used in cancer treatment is the Gerson diet, which is part of the Gerson therapy. The Gerson diet is said to cleanse the body, boost the immune system, and stimulate metabolism. The Gerson diet in general requires following a strict low-salt, low-fat, vegetarian diet containing a lot of fluids.

SCIENTIFIC EVIDENCE

NIH studies have demonstrated that a low level of salt combined with the DASH diet is effective at lowering blood pressure. The effect of this combination (at a sodium level of 1,500 milligrams per day) was an average blood pressure reduction of 8.9/4.5 millimeters of mercury (systolic/diastolic) in normal subjects. Persons in the studies who were hypertensive experienced an average reduction of 11.5/5.7 millimeters of mercury.

A low intake of saturated fats will reduce triglycerides in the blood. Studies have claimed that some diets designed for persons with cancer dramatically increase life expectancy, but many physicians counter this claim, saying that a lack of control groups means that there is insufficient scientific evidence to support those observations.

CHOOSING A PRACTITIONER

A nutritionist is the recommended professional advisor for the selection of a diet for a specific chronic condition. For persons with cancer, diets must be chosen and recommended by an oncologist.

SAFETY ISSUES

When beginning a therapeutic diet that involves a dramatically different way of eating, people should receive expert supervision so that they can avoid nutritional deficiencies. The human body, which needs carbohydrates, fats, and proteins for healthy function, burns its own reserves of energy in the absence of calorie intake. Fasting for extended periods leads to starvation, dehydration, and eventual death.

Diets based on one type of food, such as those based solely on fruits, can cause protein deficiencies, which inhibit growth and development in children. Fruit-based diets can also cause deficiencies in vitamin D, vitamin B_{12}, calcium, iron, zinc, and essential fatty acids.

Fernando J. Ferrer, Ph.D.

FURTHER READING

American Cancer Institute. "Questions and Answers About the Gerson Therapy." Available at http://www.cancer.gov/cancertopics/pdq/cam/gerson/patient/page2.

"DASH Diet Action Plan: The User-Friendly Book for the DASH Diet." Available at http://www.dashdiet.org.

Food and Nutrition Information Center. http://fnic.nal.usda.gov.

See also: Food allergies and sensitivities; Functional foods: Introduction; Functional foods: Overview; Low-carbohydrate diet; Low-glycemic index diet; Macrobiotic diet; Optimal health; Probiotics; Raw foods diet; Stanols and sterols; Supplements: Introduction; Vegan diet; Vegetarian diet.

Digoxin

RELATED TERM: Digitoxin
CATEGORY: Drug interactions

DEFINITION: A medication used for congestive heart failure and other heart conditions.
TRADE NAMES: Crystodigin, Lanoxicaps, Lanoxin
INTERACTIONS: Calcium, *Eleutherococcus senticosus*, *Ginkgo biloba*, hawthorn, horsetail, licorice, magnesium, St. John's wort, uzara

MAGNESIUM
Effect: Supplementation Possibly Helpful, but Take at a Different Time of Day

Magnesium deficiency can increase the risk of toxicity from digoxin. However, taking magnesium supplements at the same time as digoxin might impair the absorption of the drug. One should not take the magnesium supplement during the two hours before or after using digoxin.

CALCIUM
Effect: Supplementation Possibly Helpful

Although the evidence is quite weak, digoxin might cause a tendency toward calcium deficiency. Taking calcium supplements can be helpful.

HAWTHORN
Effect: Possible Interaction

The herb hawthorn is used to treat congestive heart failure. Whether it is safe to combine hawthorn with digoxin remains unclear. One small study failed to find any harmful interaction, but more research must be done before reliable conclusions can be drawn.

LICORICE
Effect: Possible Dangerous Interaction

Licorice root can lower potassium levels in the body, which can be dangerous for a person taking digoxin. The special form of licorice known as DGL (deglycyrrhizinated licorice) is a deliberately altered form of the herb that should not affect potassium levels.

ELEUTHEROCOCCUS SENTICOSUS
Effect: Possible Interaction

There has been one report of an apparent elevation in digoxin level caused by the herb *Eleutherococcus senticosus* (also known as Siberian ginseng). However, the details of the case suggest that the *Eleutherococcus* product might actually have interfered with a test for digoxin, rather than the digoxin levels themselves.

HORSETAIL

Effect: Possible Dangerous Interaction

Because horsetail can deplete the body of potassium, it may not be safe to combine this herb with digitalis drugs.

ST. JOHN'S WORT

Effect: Possible Reduction of Effectiveness of Drug

Evidence suggests that St. John's wort may interact with digoxin, possibly requiring an increased dosage to maintain the proper effect. Conversely, persons taking St. John's wort and whose digoxin dose is adjusted by their physician should note that suddenly stopping the herb could cause blood levels of the drug to rise dangerously high.

UZARA

Effect: Possible Harmful Effect

Uzara root (*Xysmalobium undulatum*) is used to treat diarrhea. It contains substances similar to digoxin and may cause false readings on tests designed to measure digoxin levels. These substances also might alter (either increase or decrease) the effectiveness of digoxin.

GINKGO BILOBA

Effect: No Interaction

One study found that simultaneous use of the herb *Ginkgo biloba* (80 milligrams three times daily of the typical standardized extract) does not change digoxin levels.

EBSCO CAM Review Board

FURTHER READING

Gurley, B. J., et al. "Gauging the Clinical Significance of P-Glycoprotein-Mediated Herb-Drug Interactions: Comparative Effects of St. John's Wort, Echinacea, Clarithromycin, and Rifampin on Digoxin Pharmacokinetics." *Molecular Nutrition and Food Research* 52, no. 7 (2008): 772-779.

Mauro, V. F., et al. "Impact of *Ginkgo biloba* on the Pharmacokinetics of Digoxin." *American Journal of Therapeutics* 10 (2003): 247-251.

Mueller, S. C., et al. "Effect of St John's Wort Dose and Preparations on the Pharmacokinetics of Digoxin." *Clinical Pharmacology and Therapeutics* 75 (2004): 546-557.

Pronsky, Z. M., and J. P. Crowe. *Food Medication Interactions.* 16th ed. Birchrunville, Pa.: Food-Medication Interactions, 2010.

Tankanow, R., et al. "Interaction Study Between Digoxin and a Preparation of Hawthorn (*Crataegus oxyacantha*)." *Journal of Clinical Pharmacology* 43 (2003): 637-642.

Thurmann, P. A., et al. "Interference of Uzara Glycosides in Assays of Digitalis Glycosides." *International Journal of Clinical Pharmacology and Therapeutics* 42 (2004): 281-284.

See also: Calcium; Congestive heart failure; *Eleutherococcus senticosus*; Food and Drug Administration; Ginkgo; Hawthorn; Heart attack; Horsetail; Magnesium; St. John's wort; Supplements: Introduction.

Diindolylmethane

CATEGORY: Functional foods
DEFINITION: Natural substance promoted as a dietary supplement for specific health benefits.
PRINCIPAL PROPOSED USE: Reducing cancer risk
OTHER PROPOSED USES: Balancing hormone levels, cervical dysplasia, female sexual function, male sexual function

OVERVIEW

Diindolylmethane (DIM) is produced when the substance indole-3-carbinol is digested. Indole-3-carbinol, found in broccoli and other vegetables, has shown considerable promise for cancer prevention. Some of its benefits in this regard may occur after it is converted by the body to DIM. Also, DIM has complex interactions with the hormone estrogen, which could lead to either positive or negative effects on cancer risk.

SOURCES

There is no dietary requirement for DIM. Good natural sources include broccoli, Brussels sprouts, cabbage, and cauliflower.

THERAPEUTIC DOSAGES

Manufacturers selling DIM products typically recommend about 500 to 1,000 milligrams daily. The optimal dose (if there is any) is not known.

THERAPEUTIC USES

Numerous test-tube and animal studies hint that DIM might help prevent various types of cancer, especially breast, cervical, prostate, and uterine cancer. However, this evidence is far too preliminary to serve as the basis for recommending that anyone use DIM. As with many proposed cancer-preventing substances, there are also circumstances in which DIM might actually increase the risk of cancer.

Some of DIM's apparent anticancer benefits appear to derive from its complex interactions with estrogen. DIM appears to alter liver function in such a manner that an increased amount of estrogen becomes metabolized into inactive forms. In addition, DIN blocks certain effects of estrogen on cells; however, it may enhance other effects of estrogen. The overall effect is far too complex and poorly understood to be described as balancing estrogen in the body, which is what many proponents say about DIM.

DIM also appears to have an antitestosterone effect, which could make it helpful for preventing or treating breast cancer. Again, this effect has been optimistically termed "balancing testosterone levels."

Preliminary evidence hints that DIM may offer benefit for diseases caused by the human papilloma virus. These diseases include cervical dysplasia and respiratory papillomatosis.

According to some manufacturers, DIM can enhance sexual function in men or women and can also enhance sports performance. However, there is no evidence that DIM actually works.

SAFETY ISSUES

DIM is thought to be a relatively nontoxic substance. However, comprehensive safety studies have not been completed. Because of DIM's complex interactions with estrogen and testosterone, it has the potential for causing hormonal disturbances. Safety in young children, pregnant or nursing women, and people with severe liver or kidney disease has not been established.

Although there are no known drug interactions with DIM, the substance has shown considerable potential for interacting with many medications. For this reason, if one uses any medication that is critical for health, one should not use DIM except under a physician's supervision.

EBSCO CAM Review Board

FURTHER READING

Dalessandri, K. M., et al. "Pilot Study: Effect of 3,3'-Diindolylmethane Supplements on Urinary Hormone Metabolites in Postmenopausal Women with a History of Early-Stage Breast Cancer." *Nutrition and Cancer* 50 (2004): 161-167.

Le, H. T., et al. "Plant-Derived 3,3'-Diindolylmethane Is a Strong Androgen Antagonist in Human Prostate Cancer Cells." *Journal of Biological Chemistry* 278 (2003): 21136-21145.

Lord, R. S., B. Bongiovanni, and J. A. Bralley. "Estrogen Metabolism and the Diet-Cancer Connection: Rationale for Assessing the Ratio of Urinary Hydroxylated Estrogen Metabolites." *Alternative Medicine Review* 7 (2002): 112-129.

See also: Cancer risk reduction; Cervical dysplasia; Indole-3-carbinol; Sexual dysfunction in men; Sexual dysfunction in women.

Dioscorides, Pedanius

CATEGORY: Biography
IDENTIFICATION: Greek physician and botanist whose work is considered foundational to pharmacology
BORN: c. 40; Anazarbus, Roman Cilicia (now in Turkey)
DIED: c. 90; unknown

OVERVIEW

Greek physician and botanist Pedanius Dioscorides' five-volume encyclopedia *De Materia Medica* (wr. late first century; *The Greek Herbal of Dioscorides*, 1655), about herbal medicine and related healing practices, has been a cornerstone of complementary and alternative medicine for more than one thousand years. The work makes him a key contributor to the early field of what came to be called pharmacology. Of note, the still-used Latin medical term *materia medica* (referring to the body of collected knowledge on the properties of any medicinal substance) was derived from the title of Dioscorides' work.

Historic records indicate that Dioscorides practiced medicine in Rome around the time of Roman emperor Nero. Dioscorides was a surgeon with the army of the emperor, a position that likely provided him the opportunity to travel far and wide. During his travels, he would have collected various plants and minerals that could be used for treating ailing persons.

In *De Materia Medica*, Dioscorides provides a thorough explanation of most medicines used by the

Medicinal Olive Oil

Pedanius Dioscorides, in his De Materia Medica, *explains medicinal uses for olive oil in these two excerpted sections.*

"New Oil from Unripe Olives"

Oil from unripe olives is the best to use for health. The best is considered that which is new, not biting, with a sweet smell. This is also effective for the preparation of ointments. It is also good for the stomach because it is therapeutic for the bowels, and when held in the mouth it contracts loose gums, strengthens the teeth and represses sweating.

"Old Olive Oil"

That which is the oldest and most fat is the most fit for bodily uses. Commonly all oil is warming and softens flesh, keeping the body from being easily chilled with cold, making it more ready to perform actions. It is good for the digestive system, and has a softening strength, dulling the strength of ulcerating medicines in mixtures. It is given against poisons, taken immediately and vomited up again. A half-pint purge, taken as a drink with the same amount of barley water or with water. Six glassfuls (boiled with rue and taken as a drink) are given effectively to those troubled with griping, and it expels worms. This is administered especially for obstruction of the intestines, but the older oil is more heating and violently dispersing. It is a good ointment to sharpen the eyesight. If there is no old oil at hand, new oil must be mixed as follows. Pour it out into the best jar at hand, and boil it until it is the thickness of honey. Then use it, for it is has an equal strength.

Romans, Greeks, and other ancient cultures. In total, Dioscorides' work discusses about six hundred different plants, seeds, fruits, and other preparations used for medicinal purposes. The encyclopedia not only contains graphic depictions and describes the uses of many of these preparations; it also outlines their ancient names and origins.

Dioscorides went on to classify many of the agents based on their medicinal properties, such as being antiseptic or anti-inflammatory. Volume 1 describes the use of aromatic oils, salves, trees, and shrubs and examines their medicinal products. Volume 2 includes medicines derived from animals and from cereals and some herbs (such as pot herbs and sharp herbs). Vol-

umes 3 and 4 detail the use of roots, juices, seeds, and other herbs. Finally, volume 5 discusses the use of various minerals and wines for medicinal purposes.

Brandy Weidow, M.S.

FURTHER READING

Dioscorides, Pedanius. *De Materia Medica: Being an Herbal with Many Other Medicinal Materials.* Translated by Tess Anne Osbaldeston and R. P. A. Wood. Johannesburg, South Africa: Ibidis, 2000.

Riddle, John M. "Dioscorides." In *Catalogus translationum et commentariorum: Mediaeval and Renaissance Latin Translations and Commentaries–Annotated Lists and Guides,* edited by F. Edward Cranz and Paul Oskar Kristeller. Washington, D.C.: Catholic University of America Press, 1984.

_____. *Dioscorides on Pharmacy and Medicine.* Austin: University of Texas Press, 1985.

Scarborough, J., and V. Nutton. "The Preface of Dioscorides' *Materia Medica*: Introduction, Translation, and Commentary." *Transactions and Studies of the College of Physicians of Philadelphia* 4, no. 3 (1982): 187-227.

See also: Herbal medicine; Traditional healing.

Diverticular disease

CATEGORY: Condition

RELATED TERMS: Acute colonic diverticulitis, acute diverticulitis, diverticulitis, diverticulosis

DEFINITION: Treatment of infected or inflamed pouches in the large intestine.

PRINCIPAL PROPOSED TREATMENTS: None

OTHER PROPOSED TREATMENTS: Fiber supplements psyllium, glucomannan, methylcellulose

INTRODUCTION

Almost one-half of all Americans older than age sixty years develop diverticulosis: small, bulging pouches (diverticula) in the colon. In most cases, these diverticula do not cause any discomfort. However, in perhaps 15 percent of people with diverticulosis, diverticula may become inflamed or infected. The result is a condition called diverticulitis. Symptoms of diverticulitis include pain, nausea, and sometimes fever.

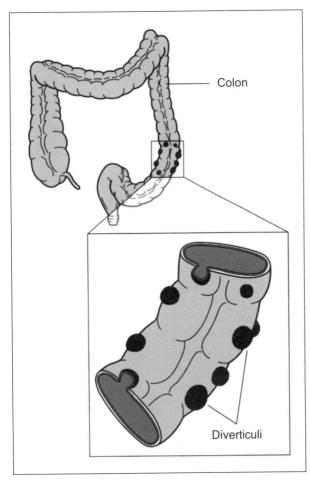

Diverticulosis occurs when multiple diverticuli (outpouchings) appear on the colon wall.

It is thought that the main cause of diverticulosis is the relatively low-fiber diet consumed in developed countries. Fiber is critical to digestion because it softens stools and makes them pass through the bowel more easily. Factors that cause diverticulitis include increased pressure in the bowel from straining to pass a hard stool, defects in the colon wall, and chronic constipation. The conventional treatment of diverticulitis includes dietary changes and antibiotics, and sometimes surgery.

PROPOSED NATURAL TREATMENTS

Fiber supplements have shown promise for both preventing and treating diverticulosis and diverticulitis. Studies suggest (but do not prove) that diets high in fiber and low in total fat and red meat may help prevent diverticular disease. Furthermore, high fiber consumption may help prevent diverticulitis from developing in people with diverticulosis. However, this has not been proven, and the results of the scant published controlled trials on the topic have been inconsistent.

Common fiber supplements used to treat the condition include psyllium, glucomannan, and methylcellulose. However, the use of fiber supplements during an active bout of diverticulitis is not advisable, because the colon needs to rest.

Contrary to some reports, there is no evidence that obesity or consumption of caffeine or alcohol increases the risk of diverticular disease. However, high levels of physical activity may reduce the risk of developing the condition.

EBSCO CAM Review Board

FURTHER READING

Aldoori, W., and M. Ryan-Harshman. "Preventing Diverticular Disease: Review of Recent Evidence on High-Fibre Diets." *Canadian Family Physician* 48 (2002): 1632-1637.

Feldman, Mark, Lawrence S. Friedman, and Lawrence J. Brandt, eds. *Sleisenger and Fordtran's Gastrointestinal and Liver Disease: Pathophysiology, Diagnosis, Management*. New ed. 2 vols. Philadelphia: Saunders/Elsevier, 2010.

Murray, C. D., and A. V. Emmanuel. "Medical Management of Diverticular Disease." *Best Practice and Research: Clinical Gastroenterology* 16 (2002): 611-620.

Ornstein, M. H., et al. "Are Fibre Supplements Really Necessary in Diverticular Disease of the Colon?" *British Medical Journal* (Clinical Research Edition) 25 (1981): 1353-1356.

Smits, B. J., A. M. Whitehead, and P. Prescott. "Lactulose in the Treatment of Symptomatic Diverticular Disease: A Comparative Study with High-Fibre Diet." *British Journal of Clinical Practice* 44 (1990): 314-318.

See also: Diet-based therapies; Gallstones; Gastritis; Gastrointestinal health; Pain management; Pancreatitis.

DMAE

CATEGORY: Herbs and supplements
RELATED TERMS: Deanol, 2-dimethylaminoethanol
DEFINITION: Natural substance promoted as a dietary supplement for specific health benefits.
PRINCIPAL PROPOSED USE: Attention deficit disorder
OTHER PROPOSED USES: Alzheimer's disease, Huntington's chorea, tardive dyskinesia

OVERVIEW

DMAE (2-dimethylaminoethanol) is a natural chemical that has been used to treat a number of conditions affecting the brain and central nervous system. Like other such treatments, it is thought to work by increasing production of the neurotransmitter acetylcholine, although this has not been proven.

SOURCES

DMAE is sold in pharmacies, in health food stores, and on the Web as a nutritional supplement.

THERAPEUTIC DOSAGES

Manufacturers' recommended dosages and those used in clinical studies vary between 400 and 1,800 milligrams (mg) daily.

THERAPEUTIC USES

Preliminary evidence suggests that DMAE may be helpful for attention deficit disorder (ADD). More widely marketed today as a memory and mood enhancer, DMAE is said to improve intellectual functioning; however, there are no clinical studies that support its use for these purposes. The basis for such claims probably stems from its purported ability to increase levels of the neurotransmitter acetylcholine. Drugs and supplements called cholinergics that increase acetylcholine have been used to treat Alzheimer's disease, tardive dyskinesia, and Huntington's chorea. Because DMAE was believed to be a cholinergic, it has been tried for all of these disorders. However, well-designed, double-blind, placebo-controlled studies have yielded almost entirely negative results. In addition, there is some controversy over whether DMAE really increases acetylcholine.

SCIENTIFIC EVIDENCE

Attention deficit disorder. There is some evidence that DMAE may be helpful for ADD, according to studies performed in the 1970s. Two such studies were reported in a review article on DMAE. Fifty children age six to twelve years who had been diagnosed with hyperkinesia (their diagnosis today would likely be ADD) participated in a double-blind study comparing DMAE with placebo. The dose was increased from 300 to 500 mg daily by the third week and was continued for ten weeks. Evaluations revealed statistically significant test score improvements in the treatment group compared with the placebo group.

Another double-blind study compared DMAE with both methylphenidate (Ritalin) and placebo in seventy-four children described as having unspecified "learning disabilities" (also probably what would be considered ADD today). The study found significant test score improvement for both treatment groups in a ten-week period. Positive results were also seen in a small open study.

Alzheimer's disease. Most people age forty years and older experience some memory loss, but Alzheimer's disease is much more serious, leading to severe mental deterioration (dementia) in the elderly. Microscopic examination of this condition shows that in the areas of the brain involved in higher thought processes, nerve cells have died and disappeared, particularly cells that release the chemical acetylcholine. Drugs such as tacrine and danazol and supplements such as huperzine A are used for Alzheimer's based on their ability to increase acetylcholine levels. Because DMAE is also thought to increase acetylcholine, trials have been performed to test its effectiveness for the same purpose. However, there is no real evidence that it works.

A double-blind, placebo-controlled study involving twenty-seven people with Alzheimer's disease tested DMAE as a treatment. Thirteen participants were placed in the group receiving DMAE; however, six of them had to drop out of the study because of side effects such as drowsiness, increased confusion, and elevated blood pressure. In those completing the trial, no differences were seen between the treatment group and those taking placebo.

An open trial enrolling fourteen persons found no improvement in memory or in cognitive function. The researchers did note improvements in symptoms of depression. However, in the absence of a placebo group, this observation means little.

Tardive dyskinesia. Tardive dyskinesia (TD) is a potentially permanent side effect of drugs used to control schizophrenia. This late-developing (tardy, or tardive) complication consists of annoying, uncontrollable movements (dyskinesias), particularly in the face.

Based on its reported cholinergic effect, DMAE has been proposed as a treatment for TD. Although some case reports and open studies seem to suggest that DMAE might be useful for this purpose, properly designed studies using double-blind methods and placebo control groups have not borne this out. Of twelve double-blind studies reviewed, only one found DMAE to be significantly effective when compared with placebo. A meta-analysis of proposed treatments for TD found DMAE to be no more effective than placebo. It seems likely, though not entirely certain, that the benefits seen in open studies and individual cases were the result of a placebo effect. However, it is also possible that some particular persons respond well to DMAE, even if most people do not.

Huntington's chorea. Huntington's chorea is a genetically inherited disease that results in personality changes and, somewhat similarly to TD, uncontrolled spastic movements. It does not usually become symptomatic until a person is in his or her late thirties or older, although about 10 percent of people with Huntington's begin to show signs of the disorder in childhood or adolescence. DMAE was not found to be an effective treatment for Huntington's chorea in double-blind, placebo-controlled trials, although mixed results have been obtained using DMAE in open trials.

SAFETY ISSUES

Although most clinical investigations using DMAE report that the participants experienced no side effects, enough researchers have found adverse reactions to suggest that some caution is appropriate in using this supplement. One study reports increased confusion, drowsiness, and elevated blood pressure; another study reports headache and muscle tension as possible adverse effects; and another study suggests that weight loss and insomnia may accompany the use of DMAE. There is also one case report of a woman who developed severe TD after taking DMAE for ten years for a hand tremor. In addition, a number of manufacturers warn against the use of DMAE by people with epilepsy or a history of convulsions. Furthermore, maximum safe dosages for young children, pregnant or nursing women, and people with severe liver or kidney disease have not been established.

EBSCO CAM Review Board

FURTHER READING

Grossman, R. "The Role of Dimethylaminoethanol in Cosmetic Dermatology." *American Journal of Clinical Dermatology* 6 (2005): 39-47.

Martorana, A., Z. Esposito, and G. Koch. "Beyond the Cholinergic Hypothesis: Do Current Drugs Work in Alzheimer's Disease?" *CNS Neuroscience and Therapeutics* 16 (2010): 235-245.

Soares, K. V., and J. J. McGrath. "The Treatment of Tardive Dyskinesia." *Schizophrenia Research* 39 (1999): 1-18.

See also: Alzheimer's disease and non-Alzheimer's dementia; Attention deficit disorder; Mental health; Schizophrenia; Tardive dyskinesia.

Dong quai

CATEGORY: Herbs and supplements

RELATED TERMS: *Angelica sinensis*, dang kwai, dang quai, dong kwai, tang quai

DEFINITION: Natural plant product used as a dietary supplement for specific health benefits.

PRINCIPAL PROPOSED USES: Dysmenorrhea, menstrual disorders, premenstrual syndrome

Probably ineffective use: Menopausal symptoms

OVERVIEW

One of the major herbs used in traditional Chinese herbal medicine, *Angelica sinensis*, or dong quai, is closely related to *A. archangelica*, a common European garden herb and the flavoring in Benedictine and Chartreuse liqueurs. The carrot-like roots of this fragrant plant are harvested in the fall after about three years of cultivation and are stored in airtight containers before processing.

Traditionally, dong quai is said to be one of the most important herbs for strengthening the *xue*. The Chinese term *xue* is often translated as "blood," but it actually refers to a complex concept in traditional Chinese medicine, of which the Western notion of blood is only a part. In the late nineteenth century, an extract of dong quai known as Eumenol became popular in Europe as a "female tonic," and this is how most people consider it in the West.

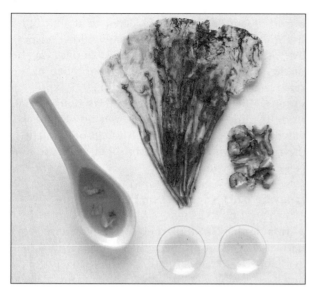

Dong quai sliced dried roots, infusion, and tincture. (Andy Crawford and Steve Gorton/Getty Images)

USES AND APPLICATIONS

Dong quai is often recommended as a treatment for menstrual cramps, premenstrual syndrome (PMS), and other problems related to menstruation, as well as for hot flashes and other menopausal symptoms. However, the scientific evidence supporting these uses is very weak, consisting primarily of test tube and animal studies and a few open studies of people. Only double-blind, placebo-controlled studies can actually show a treatment effective. A twenty-four-week study that compared the effects of dong quai with a placebo in seventy-one postmenopausal women found no benefit.

DOSAGE

It is recommended that dong quai be used under the supervision of an herbalist qualified in traditional Chinese herbal medicine. The herb is not dangerous, but it is difficult to self-prescribe Chinese herbal formulas.

A typical dosage of dong quai is ten to forty drops of dong quai tincture, one to three times daily, or one standard-size gelatin capsule, three times daily.

SAFETY ISSUES

Dong quai is generally believed to be nontoxic. According to Chinese studies, which may not have been up to current scientific standards, very large amounts have been given to rats without causing harm. Side effects are rare and primarily consist of mild gastrointestinal distress and occasional allergic reactions (such as rash).

Contrary to popular belief, dong quai does not appear to have estrogen-like actions. However, according to an article in the *Singapore Medical Journal*, a thirty-five-year-old man who used a prepared herbal formula called dong quai pills developed enlarged breasts. Such enlargement would typically result if a man used estrogen. The authors of the article blamed the dong quai itself. However, a more likely explanation is that the prepared herbal formula was "spiked" with synthetic estrogen. There are numerous reports of prepackaged Asian herb products containing unlabeled constituents, including conventional medications designed to enhance their effect.

In a test-tube study, dong quai was again found to be nonestrogenic, and yet it nonetheless stimulated the growth of breast cancer cells. Although the mechanism of this effect is not known, the results suggest that women who have had breast cancer should avoid using dong quai.

Dong quai may interact with the blood-thinning drug warfarin (Coumadin), increasing the risk of bleeding, according to one case report. Dong quai might also conceivably interact with other blood-thinning drugs, such as heparin, aspirin, clopidogrel (Plavix), ticlopidine (Ticlid), and pentoxifylline (Trental).

Certain constituents of dong quai can cause photosensitivity (increased sensitivity to the sun), but this has not been observed to occur in people using the whole herb.

Safety in young children, pregnant or nursing women, or those with severe liver or kidney disease has not been established. One case report suggests that dong quai usage by a nursing mother caused elevated blood pressure in both the mother and the child.

IMPORTANT INTERACTIONS

Dong quai might interact with blood-thinning drugs and increase the risk of bleeding.

EBSCO CAM Review Board

FURTHER READING

Amato, P., S. Christophe, and P. Mellon. "Estrogenic Activity of Herbs Commonly Used as Remedies for Menopausal Symptoms." *Menopause* 9 (2002): 145-150.

Goh, S. Y., and K. C. Loh. "Gynaecomastia and the Herbal Tonic 'Dong Quai.'" *Singapore Medical Journal* 42 (2001): 115-116.

Hirata, J. D., et al. "Does Dong Quai Have Estrogenic Effects in Postmenopausal Women?" *Fertility and Sterility* 68 (1997): 981-986.

Nortier, J. L., et al. "Urothelial Carcinoma Associated with the Use of a Chinese Herb (*Aristolochia fangchi*)." *New England Journal of Medicine* 342 (2000): 1686-1692.

Zava, D. T., C. M. Dollbaum, and M. Blen. "Estrogen and Progestin Bioactivity of Foods, Herbs, and Spices." *Proceedings of the Society for Experimental Biology and Medicine* 217 (1998): 369-378.

Zhu, D. P. "Dong Quai." *American Journal of Chinese Medicine* 15 (1987): 117-125.

See also: Dysmenorrhea; Herbal medicine; Menopause; Pain management; Premenstrual syndrome (PMS); Traditional Chinese herbal medicine; Women's health.

Double-blind, placebo-controlled studies

CATEGORY: Issues and overviews

RELATED TERMS: Evidence-based medicine, randomized double-blind, placebo-controlled trials, science-based studies

DEFINITION: Scientific trials in which a fake treatment (placebo) is used in conjunction with a real treatment and in which participants and researchers, through "blinding," do not know which participants are receiving real or placebo treatments.

OVERVIEW

The gold standard for determining whether a medical treatment works is the double-blind, placebo-controlled study. With a few exceptions, new drugs must pass a number of double-blind studies to be approved by the U.S. Food and Drug Administration (FDA). Conversely, when a drug already in use for a given purpose repeatedly fails to prove effective for that purpose in double-blind studies, that drug is eventually discredited.

Herbs and supplements do not need FDA approval, but they too are subjected to double-blind studies, and the results of those studies, whether positive or negative, can have a major impact on the public. Therefore, when an article published in the *International Journal of Epidemiology* in 2007 exposed a serious deficiency in the entire body of double-blind study literature, it struck at the very heart of evidence-based medicine. Based on the findings of this article, the results of virtually all double-blind trials are now viewed with skepticism.

HISTORY OF DOUBLE-BLIND, PLACEBO-CONTROLLED STUDIES

In a double-blind, placebo-controlled study, some participants are given the real treatment while others are given a fake treatment designed to appear as much as possible like the real treatment (the placebo control). The assignment to real or fake treatment groups is accomplished by flipping a coin or by a random-number generator. Both participants and researchers are kept from knowing who is receiving real treatment and who is receiving fake treatment and are, therefore, "blinded." The full technical name for these studies, randomized double-blind, placebo-controlled trials, is often abbreviated as RCTs, or randomized-controlled trials. However, this abbreviation leaves out both placebo and blinding and therefore is not discussed here.

The double-blind, placebo-controlled study was first conceived by German researchers in the 1950s as a way to minimize the power of suggestion and other confounding factors. By the 1960s, the medical scientific community had come to recognize that double-blind trials are the essential means of establishing treatment efficacy. However, it was not until the 1970s that pharmaceuticals were routinely required to pass meaningful double-blind studies to obtain FDA approval. (Many drugs approved before this time were "grandfathered" in.)

At about the same time, double-blind studies of herbs and supplements began to appear sporadically in the literature, but such studies remained relatively uncommon until the late 1980s. The rate of publication of double-blind studies of natural products has since grown at an astonishing pace. In the early 1990s, months could go by before a new double-blind study of a natural product was published; in the first decade of the twenty-first century, fifteen to twenty such studies were published each week. Furthermore, while the

Selected Study Definitions from ClinicalTrials.gov

- *Blind:* A randomized trial is "blind" if the participant is not told which arm of the trial he or she is on. A clinical trial is "blind" if participants are unaware of whether they are in the experimental or control arm of the study; also called masked.

- *Double-blind study:* A clinical trial design in which neither the participating individuals nor the study staff know which participants are receiving the experimental drug and which are receiving a placebo (or another therapy). Double-blind trials are thought to produce objective results, since the expectations of the doctor and the participant about the experimental drug do not affect the outcome; also called double-masked study.

- *Single-blind study:* A study in which one party, either the investigator or the participant, is unaware of what medication the participant is taking; also called single-masked study.

- *Placebo:* A placebo is an inactive pill, liquid, or powder that has no treatment value. In clinical trials, experimental treatments are often compared with placebos to assess the treatment's effectiveness.

- *Placebo-controlled study:* A method of investigation of drugs in which an inactive substance (the placebo) is given to one group of participants, while the drug being tested is given to another group. The results obtained in the two groups are then compared to see if the investigational treatment is more effective in treating the studied condition.

- *Placebo effect:* A physical or emotional change in a study participant, occurring after a substance is taken or administered, that is not the result of any special property of the substance. The change may be beneficial, reflecting the expectations of the participant and, often, the expectations of the person giving the substance.

These negative trials have been discouraging for supporters of natural medicine. However, the foregoing journal article has cast doubt on these negative results, though it also casts doubt on all positive results. This landmark 2007 article by Danish researcher Asbjorn Hróbjartsson and colleagues in the *International Journal of Epidemiology* was, essentially, a study of studies. Through extensive analysis of published studies augmented by interviews with some of the researchers who published those studies, Hróbjartsson and colleagues documented that the vast majority of researchers who perform double-blind, placebo-controlled studies fail to carry out a central, essential task: that of determining whether the blinding held firm. In other words, researchers did not check whether participants and observers remained unable to distinguish the real treatment from the fake treatment.

It would not have been difficult to answer this question; one can simply poll participants and observers and ask them to guess. If the guesses come out correct no more than about one-half the time, then it would be fair to conclude that the blinding remained intact. However, researchers generally do not conduct such a poll; therefore, they generally do not know whether the blinding remained intact. Knowing this, however, is essential to a study's validity. If blinding does not hold–that is, if most people involved in the study figure out who is taking placebo and who is taking the real treatment because, for example, the real treatment is smelly–then the validity of the study is drastically and even fatally compromised.

IMPORTANCE OF BLINDING

Suppose the researchers conducting a study want to prove that an herb or supplement does not work. Such bias does not matter much if the study is truly double-blind; because researchers cannot tell who is

typical study published in the early days of natural product testing involved ten or twenty participants, studies now commonly enroll more than one hundred participants. Some studies are even larger: Studies of vitamin E, beta-carotene, and other antioxidants, for example, have enrolled tens of thousands of participants.

As natural treatments have begun to undergo systematic testing, many have failed to prove effective. For example, in the giant studies just mentioned, vitamin E and beta-carotene proved ineffective for preventing heart disease or cancer. Others also have proved ineffective: garlic for high cholesterol, glucosamine for arthritis, and calcium supplements for osteoporosis.

getting the real treatment and who is getting the placebo, the outcome of the study is insulated from their preferences. However, once the blinding is broken, this protection disappears. For example, researchers disinclined to believe that glucosamine can help arthritis may unconsciously underestimate or under-report benefits in patients they know are taking glucosamine. This in turn could lead to a false outcome in the study, an apparent failure of a treatment that actually works.

The reverse also is true. For example, if researchers are biased in favor of the natural product (or drug) being tested, their predilections will likely cause them to see benefits not actually present; this is only human nature. However, when researchers do not know who is getting the treatment and who is getting the placebo, their bias has no effect. (Bias also can appear through manipulation of statistics or dishonesty.)

The problem of observer bias is just one of the confounding factors that double-blinding forestalls. Still, Hróbjartsson and colleagues found that most researchers do not bother to poll their study participants to see if the blinding held. Among those who did conduct such a poll, less than one-half actually found that the blinding had been maintained. This means that more than one-half of all published double-blind studies are quite possibly invalid.

In one sense this is good news for supporters of natural medicine: All the recent negative studies regarding natural products may have been flawed by a broken blinding. In another sense, the very same research deficiency identified by Hróbjartsson and colleagues means that positive studies involving natural products also may be invalid.

FURTHER READING

Hróbjartsson, A., et al. "Blinded Trials Taken to the Test: An Analysis of Randomized Clinical Trials That Report Tests for the Success of Blinding." *International Journal of Epidemiology* 36, no. 3 (2007): 654-663.

Kantor, M. "The Role of Rigorous Scientific Evaluation in the Use and Practice of Complementary and Alternative Medicine." *Journal of the American College of Radiology* 6, no. 4 (2009): 254-262.

Neutens, James J., and Laurna Rubinson. *Research Techniques for the Health Sciences*. 4th ed. San Francisco: Benjamin Cummings, 2010.

See also: CAM on Pubmed; Clinical trials; Placebo effect; Pseudoscience; Regulation of CAM; Scientific method.

Doxorubicin

RELATED DRUGS: Hydroxydaunomycin, Hydroxydoxorubicin, Liposomal doxorubicin
CATEGORY: Drug interactions
DEFINITION: A chemotherapy drug used to treat many different forms of cancer.
INTERACTION: Antioxidants
TRADE NAMES: Adriamycin, Doxil, Rubex

ANTIOXIDANTS

Effect: Possible Helpful Interactions

It is hypothesized that many of the side effects of doxorubicin occur through the production of free radicals, dangerous substances that can harm many cells. Antioxidants scavenge or quench free radicals. On this basis, a number of antioxidants have been proposed as a treatment for reducing doxorubicin toxicity. While some evidence of benefit has been seen in animal studies, at present there is inadequate supporting evidence from human trials. For example, while vitamin E has shown promise for preventing cardiac toxicity in animal studies, it has persistently failed to prove effective in people.

The supplement melatonin has also shown some promise in animal studies for reducing the cardiac toxicity of doxorubicin; however, the only human trials supporting this use fall considerably beneath modern scientific standards.

According to animal studies, lycopene might help protect the heart and also shield developing sperm cells from injury (thereby reducing male infertility); the herbal extract curcumin might help prevent damage to the heart and kidneys; N-acetylcysteine might help protect the heart and also reduce hair loss; lipoic acid and coenzyme Q_{10} might protect the heart. However, for all of these antioxidants, support from human trials is lacking. One animal study hints at potential heart- and liver-protective effects with the supplement carnitine.

EBSCO CAM Review Board

FURTHER READING

Balli, E., et al. "Effect of Melatonin on the Cardiotoxicity of Doxorubicin." *Histology and Histopathology* 19 (2004): 1101-1108.

Berthiaume, J. M., et al. "Dietary Vitamin E Decreases Doxorubicin-Induced Oxidative Stress Without Preventing Mitochondrial Dysfunction." *Cardiovascular Toxicology* 5 (2005): 257-267.

Karimi, G., M. Ramezani, and A. Abdi. "Protective Effects of Lycopene and Tomato Extract Against Doxorubicin-Induced Cardiotoxicity." *Phytotherapy Research* 19 (2005): 912-914.

Kim, C., et al. "Modulation by Melatonin of the Cardiotoxic and Antitumor Activities of Adriamycin." *Journal of Cardiovascular Pharmacology* 46 (2005): 200-210.

Oz, E., and M. N. Ilhan. "Effects of Melatonin in Reducing the Toxic Effects of Doxorubicin." *Molecular and Cellular Biochemistry* 286 (2006): 11-15.

Oz, E., et al. "Prevention of Doxorubicin-Induced Cardiotoxicity by Melatonin." *Molecular and Cellular Biochemistry* 282 (2005): 31-37.

Yilmaz, S., et al. "Protective Effect of Lycopene on Adriamycin-Induced Cardiotoxicity and Nephrotoxicity." *Toxicology* 218 (2005): 164-171.

See also: Antioxidants; Food and Drug Administration; Supplements: Introduction.

Dupuytren's contracture

CATEGORY: Condition
DEFINITION: Treatment of the thickening of tissue in the palm of the hand.
PRINCIPAL PROPOSED NATURAL TREATMENTS: None
OTHER PROPOSED NATURAL TREATMENTS: Vitamin E

INTRODUCTION

Named for a nineteenth-century French baron, Dupuytren's contracture is a thickening of tissue in the palm of the hand that causes an inability to straighten one or more fingers, usually the ring finger or little finger. The involved tissue hardens and shrinks, forming a small lump or "cord" in the palm. Discomfort is unusual. The condition can involve both hands or even the toes, and it tends to progress slowly.

Persons who have Dupuytren's contracture may wonder if the condition was caused by an injury to their hands; if injury played any role, it was probably not a major one. Although the exact cause of the condition is unknown, the disorder appears to be partially inherited. If the contracture becomes troublesome for the affected person, surgery may be useful.

PROPOSED NATURAL TREATMENTS

There are no well-documented natural treatments for Dupuytren's contracture. However, in the 1940s, a number of physicians reported attempts to treat the condition with vitamin E. Most reported some success; however, their reports were incomplete and highly subjective, leading others to question their findings.

In 1952, two different researchers added an objective measure to their investigations by examining plaster casts of patients' hands before and after treatment, but their results were conflicting. One researcher treated a group of nineteen people with 300 milligrams (mg) daily of oral vitamin E for three hundred days and reported moderate improvement in the amount of contraction. In contrast, the other researcher found no improvement among forty-six people receiving 200 mg of vitamin E daily for three months.

Because neither of these studies used a control group, the results are not particularly meaningful. Only double-blind, placebo-controlled studies can prove a treatment effective, and none have been reported for vitamin E in the treatment of Dupuytren's. In early 2010, the U.S. Food and Drug Administration approved the use of collagenase injections for Dupuytren's contracture.

EBSCO CAM Review Board

FURTHER READING

Hurst, L. C., et al. "Injectable Collagenase *Clostridium histolyticum* for Dupuytren's Contracture." *New England Journal of Medicine* 361 (2009): 968-979.

Kirk, J. E., and M. Chieffi. "Tocopherol Administration to Patients with Dupuytren's Contracture: Effect on Plasma Tocopherol Levels and Degree of Contracture." Proc Soc Exp Biol Med. 80 (1952): 565-568.

Richards, H. J. "Dupuytren's Contracture Treated with Vitamin E." *British Medical Journal* (June 21, 1952): 1328.

See also: Rolfing; Soft tissue pain; Vitamin E.

Dysmenorrhea

CATEGORY: Condition

RELATED TERMS: Cramps, menstrual cramps, menstrual pain

DEFINITION: Treatment of painful menstruation.

PRINCIPAL PROPOSED NATURAL TREATMENTS: Fish oil, magnesium, vitamin E

OTHER PROPOSED NATURAL TREATMENTS: Acupuncture, aromatherapy, black cohosh, boswellia, bromelain, calcium, chiropractic, *Coleus forskohlii*, cramp bark, dong quai, fennel, guava leaf, krill oil, magnet therapy, manganese, traditional Chinese herbal medicine, turmeric, white willow

INTRODUCTION

Medicine does not know why menstruation is uncomfortable and painful, or why it is much more uncomfortable and painful for some women than for others, or from month to month.

Occasionally, severe menstrual pain indicates the presence of endometriosis (a condition in which uterine tissue is growing in places other than the uterus) or uterine fibroids (benign tumors in the uterus). In most cases, no identifiable abnormality can be found. Natural substances known as prostaglandins seem to play a central role in menstrual pain, but their detailed actions are not fully understood.

Anti-inflammatory drugs such as ibuprofen and naproxen relieve pain and reduce levels of some prostaglandins. These drugs are the mainstay of conventional treatment for menstrual pain. Oral contraceptive treatment may also help.

PRINCIPAL PROPOSED NATURAL TREATMENTS

There is some evidence that the supplements fish oil, magnesium, and vitamin E may help reduce menstrual pain.

Fish oil. The omega-3 fatty acids in fish oil are thought to have anti-inflammatory effects. Omega-3 may relieve dysmenorrhea by affecting the metabolism of prostaglandins and other factors involved in pain and inflammation.

In a four-month study of forty-two girls and young women age fifteen to eighteen years, one-half the participants received a daily dose of 6 grams (g) of fish oil, providing 1,080 milligrams (mg) of EPA (eicosapentaenoic acid) and 720 mg of DHA (docosahexaenoic acid) daily. After two months, participants were switched to placebo for another two months. The other group received the same treatments in reverse order. The results showed that these young women experienced significantly less menstrual pain while they were taking fish oil.

Another double-blind study followed seventy-eight women, who received either fish oil, seal oil, fish oil with vitamin B_{12} (7.5 micrograms daily), or placebo for three full menstrual periods. Significant improvements were seen in all treatment groups, but the fish oil plus vitamin B_{12} proved most effective, and its benefits continued for the longest time after treatment was stopped (three months). The researchers offered no explanation why vitamin B_{12} should be helpful. Krill oil, another source of omega-3 fatty acids, also might be helpful against menstrual pain.

Vitamin E. In a double-blind, placebo-controlled trial, one hundred young women with significant menstrual pain were given either 500 international units (IU) of vitamin E or placebo for five days. Treatment began two days before and continued for three days after the expected onset of menstruation. While both groups showed significant improvement in pain during the two months of the study (because of the power of placebo), pain reduction was greater in the treatment group than in the placebo group.

In another study performed in Iran, 278 adolescents with dysmenorrhea were given either placebo or 200 IU of vitamin E twice daily on the same schedule as the foregoing study. Again, vitamin E proved more effective than placebo. It is not clear how vitamin E could affect menstrual pain.

Magnesium. Preliminary studies suggest that magnesium supplementation may be helpful for dysmenorrhea. A six-month, double-blind, placebo-controlled study of fifty women with menstrual pain found that treatment with magnesium significantly improved symptoms. The researchers reported evidence of reduced levels of prostaglandin F2 alpha, one of the prostaglandins involved in menstrual pain. Similarly positive results were seen in a double-blind, placebo-controlled study of twenty-one women.

OTHER PROPOSED NATURAL TREATMENTS

One small double-blind trial suggests that adequate amounts of calcium and manganese may help control symptoms of menstrual pain. The herb cramp bark has traditionally been used to relieve menstrual pain, but it has not received any significant scientific attention. Numerous other herbs and supplements have been suggested for relief of menstrual pain. These include boswellia, bromelain, *Coleus forskohlii*, dong quai, turmeric, and white willow. However, there is no reliable scientific support for these treatments.

One study has been reported as finding the herb fennel helpful for menstrual pain; however, a close look at the study shows that it merely found fennel less effective than the drug mefenamic acid. The study did not have a placebo control group. For this reason, it is quite possible that the relatively mild benefits seen in the fennel group simply reflect the placebo effect. Another study of fennel also failed to use a placebo.

In one study, aromatherapy massage with lavender, rose, and clary sage reduced menstrual pain to a greater extent than massage with an almond oil placebo. One seemingly substantial double-blind study reported benefits with guava leaf. However, researchers resorted to a form of statistical analysis that makes the results relatively unreliable.

A double-blind study of forty-three women found some evidence that acupuncture can be effective for control of menstrual pain. In addition, a controlled study of sixty-one women evaluated the effects of a special garment designed to stimulate acupuncture points related to menstrual pain. Researchers chose to compare treatment to no treatment, rather than to placebo treatment. For this reason, the results (which were positive) mean little. In a review of thirty controlled trials, researchers were unable to draw conclusions about the effectiveness of acupuncture and similar treatments for menstrual pain because of widespread study design problems. Similarly, in a 2008 review of thirty-nine randomized controlled trials involving 3,475 women, researchers concluded that the use of traditional Chinese herbal medicine shows some promise for the treatment of menstrual pain. However, firm conclusions were not possible because of the wide variability of study design and herbs used and because of the poor quality of many of the studies.

According to one small double-blind study, the use of magnet therapy (applying magnets to the pelvic area) might improve menstrual pain. A controlled study failed to find chiropractic spinal manipulation helpful for menstrual pain.

HERBS AND SUPPLEMENTS TO USE ONLY WITH CAUTION

Various herbs and supplements may interact adversely with drugs used to treat dysmenorrhea.

EBSCO CAM Review Board

FURTHER READING

Eccles, N. K. "A Randomized, Double-Blinded, Placebo-Controlled Pilot Study to Investigate the Effectiveness of a Static Magnet to Relieve Dysmenorrhea." *Journal of Alternative and Complementary Medicine* 11 (2005): 681-687.

Han, S. H., et al. "Effect of Aromatherapy on Symptoms of Dysmenorrhea in College Students." *Journal of Alternative and Complementary Medicine* 12 (2006): 535-541.

Modaress Nejad, V., and M. Asadipour. "Comparison of the Effectiveness of Fennel and Mefenamic Acid on Pain Intensity in Dysmenorrhoea." *Eastern Mediterranean Health Journal* 12 (2006): 423-427.

Yang, H., et al. "Systematic Review of Clinical Trials of Acupuncture-Related Therapies for Primary Dysmenorrhea." *Acta Obstetricia et Gynecologica Scandinavica* 87 (2008): 1114-1122.

Zhu X, et al. "Chinese Herbal Medicine for Primary Dysmenorrhoea." *Cochrane Database of Systematic Reviews* (2008): CD005288. Available through *EBSCO DynaMed Systematic Literature Surveillance* at http://www.ebscohost.com/dynamed.

Ziaei, S., et al. "A Randomised Controlled Trial of Vitamin E in the Treatment of Primary Dysmenorrhoea." *BJOG: An International Journal of Obstetrics and Gynaecology* 112 (2005): 466-469.

See also: Amenorrhea; Fish oil; Magnesium; Pain management; Premenstrual syndrome (PMS); Vitamin E.

Dyspepsia

CATEGORY: Condition

RELATED TERMS: Belching, bloating, gas, indigestion, nausea, poor digestion, stomach upset

DEFINITION: Treatment of digestive problems that have no identifiable physiological cause.

PRINCIPAL PROPOSED NATURAL TREATMENTS: Artichoke leaf, turmeric

OTHER PROPOSED NATURAL TREATMENTS: Astaxanthin, banana powder, betaine hydrochloride, boldo, cayenne, chamomile, essential oils of carminative herbs, herbal combinations containing candytuft (*Iberis amara*), lemon balm, melatonin, pancreatic enzymes, probiotics

INTRODUCTION

Dyspepsia includes a variety of digestive problems such as stomach discomfort, gas, bloating, belching, appetite loss, and nausea. Although many serious medical conditions can cause digestive distress, the term "dyspepsia" is used when no identifiable medical cause can be detected. In this way, dyspepsia is like a stomach version of the symptoms in the intestines called irritable bowel syndrome (IBS).

The standard medical approach to dyspepsia begins by looking for an identifiable medical condition such as gallstones, ulcers, or esophageal reflux. If none is found, various treatments are often suggested on a trial-and-error basis, including medications that reduce stomach acid and those that decrease spasm in the digestive tract. The drugs cisapride (Propulsid) and metoclopramide (Reglan) increase stomach emptying and have also been tried for dyspepsia. However, cisapride has been taken off the market and metoclopramide causes many side effects.

It is thought that stress plays a role in dyspepsia, as it does with IBS. One study of thirty people with dyspepsia found that after eight weeks of treatment with placebo, 80 percent reported their symptoms had improved. This unusually high placebo response emphasizes the emotional contribution to this condition. In Europe, it is widely believed, though without much supporting evidence, that dyspepsia is commonly caused by inadequate function of the gallbladder.

PRINCIPAL PROPOSED NATURAL TREATMENTS

Artichoke leaf. An extract of artichoke leaf has undergone considerable study as a treatment for a variety of conditions, most prominently high cholesterol. Artichoke leaf is one of many herbs thought to stimulate gallbladder function. In 2003, a large (247-participant) study evaluated artichoke leaf as a treatment for dyspepsia. In this carefully conducted study, artichoke leaf extract proved significantly more effective than placebo for alleviating symptoms of functional dyspepsia. A study of an herbal combination containing artichoke leaf is described here.

Treating Dyspepsia

There are many different terms for turmeric and for cayenne pepper, two herbs said to be helpful in treating the symptoms of dyspepsia. Some of those terms are listed here.

- *Alternative names for turmeric:* Curcuma longa, curcumin, Indian saffron, turmeric extract

- *Alternative names for cayenne pepper:* Capsaicin, *Capsicum annuum, Capsicum fruitescens, Capsicum oleoresin*, chili pepper, hot pepper, red pepper, Spanish pepper

---

Turmeric. The spice turmeric contains a substance, curcumin, that may stimulate gallbladder contractions. A double-blind, placebo-controlled study including 106 people compared the effects of 500 milligrams of curcumin four times daily with placebo (and with a locally popular over-the-counter treatment). After seven days, 87 percent of the curcumin group experienced full or partial symptom relief from dyspepsia compared to 53 percent of the placebo group.

OTHER PROPOSED NATURAL TREATMENTS

Combination herbal treatments. Several studies, enrolling six hundred participants, have found benefits with a proprietary herbal combination therapy containing bitter candytuft (*Iberis amara*) as the major active ingredient. The largest of these studies was an eight-week double-blind study of 315 people with functional dyspepsia, in which the candy-tuft product proved significantly more effective than placebo.

A double-blind trial of sixty people given either placebo or a combination of artichoke leaf, celandine, and boldo found improvements in symptoms of indigestion after fourteen days of treatment. Similarly positive effects were seen in a double-blind trial of seventy-six persons given a combination treatment containing turmeric and celandine.

Reports have raised concerns that celandine can damage the liver. In addition, boldo is dangerous for use by pregnant women and in persons with liver or kidney disease.

Essential oils of carminative herbs. Herbs believed to assist in the passing of gas are traditionally called carminatives. Classic carminatives include caraway, chamomile, dill, fennel, peppermint, spearmint, and tur-meric. Essential oils made from some of these herbs have been studied for the treatment of dyspepsia.

A double-blind, placebo-controlled study including thirty-nine persons found that an enteric-coated pep-permint-caraway oil combination taken three times daily for four weeks significantly reduced dyspepsia pain compared with placebo. Of the treatment group, 63.2 percent was pain-free after four weeks, compared to 25 percent of the placebo group.

Results from a double-blind comparative study in-cluding 118 people suggest that the combination of peppermint and caraway oil is about as effective as the standard drug cisapride, which is no longer available. After four weeks, the herbal combination reduced dys-pepsia pain by 69.7 percent, whereas the conventional treatment reduced pain by 70.2 percent.

A preparation of peppermint, caraway, fennel, and wormwood oils was compared to metoclopramide in another double-blind study enrolling sixty persons. After seven days, 43.3 percent of the treatment group was pain-free, compared to 13.3 percent of the meto-clopramide group. Metoclopramide works by reducing gastric emptying time (in other words, it speeds the passage of food from the stomach to the intestines). Some evidence suggests that peppermint oil may have the same effect.

Essential oils of herbs can present health risks. In particular, wormwood (the herb in absinthe) is dan-gerous when taken long term. Physician supervision is strongly recommended.

Cayenne. Preliminary evidence suggests that oral use of the herb cayenne can reduce the pain of dys-pepsia. This may seem like an odd use of the herb; in-tuitively, it seems that hot peppers should be hard on the stomach. However, contrary to popular belief, hot peppers do not inflame the tissues they contact; hot peppers are not even harmful for ulcers. Rather, they merely produce sensations similar to those caused by actual damage.

All hot peppers contain a substance called capsa-icin. When applied to tissues, capsaicin causes release of a chemical called substance P. Substance P is ordi-narily released when tissues are damaged; it is part of the system the body uses to detect injury. When hot peppers artificially release substance P, they trick the nervous system into thinking that an injury has oc-curred. The result is a sensation of burning pain. When capsaicin is applied regularly to a part of the

body, substance P becomes depleted in that location. This is why people who consume a lot of hot peppers gradually build up a tolerance. It is also the basis for a number of medical uses of capsaicin. When levels of substance P are reduced in an area, all pain in that area is somewhat reduced. Because of this effect, cap-saicin cream is widely used for the treatment of painful conditions such as shingles, arthritis, and diabetic neuropathy.

The oral use of capsaicin may also reduce discom-fort in the stomach. In a double-blind study, thirty people with dyspepsia were given either 2.5 grams daily of red pepper powder (divided up and taken be-fore meals) or placebo for five weeks. By the third week of treatment, the persons taking red pepper were experiencing significant improvements in pain, bloating, and nausea compared with placebo, and these relative improvements lasted through the end of the study.

Other herbs and supplements. A controlled (but not blinded) study of forty-six people suggests that ba-nana powder, a traditional Indian food, may help treat dyspepsia. After eight weeks of treatment, 75 percent of the people taking banana powder reported complete or partial symptom relief compared to 20 percent of those who received no treatment.

Herbs with a reputation for relaxing a nervous stomach, such as chamomile, valerian, and lemon balm, are also sometimes recommended for dyspepsia. Numerous other herbs that have been recommended for dyspepsia include angelica root, anise seed, bar-berry, bitter orange peel, blessed thistle, cardamom, centaury, chicory, dandelion root, cinnamon, cloves, coriander, devil's claw, dill, gentian, ginger, hore-hound, juniper, linden, milk thistle, radish, rosemary, sage, St. John's wort, star anise, and yarrow. A tea made from the "fruits" or seeds of parsley is a traditional remedy for colic, indigestion, and intestinal gas.

Reduced levels of digestive enzymes may play a role in dyspepsia. One double-blind study found that the use of pancreatic enzyme supplements improved symp-toms following consumption of a high-fat meal. How-ever, another placebo-controlled study failed to find pancreatic enzymes helpful for dyspepsia symptoms in general.

Weak evidence hints that melatonin might be helpful for dyspepsia. One study failed to find probiotics (friendly bacteria) helpful for dyspepsia in children. Two studies failed to find the carotenoid astaxanthin more effective than placebo for the treatment of stomach irritation in people with dyspepsia.

Betaine hydrochloride increases the acidity of the stomach, and on that basis it has been proposed as a digestive aid for people with inadequate stomach acid. However, there is no evidence that reduced stomach acid levels causes symptoms of indigestion.

HERBS AND SUPPLEMENTS TO USE ONLY WITH CAUTION

Various herbs and supplements may interact adversely with drugs used to treat dyspepsia.

EBSCO CAM Review Board

FURTHER READING

Bortolotti, M., et al. "The Treatment of Functional Dyspepsia with Red Pepper." *Alimentary Pharmacology and Therapeutics* 16 (2002): 1075-1082.

Gawronska, A., et al. "A Randomized Double-Blind Placebo-Controlled Trial of *Lactobacillus* GG for Abdominal Pain Disorders in Children." *Alimentary Pharmacology and Therapeutics* 25 (2007): 177-184.

Holtmann, G., et al. "Efficacy of Artichoke Leaf Extract in the Treatment of Patients with Functional Dyspepsia." *Alimentary Pharmacology and Therapeutics* 18 (2003): 1099-1105.

Inamori, M., et al. "Early Effects of Peppermint Oil on Gastric Emptying: A Crossover Study Using a Continuous Real-Time (13)C Breath Test (BreathID System)." *Journal of Gastroenterology* 42 (2007): 539-542.

Klupinska, G., et al. "Therapeutic Effect of Melatonin in Patients with Functional Dyspepsia." *Journal of Clinical Gastroenterology* 41 (2007): 270-274.

Kupcinskas, L., et al. "Efficacy of the Natural Antioxidant Astaxanthin in the Treatment of Functional Dyspepsia in Patients with or Without *Helicobacter pylori* Infection." *Phytomedicine* 15 (2008): 391-399.

Madisch, A., et al. "Treatment of Functional Dyspepsia with an Herbal Preparation." *Digestion* 69 (2004): 45-52.

Rodriguez-Stanley, S., et al. "The Effects of Capsaicin on Reflux, Gastric Emptying, and Dyspepsia." *Alimentary Pharmacology and Therapeutics* 14 (2000): 129-134.

See also: Artichoke; Candytuft; Cayenne; Diarrhea; Gas, intestinal; Gastritis; Gastroesophageal reflux disease; Gastrointestinal health; Peppermint; Turmeric; Ulcers.

E

Ear infections

CATEGORY: Condition

RELATED TERMS: Acute otitis media, infection, ear, middle ear infection, secretory otitis media

DEFINITION: Treatment of infection of the middle ear, a painful condition most common in infants and young children.

PRINCIPAL PROPOSED NATURAL TREATMENTS: Avoiding passive smoke inhalation, breast-feeding, herbal ear drop combinations containing mullein and garlic, xylitol

OTHER PROPOSED NATURAL TREATMENTS: Andrographis, cranial sacral osteopathy, echinacea, food allergen elimination, garlic, ginseng, probiotics, vitamin C, zinc

INTRODUCTION

Acute otitis media (AOM) is a painful infection of the middle ear, the portion of the ear behind the eardrum. (Another form of ear infection, otitis externa or swimmer's ear, is entirely different and is not covered here.) AOM often follows a cold, sore throat, or other respiratory illness. Although it can affect adults, AOM occurs primarily in infants and young children. It is estimated that by age seven years, up to 95 percent of all children in the United States will have experienced at least one bout of AOM, the most common reason parents take a child to the doctor.

When the Eustachian tube connecting the upper part of the throat to the middle ear is blocked by a cold's mucus and swelling, fluids pool behind the eardrum, providing an ideal place for bacteria to grow; an infection may set in, generating even more fluid. The pressure this exerts on the eardrum can be intensely painful. The eardrum turns red and bulges. Children too young to explain their discomfort will cry, fuss, and pull at their ears. They might also appear unresponsive because they cannot hear well; fluid buildup in the middle ear prevents the eardrum and small bones in the ear from moving, causing temporary hearing loss.

In addition, a complication called secretory otitis media (fluid buildup in the middle ear) may develop and cause continuous hearing loss for months. Other possible, though rare, complications of AOM include mastoiditis (an infection of the bone behind the ear) and spinal meningitis.

Without treatment, most middle ear infections resolve on their own, often through a harmless rupture of the eardrum. Some pediatricians–for example, those in the Netherlands–take a conservative approach, generally waiting twenty-four to seventy-two hours until they are certain an ear infection warrants antibiotics. Doctors in the United States, however, tend to initiate treatment early. This practice has been criticized on several grounds. First, aggressive antibiotic treatment has not been found effective in preventing complications, such as serous otitis, pneumococcal meningitis, or hearing loss. In addition, antibiotic treatment does not appear to help AOM. A double-blind, placebo-controlled trial of 240 children age six months to two years found so little benefit with antibiotic treatment that the authors recommended physician-supervised watchful waiting rather than immediate treatment.

In other published reviews, the benefits of antibiotics for AOM have also been found less than impressive. A review of thirty-three randomized trials involving 5,400 children concluded that antibiotics modestly improved the rate of recovery. An evaluation of six randomized, controlled studies concluded that early antibiotic use had only slight benefit, reducing pain and fever in a small percentage of children and helping to prevent the development of infection in the other ear, but not significantly speeding up recovery of hearing. Modest benefits were also seen in a later trial of 315 children. Another study found that children with recurrent ear infections do not appear to benefit from preventive antibiotic treatment. A meta-analysis (formal statistical review) concluded that antibiotic treatment may be helpful in children younger than two years of age who have infections in both ears and in children with drainage from the ear, but for other children it may be preferable to delay the use of antibiotics.

However, the claim (often made by proponents of alternative medicine) that early antibiotic treatment causes an increased rate of ear infection recurrence does not appear to be correct. Despite these issues, simply withholding antibiotic treatment can be dangerous. Any child who appears to have an ear infection should be seen by a physician.

When ear infections do reoccur frequently, a physician may insert a tube into the infected ear to drain fluids and relieve pressure, a procedure called tympanostomy. Nearly one million American children undergo this procedure each year; however, its usefulness is somewhat controversial.

PRINCIPAL PROPOSED NATURAL TREATMENTS

Although there is no known natural treatment for AOM, there are several promising approaches parents can take that may help prevent children from developing ear infections or reduce symptoms.

Xylitol. A natural sugar found in plums, strawberries, and raspberries, xylitol is used as a sweetener in some "sugarless" gums and candies. One of its advantages is that it inhibits the growth of *Streptococcus mutans*, a type of bacterium that causes dental cavities. Xylitol also inhibits the growth of a related bacteria species, *S. pneumoniae*, which is implicated in ear infections. Additionally, xylitol acts against *Haemophilus influenzae*, another bacterium that frequently causes ear infections.

Based on this evidence, xylitol has been tried as a preventive treatment for middle ear infections with some success. Two well-designed studies enrolling a total of 1,163 children found that when taken five times daily throughout a large portion of the cold season, chewing gum and syrup sweetened with xylitol helped prevent middle ear infections. However, xylitol has not proved effective when taken three times daily rather than five times daily, nor when it is used only after the onset of a respiratory infection.

In one of the positive studies, 857 children were given either placebo or xylitol five times daily in the form of chewing gum, syrup, or lozenges. In the two-month study period, the gum proved distinctly effective, reducing the risk of developing AOM by 40 percent. Xylitol syrup was also effective, but less so. The lozenges did not prove effective; researchers speculated that children got tired of sucking on the large

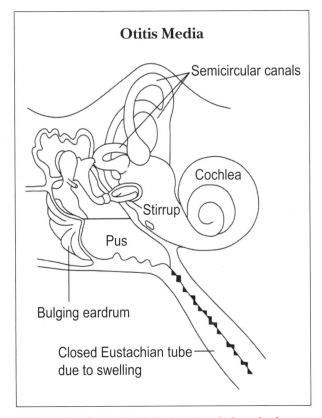

Otitis Media

Semicircular canals

Cochlea

Stirrup

Pus

Bulging eardrum

Closed Eustachian tube due to swelling

Otitis media occurs when infection spreads from the throat to the middle ear via the Eustachian tube. It is a serious condition that, left untreated, may lead to permanent ear damage and even infection of the brain.

candies and did not get the proper dose of xylitol. (In addition, the children were able to distinguish between the xylitol and placebo lozenges by taste, making that portion of the study single-blind.)

Similarly positive results had been seen in an earlier three-month double-blind study by the same researchers, evaluating about three hundred children and again using a dosing schedule requiring the use of xylitol five times daily. However, taking xylitol five times daily requires a great deal of effort. Other researchers looked at whether xylitol would still work if taken only three times daily. In their three-month, double-blind, placebo-controlled study of 663 children, no benefits were seen.

Another study, this one enrolling 1,277 children, took a different approach to simplifying the use of xylitol: They used the original dosage schedule but began treatment only after a respiratory infection had begun, rather than over a period of many months. Again, no benefits were seen.

Breast-feeding. Breast-feeding may help prevent AOM. Numerous studies tracking ear infection frequency in large groups of infants found that the infants who were breast-fed exclusively had significantly fewer middle ear infections than those fed formula. Such observational studies are not as reliable as placebo-controlled or double-blind designs, but the results do suggest that breast-feeding is a good preventive measure. Researchers are not sure how breast milk might protect infants from ear infections. Studies attempting to determine if breast milk inhibits bacteria associated with AOM have yielded mixed results.

Avoidance of cigarette smoke. Environmental conditions may predispose a child to middle ear infections. A study of 132 children in day care found that the forty-five children exposed to cigarette smoke at home had a 38 percent higher risk of middle ear infections than the eighty-seven children whose parents did not smoke.

Herbal ear drops. The herbs mullein and garlic are traditionally combined with other herbs in oily ear drops designed to reduce the pain of ear infections. One study supports this use. Two double-blind trials enrolling more than 250 children with eardrum pain caused by middle ear infection compared the effectiveness of an herbal preparation containing mullein, garlic, St. John's wort, and calendula with a standard anesthetic ear drop product (ametocaine and phenazone). The results indicated that the two treatments were equally effective. In addition, one of the studies found that the use of the antibiotic amoxicillin did not add additional benefit. However, because of the strong placebo response in pain conditions, this study would have needed a placebo group to provide truly dependable evidence that the herbs were effective.

While herbal eardrop products may relieve pain, the actual infection is on the other side of the eardrum, and it is not immediately clear how the herbs can help in this case. There is some evidence, however, that essential oils of herbs may be able to penetrate the eardrum and reach the other side. However, essential oils can be toxic and irritating to tissues.

Garlic and its oil are too harsh to introduce into the ear. Herbal drops that contain garlic use much milder extracts of the herb.

OTHER PROPOSED NATURAL TREATMENTS

Allergies. Allergies may contribute to ear infections, possibly by increasing the amount of fluid in the middle ear. There is some evidence that children allergic to pollens, dust, molds, and certain foods may be more likely to develop AOM. Weak evidence suggests that a food-allergen-elimination diet might help prevent middle ear infections.

Other herbs and supplements. Numerous natural products have been proposed for preventing or treating ear infections. These include all herbs and supplements used for colds, including echinacea, probiotics (such as acidophilus), zinc, vitamin C, andrographis, garlic, and ginseng. However, there is no direct evidence that any of these treatments are effective for AOM. In the case of echinacea, a few studies specifically found no benefit. There is mixed evidence for the effectiveness of probiotics. Cranial-sacral osteopathy has also failed to prove helpful for preventing ear infections.

EBSCO CAM Review Board

FURTHER READING

Butler, C. C., et al. "Should Children Be Screened to Undergo Early Treatment for Otitis Media with Effusion?" *Child: Care, Health, and Development* 29 (2003): 425-432.

Hatakka, K., et al. "Treatment of Acute Otitis Media with Probiotics in Otitis-Prone Children." *Clinical Nutrition* 26 (2007): 314-321.

Hautalahti, O., et al. "Failure of Xylitol Given Three Times a Day for Preventing Acute Otitis Media." *Pediatric Infectious Disease Journal* 26 (2007): 423-427.

Kristinsson, K. G., et al. "Effective Treatment of Experimental Acute Otitis Media by Application of Volatile Fluids into the Ear Canal." *Journal of Infectious Diseases* 191 (2005): 1876-1880.

Rautava, S., S. Salminen, and E. Isolauri. "Specific Probiotics in Reducing the Risk of Acute Infections in Infancy." *British Journal of Nutrition* 101 (2009): 1722-1726.

Rovers, M. M., et al. "Antibiotics for Acute Otitis Media." *The Lancet* 368 (2006): 1429-1435.

Wahl, R. A., et al. "*Echinacea purpurea* and Osteopathic Manipulative Treatment in Children with Recurrent Otitis Media." *BMC Complementary and Alternative Medicine* 8 (2008): 56.

See also: Children's health; Colds and flu; Conjunctivitis; Garlic; Hearing loss; Mullein; Tinnitus; Xylitol.

Ear infections: Homeopathic remedies

Category: Homeopathy

Related terms: Acute otitis media, infection, ear, middle ear infection, secretory otitis media

Definition: The use of highly diluted remedies to treat painful infection of the middle ear, most common in infants and young children.

Studied homeopathic remedies: *Aconitum napellus*; belladonna; *Ferrum phosphoricum*; *Pulsatilla*

Introduction

Acute otitis media (AOM) is a painful infection of the middle ear, the portion of the ear behind the eardrum. (Another form of ear infection, otitis externa or swimmer's ear, is entirely different and is not covered here.) AOM often follows a cold, sore throat, or other respiratory illness. The infection, although it can affect adults, occurs primarily in infants and young children.

The infection of the middle ear may occur when the Eustachian tube connecting the upper part of the throat to the middle ear is blocked by a cold's mucus and swelling. Fluids pool behind the eardrum, providing an ideal place for bacteria to grow. An infection will generate more fluid. Also, fluid buildup in the middle ear prevents the eardrum and small bones in the ear from moving, causing temporary hearing loss.

After the infection disappears, fluid may remain and cause a complication called secretory otitis media (fluid buildup in the middle ear), which, in turn, can cause hearing loss for months. Other possible, though rare, complications of AOM include mastoiditis (an infection of the bone behind the ear) and spinal meningitis.

Scientific Evaluations of Homeopathic Remedies

A double-blind, placebo-controlled trial of thirty-eight children and young adolescents evaluated the effectiveness of *Pulsatilla* D2 in the treatment of otitis media. However, the tested remedy failed to prove more effective than placebo.

Two studies compared homeopathic treatment to standard treatment for ear infections, but these studies were not double-blind, and for that reason alone, the results mean little. In addition, there is some contro- versy regarding whether standard treatment is much more effective than no treatment. Therefore, even if they had been performed correctly, these studies would not have provided much in the way of information.

Traditional Homeopathic Treatments

Classical homeopathy offers many possible homeopathic treatments for middle ear infections These therapies are chosen based on various specific details of the person seeking treatment.

Homeopathic belladonna is commonly recommended for ear infections that fit the following symptom picture: ear pain that varies rapidly in severity but is generally worse on the right and is accompanied by fever, facial flushing, nightmares, and sensitivity to light.

Aconitum napellus is another commonly prescribed remedy for ear infections. Its symptom picture includes ear pain that begins suddenly, often after exposure to wind and cold; pain that remains at a constant level of intensity; and pain that is accompanied by high fever, agitation, and restlessness. *Ferrum phosphoricum* is sometimes used when an ear infection has just begun and the symptoms are not yet severe.

EBSCO CAM Review Board

Further Reading

Damoiseaux, R. A., et al. "Primary Care Based Randomized, Double Blind Trial of Amoxicillin Versus Placebo for Acute Otitis Media in Children Aged Under Two Years." *British Medical Journal* 320 (2000): 350-354.

Friese, K. H., et al. "The Homeopathic Treatment of Otitis Media in Children: Comparisons with Conventional Therapy." *International Journal of Clinical Pharmacology and Therapeutics* 35 (1997): 296-301.

Haidvogl, M. "Homeopathic and Conventional Treatment for Acute Respiratory and Ear Complaints: A Comparative Study on Outcome in the Primary Care Setting." *BMC Complementary and Alternative Medicine* 7 (2007): 7.

Harrison, H. "A Randomized Comparison of Homoeopathic and Standard Treatment of Glue Ear in Children." *Complementary Therapies in Medicine* 44 (1999): 132-135.

See also: Ear infections.

Eating disorders

CATEGORY: Condition

RELATED TERMS: Anorexia nervosa, binge eating disorder, bulimia nervosa

DEFINITION: Treatment of eating disorders.

PRINCIPAL PROPOSED TREATMENTS: None

OTHER PROPOSED TREATMENTS: Dehidroepiandrosterone (DHEA), 5-hydroxytryptophan (5HTP), St. John's wort, yoga, zinc

INTRODUCTION

There are three major types of eating disorders: anorexia nervosa, bulimia nervosa, and binge eating disorder. Anorexia nervosa involves compulsive dieting and exercise to reduce weight, leading to dangerous weight loss and, in women, the absence of menstrual periods. Bulimia nervosa is characterized by binge eating followed by purging. The recently identified binge eating disorder is marked by binge eating that is not followed by purging.

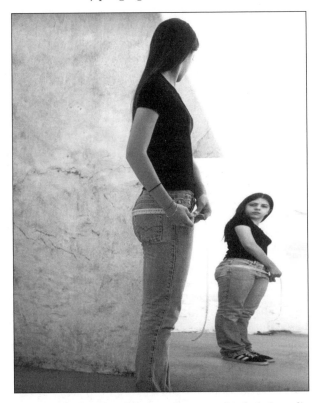

A teenage girl with anorexia nervosa sees her body in a distorted way. (Oscar Burriel / Photo Researchers, Inc.)

Eating disorders are most common in teenage girls and young adult women from the middle and upper socioeconomic classes. The causes of the various disorders are not known, but it seems indisputable that the Western emphasis on slimness as a mark of feminine attractiveness contributes greatly.

Because severe anorexia can be life-threatening, treatment generally combines a weight-gain program with psychotherapy and, sometimes, antidepressant drugs. Bulimia nervosa and binge eating disorder are both treated with psychotherapy, antidepressants, or appetite suppressants to help control binge eating.

PROPOSED TREATMENTS

While there are no well-established natural treatments for eating disorders, there is some evidence that zinc supplements, when used in conjunction with conventional medical treatments, may help people with anorexia to gain weight. Preliminary attempts to treat bulimia by altering serotonin levels are also promising. In addition, the supplement dehydroepiandrosterone (DHEA) might be helpful for protecting bone mass.

Zinc. The relationship between anorexia nervosa and zinc deficiency is controversial. The relationship also is the subject of many studies.

Symptoms of zinc deficiency, including weight loss, appetite loss, and behavior changes, resemble those of anorexia nervosa to some extent. This has led some researchers to theorize that low zinc levels may be related to the onset of the eating disorder.

Preliminary evidence, including one small double-blind trial, suggests that zinc supplements might indeed be helpful in treating anorexia nervosa, possibly enhancing weight gain and helping to stabilize mood. One frequently quoted study that has often been used to discredit the use of zinc in anorexia appears to be relatively meaningless when inspected closely.

Tryptophan. Animal and human studies suggest that when levels of the brain chemical serotonin rise, hunger decreases. People who engage in binge eating may have a different response to changes in serotonin levels. In an attempt to change binge eating behavior, some researchers have tried to alter serotonin levels. Standard antidepressant drugs are most often used for this purpose. However, it might be possible to achieve similar results with tryptophan and related supplements.

The body uses the amino acid L-tryptophan to make serotonin. Preliminary evidence from a small, double-blind, placebo-controlled study suggests that a combination of L-tryptophan and vitamin B_6 significantly reduced binge eating among people with bulimia. This evidence, however, is contradicted by results of another small study that found no significant difference between the effects of L-tryptophan and those of placebo on binge eating.

L-tryptophan is no longer sold as a supplement because of safety concerns. The dietary supplement 5-hydroxytryptophan might be a safer option; however, it has not been studied in eating disorders. The antidepressant herb St. John's wort might also raise serotonin levels.

Dehydroepiandrosterone. Women with anorexia often experience bone loss, partly because of decreases in estrogen levels. In a one-year double-blind study, women with anorexia received either dehydroepiandrosterone (DHEA) at a dose of 50 milligrams per day or standard hormone replacement therapy. The results showed equivalent bone preservation in both groups. However, because there is considerable doubt that hormone replacement therapy is truly helpful for preventing bone loss caused by anorexia, these results mean little to researchers.

Other proposed treatments. A small trial involving fifty-four adolescents with eating disorders found that adding eight weeks of yoga twice weekly to standard therapy was associated with improved eating-disorder-related thoughts and behaviors compared with standard therapy alone.

EBSCO CAM Review Board

FURTHER READING

Bakan, R., et al. "Dietary Zinc Intake of Vegetarian and Nonvegetarian Patients with Anorexia Nervosa." *International Journal of Eating Disorders* 13 (1993): 229-233.

Carei, T. R., et al. "Randomized Controlled Clinical Trial of Yoga in the Treatment of Eating Disorders." *Journal of Adolescent Health* 46, no. 4 (2010): 346.

Costin, Carolyn. *The Eating Disorder Sourcebook.* 3d ed. New York: McGraw-Hill, 2006.

Gordon, C. M., E. Grace, and S. J. Emans. "Effects of Oral Dehydroepiandrosterone on Bone Density in Young Women with Anorexia Nervosa." *Journal of Clinical Endocrinology and Metabolism* 87 (2002): 4935-4941.

Klibanski, A., et al. "The Effects of Estrogen Administration on Trabecular Bone Loss in Young Women with Anorexia Nervosa." *Journal of Clinical Endocrinology and Metabolism* 80 (1995): 898-904.

National Eating Disorders Association. http://www.nationaleatingdisorders.org.

Paterson, Anna. *Fit to Die: Men and Eating Disorders.* Thousand Oaks, Calif.: Sage, 2004.

Su, J. C., and C. L. Birmingham. "Zinc Supplementation in the Treatment of Anorexia Nervosa." *Eating and Weight Disorders* 7 (2002): 20-22.

Weltzin, T. E., et al. "Acute Tryptophan Depletion and Increased Food Intake and Irritability in Bulimia Nervosa." *American Journal of Psychiatry* 152 (1995): 1668-1671.

See also: Adolescent and teenage health; Amenorrhea; Compulsive overeating; Depression, mild to moderate; 5-Hydroxytryptophan; Obesity and excess weight; Obsessive-compulsive disorder (OCD); St. John's wort; Weight loss, undesired; Women's health; Zinc.

Echinacea

CATEGORY: Herbs and supplements

RELATED TERMS: *Echinacea angustifolia, E. pallida, E. purpurea*

DEFINITION: Herbal product promoted as a dietary supplement for specific health benefits.

PRINCIPAL PROPOSED USE: Treatment of colds and flu

OTHER PROPOSED USES: Chronic bronchitis (acute flare-ups), genital herpes

PROBABLY NOT EFFECTIVE USES: Cold and flu prevention, general immune support

OVERVIEW

The decorative plant *Echinacea purpurea,* or purple coneflower, has been one of the most popular herbal medications in both the United States and Europe for more than one century. Native Americans used the related species *E. angustifolia* for a wide variety of problems, including respiratory infections and snake bites. Herbal physicians among the European colonists quickly added the herb to their repertoire. Echinacea became tremendously popular toward the end of the nineteenth century, when businessman H. C. F.

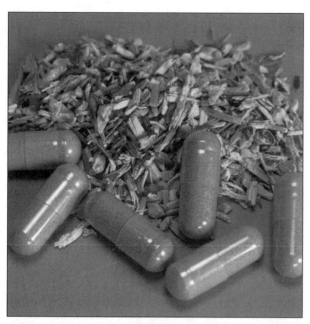

In Europe, and increasingly in the United States, echinacea products are widely used to treat colds and flu. (Carolyn A. McKeone/Photo Researchers, Inc.)

Meyer promoted an herbal concoction containing *E. angustifolia*. The garish, exaggerated, and poorly written nature of his labeling helped define the characteristics of a "snake oil" remedy.

Serious manufacturers also developed an interest in echinacea. By 1920, the respected Lloyd Brothers Pharmaceutical Company of Cincinnati, Ohio, counted echinacea as its best-selling product. In Europe, physicians took up the American interest in *E. angustifolia* with enthusiasm. Demand soon outstripped the supply coming from the United States, and in an attempt to rapidly plant echinacea locally, the German firm Madeus mistakenly purchased a quantity of *E. purpurea* seeds. This historical accident is the reason why most echinacea today belongs to the purpurea species instead of to angustifolia. Another family member, *E. pallida*, is also used.

Echinacea was the number-one cold and flu remedy in the United States until it was displaced by sulfa antibiotics. Ironically, antibiotics are not effective for colds, whereas echinacea appears to offer some real help. Echinacea remains the primary remedy for minor respiratory infections in Germany, where more than 1.3 million prescriptions for the herbal product are issued each year.

USES AND APPLICATIONS

In Europe, and increasingly in the United States, echinacea products are widely used to treat colds and flu. The best scientific evidence about echinacea concerns its ability to help one recover from colds and minor flu more quickly. It also appears to significantly reduce symptoms. Echinacea may also be able to "abort" a cold, if taken at the first sign of symptoms. However, taking echinacea regularly throughout the cold season is probably not a good idea, as evidence suggests that it does not help prevent colds.

It was earlier believed that echinacea acted by stimulating the immune system. Test-tube and animal studies had found that various constituents of echinacea can increase antibody production, raise white blood cell counts, and stimulate the activity of key white blood cells. However, later studies have tended to cast doubt on this theory. The fact that regular use of echinacea does not appear to help prevent colds (or genital herpes) also somewhat argues against an immune-strengthening effect. Thus, it can only be said that it is not understood how echinacea affects cold symptoms.

Echinacea has been proposed for the treatment and prevention of other acute infections too. One small double-blind study found that the use of an herbal combination containing echinacea enhanced the effectiveness of antibiotic treatment for acute flare-ups of chronic bronchitis. However, two other studies failed to find benefit for ear infections in children.

Finally, echinacea is frequently proposed for general immune support. However, there is some reason to think that it is not effective for this purpose.

SCIENTIFIC EVIDENCE

Reducing the symptoms and duration of colds. Double-blind, placebo-controlled studies enrolling more than one thousand people have found that various forms and species of echinacea can reduce cold symptoms and help with a faster recovery. The best evidence regards products that include the above-ground portion of *E. purpurea*.

In one double-blind, placebo-controlled trial, eighty people with early cold symptoms were given either an above-ground *E. purpurea* extract or placebo. The results showed that those who were given echinacea recovered significantly more quickly–only six days in the echinacea group versus nine days in the placebo group.

Another study found evidence that above-ground *E. purpurea* can reduce the severity of cold symptoms but that *E. purpurea* root may not be effective. In this double-blind trial, 246 people with recent onset of a respiratory infection were given either placebo or one of three *E. purpurea* preparations: two formulations of a product made of 95 percent above-ground herb (leaves, stems, and flowers) and 5 percent root, and one formulation made only from the roots of the plant. The results showed significant improvements in symptoms such as runny nose, sore throat, sneezing, and fatigue with the above-ground preparations, but the root preparation was not effective.

Symptom reduction with a whole-plant formulation of *E. purpurea* was seen in a double-blind, placebo-controlled study of 282 people. However, another double-blind, placebo-controlled study of above-ground *E. purpurea*, enrolling 120 people, failed to find benefits compared with placebo treatment. An even larger trial (407 participants) failed to find a widely used above-ground *E. purpurea* extract helpful for treating children with respiratory infections. The reasons for these negative outcomes are unclear.

In other studies, benefits were seen with a preparation of *E. pallida* root and an herbal beverage tea containing above-ground portions of *E. purpurea* and *E. angustifolia* (and some *E. purpurea* root extract). A double-blind, placebo-controlled study failed to find benefit with a dry herb product consisting largely of *E. purpurea* root and *E. angustifolia* root. Another study failed to find benefit with *E. angustifolia* root extract. The best supporting evidence for echinacea involves the above-ground portion or whole-plant extract of *E. purpurea*, but even here the results are less than fully consistent.

"Aborting" a cold. A double-blind study suggests that echinacea not only can make colds shorter and less severe but also can stop a cold that is just starting. In this study, 120 people were given *E. purpurea* or a placebo as soon as they started showing signs of getting a cold.

Participants took either echinacea or placebo at a dosage of twenty drops every two hours for one day, then twenty drops three times a day for up to ten days of treatment. The results were promising. Fewer people in the echinacea group felt that their initial symptoms actually developed into "real" colds (40 percent of those taking echinacea versus 60 percent taking the placebo actually became ill). Also, among those who did get real colds, improvement in the symptoms started sooner in the echinacea group (four days instead of eight days). Both of these results were statistically significant.

Preventing colds. Several studies have attempted to discover whether the daily use of echinacea can prevent colds from even starting, but the results have not been promising. In one double-blind, placebo-controlled trial, 302 healthy volunteers were given an alcohol tincture containing either *E. purpurea* root, *E. angustifolia* root, or placebo for twelve weeks. The results showed that *E. purpurea* was associated with perhaps a 20 percent decrease in the number of people who got sick, and *E. angustifolia* with a 10 percent decrease. However, the difference was not statistically significant. This means that the benefit, if any, was so small that it could have been caused by chance alone.

Another double-blind, placebo-controlled study enrolled 109 people with a history of four or more colds during the previous year and gave them either *E. purpurea* juice or placebo for eight weeks. No benefits were seen in the frequency, duration, or severity of colds. Similar results were seen in four other studies that enrolled more than 350 people.

A study often cited as evidence that echinacea can prevent colds actually found no benefit in the 609 participants taken as a whole. Only by looking at subgroups of participants (a statistically questionable procedure) could researchers find any evidence of benefit, and it was still slight.

Regulation of Echinacea

Because echinacea is a natural growing compound, it is covered by the U.S. Dietary Supplement Health and Education Act (DSHEA) but, like other dietary supplements, is not regulated by the U.S. Food and Drug Administration (FDA). Manufacturers and distributors do not need to register with the FDA or get FDA approval before producing or selling dietary supplements, and its use or effectiveness need not be substantiated by the FDA.

DSHEA mandates that the label of a dietary supplement must contain enough information about the composition of the product so that consumers can make informed choices. The information must be presented in the FDA-specified format. The manufacturer also is responsible for ensuring that all the dietary ingredients in a supplement are safe.

Rick Alan; reviewed by Brian Randall, M.D.

However, a later study using a combination product containing echinacea, propolis, and vitamin C did find preventive benefits. In this double-blind, placebo-controlled study, 430 children aged one to five years were given either the combination or placebo for three months during the winter. The results showed a statistically significant reduction in frequency of respiratory infections. It is not clear what components of this mixture were responsible for the apparent benefits seen.

DOSAGE

Echinacea is usually taken at the first sign of a cold and continued for seven to fourteen days. Longer-term use of echinacea is not recommended. The best (though not entirely consistent) evidence supports the use of products made from the above-ground portions of *E. purpurea* (specifically, the flowers, leaves and stems). *E. pallida* root has also shown promise, but *E. purpurea* root appears to be ineffective.

The typical dosage of echinacea powdered extract is 300 milligrams three times a day. Alcohol tincture (1:5) is usually taken at a dosage of 3 to 4 milliliters (ml) three times daily, echinacea juice at a dosage of 2 to 3 ml three times daily, and whole dried root at 1 to 2 grams three times daily. There is no broad agreement on what ingredients should be standardized in echinacea tinctures and solid extracts.

A survey of available echinacea products found many problems. In this 2003 analysis, about 10 percent had no echinacea; about one-half were mislabeled as to the species of echinacea present; more than one-half the standardized preparations did not contain the labeled amount of standardized constituents; and the total milligrams of echinacea stated on the label generally had little to do with the actual milligrams of herb present. A subsequent analysis performed in 2004 by a respected testing organization also found many problems.

Many herbalists feel that liquid forms of echinacea are more effective than tablets or capsules because they believe part of echinacea's benefit comes from the activation of the tonsils through direct contact. However, there is no real evidence to support this contention.

Finally, goldenseal is frequently combined with echinacea in cold preparations. However, there is no evidence that oral goldenseal stimulates immunity; traditional herbalists did not use it for this purpose.

SAFETY ISSUES

Echinacea appears to be generally safe. Even when taken in very high doses, it has not been found to cause any toxic effects. Reported side effects are also uncommon and usually limited to minor gastrointestinal symptoms, increased urination, and mild allergic reactions. However, severe allergic reactions have occurred occasionally, some of them life-threatening. In Australia, one survey found that 20 percent of allergy-prone people were allergic to echinacea.

Other concerns relate to echinacea's possible immune-stimulating properties. Immunity is a complex process that the body keeps under careful control; excessively strong immune reactions can be dangerous. Based on this concern, echinacea should be used only with caution (if at all) by persons with autoimmune disorders, such as multiple sclerosis, lupus, and rheumatoid arthritis.

Furthermore, a late case report strongly suggests that the use of echinacea can trigger episodes of erythema nodosum (EN), an inflammatory condition that involves tender nodules under the skin. These nodules often arise after coldlike symptoms. In this report, a forty-one-year-old man took echinacea on four separate occasions when he thought he was developing a cold, and each time he developed EN instead. When he stopped using echinacea for this purpose, he remained free of EN outbreaks for a full year of follow-up. The cause of EN is not known, but it involves increased activity of certain immune cells; echinacea has been observed to cause similar effects in the same immune cells, suggesting that the relationship is not coincidental.

One study raised questions about possible antifertility effects of echinacea. When high concentrations of echinacea were placed in a test tube with hamster sperm and ova, the sperm were less able to penetrate the ova. However, because it is not known whether this much echinacea can actually come in contact with sperm and ova when they are in the human body rather than a test tube, these results may not be meaningful in real life.

Animal studies of echinacea are supportive of safety in pregnancy. One human study found a bit of evidence that the use of echinacea during pregnancy does not increase risk of birth defects, but this evidence is not strong enough to absolutely rely on.

Furthermore, studies dating to the 1950s suggest that echinacea is safe in children. Nonetheless, the safety of echinacea in young children and pregnant or nursing women cannot be regarded as established. In addition, safety in those with severe liver or kidney disease has not been established.

Two studies suggest that echinacea might interact with various medications by affecting their metabolism in the liver, but the significance of these largely theoretical findings remains unclear. A review of the research literature found no verifiable reports of drug–herb interactions with any echinacea product.

EBSCO CAM Review Board

FURTHER READING

Cohen, H. A., et al. "Effectiveness of an Herbal Preparation Containing Echinacea, Propolis, and Vitamin C in Preventing Respiratory Tract Infections in Children." *Archives of Pediatric and Adolescent Medicine* 158 (2004): 217-221.

Cravotto, G., et al. "Phytotherapeutics: An Evaluation of the Potential of One Thousand Plants." *Journal of Clinical Pharmacy and Therapeutics* 35 (2010): 11-48.

Freeman, C., and K. Spelman. "A Critical Evaluation of Drug Interactions with *Echinacea* spp." *Molecular Nutrition and Food Research* 52 (2008): 789-798.

Goel, V., et al. "A Proprietary Extract from the Echinacea Plant (*Echinacea purpurea*) Enhances Systemic Immune Response During a Common Cold." *Phytotherapy Research* 19 (2005): 689-694.

Linde, K., et al. "Echinacea for Preventing and Treating the Common Cold." *Cochrane Database of Systematic Reviews* (2006): CD000530. Available through *EBSCO DynaMed Systematic Literature Surveillance* at http://www.ebscohost.com/dynamed.

O'Neil, J., et al. "Effects of Echinacea on the Frequency of Upper Respiratory Tract Symptoms." *Annals of Allergy, Asthma, and Immunology* 100 (2008): 384-388.

Tesche, S., et al. "The Value of Herbal Medicines in the Treatment of Acute Non-purulent Rhinosinusitis." *European Archives of Oto-Rhino-Laryngology* 265 (2008): 1355-1359.

Wahl, R. A., et al. "*Echinacea purpurea* and Osteopathic Manipulative Treatment in Children with Recurrent Otitis Media." *BMC Complementary and Alternative Medicine* 8 (2008): 56.

See also: Allergies; Bronchitis; Colds and flu; Common cold: Homeopathic remedies; Herbal medicine; Immune support; Influenza: Homeopathic remedies.

Eczema

CATEGORY: Condition

RELATED TERMS: Atopic dermatitis, atopic eczema, atopy

DEFINITION: Treatment of allergic reactions of the skin.

PRINCIPAL PROPOSED NATURAL TREATMENTS

- *Oral:* Breast-feeding (prevention), Chinese herbal medicine (treatment), probiotics (prevention)
- *Topical:* Calendula, chamomile, gamma-linolenic acid from borage oil, licorice, St. John's wort, vitamin B_{12}

OTHER PROPOSED NATURAL TREATMENTS: Burdock, *Coleus forskohlii*, combination cream containing *Mahonia aquifolium*, probiotics (treatment), quercetin, red clover, red vine leaf and licorice, sea buckthorn (*Hippophae rhamnoides*), *Viola tricolor* and *Centella asiatica*, zinc

Probably not effective treatment: Oral use of gamma-linolenic acid from evening primrose oil or borage oil

INTRODUCTION

Eczema is an allergic reaction of the skin and consists mainly of itchy, inflamed patches on the face, elbows, knees, and wrists. Eczema is most commonly found in infants and young children, and it is closely associated with asthma and hay fever. Together, these types of eczema are called atopy. Atopy tends to run in families. Medical treatment for eczema consists mainly of antihistamines and topical steroid creams.

PRINCIPAL PROPOSED NATURAL TREATMENTS

Probiotics. Probiotics are health-promoting (friendly) bacteria. The best-known probiotic is *Lactobacillus acidophilus*, which is used to make yogurt. Probiotics are thought to have immune-regulating actions. The use of probiotics during pregnancy and after childbirth may reduce the risk of childhood eczema, presumably by normalizing immune response.

The benefits of probiotics for eczema prevention were seen in a small 2001 study. Also, in a large, long-term, double-blind study, 1,223 pregnant women were given either placebo or a probiotic mixture (containing lactobacilli and bifidobacteria) beginning two to four weeks before delivery. Their newborn children then received either probiotics or placebo for six months. The results showed that the probiotics mixture markedly reduced the incidence of eczema but not of other allergic diseases.

A follow-up study of these mother-child pairs found that probiotics for mother and infant were not associated with reduced eczema, allergic rhinitis, or asthma in children followed through age five years. Another study yielded marginal results, and a third study found no benefit for the prevention of eczema. This latter study actually demonstrated a modestly increased risk of wheezing bronchitis in those infants who took the lactobacilli. Finally, researchers in another study concluded that not all probiotics are created equal. In this placebo-controlled study involving pregnant women and their infants, *L. rhamnosus* reduced the incidence of eczema in the children, but a strain of *Bifidobacterium animalis* did not.

In addition, some double-blind trials have found evidence that infants and children who already have eczema may benefit from the use of probiotics. However, in a careful review of twelve studies involving 781 children, researchers concluded that there is no convincing evidence that probiotics can effectively treat eczema.

If probiotics are beneficial for childhood eczema, they are probably more effective at preventing the condition rather than treating it. Three reviews of numerous studies cautiously conclude that probiotics may help reduce the risk of eczema in infants and children, particularly in those at high risk and when probiotics are given to both mother (before giving birth) and infant. However, in a double-blind, placebo-controlled study of 231 infants born to women with allergies, giving *L. acidophilus* to the infants failed to reduce their risk of developing eczema.

Breast-feeding. Early exposure of the infant to allergenic substances found in infant formula may play a role in the development of eczema. Breast-feeding might, therefore, help prevent this condition.

A large study lends credence to this theory. More than seventeen thousand women in the Republic of Belarus were enrolled. About one-half were entered in a program that encouraged them to breast-feed (the intervention group) while the other half was enrolled in a different program that did not instigate any particular method of infant feeding (the control group). The results showed that women encouraged to breast-feed were much more likely to do so than other women. Furthermore, children of women in the

intervention group showed almost a 50 percent reduction in the incidence of eczema.

Interpreting this study is trickier than it might appear. Technically, it does not prove that breast-feeding reduces the risk of eczema. Rather, it shows that counseling to breast-feed reduces risk of eczema. However, the implication is fairly compelling: If a woman breast-feeds her child, the child is less likely to develop eczema.

Another option might be to use special infant formulas that are less allergenic. However, it is not clear that doing so will help.

Chinese herbal medicine. A combination of traditional Chinese herbs has shown promise as a treatment for eczema. This proprietary formula contains *Ledebouriella seseloides, Potentilla chinensis, Akebia clematidis, Rehmannia glutinosa, Paeonia lactiflora, Lophatherum gracile, Dictamnus dasycarpus, Tribulus terrestris, Glycyrrhiza uralensis,* and *Schizonepeta tenuifolia.* In paired double-blind, placebo-controlled trials carried out by one research group, the mixture produced significantly better effects than placebo for both adults and children.

Each study enrolled approximately forty people and used a crossover design in which all participants received the real treatment and placebo for eight weeks each. Use of the herbal combination significantly reduced eczema symptoms compared with placebo. However, a subsequent study of similar design performed by a different research group failed to find significant benefit. The reason for this discrepancy is not clear. In a twelve-week double-blind study, a different traditional Chinese herbal formula also failed

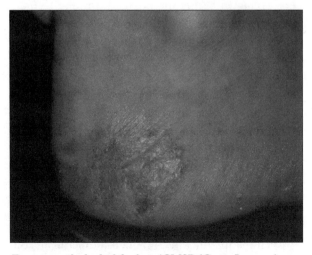

Eczema on the heel of the foot. (CMSP/Getty Images)

to prove more effective than placebo for treatment of eczema. Asian herbal creams marketed for eczema have often been found to contain high-potency corticosteroid drugs that are not listed on the label.

Topical treatments. Topical creams made from chamomile, licorice, or calendula, alone or in combination, are widely used in Europe to treat eczema. One study of 161 persons found chamomile cream just as effective as 0.25 percent hydrocortisone cream for the treatment of eczema. However, the report did not state whether doctors or study participants were blinded as to which treatment was which, so it is not clear how reliable the results may be.

A study by the same authors (also not double-blind), involving seventy-two persons with eczema, found somewhat odd results. In this trial, chamomile was not significantly more effective than placebo, but both were better than 0.5 percent hydrocortisone cream. It is difficult to interpret what these results actually mean, but they certainly cannot be taken as proof that chamomile cream is effective.

A double-blind study of thirty people compared 1 and 2 percent licorice cream with placebo cream for eczema. Both proved more effective than placebo, and the 2 percent preparation was more effective than the 1 percent preparation.

The herb St. John's wort is most often used for the treatment of depression. St. John's wort contains a substance, hypericin, that is thought to have anti-inflammatory properties, making it potentially useful in eczema too. In a double-blind study, a cream containing St. John's wort extract was compared with placebo cream in twenty-one people with mild to moderate eczema symptoms. Study participants used real cream on one arm and the placebo cream on the other. The results indicated that the use of St. John's wort cream significantly reduced symptoms.

Another placebo-controlled double-blind study, which enrolled forty-nine people with eczema, found benefit with a cream containing vitamin B_{12} at a concentration of 0.07 percent. Topical B_{12} is thought to work in eczema by affecting local levels of a substance called nitric oxide. A small study of twenty-one children age six months to eighteen years found that topical application of vitamin B_{12} for up to four weeks improved skin check scores compared with placebo.

A double-blind, placebo-controlled study of eighty-eight people with eczema tested a cream containing extracts of *Mahonia aquifolium, Viola tricolor,* and *Centella asiatica.* The results failed to show benefit overall. A post hoc (after the fact) analysis noted benefits among those participants who were not tested at the time of the year with the hottest temperatures. However, because of the mathematical laws of statistics, such retroactive evaluations are of limited meaningfulness.

Evening primrose oil and gamma-linolenic acid. Evening primrose oil, taken orally, has been widely used in Europe for the treatment of eczema. Evening primrose is a rich source of the essential fatty acid gamma-linolenic acid (GLA). Other sources of GLA include borage oil and black currant oil. However, the most recent and best-designed studies have failed to find GLA supplements helpful for eczema. More recently, topical application of GLA has been tried.

A review of all studies reported up to 1989 found that oral use of evening primrose oil reduced the symptoms of eczema after several months of use, with the greatest improvement noticeable in the level of itching. However, this review has been sharply criticized: It included studies of very poor design and also, apparently, misinterpreted the results of some of the studies it evaluated.

Later, better-designed studies have not shown promising results. A double-blind, placebo-controlled study that followed fifty-eight children with eczema for sixteen weeks found no difference in effectiveness between evening primrose oil and placebo. A twenty-four-week double-blind study of 160 adults with eczema failed to find benefit with GLA from borage oil, as did a twelve-week study of 151 adults and children. In addition, GLA from evening primrose either alone or with fish oil failed to provide benefits in a sixteen-week, double-blind, placebo-controlled study of 102 people with eczema. A fourth double-blind trial followed 39 people with hand dermatitis for twenty-four weeks. Evening primrose oil at a dosage of 6 grams daily produced no significant improvement compared with placebo. Only one double-blind trial performed subsequent to the 1989 review found therapeutic benefit with evening primrose oil, but it used very high doses of the supplement and found only marginal benefits.

The balance of the evidence suggests that GLA taken orally is probably not effective for treating eczema. However, a double-blind study tested the use of undershirts coated with borage oil for treatment of eczema. In this two-week study of thirty-two children aged one to ten years, the use of these coated undershirts appeared to reduce eczema symptoms. However, additional, higher-quality research studies need to be undertaken to establish whether or not this method of delivery really works.

OTHER PROPOSED NATURAL TREATMENTS

A cream containing red vine leaf and licorice extract has shown some promise for the treatment of eczema. Another study found that four weeks of massage therapy performed by the parents (after a one-time training session with a massage professional) significantly decreased eczema symptoms in children.

The herbs burdock, red clover, and *Coleus forskohlii* and the supplements quercetin and zinc have also been recommended for eczema, but there is no meaningful evidence that they really work. A small, thirty-day, double-blind trial failed to find vitamin B_6 at a dose of 50 milligrams (mg) daily helpful for eczema. Similarly, an eight-week double-blind trial of zinc at the high dose of 67 mg daily failed to find any benefit for eczema symptoms. Another study that tested a combination of *Eleutherococcus*, yarrow, and *Lamium album* also came up with negative results.

A widely publicized study reportedly found the oral use of the plant sea buckthorn (*Hippophae rhamnoides*) helpful for eczema, but in fact placebo treatment proved equally or more effective. Finally, although it is widely believed that food allergies are a major contributor to eczema, this assumption may be incorrect.

EBSCO CAM Review Board

FURTHER READING

Abrahamsson, T. R., et al. "Probiotics in Prevention of IgE-Associated Eczema." *Journal of Allergy and Clinical Immunology* 119 (2007): 1174-1180.

Betsi, G. I., E. Papadavid, and M. E. Falagas. "Probiotics for the Treatment or Prevention of Atopic Dermatitis." *American Journal of Clinical Dermatology* 9 (2008): 93-103.

Boyle, R. J., et al. "Probiotics for Treating Eczema." *Cochrane Database of Systematic Reviews* (2008): CD006135. Available through *EBSCO DynaMed Systematic Literature Surveillance* at http://www.ebscohost.com/dynamed.

Brand, P. L., B. J. Vlieg-Boerstra, and A. E. Dubois. "Dietary Prevention of Allergic Disease in Children: Are Current Recommendations Really Based on Good Evidence?" *Pediatric Allergy and Immunology* 18 (2007): 475-479.

Folster-Holst, R., et al. "Prospective, Randomized Controlled Trial on *Lactobacillus rhamnosus* in Infants with Moderate to Severe Atopic Dermatitis." *British Journal of Dermatology* 155 (2006): 1256-1261.

Hon, K. L., et al. "Efficacy and Tolerability of a Chinese Herbal Medicine Concoction for Treatment of Atopic Dermatitis." *British Journal of Dermatology* 157 (2007): 357-363.

Januchowski, R. "Evaluation of Topical Vitamin B(12) for the Treatment of Childhood Eczema." *Journal of Alternative and Complementary Medicine* 15 (2009): 387-389.

Kalliomaki, M., et al. "Probiotics and Prevention of Atopic Disease." *The Lancet* 361 (2003): 1869-1871.

Kanehara, S., et al. "Clinical Effects of Undershirts Coated with Borage Oil on Children with Atopic Dermatitis." *Journal of Dermatology* 34 (2007): 811-815.

Kim, J. Y., et al. "Effect of Probiotic Mix (*Bifidobacterium bifidum, Bifidobacterium lactis, Lactobacillus acidophilus*) in the Primary Prevention of Eczema." *Pediatric Allergy and Immunology* 21 (2010): e386.

Ramsay, H. M., et al. "Herbal Creams Used for Atopic Eczema in Birmingham, UK, Illegally Contain Potent Corticosteroids." *Archives of Disease in Childhood* 88 (2003): 1056-1057.

Rowlands, D., S. J. Tofte, and J. M. Hanifin. "Does Food Allergy Cause Atopic Dermatitis? Food Challenge Testing to Dissociate Eczematous from Immediate Reactions." *Dermatologic Therapy* 19 (2006): 97-103.

Takwale, A., et al. "Efficacy and Tolerability of Borage Oil in Adults and Children with Atopic Eczema." *British Medical Journal* 327 (2003): 1385.

Von Berg, A., et al. "The Effect of Hydrolyzed Cow's Milk Formula for Allergy Prevention in the First Year of Life." *Journal of Allergy and Clinical Immunology* 111 (2003): 533-534.

Woo, S. I., et al. "Effect of *Lactobacillus sakei* Supplementation in Children with Atopic Eczema-Dermatitis Syndrome." *Annals of Allergy, Asthma, and Immunology* 104 (2010): 343-348.

See also: Allergies; Children's health; Gamma-linolenic acid; Photosensitivity; Probiotics; Psoriasis; Seborrheic dermatitis; Traditional Chinese herbal medicine.

Edema

CATEGORY: Condition
RELATED TERM: Swelling
RELATED TERMS: Fluid retention, lymphedema, swelling, water retention
DEFINITION: Treatment of excessive fluid buildup, or swelling, of tissue caused by congestive heart failure, venous insufficiency, mastectomy, premenstrual syndrome, pregnancy, and other factors.
PRINCIPAL PROPOSED NATURAL TREATMENTS: None
OTHER PROPOSED NATURAL TREATMENTS: Bilberry, buchu, citrus bioflavonoids, cleavers, dandelion leaf, goldenrod, horsetail, juniper, oligomeric proanthocyanidin complexes, oxerutins, parsley, rosemary

INTRODUCTION

Many medical conditions can cause edema, or swelling. A condition related to varicose veins called chronic venous insufficiency can cause swelling in the legs. Congestive heart failure can also cause leg swelling. Numerous natural treatments have substantial supporting evidence of effectiveness for these conditions.

Women who have undergone a mastectomy for breast cancer may experience swelling in the arm near the affected breast. This condition is called lymphedema, which may be helped with natural treatments.

Women with premenstrual syndrome often experience fluid retention before the onset of menstruation, and edema frequently occurs during pregnancy. Minor injuries and also surgery may cause swelling as part of the healing process. Many of the treatments used for these conditions fall into one of two categories: bioflavonoids and diuretics. Bioflavonoids have shown promise for conditions in which edema is caused by leaky blood vessels. Bioflavonoids often used as natural treatments for edema include bilberry, citrus bioflavonoids, oligomeric proanthocyanidin complexes, and oxerutins.

Many herbs are thought to have a diuretic effect, which causes the body to increase its water excretion. Herbs with apparent diuretic effects include buchu, cleavers, rosemary, goldenrod, juniper, dandelion leaf, parsley, and horsetail.

EBSCO CAM Review Board

FURTHER READING

Bouchard, J., and R. L. Mehta. "Fluid Balance Issues in the Critically Ill Patient." *Contributions to Nephrology* 164 (2010): 69-78.

Christie, S., et al. "Flavonoids: A New Direction for the Treatment of Fluid Retention?" *Phytotherapy Research* 15 (2001): 467-475.

Favia, I., et al. "Fluid Management in Pediatric Intensive Care." *Contributions to Nephrology* 164 (2010): 217-226.

Kim, D. S., et al. "Effect of Active Resistive Exercise on Breast Cancer-Related Lymphedema." *Archives of Physical Medicine and Rehabilitation* 91 (2010): 1844-1848.

Na et al. "Evidence-Based Approaches for the Ayurvedic Traditional Herbal Formulations: Toward an Ayurvedic CONSORT Model." *Journal of Alternative and Complementary Medicine* 14 (2008): 769-776.

See also: Cancer treatment support; Congestive heart failure; Pregnancy support; Premenstrual syndrome (PMS); Varicose veins; Venous insufficiency: Homeopathic remedies

Education and training of CAM practitioners

CATEGORY: Issues and overviews
RELATED TERMS: Acupuncturist, chiropractor, homeopath, integrative medicine specialist, massage therapist, naturopath
DEFINITION: Education and training for persons seeking to practice complementary and alternative forms of therapy.

OVERVIEW

The education and training of practitioners of complementary and alternative medicine (CAM) are widely varied, as these practices encompass any type of therapy that is not considered conventional or scientifically proven. Many of these therapies, however, have a long history in other cultures. CAM education and training may involve rigorous courses of study similar to those for a medical degree or for postdoctoral training. However, some CAM education consists of only minimal training, such as a six-week course that leads to a certificate. Even within the same discipline, training and certification requirements may vary widely from state to state, because there is no national regulatory body to oversee the process.

The education and training of CAM practitioners are the focus here, so the discussion will cover only those areas of unconventional therapy with standard educational or training programs. Covered here are acupuncturists, chiropractors, homeopaths, massage therapists, naturopaths, and integrated medicine programs that combine conventional medicine with CAM practice.

Many other types of CAM practitioners, such as aromatherapists, crystal therapists, reflexologists, reiki practitioners, and native or indigenous healers, study for long periods with experienced experts in their field. However, no particular training programs, educational courses, recognized requirements, or state or national certifications are available in the United States for these practitioners.

PRACTITIONERS

Acupuncturist. Acupuncture is a standard accepted practice in the Chinese medicine tradition; however, it is relatively new in the United States and, as such, varies from state to state in education and certification requirements and venues. About forty states have established criteria for persons seeking to practice acupuncture. Nonmedical professionals, to become licensed as an acupuncturist, must take a four-year course of study and a board examination. Persons with a medical background, such as medical doctors, dentists, nurses, and chiropractors, must often complete a rigorous course of study too, including classroom study (a minimum of three hundred hours) and clinical acupuncture practice, before becoming licensed.

Courses in acupuncture focus on anatomy, physiology, and other areas that are typical for any type of medical practice. Courses also include detailed study of the nervous and vascular systems so that a practitioner has a thorough understanding of needle insertion and the body's reaction to it. A practitioner of acupuncture may also be trained in other aspects of Chinese traditional medicine.

Two bodies certify and accredit acupuncture colleges and practitioners in the United States: the Accreditation Commission for Acupuncture and Oriental Medicine and the American Board of Medical Acupuncture. These organizations provide continuing education and examinations for practitioners and oversight for educational programs in the United States. They also provide standards for acupuncturists trained in other countries who wish to practice in the United States.

Chiropractor. This branch of CAM may be one of the most highly regulated in the United States. The Council on Chiropractic Education (CCE) is an accreditation body for chiropractic schools, and its accreditation criteria are recognized by the U.S. Department of Education. CCE regulates all training programs for chiropractors. The American Chiropractic Association, a leading professional organization for chiropractors, provides continuing medical education and other resources to practitioners.

A chiropractic training program must include a minimum of 4,200 hours of class time, laboratory work, and clinical experience and must include courses in orthopedics, neurology, and physiotherapy (all with a focus on clinical practice of manipulation and spinal alignment). Chiropractors may also pursue studies in a specialty, such as orthopedics, sports medicine, or rehabilitation.

After completion of a doctor of chiropractic (D.C.) program, student practitioners must pass a four-part examination from the National Board of Chiropractic Examiners and must pass a state examination to be licensed. In some areas, the state examination takes the place of the national examination.

Homeopath. The education and training of a homeopath can take varied courses. Programs designed for medical doctors or others with medical training tend to focus on homeopathy and its application, assuming that those with a medical degree would already have a basic background in medicine and medical practice. Other courses, geared to those who do not have a medical background, focus more on medical education, such as anatomy and physiology, but also train students in homeopathy practices and principles.

A few states in the United States offer training in homeopathy (Arizona, California, Colorado, Florida, Massachusetts, and Utah, and the District of Columbia). Admission requirements for courses of study vary widely; some require a medical doctor (M.D.) or similar degree, and others enroll students with little or no medical background. Because homeopathy itself is not regulated in the United States, anyone can use the word "homeopath" to describe themselves or their type of work. However, a person cannot identify himself or herself as a homeopathic doctor or imply to the public that he or she is practicing medicine if he or she does not hold a medical license.

Several programs offer homeopathic education, but no single certification is recognized throughout the United States. Each state has its own standards for licensing this type of care. Some homeopaths are licensed in a conventional type of medicine and may hold a degree as an M.D. or as a nurse practitioner. In Arizona, Connecticut, and Nevada, M.D.'s and D.O.'s (doctors of osteopathy) can be licensed as homeopathic physicians. Homeopathic assistants, who practice under the supervision of a homeopath, are licensed in Arizona and Nevada.

Organizations such as the Council for Homeopathic Certification and the American Board of Homeotherapeutics offer certifications to homeopaths who have completed certain requirements: for example, M.D.'s or D.O.'s who pass oral and written exams in homeopathy. Upon completing these exams, the successful candidate is awarded a diplomate of homeotherapeutics (D.Ht.). Even though the Department of Education does not recognize any one organization as a certifying body, homeopathic practitioners use the standards upheld by these organizations to maintain competency and to encourage self-regulation.

Massage therapist. Most U.S. states regulate the practice of massage therapy in some way with a type of governing board providing certification or licensure. Usually, a massage therapist must complete some course of training and pass a board examination to be licensed. However, the requirements vary widely from state to state. Education provided in massage therapy schools typically requires about five hundred hours of study and involves courses in anatomy, physiology, motion and body mechanics, and clinical massage practice. Licensure also may involve passing a nationally recognized test, such as the National Certification Examination for Therapeutic Massage and Bodywork or the Massage and Bodywork Licensing Examination.

Naturopath. There are two basic types of naturopath: traditional and naturopathic physicians. Education and training for traditional naturopaths vary from nondegree certificate programs to undergraduate degree programs. After completion of a degree program, a traditional naturopath can certify with the American Naturopathic Medical Certificate Board and become a naturopathic consultant. Traditionally, these types of naturopaths do not practice medicine and thus do not require a license.

A naturopathic physician must have a doctor of naturopathic medicine (N.D., or N.M.D. in Arizona) degree from an accredited school of naturopathic medicine. Only four schools in the United States (in Washington, Oregon, Arizona, and Connecticut) are accredited for this type of education. The N.D. involves four years of graduate-level study in a standard medical curriculum, with added courses in natural therapeutics. Practitioners must then pass a state board licensing examination. (In the state of Utah, naturopathic doctors must complete a residency before starting a practice.)

Practitioners often work as primary care clinicians, but some states do not recognize the D.M. degree, so practitioners in these areas cannot legally practice medicine. Generally, they may still practice traditional naturopathic medicine. Two states, South Carolina and Tennessee, specifically prohibit the practice of naturopathy in any form.

The Council of Naturopathic Medical Education is a governing body that provides accreditation for education in naturopathy. The American Naturopathic Certification Board provides testing and continuing education for this profession.

CAM EDUCATION AND TRAINING IN MAINSTREAM INSTITUTIONS

As the practice of CAM becomes more widespread and integrated into society, many medical colleges in the United States have begun to offer courses in CAM. One area of complementary medicine that is often taught in integrative medicine courses is pain management. CAM courses often teach conventional physicians how CAM methods can be incorporated into, and can truly complement, conventional medicine.

The University of Arizona College of Medicine teaches a program of integrative medicine that critically examines branches of alternative medicine and trains clinicians in practices that it finds helpful and that cause no harm. Other such programs include Mayo Clinic Complementary and Integrative Medicine, the Integrative Medicine Program at MD Anderson Cancer Center, and University of Michigan Integrative Medicine.

Marianne M. Madsen, M.S.

FURTHER READING

Alternative Medicine. http://www.pitt.edu/~cbw/altm.html.

American Academy of Acupuncture. http://medicalacupuncture.org.

American Association of Naturopathic Physicians. http://naturopathic.org.

American Chiropractic Association. http://www.acatoday.org.

American Massage Therapy Association. http://www.amtamassage.org.

International Website for Professional Homeopathy. http://www.world-of-homeopathy.info.

National Center for Complementary and Alternative Medicine. "Selecting a Complementary and Alternative Medicine Practitioner." Available at http://nccam.nih.gov/health/decisions/practitioner.htm. Discusses choosing and evaluating a practitioner and provides questions to ask a practitioner about his or her education.

Tierney, Gillian. *Opportunities in Holistic Health Care Careers.* Rev. ed. New York: McGraw-Hill, 2007. This book addresses the job outlook, educational requirements, regulation, and salaries for many CAM practitioners.

See also: Double-blind, placebo-controlled studies; History of alternative medicine; History of complementary medicine; Integrative medicine; Licensing and certification for CAM practitioners; Popular practitioners; Regulation of CAM; Scientific method.

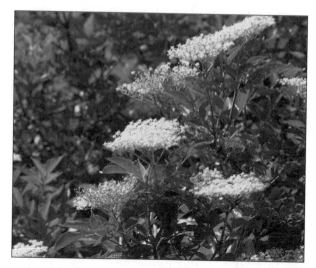

The elderberry is a plant whose bark, berries, flowers, leaves, and roots have been used medicinally for centuries. (© Anniepostma/Dreamstime.com.)

treat respiratory infections. They also used the leaves and flowers in poultices applied to wounds, and they used the bark, suitably aged, as a laxative.

THERAPEUTIC DOSAGES

Elderberry-flower tea is made by steeping 3 to 5 grams of dried flowers in 1 cup of boiling water for ten to fifteen minutes. A typical dosage is 1 cup three times daily. Standardized extracts should be taken according to the directions on the product's label.

Elderberry

RELATED TERM: *Sambucus nigra*
CATEGORY: Herbs and supplements
DEFINITION: Natural plant product used to treat specific health conditions.
PRINCIPAL PROPOSED USES: Colds, influenza
OTHER PROPOSED USES: Herpes, high cholesterol, human immunodeficiency virus infection support

OVERVIEW

The berries of the plant *Sambucus nigra* are frequently made into beverages, pies, and preserves, but they have also been used to treat arthritis. Native Americans used tea made from elderberry flowers to

THERAPEUTIC USES

A product containing elderberry, as well as small amounts of echinacea and bee propolis, has been widely marketed as a cold and flu remedy. Weak evidence suggests that this mixture may stimulate the immune system and also inhibit viral growth. In a preliminary double-blind study, this mixture was found to reduce symptoms and speed recovery from influenza A, the type of influenza for which flu shots are given. A few of the participants in this study had influenza B (a milder form of influenza), and the elderberry mixture appeared to be helpful for them as well. Another preliminary double-blind study evaluated people with influenza B and also found benefit.

Elderberry also has shown some preliminary promise for use in other viral infections, including human immunodeficiency virus and herpes. Also, based on promising results in an uncontrolled study, researchers performed a small double-blind, placebo-controlled study on the potential benefits of elderberry for improving cholesterol levels. At the dose used, no benefits were evident.

SAFETY ISSUES

Elderberry flowers are generally regarded as safe. Side effects are rare and consist primarily of occasional mild gastrointestinal distress or allergic reactions. Nonetheless, safety in young children, pregnant or nursing women, or those with severe liver or kidney disease has not been established.

EBSCO CAM Review Board

FURTHER READING

Barak, V., T. Halperin, and I. Kalickman. "The Effect of Sambucol, a Black Elderberry-Based, Natural Product, on the Production of Human Cytokines." *European Cytokine Network* 12 (2001): 290-296.

Murkovic, M., et al. "Effects of Elderberry Juice on Fasting and Postprandial Serum Lipids and Low-Density Lipoprotein Oxidation in Healthy Volunteers." *European Journal of Clinical Nutrition* 58 (2004): 244-249.

Zakay-Rones, Z., et al. "Randomized Study of the Efficacy and Safety of Oral Elderberry Extract in the Treatment of Influenza A and B Virus Infections." *Journal of International Medical Research* 32 (2004): 132-140.

See also: Cholesterol, high; Colds and flu; Herpes; HIV support; Immune support; Influenza vaccine.

Elder health

CATEGORY: Issues and overviews
RELATED TERM: Senior health
DEFINITION: Complementary and alternative medicines and therapies that are focused on the elderly.

OVERVIEW

The health and functionality of the elderly can be highly variable, but the elderly differ from younger people in that the elderly are more likely to have chronic conditions, such as high blood pressure. The elderly are increasingly using complementary and alternative medicine (CAM), but they utilize it less than younger adults. Most elderly persons who use CAM do so as a complement to standard medicine, not as a substitute for (or an alternative to) CAM.

CAM use by elders is associated with poorer overall health, although people with life-threatening conditions do not appear more likely to use CAM. Prescription medications and surgery, the main conventional treatments, are often lifesaving but have special risks for elders because of their greater tendency to have multiple chronic conditions.

Because of their higher incidence of illness, seniors can especially benefit from evidence-based medicine (EBM) instead of CAM exclusively. More research on the effectiveness of both CAM and conventional medicine in the elderly is needed.

WHY SENIORS ARE DIFFERENT

Although many seniors are physically and mentally healthy, old age is the time of life when people are most likely to suffer from chronic diseases such as arthritis, heart disease, cancer, and diabetes. Some people develop these diseases at earlier ages, are successfully treated, and live full and productive lives. Their illnesses are manageable or, in some instances, have been cured. Others have had relatively little illness throughout their lives but develop chronic conditions as they age. Some get older without having any serious conditions. Still others develop debilitating illness at relatively young ages, do not improve much with treatment or do not receive treatment, and reach their elder years already disabled and with limited mobility and ability to handle daily activities. Nonetheless, people who live to be age sixty-five and older (those who are considered elderly) are frequently healthy.

Even for healthy seniors, physical changes occur. The organs are less efficient. The kidneys take longer to filter waste from the blood, and lung capacity decreases. The immune system weakens. Variation in health among elders, however, is large. A person's chronological age does not necessarily indicate that person's level of health or functionality. Still, the elderly differ from younger people in that they are more likely to have chronic conditions. Acute diseases, such as colds and influenza, decline with age.

USING CAM

The elderly and the very young (children younger than age five years) use conventional medicine more than other age groups. It remains unclear what age group is most likely to use CAM. All age groups, however, are increasing their use of CAM, but older adults still appear somewhat less likely to use CAM. Estimates of CAM use by elders vary from 30 to 66 percent across surveys, in part because studies consider different CAM therapies. It is difficult to estimate CAM use by seniors because some research studies do not report age differences, while others use a variety of age cut-offs (such as fifty-two-plus, sixty-five-plus, and seventy-seven-plus) when studying older adults.

Seniors usually use CAM in addition to standard treatments. That is, they use complementary therapies in seeking to alleviate symptoms and pain, to manage the side effects of conventional treatment, or for finding a cure. Most seniors do not use alternative therapy alone; instead, they use alternative therapy as a complement to standard medicine. This is true for most people, regardless of age, in the United States and in other developed countries.

DEMOGRAPHICS

A 2008 study of mostly U.S.-focused research examined the demographics of CAM users. The study found that CAM users are more educated than the general population but are not necessarily higher earners. This pattern also holds for seniors. One reason why seniors use CAM less often may be that many elders are less educated than younger adults. Educated persons are often informed consumers who also tend to seek information about topics with which they are unfamiliar. For many in the United States, CAM is little known.

The importance of income in determining CAM use is less clear, and it appears to play a role independent of education level. It is also not certain if elderly women are more likely to use CAM therapies than are elderly men, although CAM use is higher among younger women. CAM use based on one's ethnicity also does not fall into a clear pattern.

CAM is often used by people with chronic conditions. Because the elderly frequently have such conditions, some will use CAM. CAM is also more likely to be used by people with multiple health problems, which many elderly experience too. CAM use is associated

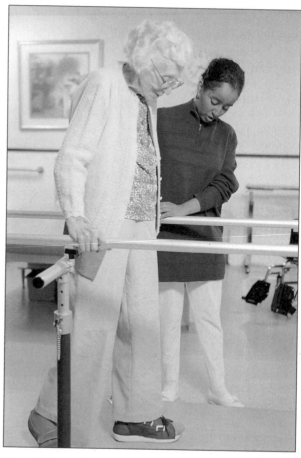

The elderly may experience mobility problems that pose a threat to safety. Falls are much more serious with advanced age, because bones and tissues do not heal as quickly or completely as they do in youth. (PhotoDisc)

with poorer overall health, in all age groups, although people with life-threatening conditions do not appear more likely to use CAM. There is no strong evidence that, for example, people with cancer are more likely to use CAM. The elderly who use only CAM tend to be younger and healthier than those using only standard medicine or a combination of standard medicine and CAM. Elderly CAM users tend to be more health conscious, or more seriously ill, than non-CAM users.

Attitudes and one's philosophy of life play only small parts in determining CAM use by the elderly, although these factors were found to be more significant for younger adults who use CAM. The elderly are more likely than younger adults to say that they want their doctors to make their health decisions. It appears that elders' use of CAM is often a pragmatic decision based on health status and the desire to alleviate symptoms, rather than on philosophy and interest in cultural alternatives.

EVIDENCE-BASED MEDICINE

Evidence-based medicine (EBM) is a growing movement focused on the use of empirical, scientific standards to evaluate treatments. EBM encourages health professionals to use treatments that have been shown by careful study to be effective. At its best, EBM promises high-quality research of CAM modalities and conventional medicine. Because seniors have more health problems, are often taking multiple medications, and are more likely than other age groups to develop conditions for which surgery is the most common treatment, evidence-based research is especially important for this age group.

For many CAM modalities, evidence of effectiveness is limited. There is also little evidence for the effectiveness of some conventional therapies. One example is chronic back pain, which affects more seniors than younger adults. Back pain is one of the most common conditions for which seniors use CAM (others conditions being arthritis, heart disease, allergy, and diabetes). Recent research suggests that back surgery may be overused and that the more invasive types of back surgery may be especially risky for seniors. Some research exists on back pain and CAM.

A 2003 study evaluated the best available evidence on several CAM treatments of back pain, finding that massage had positive outcomes. Spinal manipulation (including chiropractic) was moderately helpful. The quality of the studies on acupuncture was poor, but acupuncture appeared to be more effective than no treatment or "sham treatment" (in which a doctor simulated acupuncture treatment). The risks of all three CAM treatments for back pain were relatively low.

Another CAM modality that has received initial though inadequate study is homeopathy. A 2009 study of persons with chronic low back pain who were followed for two years found that the subjects showed significant improvement and decreased use of prescription medications. Because the elderly are more likely to have low back pain than younger persons, continued research on various treatment modalities for this health problem might have benefits for this age group.

EBM is still relatively new and sometimes meets with resistance from both conventional and CAM practitioners. The latter sometimes argue that CAM therapies are not taken seriously by conventional doctors, even when evidence of their effectiveness exists. A 2005 article on chiropractic practices suggests that EBM is mostly used to justify the use of conventional medicine. The process of determining what treatment modalities are effective can be expected to continue slowly and contentiously.

Careful evaluation of the evidence for treatment is nonetheless superior to giving treatment for which little or no evidence of effectiveness exists. The greater incidence of illness and treatment of older adults means they will especially benefit from the further development of EBM.

TREATMENT TYPES

The main conventional treatments for all persons are prescription medications and surgery. Both are often lifesaving, but each treatment modality has some special risks for the elderly. CAM could prove to be one way to address these risks.

Because they have more illnesses, the elderly are more likely to be taking multiple medications, the interactions of which are often unknown, even if there have been good studies of the individual drugs. Conventional drugs often are not tested on seniors, even though they take more of them. Thus, evidence on prescription drugs that is specific to seniors is sparse. The need for evidence-based CAM is especially important in the case of the elderly who take many medications, because CAM can reduce the chances of drug interactions, such as when massage is used instead of medication for back pain. Some CAM treatments, however, may themselves interact with conventional medications. One example is St. John's wort, an herbal preparation that is often used to treat depression. This preparation can interact with antidepressants such as alprazolam (Xanax).

The elderly are also more likely than younger adults to have conditions that are surgically treated. Surgical technologies and methods have improved significantly in a short time, increasing the chance that surgery will benefit seniors. Even the very old are increasingly considered candidates for surgical treatment.

Surgery, however, is always risky, and the elderly are at greater risk than younger people. Chronic high blood pressure, multiple chronic conditions, and a weaker immune system can make surgery more dangerous for an elderly person and can lead to a longer recuperation time. Alternatives to surgery would be of special benefit to seniors. Less healthy seniors have increased risk of complications and morbidity from surgery. The possibility of cognitive decline in seniors who are surgically treated also remains a concern, though a 2009 study indicates that surgery does not contribute to long-term cognitive decline in seniors. This issue requires further study. The effect of CAM in aiding postsurgical healing also deserves increased research.

Evidence on all medical modalities, CAM and conventional, is particularly inadequate for the elderly. The aging of the U.S. population and in societies across the world underscores the critical need for continued research.

Roxanne Friedenfels, Ph.D.

Further Reading

Aleccia, JoNel. "Surgery in the Super Old: Success at What Price?" Available at http://www.msnbc.msn.com/id/28282424. Article looking at the pros and cons of surgery on very old persons.

American Society of Anesthesiologists. "Surgery, Illness Do Not Increase Cognitive Decline for Older Patients." Available at http://www.medicalnewstoday.com/articles/168756.php. Article summarizing a study with a control group showing that surgery does not contribute to long-term cognitive decline in seniors.

Bishop, Felicity L., and G. T. Lewith. "Who Uses CAM? A Narrative Review of Demographic Characteristics and Health Factors Associated with CAM Use." *Evidence-Based Complementary and Alternative Medicine* 7, no. 1 (2008): 11-28. Available at http://ecam.oxfordjournals.org/cgi/content/full/7/1/11. Peer-reviewed article providing an overview of demographic and health factors of CAM users.

Cherkin, Daniel C., et al. "A Review of the Evidence for the Effectiveness, Safety, and Cost of Acupuncture, Massage Therapy, and Spinal Manipulation for Back Pain." *Annals of Internal Medicine* 138 (2003): 898-906. Peer-reviewed article summarizing reviews of randomized, controlled trials from research published since 1995 on massage therapy, spinal manipulation, and acupuncture as treatments for nonspecific back pain.

Cherniak, Paul, and Neil S. Cherniack. *Alternative Medicine for the Elderly.* New York: Springer, 2003. Book giving balanced, detailed, critical evaluation of CAM treatments for seniors.

Napoli, Maryann. "Is Back Surgery Worth It? An Interview with a Leading Researcher." *HealthFacts* 32 (2007): 1-3. Interview of Richard A. Deyo, a preeminent researcher on back pain treatment, which includes his comments on back surgery for seniors.

Villanueva-Russell, Yvonne. "Evidence-Based Medicine and Its Implications for the Profession of Chiropractic." *Social Science and Medicine* 60 (2005): 545-561. Peer-reviewed article examining the limitations of evidence-based medicine while supporting the development of new methodologies to evaluate the effectiveness of chiropractic and other CAM treatments.

Witt, Claudia M. "Homeopathic Treatment of Patients with Chronic Low Back Pain." *Clinical Journal of Pain* 25 (2009): 334-339. Peer-reviewed article evaluating the effect of homeopathic treatment for persons with low back pain.

See also: Aging; American Academy of Anti-Aging Medicine; Men's health; Women's health.

Elecampane

Category: Herbs and supplements
Related term: *Inula helenium*
Definition: Natural plant product used to treat specific health conditions.
Principal proposed uses: Asthma, chronic respiratory diseases, poor digestion

Overview

The Latin name of elecampane (*Inula helenium*) comes from the story of Helen of Troy, who was supposed to have carried the herb elecampane with her while being abducted from Sparta. Revered by the ancient Greeks and Romans, this herb was recommended for treating such diverse problems as indigestion, melancholy, sciatica, bronchitis, and asthma.

Therapeutic Dosages

A typical dosage of elecampane root is 1.5 to 4 grams three times daily, either in capsule form or boiled in water as tea.

THERAPEUTIC USES

Some modern herbalists regard elecampane as a long-term treatment for respiratory diseases, such as asthma and bronchitis, especially when excessive mucus is a notable feature. However, there is no real evidence that it is effective for this purpose.

Elecampane is also sometimes recommended as a daily supplement to improve general digestion. One of elecampane's constituents, alantolactone, has been used in concentrated form as a treatment for intestinal parasites, but it is not clear whether the whole herb is particularly effective for this purpose.

SAFETY ISSUES

The only reported adverse effects of elecampane are occasional allergic reactions. However, safety in young children, pregnant or nursing women, and those with severe liver or kidney disease has not been established.

EBSCO CAM Review Board

FURTHER READING

Newall, C., L. A. Anderson, and J. D. Phillipson. *Herbal Medicines: A Guide for Health-Care Professionals.* London: Pharmaceutical Press, 1996.

See also: Asthma.

Electromagnetic hypersensitivity

CATEGORY: Issues and overviews

RELATED TERMS: EMF hypersensitivity, hypersensitivity to electric and magnetic field exposure, idiopathic environmental intolerance

DEFINITION: A broad range of symptoms caused by exposure to electrical and magnetic fields in the environment.

OVERVIEW

Electromagnetic (EMF) fields, such as that of the earth, occur naturally in the environment. EMF hypersensitivity, however, is reported in association with human-made EMFs, such as those produced by power lines, appliances, and cell phone towers. Reported symptoms of EMF exposure include headaches, dizziness, fatigue, lack of concentration, depression, and anxiety. Others report dermatologic symptoms such as rashes, tingling, or a burning sensation. Issues affecting the eyes and the gastrointestinal system have also been reported. In developed countries of the world, the reported prevalence of electromagnetic hypersensitivity ranges between 3 and 10 percent, with Scandinavian countries falling on the higher end of the range.

In a well-designed study published in 2008, researchers found high rates of depression, anxiety, and somatoform disorder and higher rates of sick days, doctor visits, poorer sleep, and altered cortical excitability in EMF-sensitive persons, in comparison with age- and gender-matched controls. Those persons identified as EMF sensitive, however, were actually less able than controls to determine when they were exposed to EMFs under experimental conditions, a surprising finding that has been replicated in other studies. Some of the most convincing evidence for sensitivity to EMFs actually comes from animal studies. For instance, a 2004 study showed that deoxyribonucleic acid (DNA) strand breaks were associated with EMF exposure in a rat model.

ISSUES

EMF sensitivity is highly controversial and greatly scrutinized. The World Health Organization, among other entities, does not recognize EMF hypersensitivity as a medical diagnosis because the evidence for the condition is not strong. Gaining that evidence is difficult because of the ubiquity of electronic devices in modern culture. The wide reach of these devices makes it increasingly difficult to shield study subjects from extraneous EMFs. Also, much of the literature on this topic had poor study design, including a lack of statistical power because of low numbers of test subjects.

Most of the persons with reported EMF hypersensitivity who have been studied are self-diagnosed, leading many health experts to claim that they are misdiagnosing themselves; a physician-conducted differential diagnosis might resolve some of these issues.

Dawn M. Bielawski, Ph.D.

FURTHER READING

Del Seppia, Christina, et al. "Pain Perception and Electromagnetic Fields." *Neuroscience and Biobehavioral Reviews* 31 (2007): 619-642.

National Institutes of Health. "Electromagnetic Fields." Available at http://health.nih.gov/topic/electromagneticfields.

Lai, H., and N. P. Singh. "Magnetic-Field-Induced DNA Strand Breaks in Brain Cells of the Rat." *Environmental Health Perspectives* 112 (2004): 687-694.

Landgrebe, M., et al. "Cognitive and Neurobiological Alterations in Electromagnetic Hypersensitive Patients." *Psychological Medicine* 38 (2008): 1781-1791.

Levallois, Patrick. "Hypersensitivity of Human Subjects to Environmental Electric and Magnetic Field Exposure." *Environmental Health Perspectives* 110 (2002): 613-618.

Rubin, G. James, Rosa Nieto-Hernandez, and Simon Wessely. "Idiopathic Environmental Intolerance Attributed to Electromagnetic Fields (Formerly 'Electromagnetic Hypersensitivity'): An Updated Systematic Review of Provocation Studies." *Bioelectromagnetics* 31 (2010): 1-11.

World Health Organization. "Electromagnetic Fields and Public Health." Available at http://www.who.int/mediacentre/factsheets/fs296.

See also: Energy medicine; Photosensitivity.

Eleutherococcus senticosus

CATEGORY: Herbs and supplements
RELATED TERMS: Eleuthero, Russian ginseng, Siberian ginseng
DEFINITION: Natural plant product used as a dietary supplement for specific health benefits.
PRINCIPAL PROPOSED USES: Adaptogen, stress
OTHER PROPOSED USES: Chronic fatigue syndrome, herpes, sports performance

OVERVIEW

Eleutherococcus senticosus is only distantly related to the true ginseng species (*Panax ginseng* and *P. quinquefolius*) and possesses entirely different, unrelated chemical constituents. However, it is popularly called Russian or Siberian ginseng. The origin of this misnomer lies in the work of a Soviet scientist, I. I. Brekhman, who believed that *Eleutherococcus* has the same properties as ginseng and popularized it as a less-expensive alternative herb.

According to Brekhman, *Eleutherococcus* and ginseng are both adaptogens. This term refers to a hypothetical treatment defined as follows: An adaptogen should help the body adapt to stresses of various kinds, whether heat, cold, exertion, trauma, sleep deprivation, toxic exposure, radiation, infection, or psychological stress. Furthermore, an adaptogen should cause no side effects, be effective in treating a wide variety of illnesses, and help return an organism toward balance regardless of what may have gone wrong.

Perhaps the only indisputable example of an adaptogen is a healthful lifestyle. By eating right, exercising regularly, and generally living a life of balance and moderation, one can increase physical fitness and the ability to resist illnesses of all types. Brekhman believed that both *Eleutherococcus* and ginseng produced similarly universal benefits. However, there is little to no meaningful evidence supporting this theory. (Herbs sold under the name "ciwuja" are likely to be *Eleutherococcus*.)

USES AND APPLICATIONS

If Brekhman is right, ginseng (whether *Eleutherococcus* or *Panax*) should be the right treatment for most persons. Modern life is tremendously stressful, and if an herb could help a person withstand stress, it would be a useful herb indeed. *Eleutherococcus* is widely used for this purpose in Russia and Eastern Europe, and it is popular elsewhere as well. However, there is little meaningful evidence to support this theory. Existing evidence on the supposed adaptogenic properties falls far beneath current scientific standards.

Better-quality studies have evaluated the potential usefulness of *Eleutherococcus* for specific conditions. Most of these studies, however, have failed to find benefit. In the one unquestionably positive study, a six-month, double-blind, placebo-controlled trial of ninety-three men and women with recurrent herpes infections, treatment with *Eleutherococcus* (2 grams daily) reduced the frequency of outbreaks by approximately 50 percent.

Although *Eleutherococcus* is widely used as a sports supplement, evidence from studies is largely negative. For example, a double-blind, placebo-controlled study of twenty athletes over an eight-week period found no improvement in physical performance. In addition, a small double-blind, crossover trial found *Eleutherococcus* ineffective for improving performance in endurance exercise (prolonged cycling). Finally, in a small double-blind, placebo-controlled trial of endurance athletes, use of *Eleutherococcus* actually increased physiological signs of stress during intensive training.

One study failed to find *Eleutherococcus* helpful for chronic fatigue syndrome. Several double-blind studies enrolling about five hundred persons in total evaluated a proprietary combination therapy containing extracts of *Eleutherococcus* and the herb andrographis for the treatment of upper respiratory infections. The studies found benefit. In general, these studies reported that the use of the combination therapy may decrease both the severity and the duration of upper respiratory infections. However, it is not clear if the presence of the *Eleutherococcus* adds any benefit beyond that of the andrographis constituent, which taken alone has shown efficacy in clinical trials.

DOSAGE

The typical recommended daily dosage of *Eleutherococcus* is 2 to 3 grams whole herb or 300 to 400 milligrams of extract daily.

SAFETY ISSUES

According to studies performed primarily in the former Soviet Union, *Eleutherococcus* appears to present a low order of toxicity in both the short and long term. Human trials have not resulted in any significant side effects. Safety in pregnant or nursing women, young children, and people with severe liver or kidney disease is not known.

One report suggests that *Eleutherococcus* may alter the results of a test for the medication digoxin. However, it is not clear if it was the *Eleutherococcus* or a contaminant (such as digoxin mixed with the herb) that caused these problems.

IMPORTANT INTERACTIONS

Eleutherococcus may interfere with blood tests designed to measure digoxin level.

EBSCO CAM Review Board

FURTHER READING

Eschbach, L. F., et al. "The Effect of Siberian Ginseng (*Eleutherococcus senticosus*) on Substrate Utilization and Performance." *International Journal of Sport Nutrition and Exercise Metabolism* 10 (2000): 444-451.

Gabrielian, E. S., et al. "A Double Blind, Placebo-Controlled Study of *Andrographis paniculata* Fixed Combination Kan Jang in the Treatment of Acute Upper Respiratory Tract Infections Including Sinusitis." *Phytomedicine* 9 (2002): 589-597.

Gaffney, B. T., H. M. Hugel, and P. A. Rich. "The Effects of *Eleutherococcus senticosus* and *Panax ginseng* on Steroidal Hormone Indices of Stress and Lymphocyte Subset Numbers in Endurance Athletes." *Life Sciences* 70, no. 4 (2001): 431-442.

Hartz, A. J., et al. "Randomized Controlled Trial of Siberian Ginseng for Chronic Fatigue." *Psychological Medicine* 34, no. 1 (2004): 51-61.

Spasov, A. A., et al. "Comparative Controlled Study of *Andrographis paniculata* Fixed Combination, Kan Jang, and an Echinacea Preparation as Adjuvant, in the Treatment of Uncomplicated Respiratory Disease in Children." *Phytotherapy Research* 18 (2004): 47-53.

See also: Andrographis; Chronic fatigue syndrome; Ginseng; Herbal medicine; Herpes; Sports and fitness support: Enhancing performance; Stress.

Endometriosis

CATEGORY: Condition
DEFINITION: Treatment of the painful disease in which uterine tissue grows outside the uterus.
PRINCIPAL PROPOSED NATURAL TREATMENTS: None
OTHER PROPOSED NATURAL TREATMENTS: Acupuncture, chasteberry, crampbark, dandelion root, fish oil, magnet therapy, traditional Chinese herbal medicine

INTRODUCTION

Endometriosis is a painful, chronic disease that occurs when uterine tissue (technically, endometrial tissue) grows outside the uterus. The misplaced fragments of tissue develop and bleed in response to the hormones of the menstrual cycle. In turn, this causes inflammation and damage in nearby tissues. Symptoms of endometriosis include fatigue, infertility, and cyclic pelvic pain made worse by urination, bowel movements, or sexual intercourse.

Conventional treatment may involve anti-inflammatory medications, hormone therapies, and surgery. However, such treatment is often not fully satisfactory.

PROPOSED NATURAL TREATMENTS

Because of the limitations of conventional treatment for endometriosis, many women with this condition turn to alternative therapies. However, there is no reliable scientific evidence to indicate that any natural treatment can relieve or heal endometriosis.

Traditional Chinese herbal medicine. Traditional Chinese herbal medicine is one of the more commonly used alternative approaches to endometriosis. Chinese medical theory has its own unique way of interpreting the condition, using such concepts as blood stasis and obstructed qi. Traditional Chinese herbal medicine employs herbal combinations with acupuncture in the hopes of restoring normal health. Commonly used herbs include corydalis, conidium, bupleurum, dong quai, and perilla. No double-blind, placebo-controlled trials of Chinese herbs for endometriosis have been reported.

OTHER PROPOSED NATURAL TREATMENTS

Magnet therapy has been proposed for the treatment of many chronic pain conditions. However, a double-blind, placebo-controlled study of fourteen women with chronic pelvic pain (from endometriosis or other causes) found no significant benefit with two weeks of treatment. A larger study did find some evidence of benefit after four weeks of treatment, but a high dropout rate and other study-design problems compromised the meaningfulness of the results.

Studies in animals suggest that fish oil, a source of omega-3 fatty acids, may be helpful for endometriosis. However, human trials have not been reported. Western herbs such as crampbark, chasteberry, dandelion root, and prickly ash are sometimes suggested for the treatment of endometriosis, but there is no reliable evidence that they are helpful. Finally, some alternative practitioners associate endometriosis with chronic candida, food allergies, or immune weakness, but there is no meaningful scientific evidence to indicate that approaches based on these supposed connections provide any benefit.

EBSCO CAM Review Board

FURTHER READING

Brown, C. S., et al. "Efficacy of Static Magnetic Field Therapy in Chronic Pelvic Pain." *American Journal of Obstetrics and Gynecology* 187 (2002): 1581-1587.

Dallenbach-Hellweg, Gisela, Dietmar Schmidt, and Friederike Dallenbach. *Atlas of Endometrial Histopathology.* 3d ed. New York: Springer, 2010.

Zoorob, J. R. "CAM and Women's Health: Selected Topics." *Primary Care* 37, no. 2 (2010): 367-387.

See also: Amenorrhea; Dysmenorrhea; Infertility, female; Pain management; Premenstrual syndrome (PMS); Women's health.

Common Sites of Endometriosis

Fallopian tube

Ovary

Surface of uterus

Energy medicine

CATEGORY: Issues and overviews

RELATED TERMS: Acupuncture, cymatic therapy, electromagnetic therapy, homeopathy, intercessory prayer, light therapy, magnet therapy, polarity therapy, Prana, *qi*, qigong, spiritual healing, therapeutic touch

DEFINITION: The manipulation of energy fields to promote health and well-being.

OVERVIEW

The notion of energy medicine is an ancient one, growing out of such concepts as the traditional Chinese medicine principle *qi* (or *chi*), the life force that motivates the universe and informs all beings, and related to such modalities as acupuncture, organized around the body's electromagnetic meridians. The term "energy medicine" is, however, of recent coinage. Apparently, it had first been used as a term of art in conjunction with a 1987 conference in Madras, India, sponsored by the John E. Fetzer Foundation of Kalamazoo, Michigan, dedicated to promoting mind/body medicine. Two years later, drawing on work on psychophysiological self-regulation (also known as biofeedback) demonstrated at the Menninger Foundation in Topeka, Kansas, researchers T. M. Srinivasan, Elmer Green, and Carol Schneider founded the International Society for the Study of Subtle Energy and Energy Medicine (ISSSEEM), now based in Arvada, Colorado.

ISSSEEM, with its mission to improve human health and welfare, differentiates between therapeutic energy medicine involving tangible forces such as electromagnetic fields, acoustics, and gravity, and traditional subtle energies such as *qi*, Prana (breath of life), and homeopathic resonance, all of which operate at the level of the subtle or etheric body and are difficult to measure. The National Institutes of Health's (NIH) National Center for Complementary and Alternative Medicine (NCCAM), which recognizes energy medicine as one of five domains of complementary and alternative medicine, similarly distinguishes between "veritable" energy fields, which can be measured for diagnosis and treatment, and "putative" energy fields (also called biofields), which resist measurement by reproducible methods. NCCAM cites magnet therapy and light therapy as examples of the former and qigong and healing touch as examples of the latter.

A survey by the National Center for Health Statistics indicates that approximately 1 percent of Americans have used energy medicine techniques. It is worth noting, however, that almost one-half of all Americans use some form of alternative medicine in a given year. As energy medicine advocates emphasize, there is considerable overlap between energy medicine and NCCAM's other four domains: whole medical systems, such as homeopathy and naturopathy; mind/body medicine, such as biofeedback and meditation; biological practices involving substances such as herbs and nutraceuticals; and manipulative, body-based practices such as massage and chiropractic.

THEORY AND PRACTICE

Energy medicine as it is understood today addresses both electromagnetic energy and more subtle energies, which together make up the body's dynamic infrastructure. Physical and mental health depend upon keeping these various energies balanced and free flowing. These energies may become blocked by environmental interference from such things as toxins and electromagnetic pollution, and by internal factors such as prolonged physical or mental stress. Flow, balance, and harmony can be reestablished by manipulating specific energy points on the skin with exercises involving tapping, massaging, pinching, or twisting, or by manually tracing energy pathways over the skin. Alternatively, one can, as in certain types of yoga exercises, assume postures designed to affect the body's energies in specific ways. In addition, mental focusing exercises akin to meditation can help to realign both tangible and subtle energy.

Western medicine has long recognized and made use of the body's oscillating magnetic fields, developing sophisticated technology such as magnetic resonance imaging (MRI) scanners and bone healing electronic stimulators to help diagnose and treat physical disorders. Acupuncture, long considered a type of quackery, is now widely accepted as an effective, if still somewhat misunderstood, method for addressing pain. It is not terribly difficult, even for skeptics, to make the connection between such machines and modalities.

Acceptance of the existence of biofields, and, especially, the ability to intentionally influence them, remains profoundly controversial. However, the discovery of peptides and opiate receptors in the human brain, the molecules of emotion, has cleared the way for a burgeoning new field of inquiry: energy psychology. Considered a derivative of energy medicine, energy psychology is rooted in an assumption that mental disorders are related to disruptions in the body's energy fields. Energy psychology consists of a set of physical and cognitive procedures designed to influence emotion, cognition, and behavior.

Positive reactions to energy medicine treatment can be difficult to quantify or verify and have often been attributed to the placebo effect or to cognitive dissonance. Positive research outcomes have been similarly discounted as resulting from practitioner or publication bias. Also, energy medicine, like any medical field (particularly any alternative medicine modality), is fraught with fraud. In 2008, the U.S. Food and Drug Administration banned two devices purporting to heal with the use of energy medicine: the EPFX and the PAP-IMI.

Lisa Paddock, Ph.D.

FURTHER READING

Eden, Donna, and David Feinstein. *Energy Medicine.* New York: Tarcher, 1999. Eden, an energy medicine practitioner, and Feinstein, a psychologist, provide a comprehensive self-help guide to treating physical and emotional maladies.

International Society for the Study of Subtle Energy and Energy Medicine. http://www.issseem.org. Aims to promote energy medicine through research, publications, and conferences.

National Center for Complementary and Alternative Medicine. http://nccam.nih.gov/health/whatiscam. An overview of NCCAM's definition of "alternative and complementary medicine," including energy medicine.

Oschman, James L. *Energy Medicine: The Scientific Basis.* New York: Churchill Livingstone, 2000. This book presents scientific research supporting and explaining the concept of and various practices employed in energy medicine.

Pert, Candace B. *Molecules of Emotion: The Science Behind Mind-Body Medicine.* New York: Simon & Schuster, 1999. Pert's book describes her role in the discovery of the brain's opiate receptors and provides scientific support for mind/body medicine by linking molecules with the psyche.

See also: Acupuncture; Electromagnetic hypersensitivity; Magnet therapy; Meridians; Mind/body medicine; Qigong.

Engel, George Libman

CATEGORY: Biography
IDENTIFICATION: American psychiatrist who was a proponent of the biopsychosocial model of health and healing, also known as psychosomatic medicine
BORN: December 10, 1913; New York, New York
DIED: November 26, 1999; Rochester, New York

OVERVIEW

George Libman Engel was an American psychiatrist best known for proposing that biological, psychological, and social factors all affect health, illness, and healing. This view is known as the biopsychosocial health model, or psychosomatic medicine.

Engel completed undergraduate coursework in chemistry at Dartmouth College in 1934 and received his medical degree from Johns Hopkins University School of Medicine in 1938. He then interned in New York at Mount Sinai Hospital. Here, Engel worked among physicians who incorporated psychosomatics into clinical treatment of patients. However, at this point, he was skeptical of psychoanalysis and related medicine. Instead, he maintained that diseases could be treated with purely physical means, despite the practices of his colleagues.

After interning at Mount Sinai, Engel became a research fellow in medicine at Harvard Medical School and a graduate research assistant at the Peter Bent Brigham Hospital. While working in Boston, he met a psychiatrist, John Romano, who invited him to collaborate on research studies and later to join both the medicine and psychiatry departments of the University of Cincinnati. Engel accepted the invitation, which ultimately led to Engel's interest in integrating psychology and traditional medicine, a union that came to be known as psychosomatic medicine.

In 1946, Engel again followed Romano, this time to the University of Rochester Medical Center in New York, where he ended up spending the majority of his career. During this time, Engel held dual appointments in the departments of psychiatry and medicine. He went on to modify the classic medical school curriculum at his institution by introducing psychiatric training. At the same time, he expanded his own knowledge of and training in psychoanalysis. By the mid-1950s, Engel was considered a major figure among psychosomatic researchers.

Engel had a prominent role in the American Psychosomatic Society, which promotes the understanding of the connection between biological and psychological factors in human health. Engel edited the journal of this organization (*Psychosomatic Medicine*) for some time, and he eventually published a number of articles and books on the relationship between emotional well-being and disease. Because of his contributions at the University of Rochester Medical Center, the institution became a leading center of research and education in psychosomatic theory.

Eventually, Engel's idea of integrating psychological studies with classic medicinal techniques was termed the "biopsychosocial model." He discussed the topic at length in an article published in *Science* in 1977. This concept remains particularly important in the field of health psychology.

Engel received a number of awards and other honors for his contributions to the field. Recognition came from such institutions as the American College of Physicians and the American Psychiatric Association.

Brandy Weidow, M.S.

FURTHER READING

Cohen, Jules, and Stephanie Brown-Clark. *John Romano and George Engel: Their Lives and Work.* Rochester, N.Y.: University of Rochester Press, 2010.

Dowling, A. Scott. "George Engel, M.D. (1913-1999)." *American Journal of Psychiatry* 162 (2005). Also available at http://ajp.psychiatryonline.org/cgi/content/full/162/11/2039.

Engel, George L. "The Need for a New Medical Model: A Challenge for Biomedicine." *Science* 196 (1977): 129-136. Also available at http://www.sciencemag.org/content/196/4286/129.

See also: Integrative medicine; Mind/body medicine.

Enzyme potentiated desensitization

CATEGORY: Therapies and techniques
RELATED TERMS: Allergen injection therapy, allergy shot
DEFINITION: A therapy involving injection of substances to prevent allergies.
PRINCIPAL PROPOSED USE: Allergic rhinitis
OTHER PROPOSED USES: Hundreds of conditions

OVERVIEW

Enzyme potentiated desensitization (EPD) is an alternative form of "allergy shot" originally popularized in the United Kingdom in the 1960s by Leonard McEwan. EPD involves injection of very low levels of an allergen, combined with the naturally occurring enzyme beta glucuronidase. EPD proponents claim that this method gets to the root of allergy problems and produces permanent benefits by "retraining" the immune system. It is claimed that EPD can successfully treat hundreds of medical conditions, from rheumatoid arthritis to epilepsy. However, the evidence used to support these assertions falls considerably short of meaningful.

EPD proponents cite studies that show EPD offers cure rates approaching 85 percent for numerous illnesses. However, the evidence for this is scientifically unreliable. The cited research was of the type called an "open, uncontrolled" study. This means that researchers (or practitioners) administered EPD to people and then noted whether they saw benefit. Positive findings in this type of investigation may seem

What Are Allergy Shots?

Allergy shots, or immunotherapy, are subcutaneous (under the skin) injections of increasing concentrations of the allergen or allergens to which a person is sensitive. These injections reduce the level of immunoglobulin E (IgE) antibodies in the blood and cause the body to make a protective antibody called IgG. A series of allergy shots is the only available treatment that has a chance of reducing allergy symptoms over time.

About 85 percent of people with allergic rhinitis will see their hay fever symptoms and need for medication drop significantly within twelve months of starting immunotherapy. Those who benefit from allergy shots may continue it for three years and then consider stopping. While many are able to stop the injections with good results lasting for several years, others get worse after the shots are discontinued.

intuitively to mean something, but they are actually illusions. For most conditions, a high percentage of people given placebo will improve or appear to improve, and they often will do so dramatically.

The reasons for this fact are complicated and surprising. For researchers to actually show a treatment to be effective, they must compare it with placebo treatment. Furthermore, they must conduct the study in a double-blind fashion, meaning that neither the practitioners nor the participants know who is getting real treatment and who is getting placebo. Finally, such studies must be randomized, meaning that people are assigned to the treatment or the placebo group by random chance (such as by flipping a coin) rather than by choice. Only two such randomized, double-blind, placebo-controlled trials have been performed on EPD. One found benefit and the other did not.

In the first double-blind, placebo-controlled study, 183 people with a history of consistent hay fever were treated with EPD or placebo and followed throughout the hay fever season. The EPD preparation contained beta glucuronidase, 1,3-cyclohexanediol, protamine sulphate, and a mixed extract of allergens, including pollens, fungal spores, cat and dog dander, and dust mite. The fake treatment contained only saline. Neither the researchers administering the injections nor the study participants knew which was which. Both groups improved markedly. However, there was no difference in symptoms between the two groups, as measured by problem-free days, quality-of-life scores, or symptom severity scores.

A slightly smaller study did find benefits. In this double-blind study of 125 children, the use of a single dose of EPD reduced hay fever and asthma symptoms compared with placebo. The most that can be said about EPD is that equivocal evidence exists regarding its efficacy for allergies. Benefits for any other conditions remain entirely speculative.

A similar scientific inadequacy exists regarding claims made about how EPD works. One EPD Web site states the following:

> EPD stimulates the immune system to produce new T-suppressor cells . . . These take 3 to 4 weeks to mature before they can begin their task of disabling mis-coded T-Helper cells. Essentially, this is a re-training program so the body does not react to those substances contained in the shot. The mis-coded cells are a part of the chain that stimulates the production of histamine, the major trigger of allergic response.

While this claim may sound impressive on the surface, it succeeds only as advertising; as science, it strays much too far from established facts.

SAFETY ISSUES

Whether or not EPD is effective, it does appear to be safe. No serious adverse reactions have been associated with its use. Although in theory allergic reactions could occur in response to EPD injections, the amount of allergen used in EPD is so much lower than the amount used in a normal "allergy shot" that allergic reactions may not, in fact, occur. Finally, EPD proponents claim that there can be a temporary aggravation response that is part of the healing process; however, this has not been documented.

EBSCO CAM Review Board

FURTHER READING

Abramson, M. J., R. M. Puy, and J. M. Weiner. "Injection Allergen Immunotherapy for Asthma." *Cochrane Database of Systematic Reviews* (2010): CD001186. Available through *EBSCO DynaMed Systematic Literature Surveillance* at http://www.ebscohost.com/dynamed.

Calderon, M. A., et al. "Allergen Injection Immunotherapy for Seasonal Allergic Rhinitis." *Cochrane Database of Systematic Reviews* (2007): CD001936. Available through *EBSCO DynaMed Systematic Literature Surveillance* at http://www.ebscohost.com/dynamed.

Galli, E., et al. "A Double-Blind Randomized Placebo-Controlled Trial with Short-Term Beta-glucuronidase Therapy in Children with Chronic Rhinoconjunctivitis and/or Asthma Due to Dust Mite Allergy." *Journal of Investigational Allergology and Clinical Immunology* 16 (2006): 345-350.

Radcliffe, M. J., et al. "Enzyme Potentiated Desensitisation in Treatment of Seasonal Allergic Rhinitis." *British Medical Journal* 327 (2003): 251-254.

See also: Allergies; Asthma; Immune support; Prolotherapy; Sinusitis.

Ephedra

CATEGORY: Herbs and supplements
RELATED TERMS: *Ephedra sinica*, Ma huang
DEFINITION: Natural plant product used to treat specific health conditions.
PRINCIPAL PROPOSED USE: Asthma

OVERVIEW

The Chinese herb ma huang is a member of a primitive family of plants that look like thin, branching, connected straws. A related species, *Ephedra nevadensis*, grows wild in the American Southwest and is widely called Mormon tea. However, only the Asian species of ephedra contains the active compounds ephedrine and pseudoephedrine.

Ma huang was traditionally used by Chinese herbalists during the early stages of respiratory infections and was also used for the short-term treatment of certain kinds of asthma, eczema, hay fever, narcolepsy, and edema. Japanese chemists isolated ephedrine from ma huang at the turn of the twentieth century, and it soon became a primary treatment for asthma in the United States and abroad. Ephedra's other major ingredient, pseudoephedrine, became the decongestant Sudafed.

THERAPEUTIC DOSAGES

The dosage of ephedra should be adjusted according to the amount of the ephedrine it provides. For adults, no more than 25 milligrams (mg) should be taken at one time, and a total daily intake of 100 mg should not be exceeded. However, a survey of ephedra-containing dietary supplements found that ephedrine content as listed on the label was frequently incorrect. In addition, other chemicals were often present that could increase safety risks. For this reason, experts recommend against the use of herbal ephedra.

THERAPEUTIC USES

Although it can still be found in a few over-the-counter drugs for asthma and sinus congestion (in a safer form than the banned dietary supplements),

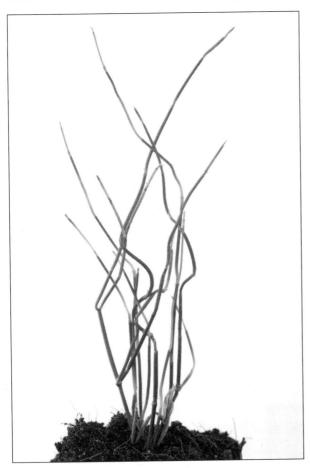

Chinese herb ephedra. (Ted Kinsman/Photo Researchers, Inc.)

physicians seldom prescribe ephedrine anymore. The problem is that ephedrine mimics the effects of adrenaline and causes symptoms such as rapid heartbeat, high blood pressure, agitation, insomnia, nausea, and loss of appetite. The newer asthma drugs are much safer and easier to tolerate.

Meaningful evidence suggests ephedrine/caffeine combinations can assist in weight loss. However, because of safety risks, experts strongly recommend that individuals seek a physician's supervision before attempting to lose weight with ephedrine/caffeine combination therapy. Experts also recommend not using herbal sources of ephedrine, which are now banned, for weight loss.

One highly preliminary study has been used to claim that ephedrine is helpful for women with sexual dysfunction. However, this trial was very small, enrolled women without sexual problems, and only examined sexual responsiveness to visual stimuli; at this time, experts recommend that women with sexual dysfunction avoid using ephedra. Another study examined the possible benefits of ephedrine for treatment of female sexual dysfunction caused by antidepressants in the selective serotonin reuptake inhibitor (SSRI) family, such as Prozac. Ephedrine failed to prove more effective than placebo.

There is no meaningful evidence that ephedra enhances sports performance. It should also be noted that persons taking ephedra or ephedrine may test positive for methamphetamine (speed) on drug screening.

SCIENTIFIC EVIDENCE

Evidence suggests that ephedrine/caffeine combinations can aid weight loss and help keep the weight off for up to six months. However, the benefits are modest.

For example, in a double-blind, placebo-controlled trial, 180 overweight persons were placed on a weight-loss diet and given either ephedrine/caffeine (20 mg/200 mg), ephedrine alone (20 mg), caffeine alone (200 mg), or placebo three times daily for twenty-four weeks. The results showed that the ephedrine/caffeine treatment significantly enhanced weight loss, resulting in a loss of more than thirty-six pounds, compared with only twenty-nine pounds in the placebo group, a seven-pound difference. Neither ephedrine nor caffeine alone produced any benefit. Contrary to some reports, participants did not develop tolerance to the treatment. For the entire six months of the trial, the treatment group maintained the same relative weight-loss advantage over the placebo group.

A few side effects were seen in this study, primarily insomnia, dizziness, and tremor, but they tended to fade away after a few weeks. Keep in mind that participants were screened prior to the study and were eliminated if they had high blood pressure or any other serious disease, or if they used medications or illegal drugs that might interact with stimulants.

Another study compared ephedrine/caffeine with the no-longer-available drug dexfenfluramine (Redux), related to fenfluramine of fen-phen fame. A total of 103 overweight individuals were enrolled in this fifteen-week, double-blind trial. All were placed on a weight-loss diet. Half were given ephedrine/caffeine at the usual dose, while the others were given 15 mg of dexfenfluramine. The results showed comparable weight loss in both groups.

Finally, a double-blind, placebo-controlled trial enrolled 225 heavy smokers who wanted to quit but were afraid of gaining weight. At twelve weeks after quitting smoking, individuals taking ephedrine and caffeine had gained significantly less weight. At that point, the dosage was gradually reduced, and the difference between the groups declined. Contrary to the hopes of the experimenters, ephedrine/caffeine use did not help individuals quit smoking. Benefits have also been seen in smaller studies using herbal sources of ephedrine.

Experts do not know exactly how ephedrine/caffeine works. However, caffeine has actions that cause fat breakdown and enhance metabolism. Ephedrine suppresses appetite and increases energy expenditure. The combination appears to produce synergistic effects, with appetite suppression probably the most important overall factor.

SAFETY ISSUES

On December 30, 2003, the U.S. Food and Drug Administration (FDA) issued a consumer alert regarding the safety of dietary supplements containing ephedra. The FDA determined that consuming these supplements poses an unnecessary risk of illness or injury, and that consumers should stop buying and using ephedra products immediately. The FDA also notified manufacturers and marketers of these dietary supplements that effective sixty days (March, 2004) after the publication of its final ruling,

the sale of all products containing ephedra in the United States would be banned. This ruling was temporarily overturned in April 2005 but was later upheld the following year, making it illegal to sell these products.

While ephedra is an herb with a long history of use in Chinese herbal medicine, Chinese tradition attaches numerous warnings: It should be used only by very robust people, for certain specific purposes, and only for a short period of time. These ancient warnings seem to have been disregarded in the transition of ephedra use from Asia to the United States, where it was often sold for continuous use by overweight, relatively unhealthy people. Herbal products containing ephedra caused the majority (64 percent) of reported adverse effects from herbs in the United States. This proportion is particularly impressive given that less than 1 percent of all herbal products sold in the United States contain ephedra. On a per-use basis, for example, ephedra has 720 times as much risk of causing harm as ginkgo biloba.

There are many reasons for this high rate of risk. While it is possible for healthy individuals under physician supervision to use ephedrine or ephedrine/caffeine combinations safely, in individuals with heart disease, and even occasionally in those with no known heart conditions, ephedrine can cause serious disturbances of the heart rhythm and possibly sudden death; strokes have also occurred. Use of herbal ephedra, as opposed to ephedrine, may present additional dangers. There is no ready way to be sure what dose of the drug ephedrine individuals are getting when they purchase the herb ephedra, which creates a potential risk of overdosage. In addition, some ephedra products contain potentially more toxic chemicals related to ephedrine, such as (+)-norpseudoephedrine.

Besides heart problems and strokes, use of ephedra has been associated with severe inflammation of the liver (in at least one case requiring a liver transplant) and of the heart. In these cases, it appears likely that ephedra (or an unidentified contaminant in the herb) triggered an autoimmune reaction.

In addition, people taking ephedra or ephedrine may develop an unusual form of kidney stones that actually contain ephedrine. Temporary psychosis has also been linked to use of ephedra. Finally, there are indications that certain preparations of ephedra may be toxic to the nervous system.

Based on the known risks of ephedrine and on the evidence described in the foregoing paragraphs, ephedra should not be taken by persons with cardiovascular disease, including angina, abnormalities of heart rhythm, hardening of the arteries, high blood pressure, high cholesterol, intermittent claudication, myocarditis, vasculitis, or history of stroke; enlargement of the prostate; diabetes; hepatitis; diseases of the nervous system; glaucoma; or hyperthyroidism.

Ephedra may be particularly risky for young children, pregnant or nursing women, people with kidney disease, and people with liver disease. Furthermore, one should never combine ephedra with monoamine-oxidase (MAO) inhibitors, such as Nardil (phenelzine), or fatal reactions may develop.

IMPORTANT INTERACTIONS

Persons taking MAO inhibitors should not take ephedra, and persons taking any stimulant drugs, including caffeine, should not take ephedra except under physician supervision.

EBSCO CAM Review Board

FURTHER READING

Bent, S., et al. "The Relative Safety of Ephedra Compared with Other Herbal Products." *Annals of Internal Medicine* 138 (2003): 468-471.

Boozer, C. N., et al. "Herbal Ephedra/Caffeine for Weight Loss." *International Journal of Obesity and Related Metabolic Disorders* 26 (2002): 593-604.

Chen, W. L., et al. "Effects of Ephedra on Autonomic Nervous Modulation in Healthy Young Adults." *Journal of Ethnopharmacology* 130, no. 2 (2010): 563-568.

Coffey, C. S., et al. "A Randomized Double-Blind Placebo-Controlled Clinical Trial of a Product Containing Ephedrine, Caffeine, and Other Ingredients from Herbal Sources for Treatment of Overweight and Obesity in the Absence of Lifestyle Treatment." *International Journal of Obesity and Related Metabolic Disorders* 28, no. 11 (2004): 1411-1419.

Levisky, J. A., et al. "False-Positive RIA for Methamphetamine Following Ingestion of an Ephedra-Derived Herbal Product." *Journal of Analytical Toxicology* 27, no. 2 (2003): 123-124.

Meston, C. M. "A Randomized, Placebo-Controlled, Crossover Study of Ephedrine for SSRI-Induced Female Sexual Dysfunction." *Journal of Sex and Marital Therapy* 30 (2004): 57-68.

Samenuk, D., et al. "Adverse Cardiovascular Events Temporally Associated with Ma Huang, an Herbal Source of Ephedrine." *Mayo Clinic Proceedings* 77 (2002): 12-16.

Shekelle, P. G., et al. "Efficacy and Safety of Ephedra and Ephedrine for Weight Loss and Athletic Performance." *Journal of the American Medical Association* 289 (2003): 1537-1545.

Skoulidis, F., G. J. Alexander, and S. E. Davies. "Ma Huang Associated Acute Liver Failure Requiring Liver Transplantation." *European Journal of Gastroenterology and Hepatology* 17 (2005): 581-584.

Walton, R., and G. H. Manos. "Psychosis Related to Ephedra-Containing Herbal Supplement Use." *Southern Medical Journal* 96 (2003): 718-720.

See also: Asthma.

Epilepsy

CATEGORY: Condition

RELATED TERMS: Generalized seizures, partial complex seizures, seizure disorder, temporal lobe epilepsy

DEFINITION: Treatment of the brain disorder that causes recurrent seizures.

PRINCIPAL PROPOSED NATURAL TREATMENTS: Ketogenic diet, nutritional support

OTHER PROPOSED NATURAL TREATMENTS: Acupuncture, electromagnetic therapy, fish oil, food allergen identification and avoidance, manganese, melatonin, *Nigella sativa*, taurine, traditional Chinese herbal remedies (saiko-keishi-to and sho-saiko-to)

HERBS AND SUPPLEMENTS TO AVOID: 5-hydroxytryptophan, ginkgo, glutamine, hyssop, ipriflavone, Japanese star anise, nicotinamide, 2-dimethylaminoethanol, white willow

INTRODUCTION

Epilepsy is a disorder of the brain that causes recurrent episodes called seizures. A seizure is sometimes described as an electrical storm in the brain leading to abnormal movements, sensations, and states of consciousness. In reality, however, the seizure is more orderly than a storm. During a seizure, nerves function in an abnormally synchronized manner, a kind of lockstep that can continue for seconds or minutes.

The results range from mild changes in awareness to violent convulsions.

Isolated seizures can occur for many reasons. The term "epilepsy" is applied when a person has recurrent seizures with no known treatable cause. If the seizure occurs in a localized part of the brain, it is called a partial complex seizure. If it affects much of brain, it is called a generalized seizure.

The most common forms of generalized seizures are absence seizures (petit mal) and tonic-clonic seizures (grand mal). Petit mal seizures involve a brief lapse of consciousness that occurs suddenly and lasts for a brief time before disappearing; there are usually no symptoms afterward. A grand mal seizure involves loss of consciousness, convulsions of the body, tongue biting, and, often, urination. A state of confusion follows the seizure.

Partial seizures come in three main varieties. They can be simple (involving just an arm, for example) or complex (involving more complicated movements and loss of consciousness). Finally, some may turn into generalized seizures. There are several medications used to treat epilepsy, generally with considerable success. Most of these drugs can cause significant side effects, some of which may be partially correctable through nutrient supplementation.

PRINCIPAL PROPOSED NATURAL TREATMENTS

There are no well-established herbs or supplements for the treatment of epilepsy. However, a number of supplements may be useful for treating nutritional deficiencies caused by anticonvulsant drugs. Besides herbs and supplements, the ketogenic diet might be helpful for controlling seizures in children.

Epilepsy is far too serious a condition for self-treatment. For this reason, none of the treatments listed here should be used without the advice and supervision of a doctor.

Ketogenic diet. Before drug treatments for epilepsy were invented, scientists noticed that fasting tends to reduce seizure frequency. Subsequent investigation pinned down a metabolic state called ketosis as the causative factor. Ketosis occurs during fasting and also while consuming a diet high in fat and very low in carbohydrates (the ketogenic diet).

When effective anticonvulsant drugs were developed, the ketogenic diet fell into disfavor, but medical interest has returned. Today, the diet is seeing increased use in the treatment of people who do not

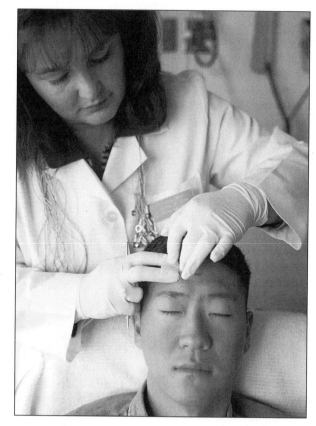

A doctor attaches electrodes to a patient's head in order to monitor his epilepsy. (PhotoDisc)

respond fully to standard medications. Most studies have involved children because they tend to accept the diet more readily than adults.

Evidence suggests that the ketogenic diet may almost completely stop seizures in about one-half of all children with epilepsy and reduce seizure frequency less dramatically in another one-third. The ketogenic diet can cause side effects, such as fatigue, nausea, reduced immunity, mental confusion, dehydration, constipation, and increased tendency to bruise. Major side effects seen occasionally with certain forms of the ketogenic diet include kidney stones, gallstones, impaired liver function, severe hypoproteinemia (dangerously low levels of protein in the blood), and kidney injury. Vitamin and mineral deficiency may also occur with some ketogenic diets, but the use of a multivitamin-multimineral supplement can easily prevent this.

Nutritional support. Many drugs can impair the body's ability to absorb or metabolize certain nutrients;

however, anticonvulsants are particular offenders. Meaningful evidence indicates that common anticonvulsants interfere with the body's handling of folate, biotin, calcium, vitamin D, and vitamin K. In addition, one anticonvulsant, valproic acid, affects the nutrient-like substance carnitine. For these reasons, it is often recommended that people using anticonvulsants take supplements that provide these nutrients.

However, there is a potential catch to correcting such "nutrient depletions." In some cases, taking the nutrient can impair the absorption or alter the metabolism of anticonvulsant drugs. In other cases, it is possible that nutrient depletion is part of how the anticonvulsant operates. For this reason, physician supervision is essential when taking any supplements.

Folate. Folate (also known as folic acid) is a B vitamin that plays an important role in many vital aspects of health. However, most drugs used for preventing seizures can reduce levels of folate in the body. In turn, low serum folate levels can cause elevated levels of homocysteine, possibly increasing the risk of heart disease.

Low folate levels are also linked to increased risk of a variety of birth defects. Because anticonvulsant drugs deplete folate, babies born to women taking anticonvulsants are at increased risk for such birth defects.

However, the case for taking extra folate is complicated by the high folate levels, which may speed up the normal breakdown of phenytoin and possibly other anticonvulsants. This could lead to breakthrough seizures. For this reason, folate supplementation during anticonvulsant therapy should always be supervised by a physician.

Biotin. Numerous anticonvulsants can reduce body levels of the essential vitamin biotin, probably by interfering with its absorption. Valproic acid may affect biotin to a lesser extent than other anticonvulsants.

It is not clear whether this biotin deficiency actually causes any problems. Nonetheless, it is not good to be short on any essential nutrient, and for this reason, biotin supplementation has been recommended during long-term anticonvulsant therapy. The action of anticonvulsant drugs may be at least partly related to their effect on biotin levels. For this reason, physician supervision is strongly advised before adding biotin to an anticonvulsant regimen.

Calcium. Many anticonvulsant drugs increase the risk of osteoporosis and other bone disorders. This is believed to be caused in part by their impairment of calcium metabolism. Effects on calcium may also increase the tendency toward seizures by lowering blood levels of calcium.

Calcium supplementation may thus be beneficial for people taking anticonvulsant drugs. However, some studies indicate that antacids containing calcium carbonate interfere with the absorption of phenytoin and perhaps other anticonvulsants. For this reason, calcium supplements and anticonvulsant drugs should be taken several hours apart.

Vitamin D. Anticonvulsant drugs may interfere with the activity of vitamin D; this may be another factor contributing to anticonvulsant-induced bone problems. Vitamin D supplementation may help prevent bone loss. Adequate sunlight exposure may also help, because sunlight aids the body in manufacturing vitamin D.

Vitamin K. Phenytoin, carbamazepine, phenobarbital, and primidone speed up the normal breakdown of vitamin K into inactive by-products, thus depriving the body of active vitamin K. The use of these anticonvulsants by pregnant women can lead to vitamin K deficiencies in their fetuses, resulting in bleeding disorders or facial-bone abnormalities in the newborns. For this reason, mothers who take these anticonvulsants may need vitamin K supplementation during pregnancy.

In other circumstances, anticonvulsants seldom deplete vitamin K enough to cause bleeding problems. However, vitamin K deficiency may contribute to anticonvulsant-induced osteoporosis.

Carnitine. Valproic acid (Depakene) and possibly other anticonvulsants may reduce the body's levels of the substance carnitine. For this reason, it has been suggested that people using these drugs should take supplemental carnitine. However, there is no evidence that taking carnitine will provide any noticeable benefit; the one study that did attempt to evaluate this possibility failed to discern any meaningful effect.

OTHER PROPOSED TREATMENTS

Herbs and supplements. The traditional Chinese herbal remedies known by the Japanese names saiko-keishi-to and sho-saiko-to have also been suggested for epilepsy, but the supporting evidence for their use remains preliminary. Both of these combination treatments consist of bupleurum, peony root, pinellia root, cassia bark, ginger root, jujube fruit,

Asian ginseng root, Asian skullcap root, and licorice root, but the proportions vary.

A double-blind study performed in Iran reportedly found that the use of an extract of the seed of the *Nigella sativa* plant helped control seizures in children. Weak evidence suggests that the amino acid taurine might offer modest, short-term benefits in epilepsy. Results are inconsistent regarding whether the use of fish oil can decrease seizure frequency in people with epilepsy. Several studies by a single research group hint that the supplement melatonin may improve quality of life in children with epilepsy. People with epilepsy have lower-than-normal levels of the mineral manganese in their blood. This suggests (but does not prove) that manganese supplements might be helpful for epilepsy

Other supplements sometimes suggested for epilepsy (but with no meaningful supporting evidence) include vitamin B_1, vitamin B_6, beta-carotene, and glycine. Herbs traditionally regarded as nervines or nerve-relaxants are also sometimes proposed. These include skullcap, lobelia, lady's slipper, valerian, kava, passionflower, and lemon balm. However, there is no meaningful evidence that they can help, and some of these herbs present significant safety concerns.

Most herbs used for epilepsy are sedatives, as are many anticonvulsant drugs. Combination treatment could lead to dangerous oversedation. People with epilepsy should therefore seek medical supervision before using any herbs or supplements.

Alternative therapies. A special form of electromagnetic therapy called rTMS (repetitive transcranial magnetic stimulation) has shown promise for epilepsy. In a double-blind, placebo-controlled trial, twenty-four participants with epilepsy localized to a specific part of the brain and not fully responsive to drug treatment were given twice daily treatment with rTMS or sham rTMS for one week. The results showed a mild reduction in seizures among the participants given real rTMS. However, the benefits rapidly disappeared when treatment was stopped.

Weak evidence hints that food allergen identification and avoidance may be helpful for people with both migraine headaches and epilepsy. Acupuncture has been proposed for the treatment of epilepsy, but there is no convincing evidence for its effectiveness. A single-blind, controlled trial of individualized acupuncture for thirty-four people with severe epilepsy found no benefit. Also, in a comprehensive review involving ten Chinese trials and one Norwegian trial, acupuncture was largely found to be ineffective.

HERBS AND SUPPLEMENTS TO AVOID

Numerous herbs and supplements have been associated with unexpected or unexpectedly severe seizures. In most cases, however, the evidence linking any particular natural product to increased seizure activity remains circumstantial. Some of the more worrisome potential "pro-seizure" agents are discussed here. Also discussed are herbs and supplements that may interact with medications used for seizures.

Ginkgo seeds contain a seizure-promoting substance called 4-methoxypyridoxine. Although ginkgo seeds are seldom used today, seizures have also been reported with the use of the more common form of the herb: ginkgo leaf extract. One possible explanation is that ginkgo leaf products may have been contaminated with ginkgo seeds. Another possibility has been proposed: Ginkgo may affect the brain in ways similar to tacrine, a drug also used to improve memory and which has been associated with seizures. Finally, it has been suggested that ginkgo might impair the effectiveness of dilantin and depakote. Regardless of the explanation, people with epilepsy should probably avoid ginkgo.

Many anti-epilepsy drugs work by blocking the effects of a substance called glutamate; for this reason, high dosages of the closely related amino acid glutamine could conceivably overwhelm these drugs and pose a risk to people with epilepsy. Manufacturers of the supplement 2-dimethylaminoethanol warn that it might increase seizure risk.

Tea made from the herb hyssop is thought to be safe, but hyssop essential oil, like most essential oils, is toxic in excessive doses. Some of the constituents of hyssop oil are thought to increase the risk of seizures. For this reason, hyssop essential oil should not be used by people with epilepsy.

Japanese star anise contains substances that can trigger seizure activity. Also, some evidence hints that the supplement 5-hydroxytryptophan could potentially exacerbate or initiate a seizure-related illness called myoclonic seizure disorder. The supplement ipriflavone might increase levels of carbamazepine and phenytoin, potentially raising the risk of side effects.

Grapefruit juice slows the body's normal breakdown of several drugs, including the anticonvulsant carbamazepine, allowing it to build up to potentially dangerous levels in the blood; this effect can continue for three days or more following the last glass of grapefruit juice.

The herb white willow, also known as willow bark, is used to treat pain and fever. White willow contains a substance closely related to aspirin known as salicin. Aspirin is known to increase phenytoin levels and toxicity during long-term use of both drugs. This raises the concern that white willow might have similar effects on phenytoin, though this has not been proven.

Nicotinamide appears to increase blood levels of carbamazepine and primidone, possibly requiring a reduction in drug dosage to prevent toxic effects. Early reports suggested the possibility that the supplement gamma-linolenic acid might worsen temporal lobe epilepsy. However, there has been no later confirmation of this.

EBSCO CAM Review Board

FURTHER READING

Akhondian, J., A. Parsa, and H. Rakhshande. "The Effect of *Nigella sativa* L. (Black Cumin Seed) on Intractable Pediatric Seizures." *Medical Science Monitor* 13 (2007): CR555-559.

Bromfield, E., et al. "A Randomized Trial of Polyunsaturated Fatty Acids for Refractory Epilepsy." *Epilepsy and Behavior* 12 (2008): 187-190.

Cheuk, D. K., and V. Wong. "Acupuncture for Epilepsy." *Cochrane Database of Systematic Reviews* (2008): CD005062. Available through *EBSCO DynaMed Systematic Literature Surveillance* at http://www.ebscohost.com/dynamed.

Gupta, M., et al. "Add-On Melatonin Improves Sleep Behavior in Children with Epilepsy." *Journal of Child Neurology* 20 (2005): 112-115.

Kajiyama, Y., et al. "Ginkgo Seed Poisoning." *Pediatrics* 109 (2002): 325-327.

Kupiec, T., and V. Raj. "Fatal Seizures Due to Potential Herb-Drug Interactions with *Ginkgo biloba*." *Journal of Analytical Toxicology* 29 (2006): 755-758.

Mikati, M. A., et al. "Two Randomized Vitamin D Trials in Ambulatory Patients on Anticonvulsants: Impact on Bone." *Neurology* 67 (2006): 2005-2014.

Theodore, W. H., et al. "Transcranial Magnetic Stimulation for the Treatment of Seizures." *Neurology* 59 (2002): 560-562.

Tyagi, A., and N. Delanty. "Herbal Remedies, Dietary Supplements, and Seizures." *Epilepsia* 44 (2003): 228-235.

Yuen, A. W., et al. "Omega-3 Fatty Acid Supplementation in Patients with Chronic Epilepsy." *Epilepsy and Behavior* 7 (2005): 253-258.

See also: Carbamazepine; Phenobarbital; Phenytoin; Primidone; Strokes; Valproic acid.

Epstein-Barr virus

CATEGORY: Issues and overviews
RELATED TERMS: Burkitt's lymphoma, chronic fatigue syndrome, infectious mononucleosis, nasopharyngeal carcinoma
DEFINITION: A disease-causing agent classified as a herpesvirus and associated with a variety of infectious illnesses.

ETIOLOGICAL AGENT OF DISEASE

Epstein-Barr virus (EBV) is the known etiological agent for several diseases, including infectious mononucleosis (IM); Burkitt's lymphoma (BL), a lymphoproliferative cancer of the lymphatic system in conjunction with the presence of malaria; and nasopharyngeal carcinoma (NPC), a cancer of the pharynx found primarily in persons of southern Chinese ancestry. The virus has been suggested as the etiological agent associated with chronic fatigue syndrome (CFS), a condition of extreme fatigue that is not relieved through sleep. As is the situation with all herpesviruses, infection by EBV establishes a lifelong carrier state of the virus.

TREATMENTS

Nutritional supplements. Infectious mononucleosis, also known as the kissing disease, is by far the most common result of infection by EBV. More serious EBV illnesses include BL and NPC, which, while life-threatening, are relatively rare and are generally associated only with certain ethnic populations. The cause of CFS is unclear, but increasingly the evidence points to the involvement of EBV.

Because EBV-related illnesses are viral infections, antibiotic treatment, which is effective against bacteria, is largely useless for other than addressing EBV illnesses with secondary bacterial infections. BL and NPC are cancers, and they are treated using the standard methods of chemotherapy utilized for many forms of the disease. Few standard treatments beyond those that are palliative have proven effective in treating either IM or CFS.

Alternative treatments for EBV disease are generally built upon the idea of improving the body's nutritional levels, with secondary improvement in the immune system. Vitamin supplements that include both vitamin C and vitamin K have been recommended, as has inclusion of minerals such as magnesium and potassium. Omega-3 oil supplements, such as those found in fish, or flaxseed oils also have been suggested as useful. Beyond the general health benefits provided by these nutritional supplements, there is minimal evidence to support their use in treatment of EBV-related illnesses.

Aromatherapy. Aromatherapy applies the volatile properties of purified plant oils for the treatment of illnesses. The oils can be delivered either as an aerosol (hence the term "aroma") or through direct application and absorption through skin. Proponents have argued that such therapy can be used to treat either bacterial or viral infections, including those caused by EBV, without the side effects associated with pharmaceuticals such as antibiotics. The oil is often delivered in the form of a spray but can be included with warm bath water. The theory for aromatherapy's efficacy as an antibacterial agent argues that the oil enters the microbe and prevents access to oxygen. As an antiviral agent, plant oils are believed to improve immune function, but to do so in an unknown manner. No controlled studies have demonstrated the effectiveness of aromatherapy in the treatment of EBV-related diseases.

Chelation therapy. Chelation therapy utilizes chelating agents such as ethylenediaminetetraacetic acid (EDTA), chemicals that bind and remove minerals that may be found in tissues or blood. The usefulness of chelation therapy dates to the 1940s, when it was found that EDTA is useful in treating lead and mercury poisoning. Intravenous use of EDTA or other chelators has been suggested for the treatment of certain cardiovascular diseases too, although there is little evidence of its effectiveness, and the treatment may even exacerbate problems.

Supplements. Certain nutritional supplements, such as vitamin C, garlic, zinc, and some amino acids, which have some chelation properties, have been tested for the treatment of chronic fatigue syndrome.

As is the case with other alternative treatments, any success has been reported anecdotally, and no controlled studies have shown their usefulness in treating EBV infections.

A variety of herbal supplements also have adherents in the treatment of EBV disease. Echinacea is allegedly an immune promoter and blood cleanser, the Chinese herb astragalus is claimed to relieve fatigue, and arsenicum is suggested for use by some holistic proponents. While available over the counter, these herbs have the potential for significant deleterious side effects and should be used only after consultation with a physician.

Usefulness of Alternative Treatments

For most persons, the use of treatments such as aromatherapy or nutritional supplements will have no undesirable side effects. If the person is nutritionally deficient, the addition of supplements may ameliorate the problem. Indeed, the mineral zinc has been shown in some studies to decrease recovery time from minor respiratory infections. Zinc also has been shown to improve immune function under some circumstances. While there is little evidence supporting its usefulness in treatment of EBV infections specifically, it is certainly possible that in boosting immune function in respiratory infections in general, this usefulness also may apply to those infections caused by EBV.

Aromatherapy and other forms of relaxation techniques may play a palliative role in decreasing stress. Chronic stress is known to produce a variety of deleterious effects, including those that affect immune function; stress hormones in particular may cause immune problems. Relaxation techniques, including those of aromatherapy, may not have a direct impact on immune function, but lowering stress levels may indirectly have a positive effect on the immune system.

Richard Adler, Ph.D.

Further Reading

Anderson, John, and Larry Trivieri, eds. *Alternative Medicine: The Definitive Guide.* 2d ed. New York: Celestial Arts/Random House, 2002.

Cohen, J. I. "Epstein-Barr Virus Infections, Including Infectious Mononucleosis." In *Harrison's Principles of Internal Medicine,* edited by Joan Butterton. 17th ed. New York: McGraw-Hill, 2008.

Freeman, Lyn. *Mosby's Complementary and Alternative Medicine: A Research-Based Approach.* 3d ed. St. Louis, Mo.: Mosby/Elsevier, 2009.

See also: Aromatherapy; Astragalus; Cancer treatment support; Chelation therapy; Chronic fatigue syndrome; Echinacea; Herbal medicine; Herpes.

Ernst, Edzard

CATEGORY: Biography
IDENTIFICATION: British medical doctor and the first professor of complementary medicine in the United Kingdom
BORN: January 30, 1948; Wiesbaden, West Germany (now in Germany)

OVERVIEW

Edzard Ernst, a German-born British medical doctor and researcher, became the first professor of complementary medicine in the United Kingdom. His work focuses on the safety and efficacy of complementary medicine. Ernst has suggested that only about five percent of techniques that fall under the umbrella of complementary and alternative medicine (CAM) are actually supported by scientific evidence, whereas the majority of CAM is either insufficiently understood or not supported by the existing evidence.

In 1993, Ernst resigned his position at the University of Vienna (in physical medicine and rehabilitation) to establish the Complementary Medicine Department at the University of Exeter in England. He is not a registered homeopath, but he has some training in homeopathy, herbalism, acupuncture, and other alternative approaches. He has been a member of the Medicines Commission of the British Medicines Control Agency, which is now part of the Medicines and Healthcare Products Regulatory Agency, a governmental agency that determines what materials may be marketed as medicinal treatments in the United Kingdom. Ernst is also a member of the Scientific Committee on Herbal Medicinal Products of the Irish Medicines Board. In addition, he was a founding member of the relatively new Institute for Science in Medicine and has been chief editor of medical journals, including *Alternative and Complementary Therapies* and *Perfusion.*

The books *Healing, Hype, or Harm? A Critical Analysis of Complementary or Alternative Medicine* (2008) and *Trick or Treatment: The Undeniable Facts About Alternative Medicine* (2008), edited and cowritten, respectively, by Ernst, present balanced views of CAM practices. The chapters in the two books are not arguments against the various approaches; they are proposals that CAM methods should be reviewed in the context of evidence supporting their worth and in the context of approved medical standards. In the preface to *Healing, Hype, or Harm?*, Ernst indicates that the purpose of the book is to critically examine "the various smoke screens" that are often used to prevent people from understanding the truth about certain medical philosophies and practices. In addition, he writes that the book's contributors come from very different backgrounds and hold quite different views, yet they are all well informed and attempt to examine the various methods associated with CAM from an objective standpoint. Finally, he indicates that the contributors had used the existing evidence to identify those particular practices whose validity should be questioned.

Brandy Weidow, M.S.

FURTHER READING

Ernst, Edzard, ed. *Healing, Hype, or Harm? A Critical Analysis of Complementary or Alternative Medicine.* Charlottesville, Va.: Imprint Academic, 2008.

Ernst, Edzard, Max H. Pittler, and Barbara Wider. *The Desktop Guide to Complementary and Alternative Medicine: An Evidence-Based Approach.* Maryland Heights, Mo.: Mosby/Elsevier, 2006.

Singh, Simon, and Edzard Ernst. *Trick or Treatment: The Undeniable Facts About Alternative Medicine.* New York: W. W. Norton, 2008.

See also: CAM on PubMed; Clinical trials; History of alternative medicine; History of complementary medicine; Integrative medicine; Pseudoscience; Regulation of CAM; Scientific method.

Essential oil monoterpenes

CATEGORY: Herbs and supplements
DEFINITION: Natural plant product used to treat specific health conditions.

PRINCIPAL PROPOSED USES: Acute bronchitis, chronic bronchitis, sinus infections

OTHER PROPOSED USES: Colds, influenza

OVERVIEW

Eucalyptus oil is a standard ingredient in cough drops and cough syrups, and an oil added to humidifiers. A standardized combination of eucalyptus oil and two other essential oils has been studied for effectiveness in a variety of respiratory conditions. This combination therapy contains cineole from eucalyptus, d-limonene from citrus fruit, and alpha-pinene from pine. Because these oils are all in a chemical family called monoterpenes, the treatment is called essential oil monoterpenes. Diindolylmethane (DIM) also has complex interactions with the hormone estrogen, which could lead to either positive or negative effects on cancer risk.

THERAPEUTIC DOSAGES

In studies, this essential oil combination was taken at a dose of 300 milligrams three to four times daily.

THERAPEUTIC USES

Most, though not all, studies indicate that oral use of essential oil monoterpenes can help acute bronchitis, chronic bronchitis, and sinus infections. For example, a double-blind, placebo-controlled trial of 676 people with acute bronchitis found that two weeks of treatment with essential oil monoterpenes was more effective than a placebo and just as effective as antibiotic treatment for reducing symptoms and aiding recovery. In addition, a three-month, double-blind, placebo-controlled trial of 246 people with chronic bronchitis found that regular use of essential oil monoterpenes helped prevent the typical worsening of chronic bronchitis that occurs during the winter. Additionally, in a double-blind, placebo-controlled study of about three hundred people, use of essential oil monoterpenes improved symptoms of acute sinusitis. One study weakly indicates that essential oil monoterpenes may be helpful for colds in children. Essential oil monoterpenes are thought to work by thinning mucus.

SAFETY ISSUES

Other than minor gastrointestinal complaints, no side effects have been reported with this essential oil combination. However, be advised that essential oils can be toxic if taken in excess. Maximum safe doses in young children, women who are pregnant or nursing, and individuals with severe liver or kidney disease have not been established.

EBSCO CAM Review Board

FURTHER READING

Behrbohm, H., O. Kaschke, and K. Sydow. "Effect of the Phytogenic Secretolytic Drug Gelomyrtol Forte on Mucociliary Clearance of the Maxillary Sinus." *Laryngorhinootologie* 74 (1995): 733-737.

Matthys, H., et al. "Efficacy and Tolerability of Myrtol Standardized in Acute Bronchitis: A Multi-Centre, Randomised, Double-Blind, Placebo-Controlled Parallel Group Clinical Trial vs. Cefuroxime and Ambroxol." *Arzneimittel-Forschung* 50 (2000): 700-711.

Meister, R., et al. "Efficacy and Tolerability of Myrtol Standardized in Long-Term Treatment of Chronic Bronchitis." *Arzneimittel-Forschung* 49 (1999): 351-358.

See also: Bronchitis; Colds and flu; Common cold: Homeopathic remedies; Herbal medicine; Sinusitis.

Estriol

CATEGORY: Herbs and supplements

RELATED TERMS: Oestriol, tri-estrogen

DEFINITION: Natural substance of the human body used as a supplement to treat specific health conditions.

PRINCIPAL PROPOSED USES: Menopausal symptoms, osteoporosis

OVERVIEW

Several forms of estrogen occur naturally in a woman's body. The ovary produces a form named estradiol, which is converted into another important estrogen called estrone. Estriol is yet another form of estrogen metabolized from estradiol, weaker than the other two but still active.

The estrogen tablets prescribed for menopausal symptoms usually contain estradiol, estrone, or a combination of the two. Some alternative medicine physicians have popularized the use of estriol as an alternative, and there is no doubt that estriol also is effective for symptoms of menopause. However, despite claims that it is safer than other forms of estrogen, the balance of evidence suggests that, in fact, estriol presents precisely the same risks.

REQUIREMENTS AND SOURCES

Estriol is manufactured in the body from estrone, estradiol, and androstenedione. When taken as a drug, it is manufactured synthetically or extracted from animal products.

THERAPEUTIC DOSAGES

The usual dose of estriol is 2 to 8 milligrams (mg) taken once daily. Estriol is also commonly sold in combination with other forms of estrogen.

THERAPEUTIC USES

Like more common forms of estrogen, estriol is used for the treatment of menopausal symptoms. Double-blind, placebo-controlled studies and other controlled trials have found oral or vaginal estriol effective for symptoms of menopause, including hot flashes, night sweats, insomnia, vaginal dryness, and

---

Estriol and Hormone Replacement Therapy

Bio-identical hormones, the components of bio-identical hormone replacement therapy (BHRT), are not recognized by the U.S. Food and Drug Administration (FDA). Sellers of compounded bio-identical hormones, including estriol, often claim that their products are identical to hormones made by the body and that these "all-natural" pills, creams, lotions, and gels are without the risks of drugs approved by the FDA for menopausal hormone therapy (MHT). FDA-approved MHT drugs provide effective relief of the symptoms of menopause such as hot flashes and vaginal dryness, and can also prevent thinning of bones. The FDA has not yet approved compounded BHRT drugs and cannot assure their safety or effectiveness.

Many marketers and consumers believe that bio-identical hormone products that contain estriol, a weak form of estrogen, are safer than FDA-approved estrogen products. However, the FDA has not approved any drug containing estriol, stating that there are no credible scientific studies that support the claims regarding its safety and effectiveness.

---

recurrent urinary tract infections. Estriol may also help prevent osteoporosis. Estriol might cause less vaginal bleeding as a side effect than other forms of estrogen, although this has not been definitively established.

Some alternative practitioners claim that estriol fights cancer, in contrast to estrogen, which increases the risk of some cancers. However, this claim is based on exaggerated interpretations of weak studies. It is more likely that estriol increases cancer risk in much the same way as other forms of estrogen.

SAFETY ISSUES

Like other forms of estrogen, oral estriol stimulates the growth of uterine tissue. This leads to the risk of uterine cancer. In a placebo-controlled study of 1,110 women, uterine tissue stimulation was seen among women given estriol orally (1 to 2 mg daily), compared with those given a placebo. Another large study found that oral estriol increased the risk of uterine cancer. In a third study of forty-eight women, estriol (1 mg twice daily) caused uterine tissue stimulation. In contrast, a twelve-month double-blind trial of oral estriol (2 mg daily) in sixty-eight Japanese women found no effect on the uterus. It may be that the high levels of soy in the Japanese diet altered the results.

To protect the uterus, estriol, like other forms of estrogen, needs to be balanced with progesterone. Additionally, one study suggests that estriol is less likely to affect the uterus when taken in a once-daily dose rather than in multiple daily doses.

However, the uterus is not the only organ at risk of cancer. Test-tube studies suggest that estriol is just as likely to cause breast cancer as any form of estrogen. While this preliminary evidence does not constitute proof, it does raise alarm bells. Until proven otherwise, estriol must be regarded as increasing breast cancer risk. As with other forms of estrogen, vaginal estriol preparations are safer than oral preparations.

EBSCO CAM Review Board

FURTHER READING

Dugal, R., et al. "Comparison of Usefulness of Estradiol Vaginal Tablets and Estriol Vagitories for Treatment of Vaginal Atrophy." *Acta Obstetricia et Gynecologica Scandinavica* 79 (2000): 293-297.

Hayashi, T., et al. "Estriol (E3) Replacement Improves Endothelial Function and Bone Mineral Density in Very Elderly Women." *Journals of Gerontology: Series*

A, Biological Sciences and Medical Sciences 55 (2000): B183-B190.

Takahashi, K., et al. "Efficacy and Safety of Oral Estriol for Managing Postmenopausal Symptoms." *Maturitas* 34 (2000): 169-177.

Vooijs, G. P., and T. B. Geurts. "Review of the Endometrial Safety During Intravaginal Treatment with Estriol." *European Journal of Obstetrics, Gynecology, and Reproductive Biology* 62 (1995): 101-106.

Weiderpass, E., et al. "Low-Potency Oestrogen and Risk of Endometrial Cancer." *The Lancet* 353 (1999): 1824-1828.

See also: Estrogen; Menopause; Osteoporosis; Women's health.

Estrogen

CATEGORY: Drug interactions

DEFINITION: Used as a component of birth control pills and for preventing osteoporosis and heart disease in menopausal women.

INTERACTIONS: Boron, chasteberry, dong quai, folate, indole-3-carbinol, ipriflavone, resveratrol, rosemary

TRADE NAMES: Medications containing a form of estrogen called estradiol include Alora, Climara, Combipatch, Delestrogen (injectable), DepGynogen (injectable), Depo-Estradiol Cypionate (injectable), Depogen (injectable), Esclim, Estrace, Estraderm, Estra-L (injectable), Estring, Fempatch, Gynogen L.A. (injectable), Vagifem, Valergen (injectable), and Vivelle

RELATED DRUGS: Premarin, Cenestin, Prempro, and Premphase contain another form of estrogen called conjugated estrogens. Other forms of estrogen and some of their brand names include diethylstilbestrol diphosphate (Stilphostrol), estrone (Kestrone-5), esterified estrogens (Estratab, Menest), estropipate (Ogen, Ortho-Est), and ethinyl estradiol (Estinyl)

FOLATE

Effect: Supplementation Possibly Helpful

Some evidence suggests that estrogen may interfere with the absorption of folate. Since folate deficiency is fairly common even among those not taking estrogen, taking a folate supplement on general principle is probably a good idea.

IPRIFLAVONE

Effect: Potential Benefits and Risks

When the two are taken together, ipriflavone may increase estrogen's ability to protect bone. This may allow one to use a lower dose of estrogen and still receive its beneficial effects. However, there may be risks involved. Although ipriflavone itself probably does not affect tissues other than bone, some evidence suggests that when it is combined with estrogen, estrogen's effects on the uterus are increased. This might mean that risk of uterine cancer would be elevated by the combination.

It should be possible to overcome this risk by taking progesterone along with estrogen, which is standard medical practice. However, this finding does make one wonder whether ipriflavone-estrogen combinations raise the risk of breast cancer as well, an estrogen side effect that has no easy solution. At present, there is no available information on this important subject.

OTHER NUTRIENTS

Effect: Supplementation Possibly Helpful

Estrogen use may decrease blood levels of magnesium, vitamin C, and zinc. This may mean that supplementation is advisable.

BORON

Effect: Theoretical Harmful Interaction

In some studies, boron has been found to elevate levels of the body's own estrogen. This might lead to an increased risk of estrogen side effects if boron is combined with estrogen therapy.

RESVERATROL

Effect: Possible Harmful Interaction

The supplement resveratrol has a chemical structure similar to that of the synthetic estrogen diethylstilbestrol and produces estrogenic-like effects. For this reason, it should not be combined with prescription estrogen products.

ROSEMARY

Effect: Possible Harmful Interaction

Weak evidence hints that the herb rosemary may enhance the liver's rate of deactivating estrogen in the body. This could potentially interfere with the activity of medications that contain estrogen.

INDOLE-3-CARBINOL

Effect: Theoretical Harmful Interaction

Indole-3-carbinol (I3C) is a substance found in broccoli that is thought to have cancer-preventive effects. One of its mechanisms of action is thought to involve facilitating the inactivation of estrogen, as well as blocking its effects on cells. The net result could be decreased effectiveness of medications containing estrogen.

CHASTEBERRY

Effect: Theoretical Harmful Interaction

Because of its effects on the pituitary gland, chasteberry might unpredictably alter the effects of estrogen-replacement therapy.

DONG QUAI

Effect: Interaction Unlikely or Probably Insignificant

The herb dong quai (*Angelica sinensis*) is used for menstrual disorders.

Because dong quai contains beta-sitosterol, a phytoestrogen, there have been concerns that taking the herb with estrogen might add to estrogen-related side effects. However, a twenty-four-week, placebo-controlled study of seventy-four postmenopausal women found no estrogen-like effects or reduction of menopausal symptoms associated with taking dong quai. Therefore, dong quai seems unlikely to increase estrogen-related side effects.

EBSCO CAM Review Board

FURTHER READING

Bradlow, H. L., et al. "Multifunctional Aspects of the Action of Indole-3-Carbinol as an Antitumor Agent." *Annals of the New York Academy of Sciences* 889 (1999): 204-213.

Meng, Q., et al. "Indole-3-Carbinol Is a Negative Regulator of Estrogen Receptor-Alpha Signaling in Human Tumor Cells." *Journal of Nutrition* 130 (2000): 2927-2931.

Pronsky, Z. M., and J. P. Crowe. *Food Medication Interactions*. 16th ed. Birchrunville, Pa.: Food-Medication Interactions, 2010.

Yuan, F., et al. "Anti-estrogenic Activities of Indole-3-Carbinol in Cervical Cells: Implication for Prevention of Cervical Cancer." *Anticancer Research* 19 (1999): 1673-1680.

See also: Boron; Chasteberry; Dong quai; Folate; Food and Drug Administration; Indole-3-carbinol; Ipriflavone; Resveratrol; Rosemary; Supplements: Introduction.

Ethambutol

CATEGORY: Drug interactions
DEFINITION: A drug used with isoniazid in the treatment of tuberculosis.
INTERACTIONS: Copper, zinc
TRADE NAME: Myambutol

COPPER AND ZINC

Effect: Take at a Different Time of Day

Ethambutol may interfere with the absorption of copper and zinc by binding to them. To avoid deficiency, one should take supplements of these essential minerals. The doses of ethambutol and the mineral supplements should be separated by a minimum of two hours.

EBSCO CAM Review Board

FURTHER READING

Mandell, G. L., and W. A. Petri. "Antimicrobial Agents: Drugs Used in the Chemotherapy of Tuberculosis, *Mycobacterium avium* Complex Disease, and Leprosy." In *Goodman and Gilman's The Pharmacological Basis of Therapeutics*, edited by Laurence L. Brunton et al. 11th ed. New York: McGraw-Hill Medical, 2011.

Solecki, T. J., et al. "Effect of a Chelating Drug on Balance and Tissue Distribution of Four Essential Metals." *Toxicology* 31, nos. 3/4 (1984): 207-216.

See also: Copper; Food and Drug Administration; Isoniazid; Zinc.

Eucalyptus

CATEGORY: Herbs and supplements
RELATED TERM: *Eucalyptus globulus*

DEFINITION: Natural plant product used to treat specific health conditions.

PRINCIPAL PROPOSED USE: Common cold

OTHER PROPOSED USES: Asthma, cough, insect repellant, periodontal disease (gingivitis), sinusitis, sore throat

OVERVIEW

The eucalyptus tree originated in Australia and Tasmania, but it has spread to all other inhabited continents. There are many different varieties of eucalyptus, with somewhat differing constituents. The most common type used medicinally is eucalyptus globules. Its essential oil contains eucalyptol (cineol or cineole).

Eucalyptus oil has a long history of use as a topical antiseptic. It also has been used as a lozenge or inhalation therapy for asthma, cough, sore throat, and other respiratory conditions.

THERAPEUTIC DOSAGES

The studied dosage of cineole is 200 mg three times daily for adults. Internal use of cineole or eucalyptus oil should be avoided in children. In the gingivitis study, chewing gum containing 0.4 and 0.6 percent eucalyptus extracts were used. For use as an insect repellent, 25 to 50 milliliters (ml) of the oil is added to 500 ml of water. One should not use in children age twelve years or younger. As an inhalant, a few drops of eucalyptus oil are added to a vaporizer.

THERAPEUTIC USES

A standardized combination of cineol from eucalyptus, d-limonene from citrus fruit, and alpha-pinene from pine has been studied for effectiveness in a variety of respiratory conditions. These oils are all in a chemical family called monoterpenes, and for this reason the combined treatment is called essential oil monoterpenes. This combination is discussed in a separate article of that name.

Eucalyptus oil or its constituents taken alone have undergone only limited study. It appears to be most promising as a treatment for the common cold. However, concerns about safety have limited its use.

In a double-blind, placebo-controlled study of 152 people, use of cineol at a dose of 200 milligrams (mg) three times daily markedly improved symptoms of the common cold. Benefits were seen in such symptoms as nasal congestion, headache, and overall malaise.

Because the participants in this study suffered, in particular, from sinus symptoms, this study has been used to indicate that cineol may be helpful for viral sinusitis. Few significant side effects were seen in this study, but the product used was of pharmaceutical grade, and not all dietary supplements of eucalyptus oil may be equally safe. A second placebo-controlled study involving 150 subjects also demonstrated favorable results for cineol, compared with a combination of five other herbal products.

In another study, thirty-two people on steroids to control severe asthma (steroid-dependent asthma) were given either placebo or cineole (200 mg three times daily) for twelve weeks. The results showed that people using cineole were able to gradually reduce their steroid dosage to a greater extent than those taking placebo. Reduction of steroid dosage should be done only under the supervision of a physician.

Cineole or eucalyptus oil applied topically also has shown some potential value for repelling mosquitoes. In one double-blind study, chewing gum containing eucalyptus extract was more beneficial for moderate gingivitis than a placebo gum.

SAFETY ISSUES

Internal use of eucalyptus oil at appropriate doses by healthy people can cause nausea, heartburn, vomiting, diarrhea, and skin rash. Excessive dosages can be fatal, especially to children. Inhalation of the oil

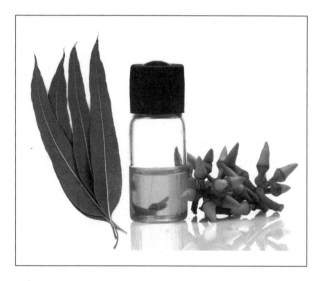

Fragrant eucalyptus leaves, oil, and flowers. (©Picstudio/ Dreamstime.com.)

can exacerbate asthma in some people. Application of cineole to the entire body resulted in severe nervous system poisoning in a six-year-old child. In general, eucalyptus oil should not be used by young children, pregnant or nursing women, or people with severe liver or kidney disease.

Although no drug interactions of eucalyptus are firmly documented, there are theoretical reasons to believe it could interact with a number of medications, either raising or lowering their levels. Therefore, people taking any oral or injected medication that is critical to their health or well-being should avoid internal use of eucalyptus until more is known.

EBSCO CAM Review Board

FURTHER READING

Juergens, U. R., et al. "Anti-Inflammatory Activity of a 1.8-Cineol (Eucalyptol) in Bronchial Asthma." *Respiratory Medicine* 97 (2003): 250-256.

Kehrl, W., U. Sonnemann, and U. Dethlefsen. "Therapy for Acute Nonpurulent Rhinosinusitis with Cineole." *Laryngoscope* 114 (2004): 738-742.

Kim, N. H., et al. "Pretreatment with 1.8-Cineole Potentiates Thioacetamide-Induced Hepatotoxicity and Immunosuppression." *Archives of Pharmacal Research* 27 (2004): 781-789.

Nagata, H., et al. "Effect of Eucalyptus Extract Chewing Gum on Periodontal Health." *Journal of Periodontology* 79 (2008): 1378-1385.

Tesche, S., et al. "The Value of Herbal Medicines in the Treatment of Acute Non-purulent Rhinosinusitis." *European Archives of Oto-Rhino-Laryngology* 265, no. 11 (2008): 1355-1359.

Traboulsi, A. F., et al. "Repellency and Toxicity of Aromatic Plant Extracts Against the Mosquito *Culex pipiens molestus*." *Pest Management Science* 61 (2005): 597-604.

See also: Asthma; Common cold: Homeopathic remedies; Cough; Herbal medicine; Insect bites and stings; Periodontal disease; Sinusitis.

Exercise

CATEGORY: Therapies and techniques
RELATED TERMS: Aerobic exercise, resistance exercise, weight training

DEFINITION: Therapeutic method involving extensive and often strenuous movement of the body for health and well-being.

PRINCIPAL PROPOSED USES: Enhancing survival in people with severe heart disease, high cholesterol and high triglycerides, hypertension, reducing falls in the elderly

OTHER PROPOSED USES: Asthma, back pain, cancer prevention, chronic fatigue syndrome, dementia, depression, diabetes (type 2), fibromyalgia, insomnia in the elderly, menopausal syndrome, osteoarthritis, osteoporosis, stroke prevention, weight loss

OVERVIEW

One of the most obvious differences between modern life and life in the past for humans can be found in the level of physical exercise. For the majority of people living in developed countries today, heavy physical exercise does not occur as a part of ordinary daily life but must be deliberately sought out. Compare this to most of human history, in which heavy daily exercise was a requirement for survival. Even among the upper classes in nineteenth-century Europe, going for a ten- to twenty-mile walk by way of recreation was not unusual.

The human body was designed to use its physical capacities. However, modern life has become a sedentary affair, in which "exercise" involves moving from couch to car to office cubicle. While decreasing strenuous exercise does have some benefits, such as reducing injuries, it also presents major drawbacks. Inadequate exercise is a major contributor to the current epidemic of obesity, which in turn leads to diabetes, heart disease, and osteoarthritis.

Conversely, increasing one's level of exercise provides a wide variety of benefits. Besides enhancing strength and endurance and improving physical attractiveness, exercise is thought to enhance overall health and to reduce symptoms in a number of specific ailments. However, while the many benefits of exercise appear self-evident, they can be quite difficult to prove in a scientific sense. The primary problem is that it is difficult, if not impossible, to design a double-blind study of exercise.

In a double-blind, placebo-controlled study, neither participants nor researchers know who is receiving a real treatment and who is receiving a placebo. Consider the following scenario: A study (technically, an observational or epidemiological study) may note that people in a given population who exercise more develop heart disease at a lower rate than those who exercise less. From this, it is tempting to conclude causality: that exercise reduces heart disease risk. However, such a conclusion might not be correct.

Observational studies show only association, not cause and effect. Studies of this type had long shown that women who used hormone replacement therapy (HRT) were less likely to develop heart disease. Furthermore, the use of HRT was known to improve one's cholesterol profile. It seemed like an obvious case. However, to researchers' surprise, when a giant double-blind study compared hormone replacement therapy with placebo, the results showed that the use of HRT actually increased heart disease risk.

It is now hypothesized that this apparent contradiction may be due to the fact that women who use HRT are generally of higher socioeconomic status than women who do not use HRT, and that it is this socioeconomic status, and not the HRT, that was responsible for the apparent benefits seen. Whatever the reason, it is now clear that HRT does not prevent heart disease, and that the conclusions drawn from observational studies were exactly backwards. Based on this, one must at least consider the possibility that people who engage in more exercise have other qualities that protect them from heart disease, and that it is these qualities, and not the exercise, that protects them. The problem here is that while it is possible to give a placebo that convincingly resembles HRT, it is difficult to conceive of a placebo form of exercise that participants and researchers would not immediately identify as different from real exercise.

Besides observational studies, other forms of scientific research involving exercise remain similarly inadequate. For example, numerous studies have attempted to prove that exercise is helpful for depression. In these studies, people who are made to exercise improve to a greater extent than those who are not interfered with. However, this finding does not prove that exercise per se aids depression. It might be, for example, that simply being enrolled in a study, and being motivated to do anything at all, might aid depression. (This suspicion is given further weight by findings that improvement in depression is not related to the intensity of the exercise done; if it were

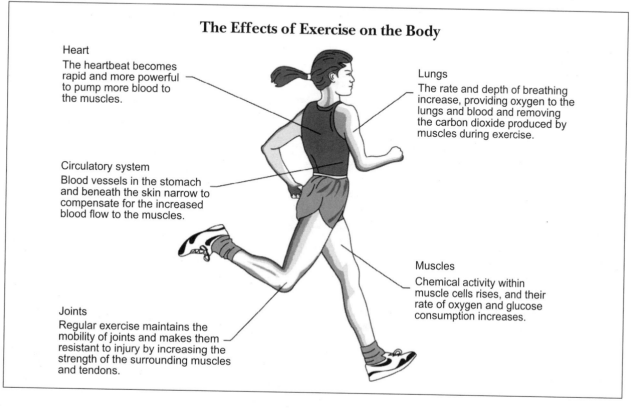

The Effects of Exercise on the Body

Heart
The heartbeat becomes rapid and more powerful to pump more blood to the muscles.

Lungs
The rate and depth of breathing increase, providing oxygen to the lungs and blood and removing the carbon dioxide produced by muscles during exercise.

Circulatory system
Blood vessels in the stomach and beneath the skin narrow to compensate for the increased blood flow to the muscles.

Muscles
Chemical activity within muscle cells rises, and their rate of oxygen and glucose consumption increases.

Joints
Regular exercise maintains the mobility of joints and makes them resistant to injury by increasing the strength of the surrounding muscles and tendons.

the exercise itself, one would think that more intense exercise would provide greater benefits.)

Double-blind, placebo-controlled studies eliminate all of these potential confounding factors and many others. However, it is not feasible to design a double-blind study in which people are unaware ("blind" to the fact) that they are exercising. Therefore, all results regarding the potential benefits of exercise must be taken with caution.

SCIENTIFIC EVIDENCE

The benefits of exercise with the most solid scientific foundation include the following: preventing falls in the elderly, slightly reducing blood pressure, mildly improving cholesterol profile, enhancing survival in people with heart disease, and improving metabolic syndrome. Regarding blood pressure, aerobic exercise has the best supporting evidence, but resistance exercise (weight training) has also shown promise. One study found that four ten-minute "snacks" of aerobic exercise per day were as effective at lowering blood pressure as forty minutes of continuous exercise. Aerobic exercise can also raise levels of HDL (good) cholesterol and reduce levels of triglycerides.

Other conditions for which exercise has some meaningful supporting evidence of benefit include asthma, depression, type 2 diabetes (improving blood sugar control, even in the absence of weight loss), fibromyalgia, and, osteoarthritis. Regarding osteoporosis, the general scientific consensus is that exercise does help, but the supporting evidence is surprisingly weak.

Inconsistent or otherwise weak evidence suggests potential benefit for back pain, chronic fatigue syndrome, cognitive impairment (mild dementia), colon cancer prevention, insomnia in the elderly, stroke prevention, and weight loss. It is widely believed that exercise improves immune function, but there is no meaningful supporting evidence for this belief. High-intensity exercise (such as marathon running) is known to temporarily weaken the immune system, increasing the likelihood of respiratory infection.

Evidence conflicts on whether exercise is helpful for reducing menopausal symptoms. However, it is known that heavy exercise causes increased calcium loss through sweat, and the body does not compensate for this by reducing calcium loss in the urine. The result can be a net calcium loss great enough to present health concerns for menopausal women. One study found that the use of an inexpensive calcium supplement (calcium carbonate), taken at a dose of 400 milligrams twice daily, is sufficient to offset this loss.

EBSCO CAM Review Board

FURTHER READING

Busch, A. J., et al. "Exercise for Fibromyalgia." *Journal of Rheumatology* 35 (2008): 1130-1144.

Elavsky, S., and E. McAuley. "Physical Activity and Mental Health Outcomes During Menopause." *Annals of Behavioral Medicine* 33 (2007): 132-142.

Elley, R., et al. "Do Snacks of Exercise Lower Blood Pressure?" *New Zealand Medical Journal* 119 (2006): U1996.

Fagard, R. H. "Exercise Is Good for Your Blood Pressure: Effects of Endurance Training and Resistance Training." *Clinical and Experimental Pharmacology and Physiology* 33 (2006): 853-856.

Hauer, K., et al. "Effectiveness of Physical Training on Motor Performance and Fall Prevention in Cognitively Impaired Older Persons." *American Journal of Physical Medicine and Rehabilitation* 85 (2006): 847-857.

Larun, L., et al. "Exercise in Prevention and Treatment of Anxiety and Depression Among Children and Young People." *Cochrane Database of Systematic Reviews* (2006): CD004691. Available through *EBSCO DynaMed Systematic Literature Surveillance* at http://www.ebscohost.com/dynamed.

Martin, B. R., et al. "Exercise and Calcium Supplementation: Effects on Calcium Homeostasis in Sportswomen." *Medicine and Science in Sports and Exercise* 39 (2007): 1481-1486.

Thomas, D. E., E. J. Elliott, and G. A. Naughton. "Exercise for Type 2 Diabetes Mellitus." *Cochrane Database of Systematic Reviews* (2006): CD002968. Available through *EBSCO DynaMed Systematic Literature Surveillance* at http://www.ebscohost.com/dynamed.

Van Uffelen, J. G., et al. "The Effect of Walking and Vitamin B Supplementation on Quality of Life in Community-Dwelling Adults with Mild Cognitive Impairment." *Quality of Life Research* 16 (2007): 1137-1146.

See also: Exercise-based therapies; Manipulative and body-based therapies; Sports and fitness support: Enhancing performance; Sports and fitness support: Enhancing recovery; Tai Chi; Yoga.

Exercise-based therapies

CATEGORY: Therapies and techniques

RELATED TERMS: Alexander technique, Feldenkrais method, Pilates, qigong, Tai Chi, Trager approach, yoga

DEFINITION: Physical activities to enhance overall health and wellness and to treat specific medical disorders.

PRINCIPAL PROPOSED USES: Anxiety, attention deficit disorder, back pain, cardiovascular fitness, depression, fatigue, flexibility, neck pain, physical conditioning, strength training

OTHER PROPOSED USES: Arthritis, asthma, osteoporosis, cancer, diabetes, fibromyalgia, gastrointestinal disorders, heart disease, high blood pressure, infertility, insomnia, menstrual pain, neuromuscular disorders, osteoporosis, sinusitis, heart disease

OVERVIEW

According to a 2008 Centers for Disease Control and Prevention (CDC) health study, 7 percent of those surveyed engaged in what is considered exercise-based complementary and alternative medicine (CAM) activities. These activities are considered outside the scope of conventional exercise practices. Although pain relief was the most common reason for its use, exercise-based CAM is used throughout the spectrum of medical conditions. A survey of the medical literature revealed seven exercise-based CAM activities, namely yoga, Tai Chi, qigong, Pilates, the Alexander technique, the Feldenkrais method, and the Trager approach.

With an estimated sixteen million participants in the United States, yoga is the most popular exercise-based CAM activity. A five-thousand-year-old practice that originated in India, yoga seeks to integrate the mind, body, and spirit through physical poses, breathing exercises, meditation, and spiritual philosophy. Pilates is another popular exercise system in the West. This one-hundred-year-old form of exercise is designed to strengthen core muscles while focusing on posture and proper breathing. Often, props and apparatus are used.

Tai Chi, originally conceived as a martial art in China five hundred years ago, is now practiced primarily for general physical fitness. Although many forms exist, in the West, Tai Chi uses a series of slow, graceful movements to enhance strength, stamina, and balance. Tai Chi is part of a larger, five-thousand-year-old system of traditional Chinese mental, spiritual, and physical training called qigong. Other components of qigong include physical poses, meditation, and breathing exercises.

The Feldenkrais method, the Alexander technique, and the Trager approach are lesser known exercise-based CAM activities. These are movement therapies in which practitioners are guided in their posture and physical actions to improve balance, reduce pain, and increase emotional well-being.

MECHANISMS OF ACTION

Four of the seven forms of exercise-based CAM can be considered forms of general physical exercise. Yoga, Pilates, Tai Chi, and qigong involve various degrees of cardiovascular, strength, and flexibility training. Thus they promote stamina, bone health, healthy weight, muscle tone, balance, and strength. Yoga, Tai Chi, and qigong also involve meditation. Although scientific research is ongoing, it appears that meditation decreases heart rate, increases blood flow to the organs, and improves mood regulation because of changes in the nervous system. No clinical data are available to determine the exact mechanism of action of the Alexander technique, the Feldenkrais method, or the Trager approach.

USES AND APPLICATIONS

Exercise-based CAM is most commonly used to improve and maintain overall fitness. Other common therapeutic uses are to reduce stress, relieve pain, and improve flexibility. Exercise-based CAM experts claim, however, that these exercise systems are helpful in treating a variety of conditions, such as asthma, osteoporosis, menstrual pain, depression, cancer, high blood pressure, diabetes, arthritis, insomnia, neuromuscular disorders, fatigue, attention deficit disorder, gastrointestinal disorders, infertility, sinusitis, and heart disease.

SCIENTIFIC EVIDENCE

Determining whether exercise-based CAM is effective in the management and prevention of illness is challenging. A limited number of well-designed clinical trials are available. The wide variety of practices within these different styles makes obtaining a consensus difficult.

In 2010, several large, well-designed studies showed that Tai Chi and qigong were beneficial in preventing

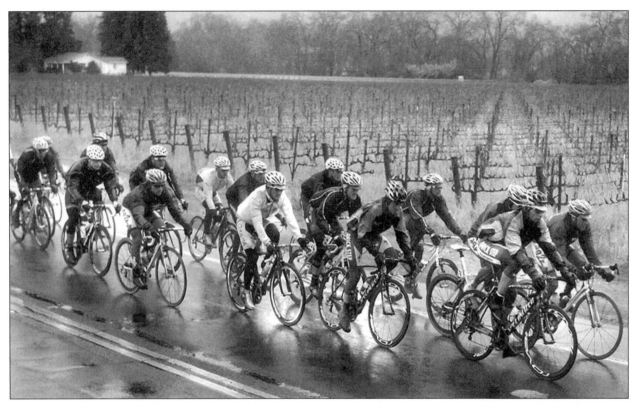

Bicycling, whether at the casual or the professional level, can significantly improve mood, alertness, and feelings of well-being, while decreasing fatigue, tension, stress, and depressed mood. (AP Photo)

osteoporosis in postmenopausal women and in treating hypertension and heart disease. Additionally, these studies suggest that Tai Chi may be effective in enhancing the immune system of the elderly.

A review of the medical literature reveals promising evidence that yoga may help treat a variety of medical conditions, including mood disorders, hypertension, insomnia, back pain, and osteoporosis, and may improve overall physical conditioning. In a 2008 randomized clinical trial in the journal *Menopause*, yoga reduced hot flashes in women by 30 percent. Furthermore, numerous studies have demonstrated that yoga diminishes sex performance anxiety and enhances female sexual desire. Many health practitioners use yoga in conjunction with conventional medicine in the treatment of cancer to reduce anxiety, pain, and insomnia, although scientists continue to debate the exact mechanisms of action involved.

A gap in the literature exists regarding the use of Pilates in treating medical conditions. Experts do agree that Pilates is effective in improving strength,

flexibility, and balance. Although experts in the Feldenkrais method, the Alexander technique, and the Trager approach claim that their movement exercises reduce pain, prevent injury, and improve balance, no well-designed clinical trials have been conducted to determine their efficacy.

With regard to other medical claims about exercise-based CAM, no well-designed randomized controlled trials are available; a review of the medical literature did not support the claims.

CHOOSING A PRACTITIONER

Hundreds of exercise-based CAM instructor-training programs have been established in the United States. None, however, include provider licensing requirements. Standards of certification for yoga instruction are largely based on the style of yoga studied and practiced. One program, the Yoga Alliance, is a nonprofit organization in the United States that maintains standards for yoga teacher-training programs. Teacher certification with this program requires a minimum of two hundred hours of training.

Several Tai Chi and qigong organizations provide teacher certification in the United States. Various levels of certification are offered based on hours of training and desired goals. Hundreds of Pilates training programs have been established in the United States too. Although licensing is not required, the Pilates Method Alliance offers a national teacher's certification program through written examination. Instructors of the Feldenkrais method, the Alexander technique, and the Trager approach are required to complete two-to-four-year training programs that encompass four hundred to sixteen hundred hours of class and fieldwork for certification.

SAFETY ISSUES

Exercise-based CAM is generally considered safe for those without serious health conditions or injuries. Persons with spine or joint disease, uncontrolled blood pressure, or severe balance abnormalities should avoid some exercise-based CAM activities. Although uncommon, spine and joint injuries have occurred during CAM exercise activities. To avoid such injuries, participants should adhere to the directions of a certified instructor. Pregnant women, who should exercise caution when considering CAM, typically require modification of certain practices. All potential participants, especially if pregnant, looking into exercised-based CAM as a form of therapy should consult with their health care providers before joining any exercise-based program. It is advisable to choose a certified provider. Typically, a national association that confers the certification will have a list of qualified providers.

Marie President, M.D.

FURTHER READING

Barnes, P. M., B. Bloom, and R. L. Nahin. "Complementary and Alternative Medicine Use Among Adults and Children: 2007 United States." *National Health Statistics Reports* 12 (December 10, 2008): 1-23.

Jahnke, R., et al. "A Comprehensive Review of Health Benefits of Qigong and Tai Chi." *American Journal of Health Promotion* 24, no. 6 (2010): 1-25.

National Center for Complementary and Alternative Medicine. http://www.nccam.nih.gov.

Yang, K. "A Review of Yoga Programs for Four Leading Risk Factors of Chronic Diseases." *Evidence-Based Complementary and Alternative Medicine* 4, no. 4 (2007): 487-491.

See also: Alexander technique; Applied kinesiology; Aston-Patterning; Dance movement therapy; Exercise; Feldenkrais method; Fibromyalgia: Homeopathic remedies; Manipulative and body-based practices; Massage therapy; Pain management; Progressive muscle relaxation; Reflexology; Rolfing; Soft tissue pain.

Eyebright

CATEGORY: Herbs and supplements
RELATED TERM: *Euphrasia officinale* L.
DEFINITION: Natural plant product used to treat specific health conditions.
PRINCIPAL PROPOSED USES: None
OTHER PROPOSED USES: Conjunctivitis, other diseases of the eye

OVERVIEW

The herb eyebright has been used since the Middle Ages as an eyewash for infection or inflammation of the eye. However, as much as one would like to believe that all traditions are wise, eyebright appears to have been selected for treating eye diseases not because it works particularly well but because its petals look bloodshot. This follows from the classic medieval philosophic view known as the Doctrine of Signatures,

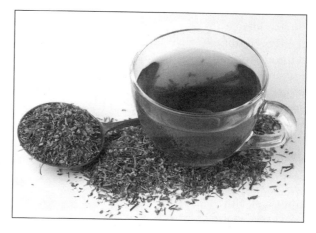

Dried herb of the eyebright plant and tea made from the herb. (TH Foto-Werbung / Photo Researchers, Inc.)

which states that herbs show their proper use by their appearance.

THERAPEUTIC DOSAGES

Traditionally, eyebright tea is made by boiling 1 tablespoon of the herb in a cup of water. This is then used as an eyewash or taken internally up to three times daily.

THERAPEUTIC USES

Like many herbs, eyebright contains astringent substances and volatile oils that are probably at least slightly antibacterial. However, there is no evidence that eyebright is particularly effective for treating conjunctivitis (pink eye) or any other eye disease; Germany's Commission E, which has evaluated the usefulness of three hundred herbs, recommends against its use. Warm compresses consisting of nothing but water (or ordinary black tea) are probably equally effective under the same conditions.

Eyebright tea is also sometimes taken internally to treat jaundice, respiratory infections, and memory loss. However, there is no evidence that it is effective for any of these conditions.

SAFETY ISSUES

Eyebright can cause tearing of the eyes, itching, redness, and many other symptoms, probably because of direct irritation. It appears to be safe when taken internally, but not many studies have been performed. Safety in young children, pregnant or nursing women, and those with severe liver or kidney disease has not been established.

EBSCO CAM Review Board

FURTHER READING

Duke, J A. *CRC Handbook of Medicinal Herbs.* Boca Raton, Fla.: CRC Press, 1985.

See also: Conjunctivitis; Herbal medicine.

F

Faith healing

CATEGORY: Issues and overviews
RELATED TERMS: Distance intercessory prayer, personal intercessory prayer, psychic healing
DEFINITION: Physical and psychic healing that occurs as a result of personal faith, assisted through a practitioner with the charismatic gift or gifts of healing.

OVERVIEW

The practice of faith healing is common to most if not all religions. Examples of faith healing include the Buddhist focus on healthy karma created by mind/body balance, the practice of Ruqya in Islam, the Zohar of Jewish mysticism, and the Christian belief that adherents may claim physical health as a benefit of salvation.

While occurring throughout history and in all societies, faith healing in Western culture may be more expressive of the individualistic nature of postmodern society. Religious meaning is increasingly found within the context of personal faith and encounter as opposed to the inclusive experience offered by institutions. Practitioners of faith healing also tend to be individual charismatic healers operating either in a religious context or in New Age and mentalist constructs of paranormal healing through the forces of nature.

Faith healing differs from more general exercises in prayer. It is intensely personal and more individualistic than group or shrine contexts, in which healing is experienced through a holy place, through a saint, or through intercessory prayer.

ISSUES

Medical analyses of faith healing have not produced any final results concerning its effectiveness. Studies devoted to the general issues of spirituality and health, or the relation of prayer to healing, have focused upon selected recipients, such as ethnic groups, religious congregations, or medical groupings. Faith healing is more difficult to isolate in that it occurs within an intensely personal and often independent context. The most prominent faith healers in contemporary American and European societies operate as independent entities. While these figures may host large meetings, the groups themselves are not expressive of any one culture or religious tradition.

The importance of the entire issue of spirituality and health is demonstrated by the creation of a number of medical centers devoted to investigating the relationship between healing and prayer. These centers include the Center for Spirituality, Theology, and Health at Duke University; the Benson-Henry Institute for Mind Body Medicine at Massachusetts General Hospital; and the George Washington Institute for Spirituality and Health.

Two primary challenges faced by researchers as they study the spectrum of faith/prayer and healing are the problem of establishing basic parameters under which the studies can be conducted and the issues of verification and falsification. At the same time, the medical community has willingly joined forces with the religious in asserting the value of positive attitudes and the exercise of faith in obtaining physical and emotional healing.

James F. Breckenridge, Th.D.

FURTHER READING

Brown, Candy Gunther, et al. "Study of the Therapeutic Effects of Proximal Intercessory Prayer (STEPP) on Auditory and Visual Impairments in Rural Mozambique." *Southern Medical Journal* 103, no. 9 (2010): 864-869.

McGuire, Meredith B. *Ritual Healing in Suburban America.* New Brunswick, N.J.: Rutgers University Press, 1998.

MacNutt, Francis. *Healing.* Reprint. London: Hodder & Stoughton, 2001.

Vellenga, Sipco J. "Hope for Healing: The Mobilization of Interest in Three Types of Religious Healing in the Netherlands Since 1850." *Social Compass* 55 (2008): 330-350.

See also: Integrative medicine; Meditation; Qigong; Reiki; Spirituality; Tai Chi; Traditional healing; Yoga.

False unicorn

CATEGORY: Herbs and supplements
RELATED TERM: *Chamaelirium luteum*
DEFINITION: Natural plant product used to treat specific health conditions.
PRINCIPAL PROPOSED USE: Dysmenorrhea
OTHER PROPOSED USES: Infertility, morning sickness, pelvic inflammatory disease, premenstrual syndrome, prevention of miscarriage

OVERVIEW

The herb false unicorn is native to North America east of the Mississippi River. It is similar in appearance, but unrelated, to true unicorn, *Aletris farinose*. The root is the portion used medicinally. Native Americans and, subsequently, European physicians believed that false unicorn stimulates the uterus, promoting menstruation. It was used for dysmenorrhea (painful menstruation), amenorrhea (absent menstruation), and irregular menstruation, and infections of the female genital tract.

THERAPEUTIC DOSAGES

A typical dose of false unicorn is 1-2 grams three times daily, or an equivalent amount in tincture form.

THERAPEUTIC USES

Some contemporary herbalists claim that false unicorn can help balance the female reproductive system, normalizing hormone levels and optimizing ovarian action. On this basis, they recommend it for preventing miscarriages and treating infertility, dysmenorrhea, premenstrual syndrome, pelvic inflammatory disease, and morning sickness. However, there is no meaningful evidence to support any of these uses.

Some herbalists support these proposed effects by referring to the presence of the hormonelike substance diosgenin in false unicorn. They claim either that diosgenin has hormonal properties or that the body can use it to create hormones. This concept, however, is based on a widespread misconception. It is true that diosgenin is used by industrial chemists as a raw material from which to economically synthesize sex hormones. This fact has been sufficient to lead to an association in people's minds between diosgenin and hormones. However, diosgenin itself does not have any hormonal properties, and while chemists can convert diosgenin into female hormones, the body does not do so.

SAFETY ISSUES

False unicorn has not undergone any meaningful safety evaluation. Even though it is traditionally recommended for use during pregnancy, its reputation as a uterine stimulant would seem to suggest it should not be taken by pregnant women. Safety in young children, nursing women, or people with severe liver or kidney disease has not been established.

EBSCO CAM Review Board

FURTHER READING

Newall, C. A., L. A. Anderson, and J. D. Phillipson. *Herbal Medicines: A Guide for Health-Care Professionals.* London: Pharmaceutical Press; 1996.

See also: Amenorrhea; Dysmenorrhea; Herbal medicine; Women's health.

Fatigue

CATEGORY: Condition
RELATED TERMS: Low energy
DEFINITION: Treatment of acute and chronic low energy.
PRINCIPAL PROPOSED NATURAL TREATMENT: Iron
OTHER PROPOSED NATURAL TREATMENTS: Adrenal extract, ashwagandha, Ayurveda, bee propolis, carnitine, chiropractic, chromium, coenzyme Q_{10}, *Cordyceps*, dehydroepiandrosterone, *Eleutherococcus*, exercise, ginseng, guarana, homeopathy, L-citrulline, maca, maitake, massage, naturopathy, nicotinamide adenine dinucleotide, pregnenolone, pyruvate, Reiki, reishi, *Rhodiola rosea*, royal jelly, schisandra, suma, Tai Chi, traditional Chinese herbal medicine, vitamin B_{12}, vitamin C, yoga

INTRODUCTION

Many people feel that they do not have as much energy as they would like. Fatigue is one of the most common complaints that people bring to their physicians. It seems that almost everyone today has low energy, is stressed, and is worn out much of the time.

There are no easy solutions to this common problem. While many medical conditions can cause fatigue, the overwhelming majority of people who experience fatigue do not have an illness that can be diagnosed. It seems most likely that the cause of this widespread problem is modern life itself.

The body was not designed for a sedentary life. Whereas today most people might consider one hour of exercise daily to be ideal, in the past, eight hours of daily exercise was not uncommon. Before modern times, humans lived much of their lives outdoors and walked many miles every day. Today, especially in developed countries, humans live indoors, sit in chairs during the workday, and seldom walk more than one mile per day. Modern humans also live in a fast-paced, noisy world with constant interruptions. This way of life simply violates the body's design principles.

Furthermore, with the invention of the electric light, the body's normal sleep habits were replaced by progressively longer periods of wakefulness. Few people today get eight hours of sleep regularly, much less the ten to twelve hours that some experts believe people ordinarily enjoyed in the past. Tiredness, in other words, is a consequence of numerous factors, and for this reason it is not easy to treat or prevent.

Persons who frequently feel tired should get a medical exam to rule out identifiable medical conditions such as hypothyroidism, depression, fibromyalgia, chronic fatigue syndrome, chronic viral hepatitis, and anemia. Problems such as these need to be addressed specifically to make any progress.

PRINCIPAL PROPOSED NATURAL TREATMENTS

Nutrient deficiencies can also cause fatigue, and for this reason it may be useful to take dietary supplements. One nutrient, iron, requires special attention. Iron deficiency can cause anemia, which in turn can cause fatigue. Certain manufacturers of iron supplements made a causal leap (that was unsupported at the time) and concluded that iron supplements were useful treatments for general fatigue. This recommendation worried many experts, because there is some evidence that taking too much iron can be harmful.

On this basis, many physicians recommended that their patients avoid iron supplements if they were not anemic. More recent evidence, however, suggests that the promoters of iron may have been partially right. Several studies indicate that marginal deficiency of iron, too slight to cause anemia, may decrease physical performance capacity.

In addition, a double-blind, placebo-controlled study of 144 women with unexplained fatigue who also had low or borderline-low levels of ferritin (a measure of stored iron) found that the use of an iron supplement enhanced energy and well-being. Nonetheless, it is not advisable to take iron simply because one feels tired. Instead, one should first get tested to check for iron deficiency and treat the deficiency under the supervision of a physician.

OTHER PROPOSED NATURAL TREATMENTS

People with inadequate energy should increase the time they give themselves to sleep, should exercise daily (as much as possible), and should reduce or eliminate bad habits, such as cigarette smoking and excessive consumption of alcohol. Cutting down on caffeine consumption may help too by improving sleep and decreasing stress. In addition, it is important not to neglect such fundamentals as enjoyable work, healthy relationships, and adequate recreation. Even very unhealthy people tend to have more energy when they love what they are doing with their lives.

Many alternative practitioners recommend reducing the intake of sugar and other simple carbohydrates or going on a low-carbohydrate diet, but there is no scientific evidence to show that this will increase a person's energy. Similarly, it is unclear whether eating organic or pesticide-free foods or becoming a vegetarian (or its opposite, going on a so-called caveman diet) will make a difference. Still, there is nothing wrong with trying these methods, and some people feel that they help.

Despite widespread claims, no herbs or supplements have been proven to enhance overall energy and

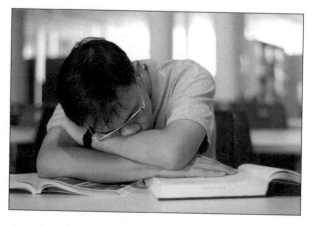

A student who is showing signs of fatigue. (©Jeffrey Koh/ Dreamstime.com)

well-being. Some of the natural products claimed to have this effect include adrenal extract, ashwagandha, bee propolis, carnitine, chromium, L-citrulline, coenzyme Q_{10}, *Cordyceps*, dehydroepiandrosterone, *Eleutherococcus*, ginseng, guarana, maca, maitake, nicotinamide adenine dinucleotide, pregnenolone, pyruvate, reishi, *Rhodiola rosea*, royal jelly, schisandra, suma, vitamin B_{12}, and vitamin C. The supplements tyrosine and nicotinamide adenine dinucleotide have shown promise for enhancing wakefulness under conditions of sleep deprivation, but they have not been investigated for treating ongoing fatigue.

Most systems of alternative medicine, including Chinese medicine, chiropractic, Ayurveda, homeopathy, and naturopathy, claim to be able to improve overall health and enhance energy. Therapies such as massage, Reiki, and therapeutic touch and exercise systems such as yoga and Tai Chi make the same claim. Furthermore, based on the theory that toxins in the environment are a major cause of illness, some alternative practitioners recommend detoxification methods. However, there is no meaningful supporting evidence to indicate that these approaches actually improve overall energy.

People who are tired because they do not sleep well might find benefit by trying natural therapies for insomnia. Similarly, people who feel overwhelmed by life may benefit from natural treatments for stress. In addition, many people with low energy report that they feel better when they use natural treatments for food allergies, candida, or low immunity; whether this is caused by the placebo effect, however, remains unclear.

In most cases, fatigue is a complex problem that does not respond to simple treatment approaches. Simply making it a priority to feel better may eventually lead to improvement.

EBSCO CAM Review Board

FURTHER READING

Adams, D., et al. "Traditional Chinese Medicinal Herbs for the Treatment of Idiopathic Chronic Fatigue and Chronic Fatigue Syndrome." *Cochrane Database of Systematic Reviews* (2009): CD006348. Available through *EBSCO DynaMed Systematic Literature Surveillance* at http://www.ebscohost.com/dynamed.

Brutsaert, T. D., et al. "Iron Supplementation Improves Progressive Fatigue Resistance During Dynamic Knee Extensor Exercise in Iron-Depleted, Nonanemic Women." *American Journal of Clinical Nutrition* 77 (2003): 441-448.

Davolos, A., et al. "Body Iron Stores and Early Neurologic Deterioration in Acute Cerebral Infarction." *Neurology* 54 (2000): 1568-1574.

Lao, T. T., K. Tam, and L. Y. Chan. "Third Trimester Iron Status and Pregnancy Outcome in Nonanaemic Women: Pregnancy Unfavourably Affected by Maternal Iron Excess." *Human Reproduction* 15 (2000): 1843-1848.

Verdon, F., et al. "Iron Supplementation for Unexplained Fatigue in Non-anaemic Women." *British Medical Journal* 326 (2003): 1124.

See also: Adrenal extract; Chronic fatigue syndrome; Fibromyalgia: Homeopathic remedies; Herbal medicine; Iron; Memory and mental function impairment; Pregnancy support; Women's health.

Feldenkrais method

CATEGORY: Therapies and techniques
DEFINITION: A self-education system focusing on the relationship between mind and body.
PRINCIPAL PROPOSED USES: Balance, coordination, and flexibility, pain relief, tension reduction
OTHER PROPOSED USES: Depression, fibromyalgia, multiple sclerosis, orthopedic problems, stroke

OVERVIEW

The Feldenkrais method of mind/body education was developed by Moshé Feldenkrais, a physicist and engineer. The basic idea of the method is that focusing on the connection between the mind and body movement causes new patterns of movement to form, restoring the body to the way it is meant to move. This reversion promotes improved movement, improved brain function, and general well-being.

MECHANISM OF ACTION

The Feldenkrais method is practiced in two different ways: by functional integration and by awareness through movement.

Functional integration involves personal, one-on-one training in which an instructor gives a student hands-on instruction in developmental movement. In this type of instruction, the teacher touches the student and helps him or her move through body awareness; the student remains fully clothed. This type of session focuses on whatever agility problems the student is experiencing but is most often focused on eliminating excess effort and on moving more easily.

Awareness through movement is a group session in which an instructor verbally guides students through developmental movement. Though the instructions are directed at a group, individuals are encouraged to discover and be aware of their own personal body movement and development.

USES AND APPLICATIONS

Through his own awareness of the body-mind connection and through his own practicing of movement, Feldenkrais came to believe that one could improve balance, coordination, and flexibility and relieve pain, tension, and stress. He also believed that a person could overcome many neurological and physical problems by focusing on this connection, which creates new neural pathways that affect movement.

SCIENTIFIC EVIDENCE

The type of hands-on instruction that helps define the Feldenkrais method is difficult to evaluate by methods such as a double-blind trial. (It would be impossible to give some people real instruction in the method while others received something else.) A few observational studies have shown, however, a relationship between Feldenkrais practice and improved balance and mobility and the relief of pain and stress, particularly in the elderly or others whose movement is limited.

CHOOSING A PRACTITIONER

Feldenkrais practitioners are certified through the Feldenkrais Guild of North America. Certification takes three to four years and involves 740 to 800 hours of training in Feldenkrais methods and a period of practice and application under supervision. Possibly the most important factor in choosing a practitioner, however, particularly for functional integration, is the person's comfort level with the instructor.

SAFETY ISSUES

The Feldenkrais method focuses on gentle movements, so there should be no pain involved in practice.

Marianne M. Madsen, M.S.

FURTHER READING

Beringer, Elizabeth, ed. *Embodied Wisdom: The Collected Papers of Moshe Feldenkrais.* Berkeley, Calif.: North Atlantic Books, 2010.

Feldenkrais Movement Institute. http://www.feldenkraisinstitute.org.

Feldenkrais, Moshe. *Awareness Through Movement: Easy-to-Do Health Exercises to Improve Your Posture, Vision, Imagination, and Personal Awareness.* San Francisco: HarperCollins, 1991.

_____. *The Elusive Obvious: Or, Basic Feldenkrais.* Cupertino, Calif.: Meta, 1981.

_____. *The Potent Self: A Study of Spontaneity and Compulsion.* Berkeley, Calif.: Frog Books, 2002.

International Feldenkrais Federation. http://www.feldenkrais-method.org.

Wyszynski, Marek. "The Feldenkrais Method for People with Chronic Pain." *Pain Practitioner* 20, no. 1 (2010): 56-61.

See also: Acupressure; Acupuncture; Alexander technique; Applied kinesiology; Aston-Patterning; Back pain; Dance movement therapy; Manipulative and body-based practices; Meridians; Metamorphic technique; Mind/body medicine; Neck pain; Pain management; Progressive muscle relaxation; Qigong; Reflexology; Relaxation therapies; Rolfing; Shiatsu; Soft tissue pain; Tai Chi; Therapeutic touch.

Feng shui

CATEGORY: Therapies and techniques
RELATED TERMS: Chi, qi, yin and yang
DEFINITION: The ancient Chinese aesthetic of designing one's environment to enhance one's qi, or energy.

OVERVIEW

Practitioners of traditional Chinese medicine believe that to feel good, one must be surrounded by good qi, or energy. The art of designing one's environment to enhance one's qi (also spelled "chi") is called feng shui (pronounced "fung shway"), and it can be practiced in rooms, buildings, offices, and neighborhoods, and even on desktops. Although these ideas may sound mystical to those who are unaccustomed to the notions of qi and yin and yang,

Domestic and Personal Feng Shui

One of the most important places for practicing good feng shui is the bedroom, where it is easy to allow the energy to be "too yin" with a lack of sunshine and fresh air—a combination that creates stagnant chi and can manifest itself in illness. To help one's chi, a person should consider the following:

- Sleeping in a room located at the end of a long hallway can cause the flow of energy in that spot to be too strong and can cause poor health.

- If possible, a bedroom door should not open directly onto a bathroom, and a bed should never be placed against a wall that is shared by a toilet.

- Bedroom doors should not open onto a staircase, which could allow bad chi to enter the room.

- Bedroom doors should not face the corner edge of another room, which can block chi and cause circulatory problems.

- Any bedroom that has been occupied by someone who was ill should be aired out, should be brightly lighted, and should get a fresh coat of paint to create a burst of positive, yang energy.

The placement of the bed is especially important. Lillian Too, in her book *Feng Shui Fundamentals: Health* (1997), outlines some taboos associated with bed placement:

- Avoid sleeping with a mirror facing the bed. "A mirror in the bedroom is one of the most harmful of feng shui features—[as it] creates health problems connected with the heart. Mirrors above the bed are equally harmful." A television counts as a mirror because it also reflects; if one must have a TV or mirror in the bedroom, one should cover it when it is not being used.

- Avoid sleeping with a water feature behind the bed. A painting of a lake or waterfall (or even an aquarium) has the same effect on the heart as a mirror.

- Avoid having the sharp edge of a corner pointing toward a sleeping person. The sharp edge of a corner is a deadly form of "poison arrow" that brings the "killing breath." One should use furniture to disguise the sharp edge.

- Avoid sleeping under an exposed overhead beam. If the beam is directly over the person's head, he or she may suffer from migraines and headaches. If the beam crosses at chest level, the person risks problems with the heart and lungs.

Kitchens, too, are important places to practice feng shui for health. If one's kitchen directly faces a bedroom, for instance, the home's yin energy (from the bedroom) and yang energy (from the kitchen) could clash and bring continuous illness to family members. The kitchen door should not be in a straight line from either the front or back door; good energy will shoot through the home without dispersing, resulting first in "annoying illness" and then progressing to more serious misfortune. One can solve this layout by hanging a mirror on one of the outside doors so that positive energy will not leave so quickly.

Many feng shui books help readers calculate the "best health direction" for their homes. The stove, for example, should always point in that best direction (as should the head of the bed). The stove, which symbolizes the fire element in feng shui, should never be located next to the sink—which would bring a clash of the fire and water elements—and should never sit in the northwest area of the room, which would be tantamount to "setting fire to heaven's gate."

Cleaning up clutter can help a person relax, and oiling doors so they do not squeak can reduce irritation. Author Patricia Santhuff offers some tips for getting "an extra boost of energy for a particular project" or if one is "having trouble decluttering":

- Add a wind chime in the room or over the work area and ring it now and then. Some feng shui practitioners say wind chimes foster clarity and creativity.

- Vacuum and dust to not only remove dirt but also freshen chi.

- Play some uplifting music.

- Add a desktop fountain to the area.

- Energetically "treat" the room by using rattles or clapping, especially in corners and closets.

To raise one's personal chi, experts suggest the following: Create something; clean house, or just a drawer; call a friend; buy oneself fresh flowers; cancel a poorly thought-out commitment; explore some part of one's city or of an unfamiliar area.

feng shui, which literally means "wind and water," has its origins in the earliest Daoist traditions of ancient China.

BASIC TENETS

There are three basic tenets of feng shui: Everything is alive, everything is connected, and everything is changing. Feng shui begins with the basic structure of one's home. For example, the placement of doors and windows can mean the difference between qi that is fresh and alive with energy and qi that is stale and damaging. A room can have too much yin, or negative energy, if it has been unoccupied and dirty for a long time; cleaning, bright lights, and uplifting music can clear the air. Happy sounds are always an effective antidote to bad energy.

According to feng shui, every object, space, and living thing has qi. "The better the quality of chi coursing through a thing, the healthier, more vibrant, or more beautiful that thing is," according to Patricia J. Santhuff, who writes about the relationship of qi to health. "When our bodies are experiencing low or blocked chi, we experience fatigue. Or, if one experiences low chi over an extended period of time," one is "more prone to develop health problems." The goal is to protect against negative energies and welcome those energies that bring health and longevity.

Mary Mihaly; reviewed by EBSCO CAM Review Board

FURTHER READING

Alexander, Skye. *The Care and Feeding of Your Chi: Feng Shui for Your Body.* Gloucester, Mass.: Fair Winds Press, 2004.

American Feng Shui Institute. http://www.amfengshui.com.

Bruun, Ole. *An Introduction to Feng Shui.* New York: Cambridge University Press, 2008.

Diamond, Kartar. *Feng Shui for Skeptics: Real Solutions Without Superstition.* Culver City, Calif.: Four Pillars, 2004.

Feng Shui Connections. http://www.fengshui connections.ca.

Geomancy.net: Center for Feng Shui Research. http://www.geomancy.net.

Too, Lillian. *Feng Shui Fundamentals: Health.* Rockport, Mass.: Element, 1997.

Traditional Chinese Medicine and Acupuncture Health Information Organization. http://tcm.health-info.org.

World of Feng Shui. http://www.wofs.ca.

See also: Energy medicine; Magnet therapy; Meridians; Polarity therapy; Qigong; Traditional Chinese herbal medicine; Traditional healing.

Fennel

CATEGORY: Herbs and supplements
RELATED TERM: *Foeniculum vulgare*
DEFINITION: Natural plant product used to treat specific health conditions.
PRINCIPAL PROPOSED USE: Infantile colic
OTHER PROPOSED USES: Dyspepsia, intestinal gas, menstrual pain

OVERVIEW

The herb fennel has a long history of use as both food and medicine. Traditionally, it is said to act as a carminative, a term that means that it helps the body expel gas. Other traditional uses include increasing breast milk production, easing childbirth, calming cough, promoting menstrual flow, soothing indigestion, and enhancing libido. Fennel is also a common ingredient in "gripe water," a traditional (and highly alcoholic) preparation used for treating infant colic.

THERAPEUTIC DOSAGES

A typical dose of fennel is 1 to 1.5 teaspoons of seeds per day, either in capsules or as tea.

THERAPEUTIC USES

Animal and test-tube studies hint at a number of potential medicinal effects of fennel or its constituents, such as relaxing smooth muscles, stimulating the flow of bile, and reducing pain. However, only double-blind, placebo-controlled studies in humans can actually show a treatment effective. Only one such study of this type has been performed for fennel.

This trial enrolled 125 infants with colic, who received either placebo or fennel seed oil at a dose of 12 milligrams (mg) daily per kilogram of body weight. The results were promising. About 40 percent of the infants receiving fennel showed relief of colic symptoms, compared with only 14 percent in the placebo group, a significant difference. Another way to view the results involves looking at hours of inconsolable crying. In the treated group, infants cried about nine hours per week, compared to twelve

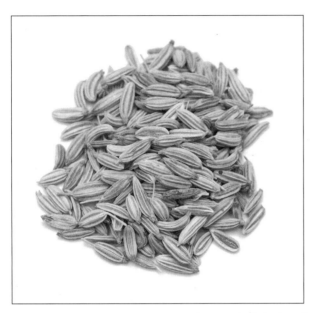

The herb fennel has a long history of use as both food and medicine. (©Brad Calkins/Dreamstime.com)

hours in the placebo group. While these are promising results, confirmation by an independent research group is necessary before the treatment can be accepted as effective. Previously, a small double-blind, placebo-controlled study found similar benefits with a tea containing fennel as well as other herbs (chamomile, vervain, licorice, and lemon balm).

No other proposed uses of fennel have undergone study in double-blind trials. One study commonly cited as evidence that fennel is helpful for menstrual pain actually proved nothing. This was an open trial that compared fennel to the drug mefenamic acid. Because participants and researchers were aware of which treatment was which, the power of suggestion had free play, making the results almost meaningless. Another study of fennel also failed to use a placebo.

At one time it was thought that fennel had estrogenlike effects, making it a phytoestrogen. However, subsequent research has tended to indicate that fennel does not have significant phytoestrogen activity.

SAFETY ISSUES

As a widely consumed food spice, fennel is thought to have a high safety factor. However, according to one placebo-controlled study with rats, fennel impairs the absorption of the antibiotic ciprofloxacin (Cipro).

Fennel might be expected to interfere similarly with other drugs in the ciprofloxacin family, the fluoroquinolone drugs. Allowing two hours between taking ciprofloxacin and fennel should reduce the potential for an interaction but may not eliminate it. For this reason, it may be advisable to avoid taking fennel during therapy with ciprofloxacin or other antibiotics in this family.

Maximum safe doses of fennel in young children, pregnant or nursing women, and people with severe liver or kidney disease have not been established. Persons taking drugs in the fluoroquinolone family, such as Cipro, should not use fennel.

EBSCO CAM Review Board

FURTHER READING

Alexandrovich, I., et al. "The Effect of Fennel (*Foeniculum vulgare*) Seed Oil Emulsion in Infantile Colic." *Alternative Therapies in Health and Medicine* 9 (2003): 58-61.

Modaress, Nejad V., and M. Asadipour. "Comparison of the Effectiveness of Fennel and Mefenamic Acid on Pain Intensity in Dysmenorrhoea." *Eastern Mediterranean Health Journal* 12 (2006): 423-427.

Namavar, J. B., A. Tartifizadeh, and S. Khabnadideh. "Comparison of Fennel and Mefenamic Acid for the Treatment of Primary Dysmenorrhea." *International Journal of Gynaecology and Obstetrics* 80 (2003): 153-157.

See also: Colic; Dyspepsia; Gas, intestinal; Herbal medicine; Pain management.

Fenugreek

CATEGORY: Herbs and supplements
RELATED TERM: *Trigonella foenumgraecum*
DEFINITION: Natural plant product used to treat specific health conditions.
PRINCIPAL PROPOSED USES: Constipation, diabetes, high cholesterol

OVERVIEW

For millennia, fenugreek has been used both as a medicine and as a food spice in Egypt, India, and the Middle East. It was traditionally recommended for increasing milk production in nursing women and for

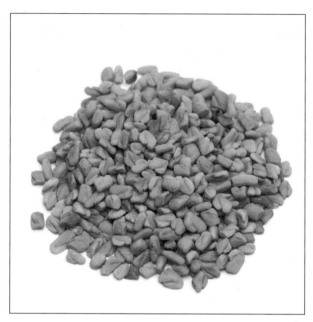

Fenugreek may have potential benefits to those with diabetes or high cholesterol. (©Corinna Gissemann/Dreamstime.com)

the treatment of wounds, bronchitis, digestive problems, arthritis, kidney problems, and male reproductive conditions.

THERAPEUTIC DOSAGES

Because the seeds of fenugreek are somewhat bitter, they are best taken in capsule form. The typical dosage is 5 to 30 grams (g) of defatted fenugreek taken three times a day with meals. The one double-blind study of fenugreek used 1 g per day of a water/alcohol fenugreek extract.

THERAPEUTIC USES

Present interest in fenugreek focuses on its potential benefits for people with diabetes or high cholesterol. Numerous animal studies and preliminary trials in humans have found that fenugreek can reduce blood sugar and serum cholesterol levels in people with diabetes. Like other high-fiber foods, it may also be helpful for constipation.

SCIENTIFIC EVIDENCE

In a two-month, double-blind study of twenty-five individuals with type 2 diabetes, use of fenugreek, 1 g per day of a standardized extract, significantly improved some measures of blood sugar control and insulin response, compared with a placebo. Triglyceride levels decreased and HDL (good) cholesterol levels increased, presumably because of the enhanced insulin sensitivity. Similar benefits have been seen in animal studies and open human trials.

SAFETY ISSUES

As a commonly eaten food, fenugreek is generally regarded as safe. The only common side effect is mild gastrointestinal distress when it is taken in high doses.

Animal studies have found fenugreek essentially nontoxic, and no serious adverse effects have been seen in two-year follow-up of human trials. However, extracts made from fenugreek have been shown to stimulate uterine contractions in guinea pigs. For this reason, pregnant women should not take fenugreek in dosages higher than are commonly used as a spice, perhaps 5 g daily. Besides concerns about pregnant women, safety in young children, nursing women, and those with severe liver or kidney disease also has not been established. Because fenugreek can lower blood sugar levels, it is advisable to seek medical supervision before combining it with diabetes medications.

IMPORTANT INTERACTIONS

If one is taking diabetes medications, such as insulin or oral hypoglycemic drugs, fenugreek may enhance their effects. This may cause excessively low blood sugar, and one may need to reduce one's dose of medication.

EBSCO CAM Review Board

FURTHER READING

Gupta, A., R. Gupta, and B. Lal. "Effect of *Trigonella foenum-graecum* (Fenugreek) Seeds on Glycaemic Control and Insulin Resistance in Type 2 Diabetes Mellitus." *Journal of the Association of Physicians of India* 49 (2001): 1057-1061.

Leung, A. Y., and S. Foster. *Encyclopedia of Common Natural Ingredients Used in Food, Drugs, and Cosmetics.* 2d ed. New York: Wiley, 1996.

See also: Constipation; Diabetes; Cholesterol, high; Herbal medicine.

Feverfew

RELATED TERM: *Tanacetum parthenium*
CATEGORY: Herbs and supplements
DEFINITION: Natural plant product used to treat specific health conditions.
PRINCIPAL PROPOSED USE: Migraine headaches
OTHER PROPOSED USES: Osteoarthritis, rheumatoid arthritis

OVERVIEW

Originally native to the Balkans, feverfew, a relative of the common daisy, was spread by deliberate planting throughout Europe and the Americas. Feverfew's feathery and aromatic leaves have long been used medicinally to improve childbirth, promote menstruation, induce abortions, relieve rheumatic pain, and treat severe headaches.

Contrary to popular belief, feverfew is not used for lowering fevers. Actually, according to one source, "feverfew" is a corruption of the name "featherfoil." Featherfoil became featherfew and ultimately feverfew. In an odd historical reversal, this name then led to a widespread belief among herbalists that feverfew could lower fevers. After a while they noticed that it did not work, and they then rejected feverfew as a useless herb. Feverfew remained unpopular until a serendipitous event occurred in the late 1970s.

At that time, the wife of the chief medical officer of the National Coal Board in England had serious migraine headaches. When workers in the industry

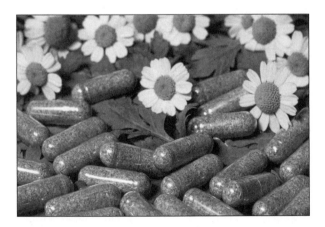

Capsules of dried feverfew are shown with the leaves and flowers of the feverfew plant. (Jeremy Burgess/Photo Researchers, Inc.)

learned of this, a sympathetic miner suggested she try a folk treatment he had used. She followed his advice and chewed feverfew leaves. The results were dramatic: Her migraines disappeared almost completely.

Her husband was impressed, too. He used his high office to gain the ear of a physician who specialized in migraine headaches, E. Stewart Johnson of the London Migraine Clinic. Johnson subsequently experimented with feverfew in his practice and seemed to observe good results. This led to the studies described here.

THERAPEUTIC DOSAGES

The tested liquid-carbon-dioxide feverfew extract is taken at a dose of 6.25 milligrams (mg) three times daily. To replicate the dosage of feverfew used in the two positive studies of whole leaf described above, one should take 80 to 100 mg of powdered whole feverfew leaf daily.

THERAPEUTIC USES

Feverfew is used primarily for the prevention of migraine headaches. For this purpose, it is taken daily. There has been no formal investigation of feverfew as a treatment for migraines that have already started, although one double-blind study evaluating feverfew as a preventive agent did find hints of possible symptom-reducing benefits.

It is important to remember that serious diseases may occasionally first present themselves as migraine-type headaches. For this reason, proper medical diagnosis is essential if one suddenly starts having migraines without a previous history or if the pattern of one's migraines changes significantly. Feverfew is sometimes recommended for osteoarthritis or rheumatoid arthritis, but there is no evidence that it works.

SCIENTIFIC EVIDENCE

Five meaningful double-blind, placebo-controlled studies have been performed to evaluate feverfew's effectiveness as a preventive treatment for migraines. The best of the positive trials used a feverfew extract made by extracting the herb with liquid carbon dioxide. Two other trials that used whole feverfew leaf also found it effective; however, two studies that used feverfew extracts did not find benefit.

In a well-conducted sixteen-week, double-blind, placebo-controlled study of 170 people with migraines, use of a feverfew extract at a dose of 6.25 mg three times daily resulted in a significant decrease in headache frequency, compared with the effect of the placebo treatment. In the treatment group, headache frequency decreased by 1.9 headaches per month, compared with a reduction of 1.3 headaches per month in the placebo group. The average number of headaches per month prior to treatment was 4.76 headaches. The extract used in this study was made utilizing liquid carbon dioxide. A previous study using the same extract had failed to find benefit, but it primarily enrolled people with less frequent migraines.

Two other studies used whole feverfew leaf and found benefit. The first followed fifty-nine people for eight months. For four months, half received a daily capsule of powdered feverfew leaf; the other half took placebo. The groups were then switched and followed for an additional four months. Treatment with feverfew produced a 24 percent reduction in the number of migraines and a significant decrease in nausea and vomiting during the headaches. A subsequent double-blind study of fifty-seven people with migraines found that use of feverfew leaf could decrease the severity of migraine headaches. This trial did not report whether there was any change in the frequency of migraines; it is possible, therefore, that this study actually showed a symptom-reducing effect rather than a preventive benefit. One study using an alcohol extract failed to find benefit.

SAFETY ISSUES

Animal studies suggest that feverfew is essentially nontoxic. In one eight-month study, there were no significant differences in side effects between the treated and control groups. There also were no changes in measurements on blood tests and urinalysis.

In a survey involving three hundred people, 11.3 percent reported mouth sores from chewing feverfew leaf, occasionally accompanied by general inflammation of tissues in the mouth. A smaller percentage reported mild gastrointestinal distress. However, mouth sores do not seem to occur in people who use encapsulated feverfew leaf powder, the usual form.

In view of its use as a folk remedy to promote abortions, feverfew should probably not be taken during pregnancy. Because feverfew might slightly inhibit the activity of blood-clotting cells known as platelets, it should not be combined with strong anticoagulants, such as warfarin (Coumadin) or heparin, except on medical advice. Feverfew might also increase the risk of stomach problems if combined with anti-inflammatory drugs, such as aspirin. Safety in young children, pregnant or nursing women, and those with severe kidney or liver disease has not been established.

IMPORTANT INTERACTIONS

If one is taking warfarin (Coumadin), heparin, aspirin, or other nonsteroidal anti-inflammatory drugs, one should use feverfew only on medical advice.

EBSCO CAM Review Board

FURTHER READING

De Weerdt, C. J., H. P. R. Bootsma, and H. Hendriks. "Herbal Medicines in Migraine Prevention: Randomized Double-Blind, Placebo-Controlled Cross-over Trial of a Feverfew Preparation." *Phytomedicine* 3 (1996): 225-230.

Diener, H., et al. "Efficacy and Safety of 6.25 mg T.I.D. Feverfew Co-extract (Mig-99) in Migraine Prevention." *Cephalalgia* 25 (2005): 1031-1041.

Newall, C., L. A. Anderson, and J. D. Phillipson. *Herbal Medicines: A Guide for Health-Care Professionals.* London: Pharmaceutical Press; 1996.

Pfaffenrath, V., et al. "The Efficacy and Safety of *Tanacetum parthenium* (Feverfew) in Migraine Prophylaxis." *Cephalalgia* 22 (2002): 523-532.

Tyler, V. E. *Herbs of Choice: The Therapeutic Use of Phytomedicinals.* New York: Pharmaceutical Products Press, 1994.

See also: Herbal medicine; Migraines; Osteoarthritis; Rheumatoid arthritis.

Fibrate drugs

CATEGORY: Drug interactions

DEFINITION: Drugs used to improve levels of cholesterol and related lipids found in the blood. Fibrates are particularly helpful for persons with high levels of triglycerides.

INTERACTIONS: B vitamins, blood-thinning supplements

DRUGS IN THIS FAMILY: Clofibrate (Atromid-S), fenofibrate (Tricor), gemfibrozil (Lopid)

B VITAMINS

Effect: Possible Helpful Interaction

Fibrate drugs are known to raise homocysteine levels in the blood. High levels of homocysteine have been associated with increased risk of heart disease, although a direct connection has not been proven.

In a double-blind, placebo-controlled trial of twenty-nine men taking fenofibrate, the use of the B vitamins folate (650 micrograms [mcg]), vitamin B_{12} (50 mcg), and vitamin B_6 (50 milligrams) once daily for six weeks restored homocysteine levels to nearly normal values.

BLOOD-THINNING SUPPLEMENTS

Effect: Possible Harmful Interaction

Fibrate drugs are known to increase the blood-thinning effects of drugs in the warfarin (Coumadin) family. Certain herbs, such as garlic, danshen, devil's claw, dong quai, papaya, PC-SPES, and red clover, may thin the blood in a manner somewhat similar to warfarin. Although no such interactions have been reported, it is theoretically possible that the combined use of these herbs and fibrate drugs could pose a risk of bleeding problems.

EBSCO CAM Review Board

FURTHER READING

Dierkes, J., et al. "Vitamin Supplementation Can Markedly Reduce the Homocysteine Elevation Induced by Fenofibrate." *Atherosclerosis* 158 (2001): 161-164.

See also: Cholesterol, high; Folate; Food and Drug Administration; Heart disease; Supplements: Overview; Vitamin B_6; Vitamin B_{12}; Vitamins and minerals.

Fibromyalgia: Homeopathic remedies

CATEGORY: Homeopathy

RELATED TERMS: Fibromyalgia syndrome, fibrositis, myofascial pain

DEFINITION: Homeopathic treatment of the chronic condition that causes severe muscle pain, fatigue, a feeling of inflammation, sensitivity to touch, and other symptoms.

STUDIED HOMEOPATHIC REMEDIES: *Arnica montana, Bryonia, Rhus tox*

INTRODUCTION

The most prominent feature of fibromyalgia, also known as fibromyalgia syndrome, myofascial pain, and fibrositis, is the chronic presence of tender, swollen, and painful muscle knots distributed throughout the body. This symptom is usually accompanied by stiffness, fatigue, nonrestorative sleep, and a general feeling of whole-body inflammation. Other symptoms include alternating diarrhea and constipation (irritable bowel syndrome), headaches, numbness and tingling, and restless legs. Also, people with fibromyalgia frequently develop prolonged pain and discomfort from injuries so mild that they would not hurt a healthy person for more than a short time.

In severe cases, people with fibromyalgia experience extreme discomfort when almost any part of the body is pressed upon, even lightly. Milder cases involve moderate to severe pain that wanders from one location to another.

SCIENTIFIC EVALUATIONS OF HOMEOPATHIC REMEDIES

Evidence regarding the use of homeopathic remedies for fibromyalgia is mixed. In a double-blind, placebo-controlled, crossover study, researchers tested the remedy *Rhus tox* 6c (centesimals) on thirty people with fibromyalgia who fit the symptom picture of *Rhus tox*, as assessed by a homeopathic physician. For one month, the participants took either *Rhus tox* 6c or placebo three times daily. For the following month, the participants took the opposite treatment; however, neither participants nor observers knew which treatment was which.

Participants experienced a statistically significant improvement when they were taking the *Rhus tox*, compared with taking placebo. The number of tender spots was reduced by 25 percent on average, and the improvement in overall pain and sleep scores was marked when participants were taking the treatment.

However, another small, double-blind, placebo-controlled study failed to find evidence of benefit. In this study, twenty-four participants with fibromyalgia were given either placebo or one of three homeopathic remedies (*Arnica, Bryonia,* or *Rhus tox*) at 6c (centesimals) potency, prescribed according to traditional homeopathic indications. Participants took remedies or placebo twice daily for three months.

The results showed no statistically significant improvements in symptoms among those participants receiving homeopathic remedies, compared with those given placebo. However, researchers found some evidence of benefit in a subgroup of participants. When the homeopathic practitioners chose the initial remedy, they noted whether the remedy was a close fit to the participant or not according to the principles of classical homeopathy. If one looks only at participants whose remedy fit well, based on the whole-person symptom picture, then some benefits were seen. This seems to indicate that properly chosen homeopathic remedies might be helpful for fibromyalgia. However, considering the small number of people involved in the study, it is impossible to draw any conclusions.

TRADITIONAL HOMEOPATHIC TREATMENTS

Classical homeopathy offers many possible homeopathic treatments for fibromyalgia. These therapies are chosen based on various specific details of the person seeking treatment.

For instance, if a person feels bruised and is physically restless, irritable, and fatigued, then that person may fit the symptom picture of *Arnica montana*. In addition, the use of *Arnica* is said to be particularly indicated when the complaints can be attributed to a previous injury. For persons who want to remain still because even a slight movement makes pain worse, and for persons who prefer cool applications to warm ones, the symptom picture may fit the remedy *Bryonia* instead.

Homeopathic *Rhus tox* is used under circumstances similar to those that indicate *Bryonia*. However, unlike the *Bryonia* recipient, who wants to lie still and is made worse by the least motion, the *Rhus tox* picture invokes a person who benefits from motion and wants to be active. In addition, the condition will worsen with exposure to cold and dampness and improve in dry, warm weather.

EBSCO CAM Review Board

FURTHER READING

Baranowsky, J., et al. "Qualitative Systemic Review of Randomized Controlled Trials on Complementary and Alternative Medicine Treatments in Fibromyalgia." *Rheumatology International* 30 (2009): 1-21.

De Silva, V., et al. "Evidence for the Efficacy of Complementary and Alternative Medicines in the Management of Fibromyalgia." *Rheumatology* 49 (2010): 1063-1068.

Fisher, P. "An Experimental Double-Blind Clinical Trial Method in Homeopathy: Use of a Limited Range of Remedies to Treat Fibrositis." *British Homeopathic Journal* 75 (1986): 143-147.

Fisher, P., et al. "Effect of Homeopathic Treatment of Fibrositis (Primary Fibromyalgia)." *British Medical Journal* 299 (1989): 365-356.

Perry, R., R. Terry, and E. Ernst. "A Systematic Review of Homoeopathy for the Treatment of Fibromyalgia." *Clinical Rheumatology* 29 (2010): 457-464.

Stevinson, C., et al. "Homeopathic *Arnica* for Prevention of Pain and Bruising." *Journal of the Royal Society of Medicine* 96 (2003): 60-65.

See also: Acupressure; Acupuncture; Back pain; Chronic fatigue syndrome; Fatigue; Homeopathy; Irritable bowel syndrome (IBS); Lupus; Massage therapy; Memory and mental function impairment; Neck pain; Pain management; Progressive muscle relaxation.

Finsen, Niels Ryberg

CATEGORY: Biography
IDENTIFICATION: Danish physician considered the founder of modern phototherapy, or light therapy
BORN: December 15, 1860; Tórshavn, Faroe Islands, Denmark
DIED: September 24, 1904; Copenhagen, Denmark

OVERVIEW

Niels Ryberg Finsen, a Danish physician, is believed to have founded modern phototherapy, or light therapy, which involves using natural or derived radiation for the treatment of various physical and psychological ailments (such as acne, seasonal affective disorder, and lupus). In 1903, Finsen received the Nobel Prize in Physiology or Medicine for his work in the early field of phototherapy.

As a young child, Finsen reportedly had initial difficulties in schooling when enrolled in a boarding school, where he was described as having "low skills and energy." As a result, he was transferred to a school attended by his father as a child, where Finsen performed much better. Finsen eventually studied medicine in Copenhagen beginning in 1882, and he received his license in 1890. In the same year, he became prosector of anatomy at the University of Copenhagen,

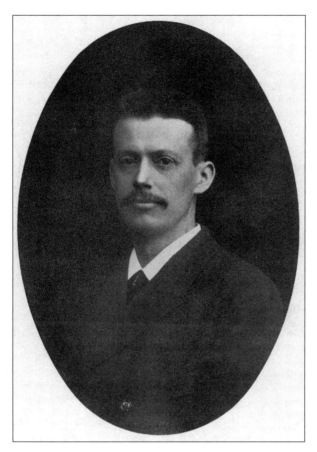

Niels Ryberg Finsen. (Hulton Archive/Getty Images)

which he left in 1893 to devote more time to his scientific research. He founded the Finsen Institute in 1896, which served as the locale for much of his research work.

Finsen had Pick's disease, which is characterized by progressive thickening of the connective tissue of certain membranes in the liver, spleen, and heart. Over the course of his disease, Finsen's symptoms worsened and eventually led him to experiment with light to treat his ailment. He initially posited that exposure to sunlight could likely improve his overall condition, which led him to further investigate alternative light sources for treatment. He eventually developed the first artificial light source for the purpose of medical treatment, using his invention to treat lupus, smallpox, and other ailments. Finsen also recognized that while some sunlight and light exposure could have beneficial effects, too much exposure could lead to negative effects, such as tissue damage.

Phototherapy has been further developed, and it continues to be used to treat a number of ailments, especially those that are related to the skin. Finsen's contributions continue to be recognized, although the field of phototherapy has declined somewhat in recent years because other treatments are now available. The Finsen Institute at Copenhagen University Hospital is named in his honor.

Brandy Weidow, M.S.

FURTHER READING

Hobday, Richard. *The Healing Sun: Sunlight and Health in the Twenty-First Century.* Forres, Scotland: Findhorn Press, 2000.

"Finsen, Niels Ryberg." In *Life Sciences in the Twentieth Century: Biographical Portraits,* by Everett Mendelsohn and Brian S. Baigrie. New York: Charles Scribner's Sons, 2001.

NobelPrize.org. Niels Ryberg Finsen Biography. Available at http://nobelprize.org/nobel_prizes/medicine/laureates/1903/finsen-bio.html#.

See also: Color therapy; Lupus; Photosensitivity; Skin, aging.

Fish oil

CATEGORY: Functional foods

RELATED TERMS: Docosahexaenoic acid, eicosapentaenoic acid, omega-3 fatty acids, omega-3 oil

DEFINITION: Natural substance essential for health that is promoted as a dietary supplement for specific health benefits.

PRINCIPAL PROPOSED USES: Heart disease prevention, rheumatoid arthritis

OTHER PROPOSED USES: Allergies, Alzheimer's disease, angina, ankylosing spondylitis, asthma, attention deficit disorder, bipolar disorder, borderline personality disorder, cancer-related weight loss, cancer treatment support, chronic fatigue syndrome, congestive heart failure, Crohn's disease, depression, diabetic neuropathy, dysmenorrhea, eczema prevention, epilepsy, gout, human immunodeficiency virus infection support, hypertension, kidney stones, liver disease, lupus, macular degeneration, male infertility, migraine headaches, multiple sclerosis, osteoporosis, postpartum depression, pregnancy support, prevention of premature birth, prostate cancer prevention, psoriasis, Raynaud's phenomenon, retinitis pigmentosa, schizophrenia, sickle-cell anemia, stroke prevention, surgery support, ulcerative colitis

OVERVIEW

Fish oil contains omega-3 fatty acids, one of the two main classes of essential fatty acids, or EFAs. (The other main type is omega-6.) Essential fatty acids are special fats that the body needs for optimum health.

Interest in the potential therapeutic benefits of omega-3 fatty acids began when studies of the Inuit (Eskimo) people found that although their diets contain an enormous amount of fat from fish, seals, and whales, they seldom have heart attacks. This is presumably because those sources of fat are very high in omega-3 fatty acids.

Subsequent investigation found that the omega-3 fatty acids found in fish oil have various effects that tend to reduce risk of heart disease and strokes. However, research into whether the use of fish oil actually prevents these diseases, while somewhat positive, remains incomplete and somewhat inconsistent. In recognition of this, the U.S. Food and Drug Administration (FDA) has allowed supplements containing fish oil or its constituents to carry a label that states "Supportive but not conclusive research shows that consumption of EPA [eicosapentaenoic acid] and DHA [docosahexaenoic acid] omega-3 fatty acids may reduce the risk of coronary heart disease."

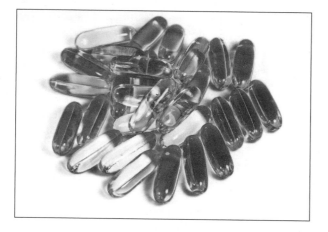

Incomplete evidence hints but does not prove that fish or fish oil might help prevent death caused by heart disease. (©Tamara Bauer/Dreamstime.com)

In addition, a slightly modified form of fish oil (ethyl-omega-3 fatty acids) has been approved by the FDA as a treatment for hypertriglyceridemia (high triglycerides). This specially processed product, sold under the trade name Omacor, is widely advertised as more effective than ordinary fish oil. However, it should be noted that Omacor has undergone relatively little study itself; the prescribing information notes only two small trials to support its effectiveness for this use. This is a far lower level of evidence than usually required for drug approval and also substantially lower than the body of evidence supporting standard fish oil as a treatment for high triglycerides.

Fish oil has also shown promise as an anti-inflammatory treatment for conditions such as rheumatoid arthritis, menstrual pain, and lupus. In addition, it may be helpful for various psychiatric conditions.

REQUIREMENTS AND SOURCES

There is no daily requirement for fish oil. However, a healthy diet should provide at least 5 grams (g) of essential fatty acids daily.

Many grains, fruits, vegetables, sea vegetables, and vegetable oils contain significant amounts of essential omega-6 and omega-3 fatty acids, but oil from cold-water fish is the richest natural source of omega-3 fats. It is commonly stated that people require a certain optimum ratio of omega-3 to omega-6 fatty acids in the diet; however, there is no real evidence that this is true, and there is some evidence that it is false.

THERAPEUTIC DOSAGES

Typical dosages of fish oil are 3 to 9 g daily, but this is not the upper limit. In one study, participants ingested 60 g daily.

The most important omega-3 fatty acids found in fish oil are called eicosapentaenoic acid (EPA) and docosahexaenoic acid (DHA). To match the dosage used in several major studies, one should take enough fish oil to supply about 2 to 3 g of EPA (2,000-3,500 milligrams [mg]) and about 1 to 2.5 g of DHA daily (1,000-2,500 mg). Far higher doses have been used in some studies; conversely, one study found blood-pressure-lowering effects with a very low daily dosage (0.7 g) of DHA.

DHA and EPA are not identical and might not have identical effects. Some evidence hints that DHA may be more effective than EPA for thinning the blood and for reducing blood pressure. The reverse may be true for reducing triglyceride levels, but study results are conflicting.

Some manufacturers add vitamin E to fish oil capsules to keep the oil from becoming rancid. Another method is to remove all the oxygen from the capsule. Also, if possible, one should purchase fish oil products certified as free of significant levels of mercury, toxic organochlorines, and polychlorobiphenyls (PCBs).

Flaxseed oil also contains omega-3 fatty acids, although of a different kind. Flaxseed oil has been suggested as a less smelly substitute for fish oil. However, it is far from clear whether flaxseed oil is therapeutically equivalent to fish oil.

THERAPEUTIC USES

Consumption of fish oil alters the body's production of certain substances in the class of chemicals called prostaglandins. Some prostaglandins increase inflammation while others decrease it. The prostaglandins whose production is enhanced by fish oil fall into the anti-inflammatory category. Based on this, fish oil has been tried as a treatment for early stages of rheumatoid arthritis, with positive results. It is thought to significantly reduce symptoms without causing side effects and may magnify the benefits of standard arthritis drugs. However, while some standard medications can slow the progression of the disease, there is no evidence that fish oil can do this. Much weaker evidence hints that fish oil might be helpful for the related disease ankylosing spondylitis.

Fish oil's apparent anti-inflammatory properties are the likely explanation for its apparent benefit in dysmenorrhea (menstrual pain), as seen in two studies. Similarly, fish oil may be helpful for the autoimmune disease lupus. (However, two studies failed to find fish oil helpful for kidney disease caused by lupus.) Evidence has been mixed regarding whether fish oil is beneficial for Crohn's disease or ulcerative colitis, conditions in which parts of the digestive tract are highly inflamed. More recently, however, two well-designed trials enrolling a total of 738 persons convincingly failed to find any benefit for omega-3 fatty acid supplementation in the prevention of Crohn's disease relapse.

Incomplete evidence hints but does not prove that fish or fish oil might help prevent death caused by heart disease. This effect seems to result from several separate actions. The best documented involves

reducing high triglyceride levels; studies enrolling more than two thousand people have substantiated this use. In addition, fish oil might raise HDL (good) cholesterol levels, thin the blood, lower levels of homocysteine, prevent dangerous heart arrhythmias, slow heart rate, improve blood vessel tone, and decrease blood pressure. These effects also support findings that fish oil may help prevent strokes. However, results are conflicting on whether people with angina should take fish oil or increase intake of fatty fish; one large study actually found that fish oil increased risk of sudden death.

For a number of theoretical reasons, it has been suggested that fish oil and its constituents (especially a slightly modified form of EPA called ethyl-EPA) might have positive effects on various psychiatric disorders, most notably depression. However, there is no convincing evidence that low levels of omega-3 fatty acids in the bloodstream lead to even mild depression. Moreover, larger trials have generally failed to demonstrate a beneficial effect of fish oil-related products in depressed persons. Preliminary, and not altogether consistent, evidence hints that high doses of fish oil may produce benefits in bipolar disorder, reducing risk of relapse and improving emotional state.

Other preliminary, and again not altogether consistent, evidence hints that fish oil might enhance the effectiveness of standard drugs (such as phenothiazines) for schizophrenia. One trial of eighty-one adolescents and young adults (considered at very high risk) found that daily omega-3 fatty acid supplements for twelve weeks delayed transition to a first full psychotic episode (such as schizophrenia) within one year.

Fish oil has also shown a bit of promise for borderline personality disorder. In one study, DHA failed to augment the effectiveness of standard therapy for attention deficit disorder (ADD). However, two studies that evaluated the potential benefits of fish oil combined with omega-6 fatty acids found some evidence of benefit for this condition. Finally, one small trial found evidence that the use of fish oil might decrease anger and aggressiveness in people with a history of aggressive behaviors, substance abuse, and problems with the law.

Small studies also suggest that fish oil may be helpful in Raynaud's phenomenon (a condition in which a person's hands and feet show abnormal sensitivity to cold temperatures), sickle cell anemia, and a form of kidney disease called IgA nephropathy. Also, according to some studies, but not all, fish oil may help treat the undesired weight loss often experienced by people with cancer. In addition, highly preliminary evidence hints that DHA might enhance the effects of the cancer chemotherapy drug doxorubicin and decrease side effects of the chemotherapy drug irinotecan.

Use of fish oil by pregnant women might help prevent premature birth, although evidence is somewhat inconsistent. In addition, the use of fish oil by pregnant women may support healthy brain function and help prevent eczema and allergies in offspring.

Intriguing, but unreliable, evidence hints that fish oil, or its constituents, might be helpful for treating kidney stones or alleviating the symptoms of chronic fatigue syndrome, and for reducing the risk of prostate cancer. Results are inconsistent regarding whether the use of fish oil can decrease seizure frequency in people with epilepsy.

One study found that insulin metabolism in 278 young, overweight persons improved on a calorie-restricted diet rich in fish oil from seafood or supplements compared with those on a diet low in fish oil, suggesting that fish oil may help delay the onset of diabetes in susceptible persons. Fish oil has also been proposed as a treatment for many other conditions, including diabetic neuropathy, allergies, and gout, but there has been little real scientific investigation of these uses.

Some studies suggest that fish oil combined with omega-6 essential fatty acids may augment the effectiveness of calcium in the treatment of osteoporosis. One promising, but highly preliminary, double-blind, placebo-controlled study suggests that the same combination therapy may improve symptoms of the severe neurological illness called Huntington's disease.

Use of a fish oil product as part of a total parenteral (intravenous feeding) nutrition regimen may help speed recovery after major abdominal surgery. For several other conditions, the current balance of the evidence suggests that fish oil is not effective.

For example, despite widely publicized claims that fish oil helps asthma, most preliminary studies have failed to provide evidence that it is effective, and one study found that fish oil can actually worsen aspirin-related asthma. However, there is some evidence that the use of fish oil could help prevent exercise-induced asthma in athletes. In a randomized-controlled trial with long-term follow-up, women who took fish-oil during late pregnancy reduced the risk of asthma in their children up to sixteen years later.

One study found that fish oil did not benefit the lung function of persons with cystic fibrosis. Similarly, a sixteen-week, double-blind, placebo-controlled study of 167 persons with recurrent migraine headaches found that fish oil did not significantly reduce headache frequency or severity. Conflicting results have been seen in other, much smaller trials of fish oil for migraines.

One study found weak evidence that the use of fish oil might decrease aggressive behavior in young girls (but, in this study, not in young boys). Another study found benefit in developmental coordination disorder (a condition in which children display a lack of physical coordination and problems with learning and behavior).

Fish oil is also sometimes recommended for enhancing immunity in human immunodeficiency virus (HIV) infection. However, one six-month, double-blind study found that a combination of the omega-3 fatty acids in fish oil plus the amino acid arginine was no more effective than placebo in improving immune function in people with HIV. Fish oil, however, might help persons with HIV gain weight.

In one large, randomized-controlled trial, diets rich in fish and omega-3 fatty acids from fish were associated with a significant reduction in the risk of developing colorectal cancer among men in a twenty-two-year period. Another study provides preliminary evidence for the benefits of fish oil in reducing the risk of prostate cancer. On balance, there is still relatively little evidence that the consumption of fish oil reduces cancer risk.

Preliminary studies have suggested that fish oil could help symptoms of multiple sclerosis; however, the largest double-blind study on the subject found no difference between people taking fish oil and those taking olive oil (used as a placebo). Although one study found fish oil somewhat helpful in psoriasis, a much larger study found no benefit.

DHA has been evaluated as a possible treatment for male infertility, but a double-blind trial of twenty-eight men with impaired sperm activity found no benefit. Combination therapy with gamma-linolenic acid (GLA) and fish oil failed to prove effective for cyclic breast pain.

One study failed to find fish oil more effective than placebo for treating stress. DHA also has been tried for slowing the progression of retinitis pigmentosa (a condition in which the retina gradually degenerates), but without much success. In observational studies, people who happen to consume a diet rich in omega-3 fatty acids seem to lower their risk of age-related macular degeneration (the most common cause of blindness in the elderly). However, in the absence of randomized-controlled trials, it is not possible to say whether or not it is omega-3 that produces this benefit.

Studies of fish oil have failed to find it helpful for Alzheimer's disease, whether for slowing its progression or improving symptoms. Also, one well-designed study failed to find any benefit of fish oil for enhancing memory and mental function in older adults without dementia in a twenty-six-week period. Use of essential fatty acids in the omega-3 family has also shown some promise for the treatment of nonalcoholic fatty liver.

SCIENTIFIC EVIDENCE

Heart disease prevention. Studies on fish or fish oil for preventing cardiovascular disease, slowing the progression of cardiovascular disease, and preventing heart-related death have returned somewhat contradictory results. A major review published in 2004 failed to find trustworthy evidence of benefit, and a subsequent study actually found that the use of fish oil increases risk of sudden death in people with stable heart disease. A 2008 systematic review found that fish oil was associated with modestly reduced cardiac mortality, but not sudden cardiac death, in eleven studies with more than thirty-two thousand participants.

The reliability of these results is limited by the inclusion of trials that were of low to moderate in quality. Though not entirely consistent, on balance the evidence does suggest that regularly consuming oily fish or taking omega-3 fatty acid supplements can reduce the risk of cardiovascular events (such as heart attacks) and deaths.

A 2009 review pooled data from eight trials examining the effect of omega-3 fatty acids on prevention of cardiac death in almost twenty-one thousand persons with coronary heart disease. This review separated persons into two general groups (those with previous myocardial infarction versus those with angina history) and found that omega-3 supplementation reduced risk of sudden cardiac death in persons with previous myocardial infarction, but increased risk in persons with angina. Though compelling, this finding may be limited because it was derived from a retrospective analysis of original data reorganized into subgroups.

A gigantic study (more than eighteen thousand participants) published in 2007 was widely described in the media as finally proving that fish oil helps prevent heart problems. However, this study lacked a placebo group; therefore, it failed to provide reliable evidence.

As noted, fish oil is hypothesized to exert several separate effects that act together to help protect the heart. The most important action of fish oil may be its apparent ability to reduce high triglyceride levels. Like cholesterol, triglycerides are a type of fat in the blood that tends to damage the arteries, leading to heart disease. According to most studies, fish oil supplements can reduce triglycerides by as much as 25 to 30 percent. In a detailed review of forty-seven randomized trials, researchers concluded that fish oil can significantly reduce triglyceride levels with no change in total cholesterol levels and only slight increases in HDL (good) cholesterol and LDL (bad) cholesterol.

A slightly modified form of fish oil (ethyl-omega-3 fatty acids) has been approved by the FDA as a treatment for elevated triglycerides. However, in some studies, the use of fish oil has markedly raised LDL cholesterol, which might offset some of the benefit. A 2009 review of thirty trials involving about fifteen hundred persons with type 2 diabetes demonstrated that marine-derived omega-3 polyunsaturated fatty acids (mean dose 2.4 g per day) lowered triglyceride levels but increased LDL cholesterol after an average twenty-four weeks of treatment.

Stanols and sterols (or phytosterols) are naturally occurring substances found in various plants that can help to lower cholesterol in persons with normal or mildly to moderately elevated levels. A study investigating the possible benefit of combining a phytosterol with fish oil found that together they significantly lowered total cholesterol, LDL-cholesterol, and triglycerides, and raised HDL (good) cholesterol in persons with undesirable cholesterol profiles.

Fish oil has been specifically studied for reducing triglyceride levels in people with diabetes, and it appears to do so safely and effectively. It also seems to remain effective in persons who are already using statin drugs to control lipid levels (people both with and without diabetes). However, one study found that the standard drug gemfibrozil is more effective than fish oil for reducing triglycerides.

Some but not all studies suggest that fish, fish oil, or EPA or DHA separately may also raise the level of HDL (good) cholesterol and possibly improve other aspects of cholesterol profile. This too should help prevent heart disease. Additionally, fish oil may help the heart by thinning the blood and by reducing blood levels of homocysteine, though not all studies have found a positive effect.

Studies contradict one another on whether fish oil can lower blood pressure, but on balance the supplement does seem to exert a modest positive effect. A six-week, double-blind, placebo-controlled study of fifty-nine overweight men suggests that the DHA in fish oil, not the EPA, is responsible for this benefit.

Evidence is conflicting on whether fish oil helps prevent heart arrhythmias. A large Italian trial involving almost seven thousand participants found that fish oil may modestly reduce the risk of death or admission to the hospital for cardiovascular reasons in persons with congestive heart failure. Finally, fish oil may slightly reduce heart rate. This effect could contribute to preventing heart attacks and other heart problems.

Rheumatoid arthritis. The results of numerous small, double-blind trials indicate that omega-3 fatty acids in fish oil can help reduce the symptoms of rheumatoid arthritis. One small study suggests that it may help persons with rheumatoid arthritis to lower their dose of nonsteroidal anti-inflammatory medication (such as ibuprofen). The benefits of the fish oil effect may be enhanced by a vegetarian diet. Simultaneous supplementation with olive oil (about two teaspoons daily) may further increase the benefits. However, unlike some conventional treatments, fish oil probably does not slow the progression of rheumatoid arthritis.

Menstrual pain. The regular use of fish oil may reduce the pain of menstrual cramps. In a four-month study of forty-two young women age fifteen to eighteen years, one-half the participants received a daily dose of 6 g of fish oil, providing 1,080 mg of EPA and 720 mg of DHA daily. After two months, they were switched to placebo for another two months. The other group received the same treatments in reverse order. The results showed that these young women experienced significantly less menstrual pain while they were taking fish oil.

Another double-blind study followed seventy-eight women, who received either fish oil, seal oil, fish oil with vitamin B$_{12}$ (7.5 mcg [micrograms] daily), or placebo for three full menstrual periods. Significant improvements were seen in all treatment groups, but the combination of fish oil and vitamin B$_{12}$ proved most effective, and its benefits continued for the longest time after treatment was stopped (three months). The researchers offered no explanation why vitamin B$_{12}$ should be helpful.

Bipolar disorder. A four-month, double-blind, placebo-controlled study of thirty people suggests that fish oil can enhance the effects of standard treatments for bipolar disorder, reducing risk of relapse and improving emotional state. Eleven of the fourteen persons who took fish oil improved or remained well during the course of the study, while only six of the sixteen given placebo responded similarly. Another small study found that ethyl-EPA (a modified form of EPA) is helpful for the depressive phase of bipolar disease.

Depression. A four-week, double-blind, placebo-controlled trial evaluated the potential benefits of fish oil in twenty persons with depression. All but one participant were also taking standard antidepressants and had been taking them for at least three months. By week three, the level of depression had improved to a significantly greater extent in the fish oil group than in the placebo group. Six of ten participants given fish oil, but only one of ten given placebo, showed at least a 50 percent reduction in depression scores by the end of the trial. (A reduction of this magnitude is considered a cure.)

A double-blind, placebo-controlled study of seventy people who were still depressed despite standard drug therapy (such as selective serotonin reuptake inhibitors) found that additional treatment with ethyl-EPA improved symptoms. Similar add-on benefits were seen in other double-blind studies of ethyl-EPA or mixed essential fatty acids. However, one study failed to find benefit with fish oil as an add-on treatment. Another double-blind study failed to find DHA alone helpful for depression. A third, relatively large placebo-controlled study found no benefit for fish oil in improving mental well-being among 320 older adults without a diagnosis of depression.

Postpartum depression. The effectiveness of fish oil supplementation in treating or preventing perinatal (including postpartum) depression is unclear. A small preliminary study of women found that fish oil was significantly more effective than placebo at alleviating postpartum depression. However, another small, placebo-controlled study was unable to show a benefit in women with depression, whether before or after delivery. In addition, a 2009 trial of 182 pregnant women with suspected low intake of DHA found that daily DHA supplementation (with or without arachidonic acid) did not reduce risk of postpartum depression, compared with placebo. Also, in another, much larger study involving 2,399 women, researchers found that fish oil capsules (a combination of DHA 800 mg per day and EPA 100 mg per day) did not prevent postpartum depression. It also did not improve the cognitive and language development in their children up to four years after their birth.

Raynaud's phenomenon. In small, double-blind studies, fish oil has been found to reduce the severe finger and toe responses to cold temperatures that occur in Raynaud's phenomenon. However, these studies suggest that a higher-than-usual dosage must be used to get results, perhaps 12 g daily.

Osteoporosis. There is some evidence that essential fatty acids may enhance the effectiveness of calcium in osteoporosis. In one study, sixty-five postmenopausal women were given calcium with either placebo or a combination of omega-6 fatty acids (from evening primrose oil) and omega-3 fatty acids (from fish oil) for eighteen months. At the end of the study period, the group receiving essential fatty acids had higher bone density and fewer fractures than the placebo group. However, a twelve-month, double-blind trial of forty-two postmenopausal women found no benefit.

The explanation for the discrepancy may lie in the differences between the women studied. The first study involved women living in nursing homes, while the second study looked at healthier women living on their own. The latter group of women may have been better nourished and already receiving enough essential fatty acids in their diet.

Lupus. Lupus is a serious autoimmune disease that can cause numerous problems, including fatigue, joint pain, and kidney disease. One small, thirty-four-week, double-blind, placebo-controlled crossover study compared placebo with daily doses of EPA (20 g) from fish oil. Seventeen persons completed the trial. Of these, fourteen showed improvement when taking EPA, while only four did so when treated with placebo. Another small study found similar benefits with fish oil in a twenty-four-week period. However, two small studies failed to find fish oil helpful for lupus nephritis (kidney damage caused by lupus).

Attention deficit disorder (ADD). Based on evidence that essential fatty acids are necessary for the proper development of brain function in growing children, essential fatty acids have been tried for the treatment of ADD and related conditions. A preliminary double-blind, placebo-controlled trial found some evidence that a supplement containing fish oil and evening primrose oil might improve ADD symptoms. However, a high dropout rate makes the results of this trial somewhat unreliable. Another small study examined fish oil in children with ADD who had thirst and skin problems. Benefits were seen with fish oil, but the benefits also occurred with placebo and did so to about the same extent.

Safety Issues

Fish oil appears to be generally safe. The most common problem is fishy burps. However, there are some safety concerns to consider.

For example, it has been suggested that some fish oil products contain excessive levels of toxic substances such as organochlorines and PCBs. If possible, one should try to purchase fish oil products certified not to contain significant levels of these contaminants. Various types of fish contain mercury, but this has not been a problem with fish oil supplements, according to some reports.

Fish oil has a mild blood-thinning effect; in one case report, it increased the effect of the blood-thinning medication warfarin (Coumadin). Fish oil does not seem to cause bleeding problems when it is taken by itself or with aspirin. Nonetheless, people who are at risk of bleeding complications for any reason should consult a physician before taking fish oil.

Fish oil does not appear to raise blood sugar levels in people with diabetes. Nonetheless, persons with diabetes should not take any supplement except on the advice of a physician.

Fish oil may modestly increase weight and lower total cholesterol and HDL (good) cholesterol levels. It may also raise the level of LDL (bad) cholesterol; however, this effect may be short-lived.

Persons deciding to use cod liver oil while finishing their fish oil supplement should avoid exceeding the safe maximum intake of vitamins A and D. These vitamins are fat soluble, which means that excess amounts tend to build up in the body, possibly reaching toxic levels. The official maximum daily intake of vitamin A is 3,000 mcg for pregnant women and other adults.

The bottle label will help one determine how much vitamin A one is receiving. (It is less likely that a person will get enough vitamin D to produce toxic effects.)

EBSCO CAM Review Board

FURTHER READING

Amminger, G. P., et al. "Long-Chain Omega-3 Fatty Acids for Indicated Prevention of Psychotic Disorders." *Archives of General Psychiatry* 67, no. 2 (2010): 146.

Chong, E. W., et al. "Dietary Omega-3 Fatty Acid and Fish Intake in the Primary Prevention of Age-Related Macular Degeneration." *Archives of Ophthalmology* 126 (2008): 826-833.

Damsgaard, C. T., et al. "Fish Oil in Combination with High or Low Intakes of Linoleic Acid Lowers Plasma Triacylglycerols but Does Not Affect Other Cardiovascular Risk Markers in Healthy Men." *Journal of Nutrition* 138 (2008): 1061-1066.

Hall, M. N., et al. "A Twenty-Two-Year Prospective Study of Fish, N-3 Fatty Acid Intake, and Colorectal Cancer Risk in Men." *Cancer Epidemiology, Biomarkers, and Prevention* 17 (2008): 1136-1143.

Hartweg, J., et al. "Potential Impact of Omega-3 Treatment on Cardiovascular Disease in Type 2 Diabetes." *Current Opinion in Lipidology* 20 (2009): 30-38.

Itomura, M., et al. "The Effect of Fish Oil on Physical Aggression in Schoolchildren." *Journal of Nutritional Biochemistry* 16 (2005): 163-171.

Lin, P. Y., and K. P. Su. "A Meta-Analytic Review of Double-Blind, Placebo-Controlled Trials of Antidepressant Efficacy of Omega-3 Fatty Acids." *Journal of Clinical Psychiatry* 68 (2007): 1056-1061.

Makrides, M., et al. "Effect of DHA Supplementation During Pregnancy on Maternal Depression and Neurodevelopment of Young Children." *Journal of the American Medical Association* 304, no. 15 (2010): 1675-1683.

Mozaffarian, D. "Fish and N-3 Fatty Acids for the Prevention of Fatal Coronary Heart Disease and Sudden Cardiac Death." *American Journal of Clinical Nutrition* 87 (2008): 1991S-1996S.

Olsen, S. F., et al. "Fish Oil Intake Compared with Olive Oil Intake in Late Pregnancy and Asthma in the Offspring." *American Journal of Clinical Nutrition* 88 (2008): 167-175.

Rees, A. M., M. P. Austin, and G. B. Parker. "Omega-3 Fatty Acids as a Treatment for Perinatal Depression." *Australian and New Zealand Journal of Psychiatry* 42 (2008): 199-205.

Schubert, R., et al. "Effect of N-3 Polyunsaturated Fatty Acids in Asthma After Low-Dose Allergen Challenge." *International Archives of Allergy and Immunology* 148 (2009): 321-329.

Su, K. P., et al. "Omega-3 Fatty Acids for Major Depressive Disorder During Pregnancy." *Journal of Clinical Psychiatry* 69 (2008): 644-651.

Van de Rest, O., et al. "Effect of Fish-Oil Supplementation on Mental Well-Being in Older Subjects." *American Journal of Clinical Nutrition* 88 (2008): 706-713.

Zhao, Y. T., et al. "Prevention of Sudden Cardiac Death with Omega-3 Fatty Acids in Patients with Coronary Heart Disease." *Annals of Medicine* 41 (2009): 301-310.

See also: Asthma; Atherosclerosis and heart disease prevention; Attention deficit disorder; Bipolar disorder; Cancer risk reduction; Cholesterol, high; Congestive heart failure; Dysmenorrhea; Gamma-linolenic acid (GLA); Heart attack; Hypertension; Lupus; Macular degeneration; Mental health; Pregnancy support; Rheumatoid arthritis; Stanols and sterols; Strokes; Vitamin B_{12}.

Fitzgerald, William H.

CATEGORY: Biography

IDENTIFICATION: American medical doctor who introduced zone therapy, later known as reflexology, to the United States

BORN: 1872

DIED: 1942

OVERVIEW

William H. Fitzgerald was an American ear, nose, and throat specialist who, with Edwin Bowers, introduced an early form of what is now known as reflexology to the United States in 1913. Fitzgerald claimed that applying pressure to certain parts of the body (especially the hands and feet) had an anesthetic effect on other areas of the body. Fitzgerald graduated with a medical degree from the University of Vermont in 1895, worked at Boston City Hospital for about two years, then worked as a physician at a nose and throat hospital in London, and later became the head of the nose and throat department at St. Francis in Hartford, Connecticut.

Fitzgerald commonly recommended, for example, the use of clothes pins or rubber bands to pinch certain regions, or zones, of the extremities to overcome or cope with pain in other areas of the body. Such practices were said to have helped persons undergoing dental surgery, minor ear or nose surgeries, and even childbirth. In addition, he reported that electrical shock and lasers could be useful treatments for certain ailments. He posited that such therapy not only could provide an anesthetic effect but also could sometimes remedy the underlying cause of the pain or ailment.

With Edwin Bowers, Fitzgerald published the book *Zone Therapy* (1917), the name by which reflexology was known until the early 1960s. This book was intended to instruct persons on self-treatment between clinical visits, and it thus received much public attention, especially from "working men," after its publication. It is believed that reflexology had received a large amount of attention because it was based on a noninvasive healing method that could be carried out in the home.

Fitzgerald's practices were advocated by a number of esteemed colleagues during his lifetime, including Benedict Lust (the founder of naturopathy in the United States), and were further developed by other influential reflexologists, such as Eunice D. Ingham, who brought the field closer to its current state. Fitzgerald and the practice of reflexology have also received criticism from other clinicians, especially those rooted in more traditional modern medicine. However, Fitzgerald's and Bowers's ideas and practices continue to be used and expanded upon.

Brandy Weidow, M.S.

FURTHER READING

Issel, Christine. *Reflexology: Art, Science, and History*. 4th ed. Frenchs Forest, N.S.W.: New Frontier, 1990.

Fitzgerald, William H., and Edwin Frederick Bowers. *Zone Therapy: Or, Relieving Pain at Home*. Reprint. Whitefish, Mont.: Kessinger, 2007.

Marquardt, Hanne. *Reflex Zone Therapy of the Feet: A Textbook for Therapists*. Rochester, Vt.: Healing Arts Press, 1988.

See also: Acupressure; Bowers, Edwin; Lust, Benedict; Manipulative and body-based practices; Massage therapy; Pain management; Reflexology.

5-Hydroxytryptophan

CATEGORY: Herbs and supplements
RELATED TERM: 5-HTP
DEFINITION: Natural plant product used as a dietary supplement for specific health benefits.
PRINCIPAL PROPOSED USES: Depression, migraines, and other types of headaches
OTHER PROPOSED USES: Anxiety, fibromyalgia, insomnia, weight loss

OVERVIEW

Many antidepressant drugs work by raising serotonin levels. The supplement 5-hydroxytryptophan (5-HTP) has been tried in cases of depression for a similar reason: The body uses 5-HTP to make serotonin, so providing the body with 5-HTP might, therefore, raise serotonin levels.

As a supplement, 5-HTP has also been proposed for the same uses as other antidepressants, including aiding weight loss, preventing migraine headaches, decreasing the pain and discomfort of fibromyalgia, improving sleep quality, and reducing anxiety.

SOURCES

The supplement 5-HTP is not found in foods to any appreciable extent. For use as a supplement, it is manufactured from the seeds of an African plant called *Griffonia simplicifolia*.

THERAPEUTIC DOSAGES

A typical dosage of 5-HTP is 100 to 300 milligrams (mg) three times daily. Once 5-HTP starts to work, it may be possible to reduce the dosage significantly and still maintain good results.

THERAPEUTIC USES

The primary use of 5-HTP is for depression. Several small, short-term studies have found that it may be as effective as standard antidepressant drugs. Because standard antidepressants are also used for insomnia and anxiety, 5-HTP has also been suggested as a treatment for those conditions, but there is only preliminary evidence that it works.

Similarly, antidepressant drugs are often used for migraine headaches. Some studies suggest that the regular use of 5-HTP may help reduce the frequency and severity of migraines and may help other types of headaches. Additionally, preliminary evidence suggests that 5-HTP can reduce symptoms of fibromyalgia and perhaps help a person lose weight.

SCIENTIFIC EVIDENCE

Depression. Several small studies have compared 5-HTP to standard antidepressants. The best trial was a six-week study of sixty-three people given either 5-HTP (100 mg three times daily) or an antidepressant in the Prozac family (fluvoxamine, 50 mg three times daily). Researchers found equal benefit with the supplement and with the drug. However, 5-HTP caused fewer and less severe side effects.

Migraine and other headaches. There is some evidence that 5-HTP may help prevent migraines when taken at a dosage of 400 to 600 mg daily. Lower doses may not be effective.

In a six-month trial of 124 people, 5-HTP (600 mg daily) proved just as effective as the standard drug methysergide. The most dramatic benefits observed were reductions in the intensity and duration of migraines. Because methysergide has been proven better than placebo for migraine headaches in earlier studies, the study results provide meaningful, although not airtight, evidence that 5-HTP is also effective.

Similarly good results were seen in another comparative study, using a different medication and 5-HTP (at a dose of 400 mg daily). However, in another study, 5-HTP (up to 300 mg daily) was less effective than

the drug propranolol. Also, in a study involving children, 5-HTP failed to demonstrate benefit. Other studies that are sometimes quoted as evidence that 5-HTP is effective for migraines actually enrolled adults or children with many different types of headaches (including migraines).

Putting all this evidence together, it appears likely that 5-HTP can help people with frequent migraine headaches if taken in sufficient doses, but further research needs to be done. In particular, what is needed is a large double-blind study that compares 5-HTP with placebo over a period of several months.

Finally, an eight-week, double-blind, placebo-controlled trial of sixty-five people (mostly women) with tension headaches found that 5-HTP at a dose of 100 mg three times daily did not significantly reduce the number of headaches experienced; however, it did reduce participants' need to use other pain-relieving medications.

Obesity (weight loss). The drug fenfluramine (with phentermine) made up the infamous Fen-Phen for weight loss. Although successful for weight loss, fenfluramine was later associated with damage to the valves of the heart and was removed from the market. Because fenfluramine raises serotonin levels, it seems reasonable to believe that other substances that affect serotonin might also be useful for weight reduction.

Four small, double-blind, placebo-controlled clinical trials examined whether 5-HTP can aid weight loss. The first, a double-blind crossover study, found that the use of 5-HTP (at a daily dose of 8 mg per kilogram of body weight) reduced caloric intake even though the nineteen participants made no conscious effort to eat less. Participants given placebo consumed about 2,300 calories per day, while those taking 5-HTP ate only 1,800 calories daily. The use of 5-HTP appeared to lead to a significantly enhanced sense of satiety after eating. In five weeks, women taking 5-HTP effortlessly lost more than three pounds of body weight.

A follow-up study by the same research group enrolled twenty overweight women who were trying to lose weight. Participants received either 5-HTP (900 mg per day) or placebo for two consecutive six-week periods. During the first period, there was no dietary restriction, while during the second period, participants were encouraged to follow a defined diet expected to lead to weight loss.

Participants receiving placebo did not lose weight during either period. However, those receiving 5-HTP

What Is a Dietary Supplement?

A dietary supplement, including the herbal product 5-hydroxytryptophan, as defined in the Dietary Supplement Health and Education Act (DSHEA) of 1994, is a product taken by mouth that contains a "dietary ingredient" intended to supplement the diet. The dietary ingredients in these products may include vitamins, minerals, herbs or other botanicals, amino acids, and substances such as enzymes, organ tissues, glandulars, and metabolites. Dietary supplements can also be extracts or concentrates, and they may be found in many forms, such as tablets, capsules, soft gels, gel caps, liquids, and powders. DSHEA places dietary supplements in a special category under the general umbrella of "foods," not drugs, and requires that every supplement be properly labeled.

lost about 2 percent of their initial body weight during the no-diet period and an additional 3 percent while on the diet. Thus, a woman with an initial weight of 170 pounds lost about 3.5 pounds after six weeks of using 5-HTP without dieting and another 5 pounds while dieting. Once again, participants taking 5-HTP experienced quicker satiety.

Similar benefits were seen in a double-blind study of fourteen overweight women given 900 mg of 5-HTP daily. Finally, a double-blind, placebo-controlled study of twenty overweight people with type 2 diabetes found that the use of 5-HTP (750 mg per day) without intentional dieting resulted in about a 4.5-pound weight loss in two weeks. The use of 5-HTP reduced carbohydrate intake by 75 percent and fat intake to a lesser extent.

Fibromyalgia. Antidepressants are the primary conventional treatment for fibromyalgia, a little-understood disease characterized by painful and tender muscles, fatigue, and disturbed sleep. One study suggests that 5-HTP also may be helpful for fibromyalgia. In this double-blind trial, fifty persons with fibromyalgia were given either 100 mg of 5-HTP or placebo three times daily for one month. Those receiving 5-HTP experienced significant improvements in all symptom categories, including pain, stiffness, sleep patterns, anxiety, and fatigue.

Anxiety. An eight-week, double-blind, placebo-controlled study compared 5-HTP and the drug clomipramine in forty-five people suffering from anxiety disorders. The results showed that 5-HTP was effective, but clomipramine was more effective.

SAFETY ISSUES

No significant adverse effects have been reported in clinical trials of 5-HTP. Side effects appear to be generally limited to short-term, mild digestive distress and possible allergic reactions.

One potential safety issue with 5-HTP involves an interaction with a medication used for Parkinson's disease: carbidopa. Several reports suggest that the combination can create skin changes similar to those that occur in the disease scleroderma.

According to several reports, dogs that have consumed excessive amounts of 5-HTP have developed signs of excess serotonin. In humans, this so-called serotonin syndrome includes such symptoms as confusion, agitation, rapid heart rate, high blood pressure, muscle jerks, loss of coordination, sweating, shivering,

and fever; rapid breathing, coma, and death are possible. Serotonin syndrome might also occur if 5-HTP is combined with drugs that raise serotonin levels, such as selective serotonin reuptake inhibitors (including Prozac), other antidepressants, or the pain medication tramadol.

There are some reasons for concern that 5-HTP could increase the risk of "infantile spasms" (technically, massive myoclonic seizure disorder) in developmentally disabled children. Although safety in children in general has not been proven, children have been given 5-HTP in studies without any apparent harmful effects. Safety in pregnant or nursing women and those with liver or kidney disease has not been established.

Peak X. One report in 1998 raised a potential safety concern with 5-HTP. Researchers discovered evidence of an unidentified substance called peak X in a limited number of 5-HTP products.

Peak X has a frightening history involving a supplement related to 5-HTP: tryptophan. The body turns tryptophan into 5-HTP, and the two supplements have similar effects in the body. Until the late 1980s, tryptophan was widely used as a sleep aid. However, it was taken off the market when thousands of people using tryptophan developed a disabling and sometimes fatal blood disorder called eosinophilia myalgia. Peak X, introduced through a manufacturer's mistake, is thought to have been the cause, although not all experts agree.

Despite this one report, it seems unlikely that 5-HTP could present the same risk as tryptophan. It is manufactured completely differently; peak X has not been seen again in 5-HTP samples, and no epidemic of eosinophilia myalgia has occurred with 5-HTP use.

IMPORTANT INTERACTIONS

Persons should not take 5-HTP, except on a physician's advice, if also taking prescription antidepressants (including selective serotonin reuptake inhibitors, monoamine oxidase inhibitors, or tricyclics), the pain drug tramadol, or migraine drugs in the triptan family (such as sumatriptan). One also should avoid taking the Parkinson's disease medication carbidopa at the same time as 5-HTP; the two together could cause skin changes similar to those that develop in the disease scleroderma.

EBSCO CAM Review Board

FURTHER READING

Cangiano, C., et al. "Effects of Oral 5-Hydroxy-Tryptophan on Energy Intake and Macronutrient Selection in Non-insulin-Dependent Diabetic Patients." *International Journal of Obesity and Related Metabolic Disorders* 22 (1998): 648-654.

Das, Y. T., et al. "Safety of 5-Hydroxy-L-Tryptophan." *Toxicology Letters* 150 (2004): 111-122.

Ribeiro, C. A. F. "L-5-Hydroxytryptophan in the Prophylaxis of Chronic Tension-Type Headache." *Headache* 40 (2000): 451-456.

See also: Anxiety and panic attacks; Depression, mild to moderate; Fibromyalgia: Homeopathic remedies; Headache, cluster; Headache, tension; Insomnia; Migraines.

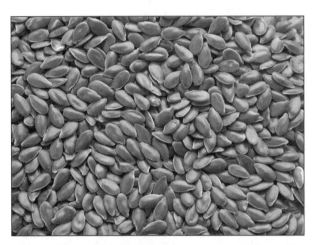

Flaxseeds contain a type of omega-3 fatty acid similar to that found in fish oil and can offer some of the same benefits. (©Picsfive/Dreamstime.com)

Flaxseed

CATEGORY: Functional foods

RELATED TERM: Linseed

DEFINITION: Plant product consumed for specific health benefits.

PRINCIPAL PROPOSED USES: Constipation, heart disease, high cholesterol

OTHER PROPOSED USES: Benign prostatic hyperplasia, cancer prevention, diverticulitis, dyspepsia, high cholesterol, irritable bowel syndrome, liver disease, lupus nephritis, menopausal symptoms, skin inflammation

OVERVIEW

Flaxseed is the hard, tiny seed of *Linum usitatissimum*, the flax plant, which has been widely used for thousands of years as a source of food and clothing. There are a minimum of three flaxseed components with potential health benefits. The first is fiber, valuable in treating constipation. Flaxseed also contains alpha-linolenic acid, a type of omega-3 fatty acid similar to the omega-3 fatty acids found in fish oil but significantly different in other ways and perhaps offering some of the same benefits. Finally, substances called lignans in flaxseed have phytoestrogenic properties, making them somewhat similar to the isoflavones in soy. The oil made from flaxseed has no appreciable amounts of lignans, but it does contain alpha-linolenic acid.

THERAPEUTIC DOSAGES

According to the European Scientific Cooperative on Phytotherapy, the usual dose of flaxseed for constipation is 5 grams (g) of whole, cracked, or freshly crushed seeds soaked in water and taken with a glassful of liquid three times a day. Effects begin in eighteen to twenty-four hours. Because of this time delay, it is recommended to take flaxseed for a minimum of two to three days. Children age six to twelve years should be given one-half the adult dose, while children younger than age six years should be treated only under the guidance of a physician.

To soothe an upset stomach, one should soak 5 to 10 g of whole flaxseed in one-half cup of water, strain after twenty to thirty minutes, then drink. For painful skin inflammations, the recommended dose is 30 to 50 g of crushed or powdered seed applied externally as a warm poultice or compress.

Like other sources of fiber, flaxseed should be taken with plenty of fluids, or it may actually worsen constipation. Also, it is best to start with smaller doses and then increase.

USES AND APPLICATIONS

The fiber in flaxseed binds with water, swelling to form a gel that, like other forms of fiber, helps soften the stool and move it along in the intestines. One study found that flaxseed can help with chronic constipation in irritable bowel disease. German health authorities approve of the use of flaxseed for various digestive problems, such as chronic constipation, irritable bowel syndrome, diverticulitis, and general stomach discomfort.

Flaxseed may be slightly helpful for improving cholesterol profile, according to some studies. Purified alpha linolenic acid or lignans alone have not consistently shown benefits. It may be the generic fiber and not the other specific ingredients in flaxseed that improve cholesterol levels.

Flaxseed, its lignans, and its oil have undergone a small amount of investigation for potential cancer prevention or cancer treatment possibilities. Flaxseed has shown some promise for treating kidney disease associated with lupus (lupus nephritis). Because it is believed to have soothing properties, flaxseed is sometimes used for symptomatic relief of stomach distress and is applied externally for inflammation of the skin. However, research on these potential uses is essentially nonexistent.

Although flaxseed is often advocated for the treatment of symptoms related to menopause, a sizable twelve-month study failed to find it more helpful than wheat germ placebo. Besides failing to improve immediate symptoms such as hot flashes, flaxseed did not appear to provide any protection against loss of bone density. An earlier, much smaller study by the same researchers found it equally effective for menopausal symptoms as hormone replacement therapy, but because of the absence of a placebo group and the high rate of placebo response in menopausal symptoms, these results cannot be taken as indicating much. Another study tested flaxseed without comparing it with placebo and reported a 50 percent reduction in hot flashes. The researchers went on to state that this reduction in hot flashes was "greater than what would be expected with placebo," a rather curious claim because menopausal women given placebo typically experience almost exactly a 50 percent decrease in hot flashes.

In a preliminary double-blind trial of seventy-eight older men, flaxseed extract modestly improved the urinary symptoms associated with benign prostatic hyperplasia (prostate enlargement) after four months of treatment. The use of essential fatty acids in the omega-3 family has also shown some promise for the treatment of nonalcoholic fatty liver.

SCIENTIFIC EVIDENCE

Constipation. In a double-blind study, fifty-five people with chronic constipation caused by irritable bowel syndrome received either ground flaxseed or psyllium seed (a well-known treatment for constipation) daily for three months. Those taking flaxseed had significantly fewer problems with constipation, abdominal pain, and bloating than those taking psyllium. The flaxseed group had even further improvements in constipation and bloating while continuing their treatment in the three months after the double-blind part of the study ended. The researcher concluded that flaxseed relieved constipation more effectively than psyllium.

Cholesterol and atherosclerosis. Some human studies have found that flaxseed improves cholesterol profile. However, the benefits, if they do exist, are very modest. For example, in a double-blind study of about two hundred postmenopausal women, the use of flaxseed at a dose of 40 g daily produced measurable improvements in cholesterol profile, but the improvements were so small that the researchers considered them "clinically insignificant." It has been claimed that flaxseed might also have a direct effect in helping to prevent atherosclerosis based on its lignan ingredients, but the evidence upon which these claims are based is limited to studies in rabbits.

Cancer. Some evidence hints that flaxseed or its lignan components might have cancer-preventive properties. Observational studies and other forms of preliminary evidence suggest that people who eat more lignan-containing foods have a lower incidence of breast cancer and perhaps colon cancer.

The lignans in flaxseed are phytoestrogens, plant chemicals mimicking the effects of estrogen in the body: Phytoestrogens hook onto the same spots on cells where estrogen attaches. If there is little estrogen in the body, for example after menopause, lignans may act like weak estrogen. However, when natural estrogen is abundant, lignans may reduce the hormone's effects by displacing it from cells; displacing estrogen in this manner might help prevent those cancers that depend on estrogen, such as breast cancer, from starting and developing. (This is also, in part, how soy is believed to work in breast cancer prevention, although the phytoestrogens in soy are isoflavones.)

Some preliminary research indicates that these lignans may also fight cancer in other ways, perhaps by acting as antioxidants. Animal studies using flaxseed and its lignans offer supporting evidence for a potential cancer-preventive or even cancer-treatment effect; several found that one or the other inhibited breast and colon cancer in animals and reduced metastases from melanoma (a type of skin cancer) in mice. Test-tube studies have found that flaxseed or one of its lignans inhibited the growth of human breast cancer cells, and that the lignans enterolactone and enterodiol inhibited the growth of human colon tumor cells. This preliminary research is promising, but much more is needed before any conclusions can be drawn. Although much of this anticancer work has focused on the lignans in flaxseed, one study also found that flaxseed oil, which contains no appreciable amounts of lignans, slowed the growth of malignant breast tumors in rats.

SAFETY ISSUES

Flaxseed is generally believed to be safe. However, there are some potential risks to consider. As with many substances, there have been reports of life-threatening allergic reactions to flaxseed.

Because of its potential effects on estrogen, pregnant or breast-feeding women should probably avoid flaxseed. One study found that pregnant rats who ate large amounts of flaxseed (5 or 10 percent of their diet) or one of its lignans, gave birth to offspring with altered reproductive organs and functions (in humans, eating 25 g of flaxseed per day amounts to about 5 percent of the diet). Lignans were also found to be transferred to baby rats during nursing. Additionally, a study of postmenopausal women found that the use of flaxseed reduced estrogen levels and increased levels of prolactin. This suggests hormonal effects that could be problematic in pregnancy.

Flaxseed may not be safe for women with a history of estrogen-sensitive cancer, such as breast or uterine cancer. A few test-tube studies suggest that certain cancer cells can be stimulated by lignans such as those present in flaxseed. Other studies found that lignans inhibit cancer cell growth. As with estrogen, lignans' positive or negative effects on cancer cells may depend on dose, type of cancer cell, and levels of hormones in the body. Persons with a history of cancer, particularly breast cancer, should consult a doctor before consuming large amounts of flaxseed.

Flaxseed (like other high-fiber foods) may delay glucose absorption. This may lead to better blood sugar control but it also may increase the risk of hypoglycemic reactions. Persons with diabetes should consult a doctor about appropriate use.

Finally, flaxseed contains tiny amounts of cyanide-containing substances, which can be a problem among livestock eating large amounts of flax. While normal cooking and baking of whole flaxseed or flour eliminates any detectable amounts of cyanide, it is theoretically possible that eating huge amounts of raw or unprocessed flaxseed or flaxseed meal could pose a problem. However, most authorities do not think this presents much of a risk in real life.

EBSCO CAM Review Board

FURTHER READING

Bloedon, L. T., et al. "Flaxseed and Cardiovascular Risk Factors." *Journal of the American College of Nutrition* 27 (2008): 65-74.

Dodin, S., et al. "The Effects of Flaxseed Dietary Supplement on Lipid Profile, Bone Mineral Density, and Symptoms in Menopausal Women." *Journal of Clinical Endocrinology and Metabolism* 90 (2005): 1390-1397.

Pruthi, S., et al. "Pilot Evaluation of Flaxseed for the Management of Hot Flashes." *Journal of the Society for Integrative Oncology* 5 (2007): 106-112.

Stuglin, C., and K. Prasad. "Effect of Flaxseed Consumption on Blood Pressure, Serum Lipids, Hemopoietic System, and Liver and Kidney Enzymes in Healthy Humans." *Journal of Cardiovascular Pharmacology and Therapeutics* 10 (2005): 23-27.

Thompson, L. U., et al. "Dietary Flaxseed Alters Tumor Biological Markers in Postmenopausal Breast Cancer." *Clinical Cancer Research* 11 (2005): 3828-3835.

Zhang, W., et al. "Effects of Dietary Flaxseed Lignan Extract on Symptoms of Benign Prostatic Hyperplasia." *Journal of Medicinal Food* 1 (2008): 207-214.

See also: Cetylated fatty acids; Cholesterol, high; Flaxseed oil; Functional foods: Introduction; Hypertension; Lignans.

Flaxseed oil

CATEGORY: Functional foods
RELATED TERMS: Alpha-linolenic acid, linseed oil
DEFINITION: Plant product consumed for specific health benefits.
PRINCIPAL PROPOSED USES: None
OTHER PROPOSED USES: Bipolar disorder, cancer prevention, heart disease prevention, high blood pressure, high cholesterol, pregnancy support, rheumatoid arthritis, Sjögren's syndrome

OVERVIEW

Flaxseed oil, which is derived from the hard, tiny seeds of the flax plant, has been proposed as a less smelly alternative to fish oil. Like fish oil, flaxseed oil contains omega-3 fatty acids, a type of fat the body needs as much as it needs vitamins.

However, it is important to realize that the omega-3 fatty acids in flaxseed oil are not identical to those in fish oil. Flaxseed oil contains alpha-linolenic acid (ALA), while fish oil contains eicosapentaenoic acid and docosahexaenoic acid. The effects and potential benefits may not be the same.

Whole flaxseed contains another important group of chemicals known as lignans. Lignans are being studied for use in preventing cancer. However, flaxseed oil contains no lignans.

REQUIREMENTS AND SOURCES

Flaxseed oil contains both omega-3 and omega-6 fatty acids, which are essential to health. Although the exact daily requirement of these essential fatty acids is not known, deficiencies are believed to be fairly common. Flaxseed oil may be an economical way to ensure that one gets enough essential fatty acids in the diet.

The essential fatty acids in flax can be damaged by exposure to heat, light, and oxygen (essentially, they become rancid). For this reason, one should not cook with flaxseed oil. A good product should be sold in an opaque container, and the manufacturing process should keep the temperature under 100° Fahrenheit. Some manufacturers combine the product with vitamin E because it helps prevent rancidity.

THERAPEUTIC DOSAGES

A typical dosage is 1 to 2 tablespoons of flaxseed oil daily. It can be taken in capsule form or made into salad dressing. Some people find the taste pleasant, although others would disagree. For whole flaxseed, a typical dose is 1 tablespoon of the seed (not ground) with plenty of liquid two to three times daily.

THERAPEUTIC USES

The best use of flaxseed oil is as a general nutritional supplement to provide essential fatty acids. There is little evidence that it is effective for any specific therapeutic purpose.

Flaxseed oil has been proposed as a less smelly alternative to fish oil for the prevention of heart disease. However, there is no consistent evidence that it works. One double-blind study of fifty-six people failed to find that flax oil improved cholesterol profile. Other studies did find improvements in cholesterol or blood pressure (or both), but these were small trials and they had serious problems in study design.

One study found that a diet high in ALA (from sources other than flaxseed oil) was associated with a reduced risk of heart disease. However, there were so many other factors involved that it is hard to say what caused what.

Sjögren's syndrome is an autoimmune condition in which the immune system destroys moisture-producing glands, such as tear glands and salivary glands. It can occur by itself or with other autoimmune diseases, such as lupus. One small double-blind study found preliminary evidence that the use of flaxseed oil at a dose of one to two grams daily can improve dry eye symptoms in Sjögren's syndrome.

One preliminary study hints that flaxseed oil may enhance the effects of conventional treatments for bipolar disorder when combined with conventional medications. It has been suggested that flaxseed oil may have anticancer effects because of its ALA and lignan content. However, the supporting evidence for this belief is incomplete and somewhat contradictory (some studies actually found weak evidence of increased cancer risk with higher ALA intake). Although fish oil appears to be effective for reducing symptoms of rheumatoid arthritis, one study failed to find flaxseed oil helpful for this purpose. Another study failed to find flaxseed oil helpful for preventing premature birth. One small randomized trial found flaxseed oil ineffective for reducing blood sugar in people with type 2 diabetes.

SAFETY ISSUES

Flaxseed oil appears to be a safe nutritional supplement when used as recommended. However, because of the contradictory evidence regarding its effects on cancer, persons at high risk of cancer should not take flaxseed oil except on the advice of a physician.

EBSCO CAM Review Board

FURTHER READING

Barre, D. E., et al. "High Dose Flaxseed Oil Supplementation May Affect Fasting Blood Serum Glucose Management in Human Type 2 Diabetics." *Journal of Oleo Science* 57 (2008): 269-273.

Maillard, V., et al. "N-3 and N-6 Fatty Acids in Breast Adipose Tissue and Relative Risk of Breast Cancer in a Case-Control Study in Tours, France." *International Journal of Cancer* 98 (2002): 78-83.

Neukam, et al. "Supplementation of Flaxseed Oil Diminishes Skin Sensitivity and Improves Skin Barrier Function and Condition." *Skin Pharmacology and Physiology* 24 (2010): 67-74.

Paschos, G. K., et al. "Dietary Supplementation with Flaxseed Oil Lowers Blood Pressure in Dyslipidaemic Patients." *European Journal of Clinical Nutrition* 61 (2007): 1201-1206.

See also: Cetylated fatty acids; Cholesterol, high; Flaxseed; Functional foods: Introduction; Hypertension; Lignans.

Fluoride

CATEGORY: Herbs and supplements

RELATED TERMS: Sodium fluoride, sodium hexafluorosilicate, sodium monofluorophosphate, stannous fluoride, water fluoridation

DEFINITION: Chemical compound used to prevent specific medical conditions and diseases.

PRINCIPAL PROPOSED USE: Cavity prevention

OTHER PROPOSED USE: Osteoporosis prevention

OVERVIEW

While conventional dentistry tends to regard the use of fluoride to prevent cavities as a remarkable triumph of preventive medicine, proponents of alternative medicine have long taken the opposite view. To them, water fluoridation, in particular, is a form of medically sanctioned environmental pollution. These strongly emotional and diametrically opposed views have created a murky world of charges and countercharges. This article is limited to the current scientific evidence regarding fluoride and cavities and avoids delving into the numerous myths, rumors, exaggerations, and conspiracy theories associated with the topic.

THERAPEUTIC USES

Fluorine is an element in the family of chlorine, bromine, and iodine. A "fluoride" is a certain type of chemical compound containing fluorine. The most common forms of fluoride used to prevent cavities

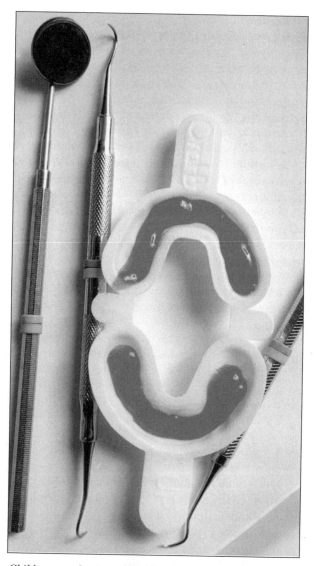

Children may be given fluoride treatments as a gel in a foam mouthpiece in order to protect against the formation of cavaties. (AP Photo)

are sodium fluoride (analogous to sodium chloride, or common salt), sodium monofluorophosphate, and sodium hexafluorosilicate. Stannous fluoride, a compound containing tin, was once popular, but it is now seldom used.

The use of fluorine for preventing cavities originally derived, at least in part, from the observation that people who grow up drinking water that is high in fluorides, but not too high, have a much reduced incidence of cavities. This observation led dental researchers to conclude that if fluoride is present during the initial stages of tooth formation, those teeth will emerge with stronger enamel. Direct application of fluoride to teeth also was thought to provide benefit, but to a lesser extent. Therefore, it became common practice to recommend that infants and young children receive fluoride supplementation, through either the water supply or fluoride supplements.

However, subsequent evidence has shown that these early researchers had it backward. It appears that fluoride acts only on teeth that have already erupted. When fluoride comes in direct contact with tooth enamel, it replaces some of the calcium in the enamel, forming a surface that is more resistant to cavities. The only dental value of fluoridated water, therefore, occurs during the process of drinking it, when the fluoride in the water bathes the surface of the teeth.

However, there are more direct ways of bringing fluoride into contact with tooth enamel. The most common of these is the use of fluoride toothpastes. Very strong evidence shows that such toothpastes help prevent cavities. These toothpastes are so widely used, in fact, that water fluoridation is probably of little to no value except in poorer, less-developed countries, where use of fluoride toothpastes is not so universal.

Fluoride mouth rinses, available over the counter, may offer additional benefit to fluoride toothpastes. However, there is little to no scientific support for the use of the much more expensive, professionally applied fluoride varnishes.

Just as fluoride replaces some of the calcium in dental enamel, fluoride can also replace calcium in bone. This has led to the hypothesis that fluoridated water may prevent osteoporosis. On the other hand, when too much calcium is replaced by fluoride, bone strength decreases. For this reason, it has been suggested that water fluoridation may increase the risk of osteoporosis. However, a judicious examination of the evidence suggests that neither of these outcomes occurs in real life: Water fluoridation appears to have little or no effect on osteoporosis rates, one way or the other.

EBSCO CAM Review Board

FURTHER READING

Demos, L. L., et al. "Water Fluoridation, Osteoporosis, Fractures: Recent Developments." *Australian Dental Journal* 46 (2001): 80-87.

Pizzo, G., et al. "Community Water Fluoridation and Caries Prevention." *Clinical Oral Investigations* 11 (2007): 189-193.

See also: Cavity prevention; Children's health; Osteoporosis.

Fluoroquinolones

CATEGORY: Drug interactions
DEFINITION: Types of antibiotics used to treat urinary tract infections and other infectious diseases.
INTERACTIONS: Dong quai, fennel, minerals, St. John's wort
DRUGS IN THIS FAMILY: Ciprofloxacin (Cipro), enoxacin (Penetrex), grepafloxacin (Raxar), levofloxacin (Levaquin), lomefloxacin (Maxaquin), norfloxacin (Noroxin), ofloxacin (Floxin), sparfloxacin (Zagam), trovafloxacin/alatrofloxacin (Trovan)

MINERALS

Effect: Take at a Different Time of Day

The minerals calcium, iron, magnesium, and zinc can interfere with the absorption of fluoroquinolones (and vice versa). Therefore, persons taking supplements of these minerals should take them a minimum of two hours before or after taking the dose of fluoroquinolone.

FENNEL

Effect: Possible Harmful Interaction

The herb fennel appears to reduce blood levels of ciprofloxacin, possibly impairing its effectiveness. This finding comes from a placebo-controlled study in rats. Fennel might be expected to interfere similarly with other fluoroquinolone antibiotics.

Allowing two hours between taking ciprofloxacin and fennel should reduce the potential for an interaction but may not eliminate it. For this reason, it may be advisable to avoid fennel supplementation during therapy with ciprofloxacin or other antibiotics in this family.

DONG QUAI, ST. JOHN'S WORT

Effect: Possible Harmful Interaction

Fluoroquinolone antibiotics have been reported to cause increased sensitivity to the sun, amplifying the risk of sunburn or skin rash. Because St. John's wort and dong quai may also cause this problem, taking these herbal supplements during treatment with fluoroquinolone drugs might add to the risk. One should use sunscreen or wear protective clothing during sun exposure if also taking one of these herbs with a fluoroquinolone antibiotic.

EBSCO CAM Review Board

FURTHER READING

Campbell, N. R., and B. B. Hasinoff. "Iron Supplements: A Common Cause of Drug Interactions." *British Journal of Clinical Pharmacology* 31, no. 3 (1991): 251-255.

Lim, D., and M. McKay. "Food-Drug Interactions." *Drug Information Bulletin* 15, no. 2 (1995).

See also: Antibiotics, general; Dong quai; Fennel; Food and Drug Administration; St. John's wort; Supplements: Overview; Vitamins and minerals.

Folate

CATEGORY: Herbs and supplements
RELATED TERMS: Folacin, folic acid
DEFINITION: Essential natural substance used as a dietary supplement for specific health benefits.
PRINCIPAL PROPOSED USES: Cancer prevention, depression, heart disease prevention, prevention of birth defects and disorders, reduction of methotrexate side effects
OTHER PROPOSED USES: Bipolar disorder, enhancing memory and mental function, hearing loss, gout, improving action of drugs in the nitroglycerin family, migraine headaches, nutritional support for cigarette smokers, osteoarthritis, osteoporosis, periodontal disease, restless legs syndrome, rheumatoid arthritis, seborrheic dermatitis, stroke prevention, vitiligo

OVERVIEW

Folate, a B vitamin, plays a critical role in many biological processes. It participates in the crucial biological process known as methylation and plays an important role in cell division: Without sufficient amounts of folate, cells cannot divide properly. Adequate folate intake can reduce the risk of heart disease and prevent

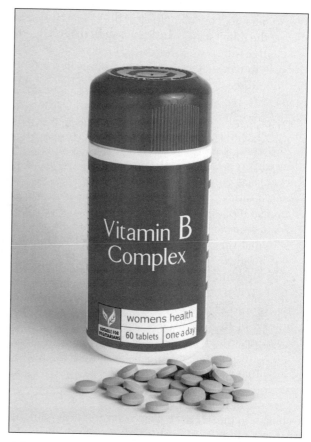

A bottle and pills containing vitamin B complex supplements. (Cordelia Molloy/Photo Researchers, Inc.)

serious birth defects and disorders, and it may lessen the risk of developing certain forms of cancer.

REQUIREMENTS AND SOURCES

Folate requirements rise with age. The official U.S. and Canadian recommendations for daily intake of folate (in micrograms) are as follows: infants to six months of age (65) and seven to twelve months of age (80); children age one to three years (150) and four to eight years (200); children age nine to thirteen years (300); children and adults age fourteen and older (400); pregnant females (600); and nursing females (500).

Folate deficiency was fairly common in the developed world, causing thousands of children to be born with preventable birth defects. However, in 1998, widespread fortification of cereal products began in Canada and the United States. As a result, the prevalence of folate deficiency is decreasing in these countries.

Folate for Enhancing Mental Function in the Elderly

Homocysteine is a substance found in the blood. Some evidence suggests that high levels of homocysteine might be an important risk factor for heart disease. Because homocysteine levels can be reduced without drugs—adequate intake of folate, vitamin B_{12}, and vitamin B_6 will suffice—in the late 1990s some public-health researchers seized on the homocysteine hypothesis as a possible way to prevent major killers through simple nutritional supplementation.

Numerous large studies were designed and conducted to determine whether homocysteine reduction can reduce heart disease, strokes, and other cardiovascular diseases. The results have been disappointing. Completed trials suggest that homocysteine reduction does not have a marked effect on heart disease and related conditions. However, some of these large studies have, in passing, noted unexpected benefits among those given homocysteine-reducing supplements.

One of these possible "positive side effects" is discussed in an article published in 2007 by the prestigious journal *The Lancet*. Researchers in this article analyzed results of a study that enrolled 818 people with high homocysteine. Participants in this study were given either folate (800 micrograms daily) or placebo for three years. All were given a great number of medical tests as the study progressed, some of which involved evaluation of mental function. The results of the mental function tests indicated that those who were given folate showed improvement in areas of cognitive function that typically decline with age; in comparison, those given placebo did not improve.

This finding suggests that the use of folate may help enhance mental function in the elderly. One should note, however, that the foregoing study was not designed to look at effects on mental function. The laws of probability ensure that if enough variables are measured, some will come out better in the treatment group of a double-blind study, just by chance. Only if benefit is shown in repeat studies, designed in advance to evaluate folate's effect on mental function, will there be reliable evidence that it actually works.

Steven Bratman, M.D.

Deficiency appears to be most common today among African Americans, Hispanics, Asians, and Pacific Islanders, and among younger people and persons who are overweight.

Various drugs may impair the body's ability to absorb or utilize folate. These drugs include antacids, bile acid sequestrants (such as cholestyramine and colestipol), H_2 blockers, methotrexate, oral medications used for diabetes, various antiseizure medications (carbamazepine, phenobarbital, phenytoin, primidone, and valproate), sulfasalazine and possibly other nonsteroidal-anti-inflammatory-type drugs, high-dose triamterene, nitrous oxide, and the antibiotic trimethoprim-sulfamethoxazole. In addition, some of these drugs might put pregnant women at higher risk of giving birth to children with various kinds of birth defects; taking folate supplements may help reduce this risk.

Oral contraceptives may also affect folate slightly, but there appears to be no need for supplementation. Good sources of folate include dark green leafy vegetables, oranges, other fruits, rice, brewer's yeast, beef liver, beans, asparagus, kelp, soybeans, and soy flour.

THERAPEUTIC DOSAGES

For most uses, folate should be taken at nutritional doses, about 400 mcg daily for adults. However, higher dosages, up to 10 milligrams (mg) daily, have been used to treat specific diseases. Before taking more than 400 mcg daily, it is important to make sure that one does not have a vitamin B_{12} deficiency.

A particular kind of digestive enzyme taken as a supplement, pancreatin, may interfere with the absorption of folate. A person can avoid this by taking the two supplements at different times of the day.

THERAPEUTIC USES

The use of folate supplements by pregnant women dramatically decreases the risk that their children will be born with a serious condition called neural tube defect, which consists of problems with the brain or spinal cord. Folate supplements may also help prevent other types of birth disorders, such as defects of the heart, palate, and urinary tract; conversely, drugs that impair folate action may increase the risk of birth defects. An observational study suggests that folate supplements may reduce this risk in pregnant women taking such drugs.

Folate also lowers blood levels of homocysteine, which in turn has been hypothesized to reduce the risk of heart disease and other conditions. Studies conflict on the optimum dose of folate for this purpose; 100 to 400 mcg may produce some homocysteine-lowering effects, while 800 mcg daily may lead to maximum effects. Note, however, that there is no meaningful evidence that reducing homocysteine is beneficial and considerable evidence that it is not. Overall, studies of folate supplementation for reducing cardiovascular risk have failed to show benefit. On a more positive note, a double-blind, placebo-controlled study of 728 Danish elderly people with high homocysteine and relatively low folate intake found that the use of folate supplements slowed the progression of age-related hearing loss. Folate supplementation might also improve mental function in elderly persons with high homocysteine levels.

Based on preliminary evidence, folate has been suggested as a treatment for depression. One double-blind, placebo-controlled trial found that folate supplements at a dose of 500 mcg daily may help antidepressants work more effectively in women, but perhaps not in men. However, another study randomized 909 older adults with mild depression to different treatment groups, which included a group that took folate (400 mcg) and vitamin B_{12} (100 mcg) daily for two years. Folate and vitamin B_{12} were no better than placebo at improving depressive symptoms.

Observational studies hint that a deficiency in folate might predispose people to develop cancer of the cervix, colon, lung, breast, pancreas, and mouth, and that folate supplements may help prevent colon cancer, especially when taken for many years or by people with ulcerative colitis. However, observational studies are notoriously unreliable; large double-blind, placebo-controlled studies are needed to prove a treatment effective. One such study performed on folate for cancer prevention among one thousand people for five years found folate ineffective for preventing early colon cancer. However, a much smaller study involving ninety-four persons with colon polyps (a precancerous condition) found that folate may reduce the risk of recurrent polyps in a three-year period.

High-dose folate (10 mg daily) might be helpful for normalizing abnormalities in the appearance of the cervix (as seen under a microscope) in women taking oral contraceptives, but it does not appear to reverse actual cervical dysplasia. Also, some evidence suggests

that folate supplements might reduce risk of stroke. Folate deficiency may also increase the risk of Alzheimer's disease, although this has not been proven.

Folate supplements may reduce drug side effects in persons taking the drug methotrexate for certain conditions. Folate may also reduce side effects of the antiseizure drug carbamazepine.

Folate supplements may help medications in the nitroglycerin family remain effective. Folate supplementation may reduce blood arsenic levels in people who have been exposed to this toxic substance.

Very high dosages of folate may be helpful for gout, although some authorities suggest that it was actually a contaminant of folate that caused the benefit seen in some studies. Furthermore, other studies have found no benefit.

Based on intriguing but not definitive evidence, folate in various dosages has been suggested as a treatment for bipolar disorder, osteoarthritis (in combination with vitamin B_{12}), osteoporosis, restless legs syndrome, rheumatoid arthritis, seborrheic dermatitis, and vitiligo (splotchy loss of skin pigmentation). Other conditions for which folate has been suggested include migraine headaches and periodontal disease. Finally, folate does not appear to be helpful for enhancing mental function in the elderly.

SCIENTIFIC EVIDENCE

Birth defects and disorders. Strong evidence shows that the regular use of folate by pregnant women can reduce the risk of neural tube defect by 50 to 80 percent. Less direct evidence suggests that folate can help prevent other kinds of birth defects and disorders, especially among women using medications that interfere with folate.

Depression. One study found that people with depression who do not respond well to antidepressants are likely to have low levels of folate. A ten-week, double-blind, placebo-controlled trial of 127 persons with severe major depression found that folate supplements at a dose of 500 mcg daily significantly improved the effectiveness of fluoxetine (Prozac) in female participants. Improvement in male participants was not significant, but blood tests taken during the study suggested that higher intake of folate might be necessary for men.

Methotrexate side effects. Methotrexate is used in cancer chemotherapy and in treating inflammatory diseases such as rheumatoid arthritis and psoriasis.

While often highly effective, methotrexate can produce a number of severe side effects. These include liver toxicity and gastrointestinal distress. In addition, the use of methotrexate is thought to raise levels of homocysteine, potentially increasing the risk of heart disease.

Supplementation with folate may help. Methotrexate is called a "folate antagonist" because it prevents the body from converting folate to its active form. This inactivation of folate plays a role in methotrexate's therapeutic effects. This leads to a dilemma: Methotrexate use can lead to folate deficiency, but taking extra folate could theoretically prevent methotrexate from working properly.

However, evidence suggests that people who take methotrexate for rheumatoid arthritis, juvenile rheumatoid arthritis, or psoriasis can safely use folate supplements. Not only does the methotrexate continue to work properly; its usual side effects may decrease too.

For example, in a 48-week, double-blind, placebo-controlled trial of 434 persons with active rheumatoid arthritis, the use of folate helped prevent liver inflammation caused by methotrexate. This effect allowed more participants to continue methotrexate therapy; the development of liver inflammation often requires people to stop using the drug. A slightly higher dose of methotrexate was needed to reach the same level of benefit as taking methotrexate alone, but researchers felt doing so was worth it.

In the foregoing study, folate supplements did not reduce the incidence of mouth sores and nausea. However, in other studies, folate supplements did reduce these side effects, both in persons receiving methotrexate for rheumatoid arthritis and in those with psoriasis. In addition, two studies of people with rheumatoid arthritis found that the use of folate supplements corrected the methotrexate-induced rise in homocysteine without affecting disease control.

Folate supplements have been found safe only as supportive treatment in the specific conditions noted. It is not known, for example, whether folate supplements are safe for use by persons taking methotrexate for cancer treatment.

SAFETY ISSUES

Folate at nutritional doses is extremely safe. The only serious potential problem is that folate supplementation can mask the early symptoms of vitamin B_{12} deficiency (a special type of anemia), potentially allowing more irreversible symptoms of nerve damage to develop. For this reason, when taking more than 400 mcg daily, it is important check one's B_{12} level.

Very high dosages of folate, greater than 5 mg (5,000 mcg) daily, can cause digestive upset. The maximum recommended dosage of folate for pregnant or nursing women is 1,000 mcg daily (800 mcg if eighteen years of age or younger).

Media reports that the use of folate by pregnant women may increase their risk of breast cancer are based on a single study of highly questionable validity. This report is not considered a significant concern, but further research is needed.

As mentioned, the antiseizure drug phenytoin may interfere with folate absorption. However, folate may reduce the effectiveness of phenytoin. Persons taking phenytoin should consult with a physician about the proper dosage of folate.

Persons who are taking the drug methotrexate for rheumatoid arthritis, juvenile rheumatoid arthritis, or psoriasis can safely take folate supplements at the same time. However, if one is taking methotrexate for any other purpose, one should not take folate except on the advice of a physician.

IMPORTANT INTERACTIONS

Persons may need to take extra folate if also using aspirin and other anti-inflammatory medications, drugs that reduce stomach acid (such as antacids, H_2 blockers, and proton pump inhibitors), bile acid sequestrants (such as cholestyramine and colestipol), carbamazepine, estrogen replacement therapy, nitrous oxide, oral contraceptives, oral hypoglycemic drugs, phenobarbital, primidone, sulfa antibiotics, triamterene, valproic acid, or the antibiotic trimethoprim-sulfamethoxazole.

Persons taking phenytoin may need more folate. However, too much folate can interfere with this medication and can cause seizures. Physician supervision is essential.

Folate may boost the effectiveness of drugs in the nitroglycerin family. For persons taking pancreatin (a proteolytic enzyme), it may be advisable to separate the dose of pancreatin from the dose of folate by a minimum of two hours to avoid absorption problems.

For persons taking methotrexate for rheumatoid arthritis, juvenile rheumatoid arthritis, or psoriasis: Evidence suggests that folate supplements may reduce side effects of the drug without decreasing its benefits. Nonetheless, physician supervision is highly recommended. Note that for persons taking methotrexate for other conditions, folate might decrease the drug's effectiveness. Finally, green tea and black tea may decrease the absorption of folic acid into the bloodstream.

EBSCO CAM Review Board

FURTHER READING

Durga, J., M. P. van Boxtel, et al. "Effect of Three-Year Folic Acid Supplementation on Cognitive Function in Older Adults in the FACIT Trial." *The Lancet* 369 (2007): 208-216.

Durga, J., P. Verhoef, et al. "Effects of Folic Acid Supplementation on Hearing in Older Adults." *Annals of Internal Medicine* 146 (2007): 1-9.

Ebbing, M., et al. "Mortality and Cardiovascular Events in Patients Treated with Homocysteine-Lowering B Vitamins after Coronary Angiography." *Journal of the American Medical Association* 300 (2008): 795-804.

Gamble, M. V., et al. "Folic Acid Supplementation Lowers Blood Arsenic." *American Journal of Clinical Nutrition* 86 (2007): 1202-1209.

Gilbody, S., T. Lightfoot, and T. Sheldon. "Is Low Folate a Risk Factor for Depression? A Meta-analysis and Exploration of Heterogeneity." *Journal of Epidemiology and Community Health* 61 (2007): 631-637.

Lawrence, J. M., et al. "Do Racial and Ethnic Differences in Serum Folate Values Exist After Food Fortification with Folic Acid?" *American Journal of Obstetrics and Gynecology* 194 (2006): 520-526.

Walker, J. G., et al. "Mental Health Literacy, Folic Acid and Vitamin B12, and Physical Activity for the Prevention of Depression in Older Adults." *British Journal of Psychiatry* 197 (2010): 45-54.

Wang, X., et al. "Efficacy of Folic Acid Supplementation in Stroke Prevention." *The Lancet* 369 (2007): 1876-1882.

See also: Cancer risk reduction; Depression, mild to moderate; Homocysteine; Pregnancy support; Strokes; Vitamin B$_{12}$.

Folk medicine

CATEGORY: Therapies and techniques
RELATED TERMS: Acupuncture, acupressure, alternative medicine, complementary medicine, Eastern medicine, folk remedies, herbal medicine, holistic/wholistic medicine, Native, indigenous, or traditional medicine and healing, naturopathic medicine, shamanism
DEFINITION: Beliefs and practices that include home remedies, herbal therapies, and traditional healing.
PRINCIPAL PROPOSED USES: Anxiety, arthritis, back pain, cancer, depression, digestive disorders, heart disease, headaches, stress
OTHER PROPOSED USES: Acquired immunodeficiency syndrome, allergies, human immunodeficiency virus infection, poor circulation, premenstrual syndrome, sexual dysfunction, weight loss

OVERVIEW

At the beginning of the twentieth century in the United States, different forms of medical care were widely patronized. In 1910, Abraham Flexner published an influential report that advocated for the use of medical practices based on scientific evidence; he anticipated that folk medicine, which was presumably not evidence-based, would die out in time. A century later, however, alternative medicine is very much alive and thriving. With the advent of the Internet and the Web, and with the growing scope of immigration and travel, alternative medical practices from a wide range of cultures have been introduced in the United States. Furthermore, the number of rigorous clinical studies comparing the efficacy of alternative medical practices with conventional medicine continues to increase.

Besides treating a specific disease, many types of folk medicine aim to treat and promote well-being in the whole person, including a person's physical, emotional, mental, and spiritual aspects. Some practices evoke the occult and witchcraft and aim to remove or neutralize evil spirits to cure physical ailments. Other practices take into account a person's character traits and predispositions before making a diagnosis or creating a treatment plan.

There are many types of folk medicine, but all can be roughly classified into several categories. The first category involves natural products, which are ingested, inhaled, or applied to parts of the body. Over centuries and even millennia of empirical testing, many cultures have derived combinations of natural substances such as plant and animal materials for treating disease. Plant material includes leaves, fruits, seeds, bark, stems, and roots.

Another category of folk medicine is mind/body medicine, which involves using the power of the mind to heal the body. Yoga, meditation, and acupuncture can be classified under this category. A popular example of mind/body medicine is acupuncture, in which thin metal needles are inserted through the skin at specific pressure points along "meridians," or pathways, on the body to clear blockages in the flow of qi (energy). Acupressure stimulates these pressure points manually, using the hands instead of needles.

A third category of folk medicine, manipulative and body-based practices, encompasses therapies that address the bones and joints, soft tissues, and the circulatory and lymphatic systems. One example is spinal manipulation, which involves applying force to a part of the spine, causing it to move beyond its passive range of motion. Another example is massage, which involves rubbing and pressing muscles to stimulate blood and oxygen flow through the muscles.

Finally, other practices, such as movement therapies and energy therapies, can also be considered folk medicines. Energy therapies include those that exploit electromagnetic fields for healing purposes and practices, such as Reiki, which involve the transmission of "universal" energy (believed to be present in every person) from the practitioner to the patient by placing of hands on or near the patient or by transmission from a distance.

MECHANISM OF ACTION

Natural products that are used as medicines have many different modes of action. For example, fish, seeds, and oils rich in omega-3 fatty acids act by reducing the level of cholesterol in the blood, reducing inflammation, and reducing cardiac arrhythmias (irregular heartbeat). The biological effects of Asian herbal medicines range from promoting circulation and dilating blood vessels to stimulating digestion and increasing skin elasticity. Natural products, such as herbs, are used in both Asian and Hispanic traditional medical practices to restore balance between "hot" and "cold" humors or conditions. In Hispanic folk medicine, for example, hot states are associated with vasodilation and a high metabolic rate, while cold states are associated with vasoconstriction and a low metabolic rate. A hot condition would be treated with herbal therapies that are considered cold treatments; conversely, cold conditions would be treated with hot therapies. Similar principles are used in Asian folk medicine.

Mind/body medicine such as meditation, yoga, and acupuncture uses the power of the mind to improve physical and mental health. The idea is that the mind and body are inextricably connected and influence health as an inseparable whole. Meditation and yoga improve health by reducing stress and increasing calmness and relaxation, which in turn boosts the immune system and promotes physical health. According to Chinese medical concepts, acupuncture releases qi blockages in the body, allowing qi to flow freely, and corrects imbalance between the yin ("cold") and yang ("hot") forces. Although the positive effects of acupuncture are becoming accepted among a growing number of laypersons and clinicians, the mechanism of action cannot be readily explained in conventional or Western medical terms. Faith healing can also be thought of as mind/body medicine and is thought to work through the actions of a spiritual power.

Manipulative and body-based practices work by applying force on parts of the body such as muscles and bone. Massage therapy soothes muscle tension and stimulates blood and oxygen circulation in the muscles. Spinal manipulation increases flexibility and range of motion of the spinal vertebrae. The mechanisms of action of energy therapies such as Reiki therapy are challenging to characterize in scientific terms.

USES AND APPLICATIONS

The uses of natural products are wide-ranging. They can be used to improve blood circulation throughout the body, treat headaches, and promote weight loss; they are also used to treat arthritis, diabetes, cancer, and heart disease. Mind/body techniques such as yoga and meditation are often used to treat illnesses related to anxiety, stress, and depression. Yoga, meditation, and acupuncture can be helpful in alleviating chronic pain. Acupuncture is also used to treat a wide range of disorders, from headaches to cancer. Manipulative and body-based practices treat back, neck, and shoulder pain, as well as spinal problems. Spinal manipulation is especially useful for treating lower back pain, a common ailment.

SCIENTIFIC EVIDENCE

Many scientific studies support the use of different types of oils in treating and preventing disease. This includes the use of fish oil in reducing cardiac arrhythmias, sunflower seed oil and olive oil in reducing cholesterol in the blood, and red palm oil in protecting against ischemia-reperfusion injury, which refers to damage to the heart when blood flow is restored (reperfusion) following a period without blood flow (ischemia).

Among mind/body traditional practices, acupuncture is one of the most widely studied. A National Institutes of Health (NIH) consensus panel reviewed the scientific literature about acupuncture to assess its clinical efficacy and biological effects. According to the NIH panel, scientific evidence shows that only dental pain and nausea (related to surgery, chemotherapy, or pregnancy) have been effectively treated by acupuncture. More scientific studies are needed to determine if acupuncture is effective for other conditions. Several studies sponsored by the National Center of Complementary and Alternative Medicine are underway to explore the use of acupuncture therapy in treating high blood pressure and advanced colorectal cancer. However, the National Cancer Institute Web site provides a summary of studies that show the efficacy of acupuncture in boosting immune function and in reducing some of the side effects of chemotherapy, including nausea, weight loss, and depression. Acupuncture also appears to reduce cancer-related fatigue.

Choosing a Practitioner

One should choose a practitioner only after carefully researching his or her training, qualifications, and experience. In some types of alternative medicine, certification by an accreditation board can help in selecting a practitioner. For example, forty-one states in the United States require acupuncturists to be certified by the National Certification Commission for Acupuncture and Oriental Medicine before they are issued a license to practice. Certification requires passing of exams in oriental medicine, acupuncture, and Western biomedicine, usually after completion of master's-level educational programs that involve three to four years of course work and clinical experience. If candidates pass these exams, they are awarded a diplomate in acupuncture.

As with conventional health-care practitioners, certified acupuncturists must earn sufficient continuing education credits to renew this certification every four years. Some physicians and dentists are certified and licensed to practice acupuncture. There are also advanced degree programs in naturopathy and com-

plementary medicine in the United States, focusing on holistic healing using alternative and conventional medical practices. Several schools offer the doctor of naturopathy (N.D.) degree, which takes four to six years to complete, and fourteen states license N.D.'s; licensing requires successful completion of the naturopathic licensing examination.

Safety Issues

The safety of alternative medicine depends on the practitioner and on the nature of the therapy and the context in which the therapy is applied. In addition to choosing a qualified, well-established practitioner, one should take care when initiating new alternative therapies. For example, when starting a new diet regimen or adding dietary supplements, one should be alert to possible interactions with medications or other supplements. Also, because many supplements are not regulated by the U.S. Food and Drug Administration and can be purchased without a prescription, one should research possible side effects and interactions thoroughly before adding these substances to one's diet.

For therapies that involve body manipulation, such as massage and spinal manipulation, possible side effects from poor treatment include sore muscles and muscle and ligament injury. Acupuncture has several side effects; these are mainly associated with the needle puncture site and include the puncture of organs, nerves, or blood vessels; infection (avoidable by using safe-needle techniques); puncture site pain; bleeding; hematoma; and the so-called needle shock reaction, which manifests as excessive sweating and a feeling of faintness after needle puncture.

Ing-Wei Khor, Ph.D.

Further Reading

Bester, D., et al. "Cardiovascular Effects of Edible Oils: A Comparison Between Four Popular Oils." *Nutrition Research Reviews* (2010): 1-15. Review article of the efficacy of fish, sunflower seed, olive, and red palm oils in treating and preventing heart disease.

Brady, E., ed. *Healing Logics: Culture and Medicine in Modern Health Belief Systems.* Logan: Utah State University, 2001. Overview of the traditional medical practices of various cultures.

Hadady, L. *Asian Health Secrets: The Complete Guide to Asian Herbal Medicine.* New York: Three Rivers Press, 1996. Comprehensive and user-friendly guide to the use of Asian herbal medicine in the diagnosis and treatment of a range of diseases.

Kirkland, H. F., et al., eds. *Herbal and Magical Medicine: Traditional Healing Today*. Durham, N.C.: Duke University Press, 1992. Discusses the use of traditional herbal medicines in disease treatment.

National Cancer Institute. "Acupuncture." Available at http://www.cancer.gov/cancertopics/pdq/cam/acupuncture/healthprofessional. A summary of clinical studies examining the efficacy of acupuncture for cancer symptoms and chemotherapy-related side effects.

National Center for Complementary and Alternative Medicine. http://nccam.nih.gov. A comprehensive U.S. government resource for news articles, scientific studies, and general consumer information about complementary and alternative medicine.

See also: Alternative versus traditional medicine; Ayurveda; Chinese medicine; Herbal medicine; Home health; Naturopathy; Traditional Chinese herbal medicine; Traditional healing.

Food allergies and sensitivities

CATEGORY: Condition

DEFINITION: Treatment of food allergies and sensitivities to food.

PRINCIPAL PROPOSED NATURAL TREATMENTS: Elimination diet, hypoallergenic infant formula

OTHER PROPOSED NATURAL TREATMENTS: Bromelain, probiotics, proteolytic enzymes, thymus extract

INTRODUCTION

A food allergy is an abnormal immune reaction caused by the ingestion of a food or food additive. The most dramatic form of food allergy reaction occurs within minutes, usually in response to certain foods such as shellfish, peanuts, or strawberries. The effects are similar to those of a bee sting allergy, involving hives, itching, swelling in the throat, and difficulty breathing; this immediate type of allergic reaction can be life-threatening.

Other food allergy reactions are more delayed, causing relatively subtle symptoms over days or weeks. These symptoms include gastrointestinal problems (constipation, diarrhea, gas, cramping, and bloating), rashes, and headaches. However, because such delayed reactions are relatively vague and can have other causes, they have remained a controversial subject in medicine.

Some reactions that are similar to those from food allergies, but do not actually involve the immune system, are termed "food sensitivities" (or "food intolerance"). In most cases, the cause of such sensitivities is unknown.

Delayed-type food allergies and sensitivities might play a role in many diseases, including asthma, attention deficit disorder, rheumatoid arthritis, vaginal yeast infection, canker sores, colic, ear infection, eczema, irritable bowel syndrome, migraine headache, psoriasis, chronic sinus infection, ulcerative colitis, Crohn's disease, and celiac disease. However, not all experts agree; practitioners of natural medicine tend to be more enthusiastic about the food allergy theory of disease than conventional practitioners.

Conventional treatment for immediate-type food allergy reactions includes desensitization (allergy shots), emergency epinephrine (adrenaline) kits for self-injection, and the antihistamine diphenhydramine (Benadryl). Delayed-type food allergies are much more difficult to identify and treat. Although skin and blood tests are sometimes used, their reliability is questionable. A particular blood test called ALCAT has shown some promise, but much more study is necessary to establish its accuracy.

The double-blind food challenge is the only truly reliable way to identify delayed-type food allergies. This method uses some means of disguising the possibly allergenic food, usually by mixing it with other, nonallergenic foods. Persons are randomly given either the possibly allergenic food or placebo on a number of occasions separated by one or more days. Neither the physician nor the participant knows what food is truly allergenic and what is not. Evaluation of the response can then determine whether an allergic response is present. Studies suggest that perhaps only one-third of people who believe they are allergic to a given food actually experience an allergic reaction when they are given it in a double-blind fashion; in addition, reactions are often milder than persons believe.

Although it is the most accurate way of determining food allergies, the double-blind food challenge is still mostly used in research. The elimination diet with food challenges is the most common technique in use.

Another conventional approach for delayed-type food allergies is oral cromolyn (a drug sometimes used in an inhaled form for treating asthma and other allergic illnesses). A double-blind, placebo-controlled study of fourteen children with milk and other food allergies found that cromolyn was effective in preventing allergic reactions in eleven of thirteen cases, whereas placebo was effective in only three of nine cases. In another study, thirty-two persons were given cromolyn one-half hour before meals and at bedtime. If their food allergy symptoms were prevented, the participants were entered into a double-blind, placebo-controlled crossover study using cromoglycate. Of the thirty-one people who completed the study, twenty-four experienced relief of gastrointestinal symptoms when taking cromolyn compared with two when taking placebo. In addition, systemic allergic reactions were blocked with the cromolyn. The drug also had many side effects.

PRINCIPAL PROPOSED NATURAL TREATMENTS

There are no well-documented natural treatments for food allergies. The most obvious approach would be to remove known allergenic foods from the diet. Some alternative practitioners offer laboratory tests to identify such allergens. However, no lab tests have been proven accurate for this purpose.

The elimination diet is another approach for identifying allergenic foods. This method involves starting with a highly restricted diet consisting only of foods that are seldom allergenic, such as rice, yams, and

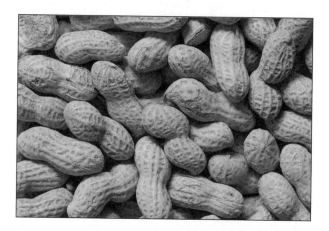

An allergic reaction to peanuts usually occurs within minutes of ingesting the peanuts. (©Brad Calkins/Dreamstime.com)

turkey. If dietary restriction leads to resolution or improvement of symptoms, foods are then reintroduced one by one to see which, if any, will trigger reactions. There is some evidence that the elimination diet may be effective for chronic or recurrent hives; it has been tried for many other conditions too, including irritable bowel syndrome, asthma, chronic ear infections, reflux esophagitis, and Crohn's disease.

Still another method involves simply eliminating the most common allergens. Cow's milk protein intolerance is thought to be the most common childhood allergy, followed by allergies to eggs, peanuts, nuts, and fish. Some evidence indicates that the use of special hypoallergenic infant formulas rather than cow's milk formula may help prevent eczema, urticaria, and food-induced digestive distress. In addition, eliminating cow's milk from the diets of breast-feeding infants and their nursing mothers might reduce symptoms of infantile colic, although not all studies have found benefit.

In hopes of preventing food allergies and diseases related to them, some experts recommend that pregnant women and women who are breast-feeding (and their children) should avoid allergenic foods. However, it is not clear if this method actually provides any benefit. For example, one study evaluated 165 children at high risk of developing allergic symptoms. Careful avoidance of allergenic foods in the diets of the mothers and infants did not reduce the later development of eczema, asthma, hay fever, or food allergy symptoms.

OTHER PROPOSED TREATMENTS

Digestive enzymes such as bromelain and other proteolytic enzymes have been proposed as a treatment for food allergies, based on the reasonable idea that digesting offending proteins will reduce allergic reactions to them. However, there is no real evidence that they are effective against food allergies.

Thymus extract is a supplement derived from the thymus gland of cows. Preliminary evidence suggests that by normalizing immune function, thymus extracts may be helpful for food allergies. However, there are significant safety issues, and this study did not prove the supplement to be effective.

Probiotics (such as *Lactobacillus* species) are friendly bacteria that have been studied for their ability to prevent or treat respiratory allergies and various gastrointestinal symptoms, most notably diarrhea. However, at least one study found that probiotics were not helpful in treating cow's milk allergy among infants.

EBSCO CAM Review Board

FURTHER READING

Arvola, T., and D. Holmberg-Marttila. "Benefits and Risks of Elimination Diets." *Annals of Medicine* 31 (1999): 293-298.

Bindslev-Jensen, C., et al. "Food Allergy and Food Intolerance: What Is the Difference?" *Annals of Allergy* 72 (1994): 317-320.

Carroccio, A., et al. "Evidence of Very Delayed Clinical Reactions to Cow's Milk in Cow's Milk-Intolerant Patients." *Allergy* 55 (2000): 574-579.

Dainese, R., et al. "Discrepancies Between Reported Food Intolerance and Sensitization Test Findings in Irritable Bowel Syndrome Patients." *American Journal of Gastroenterology* 94 (1999): 1892-1897.

Drisko, J., et al. "Treating Irritable Bowel Syndrome with a Food Elimination Diet Followed by Food Challenge and Probiotics." *Journal of the American College of Nutrition* 25 (2006): 514-522.

Geha, R. S., et al. "Multicenter, Double-Blind, Placebo-Controlled, Multiple-Challenge Evaluation of Reported Reactions to Monosodium Glutamate." *Journal of Allergy and Clinical Immunology* 106 (2000): 973-980.

Hill, D. J., et al. "Role of Food Protein Intolerance in Infants with Persistent Distress Attributed to Reflux Esophagitis." *Journal of Pediatrics* 136 (2000): 641-647.

Hol, J., et al. "The Acquisition of Tolerance Toward Cow's Milk Through Probiotic Supplementation." *Journal of Allergy and Clinical Immunology* 121, no. 6 (2008): 1448-1454.

Kim, T. E., et al. "Comparison of Skin Prick Test Results Between Crude Allergen Extracts from Foods and Commercial Allergen Extracts in Atopic Dermatitis by Double-Blind Placebo-Controlled Food Challenge for Milk, Egg, and Soybean." *Yonsei Medical Journal* 43 (2002): 613-620.

Metcalfe, D. D. "Food Allergy." *Primary Care* 25 (1998): 819-829.

Niggemann, B., et al. "Prospective, Controlled, Multicenter Study on the Effect of an Amino-Acid-Based Formula in Infants with Cow's Milk Allergy/Intolerance and Atopic Dermatitis." *Pediatric Allergy and Immunology* 12 (2001): 78-82.

Rodriguez, J., et al. "Randomized, Double-Blind, Crossover Challenge Study in Fifty-Three Subjects Reporting Adverse Reactions to Melon (*Cucumis melo*)." *Journal of Allergy and Clinical Immunology* 106 (2000): 968-972.

Zeiger, R. S. "Dietary Aspects of Food Allergy Prevention in Infants and Children." *Journal of Pediatric Gastroenterology and Nutrition* 30, suppl. (2000): S77-S86.

See also: Allergies; Breast-feeding support; Bromelain; Children's health; Colostrum; Eating disorders; Gas, intestinal; Gastritis; Gastrointestinal health; Immune support; Irritable bowel syndrome (IBS); Lactose intolerance; Nondairy milk; Probiotics; Proteolytic enzymes; Thymus extract.

Food and Drug Administration (FDA)

CATEGORY: Organizations and legislation

DEFINITION: A U.S. government agency that oversees regulations and inspections of the safety and quality of pharmaceuticals and nutritional resources, including food and food products.

DATE: Established in 1906

OVERVIEW

Since its creation, the U.S. Food and Drug Administration (FDA) has addressed the marketing of manufactured foods and drugs to consumers. Legislation and policies developed in the twentieth and twenty-first centuries defined specific roles and powers that the federal agency, part of the U.S. Department of Health and Human Services, can practice to protect consumers from hazardous products.

The FDA had earlier regulated complementary and alternative medicine (CAM) precursors, evaluating the quality, safety, and factual labeling of additives and supplements based on legislation, including the 1938 Federal Food, Drug, and Cosmetic Act, the 1944 Public Health Service Act, and the 1990 Nutritional Labeling and Education Act.

LEGISLATIVE RESTRICTIONS

During the 1980s, CAM products became popular consumer goods, with the quantity of CAM merchandise and therapies available to consumers expanding in the following decade. The FDA expressed concern regarding the regulation of minerals, vitamins, dietary supplements, and products consisting of herbs and biological ingredients, wanting them to be evaluated with clinical trials and scientific studies similar to those utilized to test and approve pharmaceuticals. Concerned about potential economic losses associated with such testing, the supplements industry lobbied to reduce FDA interference.

In October 1994, U.S. president Bill Clinton approved the Dietary Supplement Health and Education Act (DSHEA). That legislation restricted the FDA from intervening before the marketing of CAM products and, thus, from insisting that manufacturers test herbal and dietary supplement products before selling them. The FDA could act only if products were proven to be hazardous. The agency asked consumers who experienced toxic supplements and herbal products to contact them to report such issues and it began to routinely issue alerts, warning consumers about using some CAM products, especially those marketed for weight loss or as cold remedies.

The FDA and the National Institutes of Health's (NIH) Office of Alternative Medicine cooperated in an attempt to improve CAM policies. The 1997 Food and Drug Administration Modernization Act (FDAMA) addressed some CAM topics. That year, the FDA and NIH agreed that acupuncture, a CAM technique, could be incorporated in traditional medical practices.

GUIDANCE

Increased CAM demand and supply in the twenty-first century led the FDA to assess its legal authority and responsibility to regulate CAM products and services. Many CAM manufacturers, distributors, and practitioners were unsure if they had to comply with FDA rules associated with drugs and foods. The agency also rethought its role in regulating CAM imports arriving in U.S. markets and in regulating CAM products advertised and sold on the Internet. In 2005, an Institute of Medicine report, "Complementary and Alternative Medicine in the United States," asserted the need for regulation of CAM products that were equivalent to traditional medical drugs.

On December 26, 2006, the FDA released a draft of its "Guidance for Industry on Complementary and Alternative Medicine Products and Their Regulation by the Food and Drug Administration." These guidelines

---

Regulating CAM

The "Guidance for Industry on Complementary and Alternative Medicine Products and Their Regulation by the Food and Drug Administration" (2006) makes the following two fundamental points:

Depending on the CAM therapy or practice, a product used in a CAM therapy or practice *may* be subject to regulation as a biological product, cosmetic, drug, device, or food (including food additives and dietary supplements) under the [1938 Federal Food, Drug, and Cosmetic] Act or the PHS [1944 Public Health Service] Act. For example, the PHS Act defines "biological product" and the Act defines (among other things) the terms "cosmetic," "device," "dietary supplement," "drug (as well as "new drug" and "new animal drug"), "food," and "food additive."

Neither the Act nor the PHS Act exempts CAM products from regulation. This means, for example, [that] if a person decides to produce and sell raw vegetable juice for use in juice therapy to promote optimal health, that product is a food subject to the requirements for foods in the Act and FDA regulations, including the hazard analysis and critical control point system requirements for juices. If the juice therapy is intended for use as part of a disease treatment regimen instead of for general wellness, the vegetable juice would also be subject to regulation as a drug under the Act.

---

were later printed in the *Federal Register* of February 27, 2007. FDA personnel who helped compile this document consulted with experts and researchers focusing on food safety, applied nutrition, biologics and drug evaluation, radiological health, and health care devices. The guidelines outlined how the FDA proposed to add CAM items to existing regulation categories.

Some groups, including the Natural Solutions Foundation, American Holistic Nurses Association, and American Chiropractic Association, reacted to the guidelines as a potential threat. The organizations feared they would no longer have access to herbs and other natural alternative medicines and devices. Many critics thought the FDA would prohibit anything associated with CAM. The American Herbal Products Association and the United Natural Products Alliance, concerned about wording describing biological substances, demanded the guidelines be withdrawn.

Not considering the guidelines detrimental, National Health Foundation lobbyist Lee Bechtel reassured CAM advocates that the guidelines would not give the FDA unlimited legal authority to block use of CAM products.

INSPECTION AND REGULATION

In June 2007, the FDA announced that dietary supplement manufacturers would be required to follow stricter good-manufacturing practices as described in the U.S. Code of Federal Regulations. The FDA scheduled inspections of manufacturers to determine how well they were meeting the more demanding manufacturing standards and to determine whether they were committing violations, especially concerning the quality of ingredients.

In 2008, FDA inspectors began examining manufacturers who had more than five hundred employees. Starting on June 25, 2009, the FDA inspected manufacturing sites with between twenty and five hundred employees. Inspectors evaluated small companies with fewer than twenty employees beginning in the summer of 2010. They assessed manufacturers' testing of botanical materials used to produce supplements and examined physical plant maintenance, operating procedures, employee training, the documentation of details for all aspects of manufacturing, preventive methods against contamination by allergens and toxins, factual labeling, and the company's response to criticism from consumers.

In 2010, the FDA wrote its initial warning letters regarding violations of the new manufacturing practices and regarding scientifically unsubstantiated health claims. Several companies, including Coats International Holdings and POM Wonderful, were ordered to revise labels and marketing information. The FDA planned a second round of inspections after 2010 to evaluate how manufacturers responded to the agency's reports of violations.

Elizabeth D. Schafer, Ph.D.

FURTHER READING

Carpenter, Daniel P. *Reputation and Power: Organizational Image and Pharmaceutical Regulation at the FDA.* Princeton, N.J.: Princeton University Press, 2010. Comprehensive study by a leading FDA historian incorporates examination of how this federal agency has historically dealt with the monitoring of supplements.

Czap, Al. "Some (Abbreviated) Facts About GMP Compliance." *Alternative Medicine Review* 15, no. 1 (2010): 1-2. Editorial comments about factors FDA inspectors surveyed at dietary supplement manufacturers from 2008 through 2010 and inspections' potential effectiveness to reform dangerous CAM production.

Daemmrich, Arthur, and Joanna Radin, eds. *Perspectives on Risk and Regulation: The FDA at 100.* Philadelphia: Chemical Heritage Foundation, 2007. Several chapters discuss FDA policies regarding dietary supplements and legislation regulating that industry.

"FDA Rule on Supplements: 'Only a First Step,' Urologists Say." *Urology Times* 35, no. 9 (2007): 1, 13. Critical of FDA attempts to enforce manufacturing practices. Suggests how manufacturers can assess raw materials and improve quality control procedures.

Hickmann, Meredith A. ed. *The Food and Drug Administration (FDA).* Hauppauge, N.Y.: Nova Science, 2003. Explains how the FDA is responsible for ensuring the safety of CAM and foods, drugs, medical devices, cosmetics, and other products.

Jiang, Tao. "Re-thinking the Dietary Supplement Laws and Regulations Fourteen Years After the Dietary Supplement Health and Education Act Implementation." *International Journal of Food Sciences and Nutrition* 60, no. 4 (2009): 293-301. Describes worldwide legislation impacting CAM quality, revealing how laws favoring manufacturers can result in hazardous products reaching consumers.

O'Reilly, James T. *Food and Drug Administration.* 2d ed. St. Paul, Minn.: Thomson/West, 2005. This authoritative guide explains the practice of law within the FDA.

See also: Codex Alimentarius Commission; Dietary Supplement Health and Education Act; Functional foods: Introduction; Functional foods: Overview; Herbal medicine; National Center for Complementary and Alternative Medicine; Office of Dietary Supplements; Regulation of CAM; Supplements: Introduction; Vitamins and minerals.

Fructo-oligosaccharides

CATEGORY: Herbs and supplements

RELATED TERMS: FOS, galacto-oligosaccharides (GOS), inulin, prebiotics

DEFINITION: Natural substance used to treat specific health conditions.

PRINCIPAL PROPOSED USES: None

OTHER PROPOSED USES: Diabetes (blood sugar control), high cholesterol, irritable bowel syndrome, travelers' diarrhea

OVERVIEW

Fructo-oligosaccharides (FOS) are starches that the human body cannot fully digest. Inulin and galacto-oligosaccharides (GOS) are similar substances also discussed. When a person consumes FOS, the undigested portions provide nourishment for bacteria in the digestive tract. "Friendly" bacteria (probiotics) may respond particularly well to this nourishment. Because FOS feed probiotics, they are sometimes called prebiotics.

Low doses of FOS are often provided along with probiotic supplements to aid their growth. High doses of FOS (and related substances) have been advocated for a variety of health conditions. However, currently, the available scientific evidence on benefit remains more negative than positive.

REQUIREMENTS AND SOURCES

There is no daily requirement for FOS. FOS and related substances are found in asparagus, Jerusalem artichokes, leeks, onions, and soybeans, among other foods.

THERAPEUTIC DOSAGES

When taken simply for promoting healthy bacteria, FOS are often taken at a dose of 4-6 grams (g) daily. When used for therapeutic purposes, the typical dose of FOS is 10-20 g daily, divided into three doses and taken with meals. Side effects are common at a daily intake of 15 g or more.

THERAPEUTIC USES

Animal studies hint that FOS, GOS, and inulin can significantly improve cholesterol profile; however, study outcomes in humans have been inconsistent at best. One study found that while inulin might produce a short-term benefit, any such benefit disappears after six months of use.

At most, it appears that FOS might improve cholesterol profiles by 5 percent, an amount too small to make much of a difference in most circumstances. These relatively poor results might be because of the fact that humans cannot tolerate doses of FOS much above 15 g daily without developing gastrointestinal side effects.

FOS has also been suggested for preventing travelers' diarrhea. However, in a large (244-participant) double-blind study, FOS at a dose of 10 g daily again offered only minimal benefits. Probiotics themselves might be a better bet.

Another study found that use of FOS might help reduce incidents of diarrhea, flatulence, and vomiting in preschoolers. According to most studies, FOS at 10 to 20 g daily do not improve blood sugar control in people with type 2 diabetes.

FOS have been advocated as a treatment for irritable bowel syndrome. However, research results are inconsistent at best. For example, a six-week, double-blind study of 105 people with mild irritable bowel syndrome compared 5 g of fructo-oligosaccharides daily against placebo and returned conflicting results. According to some measures of symptom severity employed by the researchers, use of FOS led to an improvement in symptoms. However, according to other measures, FOS worsened symptoms. Conflicting results, though of a different kind, were also seen in a twelve-week, double-blind, placebo-controlled study of ninety-eight people. Treatment with FOS at a dose of 20 g daily initially worsened symptoms, but over time this negative effect wore off. At no time in the study were clear benefits seen, however. On a positive note, one study did find benefit with a combination prebiotic-probiotic formula, and another study found the combination beneficial for women with constipation when taken in yogurt.

Small double-blind studies found that FOS at a dose of 10 g daily may improve magnesium absorption in postmenopausal women. Whether this is beneficial remains unclear, since magnesium deficiency is not believed to be a widespread problem. FOS may also slightly increase copper absorption but does not appear to affect absorption of calcium, zinc, or selenium.

A randomized, placebo-controlled trial, involving 134 infants less than six months old whose parents suffered from allergies found that those fed a prebiotic combination of FOS/GOS experienced a significant reduction in both allergy symptoms and minor infections that lasted at least through age two. The researchers suggested that the favorable effects of prebiotics on intestinal bacteria early in life may produce lasting benefits to the immune system. One study found that use of inulin promoted growth of probiotic bacteria in the bifidobacteria family.

SAFETY ISSUES

FOS appear to be generally safe. However, they can cause bloating, flatulence, and intestinal discomfort, especially when taken at doses of 15 g or higher daily. People with lactose intolerance may particularly suffer from these side effects.

EBSCO CAM Review Board

FURTHER READING

Arslanoglu, S., et al. "Early Dietary Intervention with a Mixture of Prebiotic Oligosaccharides Reduces the Incidence of Allergic Manifestations and Infections During the First Two Years of Life." *Journal of Nutrition* 138 (2008): 1091-1095.

Bittner, A. C., et al. "Prescript-Assist Probiotic-Prebiotic Treatment for Irritable Bowel Syndrome." *Clinical Therapeutics* 27 (2005): 755-761.

Bouhnik, Y., et al. "Prolonged Administration of Low-Dose Inulin Stimulates the Growth of Bifidobacteria in Humans." *Nutrition Research* 27 (2007): 187-193.

De Paula, J. A., E. Carmuega, and R. Weill. "Effect of the Ingestion of a Symbiotic Yogurt on the Bowel Habits of Women with Functional Constipation." *Acta Gastroenterologica Latinoamericana* 38 (2008): 16-25.

Forcheron, F., and M. Beylot. "Long-term Administration of Inulin-Type Fructans Has No Significant Lipid-lowering Effect in Normolipidemic Humans." *Metabolism* 56 (2007): 1093-1098.

Paineau, D., et al. "The Effects of Regular Consumption of Short-Chain Fructo-Oligosaccharides on Digestive Comfort of Subjects with Minor Functional Bowel Disorders." *British Journal of Nutrition* 99, no. 2 (2008): 311-318.

Waligora-Dupriet, A. J., et al. "Effect of Oligofructose Supplementation on Gut Microflora and Well-Being in Young Children Attending a Day Care Centre." *International Journal of Food Microbiology* 1, no. 113 (2007): 108-113.

See also: Cholesterol, high; Diabetes; Diarrhea; Gastrointestinal health; Irritable bowel syndrome (IBS); Probiotics.

Functional beverages

CATEGORY: Functional foods

DEFINITION: Juices, waters, and sodas to which natural additives such as ginseng and ginkgo or other alternative ingredients are introduced to improve health.

PRINCIPAL PROPOSED USES: Memory enhancement, muscle building, relaxation

OTHER PROPOSED USES: Immune system enhancement, increased alertness and energy, stress relief

OVERVIEW

To avoid entanglement with the U.S. Food and Drug Administration (FDA), which has strict guidelines about product health claims, most manufacturers of functional beverages carefully refrain from making direct promises about curing diseases. However, product labels list ingredients and often outline the general benefits of these ingredients, leaving consumers to draw their own conclusions about the potential health effects of the drink.

USES AND APPLICATIONS

Common herbal ingredients used in functional drinks (and their claimed associated benefits), as listed by the manufacturers, include ginseng (enhances energy), ginkgo (enhances memory and mental alertness), guarana (enhances energy), gotu kola (enhances alertness), echinacea (stimulates the body's defenses), St. John's wort (enhances mood), and kava (promotes relaxation).

SAFETY ISSUES

Questions have been raised about the possible risks and benefits of adding herbs to beverages. Herbs are not essential nutrients. Therefore, a person cannot be deficient in ginseng or echinacea, as one can be deficient in, for example, iron. Foods that are fortified with essential nutrients can benefit people who do not consume enough of these nutrients.

In some cultures, herbs are prescribed in specific quantities and combinations to treat certain medical conditions. However, how effective is a miniscule amount of ginseng that has been added to diet iced tea? What are the long-term effects of consuming these products?

Paul LaChance, executive director of the Nutraceuticals Institute at Rutgers University in New Jersey,

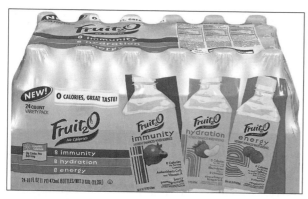

These beverages contain additives to promote immunity, hydration, and energy. (PR Newswire)

believes these questions have yet to be answered by scientific research. "Herbally-enhanced beverage products are developed by marketing departments, not scientists," he noted. However, he added, consumers are probably at little risk because "the amount of ingredients in these products is quite minimal."

Researchers are not sure what the benefits, risks, or long-term effects (if any) will be from drinking functional beverages. For now, one should consider the following before drinking these types of beverages:

Moderation. Though the amount of added ingredients is very small, one should not overdo the consumption of functional beverages. Drinking excessive amounts or consuming them regularly over a long period of time may lead to problems.

Allergies. Persons allergic to a given herb may have an allergic reaction regardless of the amount of that herb in a drink.

Extra calories. Some functional beverages, particularly sodas and juices, may contain several hundred calories in a bottle. Persons wanting to consume flavored drinks should try the flavored waters, which have fewer calories.

Kava. This herb has been taken off the market in Canada, Australia, and Germany because it unexpectedly caused severe liver damage in a number of previously healthy people. Researchers do not know how kava causes this damage, nor do they know at what levels damage occurs. It is possible that even small amounts can cause harm.

Michelle Badash, M.S.;
reviewed by Brian Randall, M.D.

FURTHER READING

American Dietetic Association. "Functional Beverages." Available at http://www.eatright.org/about/content.aspx?id=7519.

Barnes, J., and G. Winter. "Stressed Out? Bad Knee? Relief Promised in a Juice." *The New York Times,* May 27, 2001.

Council for Responsible Nutrition. http://www.crnusa.org.

Jacobson, M., B. Silverglade, and I. Heller. "Functional Foods: Health Boon or Quackery?" *Western Journal of Medicine* 172, no. 1 (2000): 8-9.

U.S. Food and Drug Administration. http://www.fda.gov.

See also: Echinacea; Fatigue; Functional foods: Introduction; Ginkgo; Ginseng; Gotu kola; Guarana; Herbal medicine; Kava; Memory and mental function impairment; Relaxation therapies; St. John's wort; Stress.

Functional foods: Introduction

CATEGORY: Functional foods
DEFINITION: Foods marketed as having specific health-promoting benefits.

OVERVIEW

Increasingly, foods sold in supermarkets come with health claims on their labels. Labels claim that oatmeal and soy help prevent heart disease, that milk and calcium-fortified orange juice fight osteoporosis, and that folate-enriched flour prevents birth defects and disorders. These foods are all functional foods, that is, foods marketed as offering specific health benefits.

There are two main categories of functional foods. The first, and largest, category consists of ordinary foods that contain health-promoting substances. This category essentially includes all fruits, vegetables, and whole grains, soy and other legumes, and numerous other foods such as herbal teas, yogurt, and cold-water fish. When these foods are presented as functional foods, their specific health benefits and healthy constituents are highlighted, constituents such as fiber, vitamins, minerals, and non-nutrient chemicals with potential health benefits.

The second category of functional foods consists of foods that have been enriched with a potentially health-promoting ingredient. Examples include margarine containing stanol esters, orange juice enriched with calcium and other nutrients, and beverages to which echinacea and other herbs have been added.

Some of these functional food products are based on good, solid science. For others, the supporting evidence is weak or speculative. Furthermore, the requirement for good taste sometimes forces manufacturers to limit the amount of herbs and other additives to a level so low that they are unlikely to have any effect.

The following is a list, by condition treated, of some of the more promising functional foods and natural products that are added to food products to create functional foods.

- *Cancer prevention.* Diindolylemethane (found in broccoli-family vegetables), fish oil (found in salmon and other cold-water fish), flaxseed (contains lignans), folate, garlic, green tea, I3C (found in vegetables in the broccoli family), IP6 (found in nuts, seeds, beans, whole grains, cantaloupe, and citrus fruits), lycopene (found in tomatoes), resveratrol (found in grape skin), selenium, soy foods, turmeric (added to many foods as a preservative), vitamin C, and vitamin E
- *Cataracts.* Lutein (found in dark-green vegetables)
- *Cavities.* Xylitol (added to chewing gum and candy)
- *Colds and flu.* Echinacea (herbal tea) and garlic
- *Diabetes.* Chromium (whole grains, brewer's yeast, fortified nutritional yeast, liver) and evening primrose oil
- *Diarrhea and other digestive problems.* Probiotics (friendly bacteria) found in yogurt
- *Ear infections.* Xylitol (added to chewing gum and candy)
- *Easy bruising.* Bioflavonoids (found in citrus fruits, buckwheat, and most fruits and vegetables)
- *Eczema.* Probiotics (friendly bacteria) found in yogurt
- *General nutrition.* Fortified grains and beverages
- *Heart disease prevention.* Alpha-linolenic acid (found in flaxseed oil), calcium (added to beverages; found in milk and other dairy products), garlic, fish oil (found in salmon and other cold-water fish), potassium (found in orange juice, bananas, and other foods), soy products, stanols-sterols (added to margarine and other spreads), fiber (such as in oats), wine and other alcoholic beverages (in moderation)
- *High cholesterol.* Fiber (found in whole grains and fruits, legumes, and vegetables), garlic, krill oil, soy products, stanols (added to margarine and other spreads)
- *Menopausal symptoms.* Soy products
- *Nausea.* Ginger (beverages)
- *Osteoporosis.* Calcium (added to beverages; found in milk and other dairy products), vitamin D (added to butter, milk, and other beverages), soy foods
- *Premenstrual syndrome.* Calcium (added to beverages; found in milk and other dairy products) and krill oil
- *Ulcerative colitis.* Probiotics (friendly bacteria; found in yogurt)
- *Urinary tract infection.* Cranberry juice
- *Vaginal infection.* Probiotics (friendly bacteria) found in yogurt

A Note About Labeling

The U.S. Food and Drug Administration (FDA) allows labels on foods similar to those used on dietary supplements. These labels do not require very much scientific validation, and they formally state that the claims made are not approved by the FDA.

In some cases, however, the FDA has specifically authorized higher-level health claims such as "heart healthy." These claims may be taken as representing scientific consensus. Because food supplementation is such a rapidly growing area, an increasing number of these labels should be expected.

EBSCO CAM Review Board

Further Reading

American Dietetic Association. "Functional Foods." Available at http://www.eatright.org/public.

Bratman, S., and A. Girman, eds. *Mosby's Handbook of Herbs and Supplements and Their Therapeutic Uses.* St. Louis, Mo.: Mosby, 2003.

Carlsen, M. H., et al. "The Total Antioxidant Content of More than 3,100 Foods, Beverages, Spices, Herbs, and Supplements Used Worldwide." *Nutrition Journal* 9 (2010): 3.

Gobbetti, M., R. D. Cagno, and M. De Angelis. "Functional Microorganisms for Functional Food Quality." *Critical Reviews in Food Science and Nutrition* 50 (2010): 716-727.

Lipski, E. "Traditional Non-Western Diets." *Nutrition in Clinical Practice* 25 (2010): 585-593.

Roberfroid, Marcel. "Concepts and Strategy of Functional Food Science: The European Perspective." *American Journal of Clinical Nutrition* 71 (2000): 1660-1664.

Tapsell, L. C., et al. "Health Benefits of Herbs and Spices: The Past, the Present, the Future." *Medical Journal of Australia* 185, suppl. 4 (2006): S4-S24.

See also: Carotenoids; Diet-based therapies; Food allergies and sensitivities; Functional foods: Overview; Low-carbohydrate diet; Low-glycemic index diet; Macrobiotic diet; Probiotics; Raw foods diet; Stanols and sterols; Supplements: Introduction; Vegan diet; Vegetarian diet.

Functional foods: Overview

CATEGORY: Issues and overviews

DEFINITION: A natural or modified food or food component that provides a health benefit beyond basic nutrition.

OVERVIEW

Functional foods are whole foods that naturally contain health-promoting substances or contain added health-promoting substances. Also, functional foods can act in concert with herbal supplements and drugs in the prevention and treatment of disease. In contrast, neutraceuticals are active ingredients isolated from foods and prepared in a medicinal form, and phytochemicals are chemical substances obtained from plants that are biologically active but not nutritive.

The concept of functional foods is not new, as the medical and physiological benefits of some foods have been known for ages. The enhanced interest in functional foods is driven by a confluence of three factors: a greater understanding of the way functional food components exert medical benefits, the desire and capability of the food industry to produce new products based on these concepts, and interest and acceptance by the consumer. The new discipline of functional food science places emphasis in gaining knowledge of how functional food components can affect certain body functions related to health and disease.

Several methods exist to modify a natural (unmodified) food to be a functional food. Any natural food with an active ingredient can be modified to improve its effectiveness as a functional food. For example, the concentration of a particular component that is naturally present in the particular food could be increased to produce beneficial effects. Similarly, a component known to cause a detrimental health effect could be removed. A component not normally found in a particular food but known to produce a beneficial effect could be added. A component whose intake is usually excessive and could cause deleterious health effects can be replaced by a component with beneficial health effects. Finally, the bioavailability or stability of a component known to reduce the disease-risk potential of a particular food could be improved.

The value of functional foods has been recognized by the American Dietetic Association and many other organizations. However, consumers should carefully weigh the health claims and overall value of functional food products. The U.S. Food and Drug Administration (FDA) considers functional foods as foods, not drugs, so manufacturers cannot claim that a functional food can cure, mitigate, treat, or prevent any disease. The Nutrition Labeling and Education Act (1990) does permit some exceptions, known as

List of Common Functional Foods and Food Components

- Ascorbic acid
- Bioflavonoids
- Black tea
- Calcium
- Carob
- Carotenoids
- Cherries
- Chocolate
- Cocoa
- Coconut oil
- Cranberry juice
- Echinacea
- Evening primrose oil
- Fish oil
- Flaxseed
- Flaxseed oil
- Garlic
- Ginger
- Green tea
- Honey
- Krill oil
- Acidophilus
- Lycopene
- Omega-3 fatty acids
- Palm oil
- Potassium
- Probiotics
- Pumpkin seed
- Rhubarb
- Saffron
- Soy
- Turmeric
- Vitamin C
- Vitamin D
- Vitamin E
- Whey protein

health claims, which state that a substance included in the diet on a regular basis "may help reduce the risk" of a certain disease. Most companies, however, prepare label claims based on maintaining a normal, healthy structure or function of the human body. Although so-called structure/function statements do not need approval from the FDA, the label must show a disclaimer statement to this effect. An example of a structure/function claim is the statement "helps build strong bones."

FUNCTIONAL FOOD TYPES

In general, foods in their natural state, such as fruits and vegetables, oily fish, whole grains, and nuts and seeds, are among the best functional foods. They have active ingredients and a fine overall nutritional balance.

Probiotics and prebiotics. Probiotics are beneficial bacteria added to dairy products such as yogurt to improve gastrointestinal health. Prebiotics (oligosaccharide carbohydrates that are abundantly found in artichokes, shallots, and onions) are growth media for beneficial bacteria.

Polyphenols, anthocyanidins, flavones, and tannins. Polyphenols are found in a variety of foods. They have an antioxidant effect, thought to reduce the incidence of cancer and coronary heart disease. Anthocyanidins are found in fruits, catechins in tea, and flavones in citrus. Flavones are widely distributed in fruits and vegetables, and lignans are found in flax, rye, and some vegetables. Tannins are found in cranberries and cocoa.

Dietary fibers. Dietary fibers, those food components obtained from plants that cannot be digested by the body, are classified as either insoluble or soluble. Insoluble fiber consists of plant cell-wall components, particularly cellulose, which form bulk in the diet and promote the regularity of bowel movements. Soluble fiber dissolves in water and thickens to form gels. Soluble fiber consistently has been shown to reduce total cholesterol and LDL (low-density lipoprotein), or bad cholesterol, in the blood. This reduction occurs through the reduced dietary fat and cholesterol uptake of the intestine and through increased fecal excretion of bile acids (which are derived from cholesterol).

Oats and barley contain an important fiber known as beta-glucan, a complex carbohydrate made of glucose units. Oatmeal has become a popular cereal for this reason, and oat bran too is marketed as a cereal or as an ingredient in other foods. Guar gum, pectin, and psyllium also contain abundant soluble fiber.

Omega-3 fatty acids. Omega-3 fatty acids have been found to be beneficial for the prevention of heart disease. (Omega-3 refers to chemical structure.) The omega-3 fatty acids eicosapentaenoic acid and docosapentaenoic acid are found in abundance in fatty fish, such as herring, anchovies, mackerel, salmon, and sardines. Another omega-3 fatty acid, linolenic acid, is found in walnut, soybean, and canola oils. The fish oils have a more protective effect than the plant oils. Omega-3 fatty acids are converted to biologically active compounds such as prostaglandins and leukotrienes, which have anti-inflammatory, antithrombic, antiarrythmic, and vasodilatory effects.

Plant sterols. Plant sterols are similar in structure to cholesterol and are found in the diet as sitosterol, stigmasterol, and campesterol. A compound made from sitosterol, known as stanol ester, is incorporated into a commercial margarine as a cholesterol-reducing agent. Nuts act as antioxidants and have a cholesterol-lowering effect.

Carotenoids. Carotenoids represent a large group of natural pigments found in plants (including yellow and orange fruits and vegetables such as carrots, apricots, squash, and sweet potatoes) and in dark green vegetables such as spinach, kale, and collard greens. The most common dietary carotenoids are alpha-carotene, beta-carotene, and lutein. Because of the nature of their molecules, carotenoids have strong antioxidant activity. Evidence shows that carotenoids have a protective effect against heart disease and some cancers.

RESEARCH

Most studies on functional foods have been observational; the great time and expense involved in clinical trials make observational studies the best option. Although there are many types of observational studies of functional foods, all attempt to relate the incidence of disease in a population with the dietary intake of a particular food. Observational studies can provide data from a large number of people in a relatively short period of time at low cost; however, these studies have been criticized for not controlling variables and for being subject to bias. Observational studies, however, can provide a strong indication of trends.

Intervention studies involve assigning participants to control or treatment groups, marked by various types and amounts of functional food components. The groups are followed over time, and researchers note the incidence of disease among groups. In a clinical trial, the groups are randomly assigned. Randomization reduces biases in evaluation of treatment and control groups by making the groups equal in all respects except for the treatments applied.

Before beginning a study, researchers start with basic scientific knowledge regarding functions that are sensitive to modification by food components. These functions could be genetic, cellular, biochemical, or physiologic. Quite often, instead of examining the effect of the component on an outcome, researchers may use a marker that is related to the outcome. For example, researchers could study the effect of an ingredient on cholesterol levels instead of waiting for heart disease to develop. Markers must be able to predict the beneficial or detrimental effects of a food component. The body could respond to the intake of a food component through changes in body fluid levels of certain metabolites or enzymes. Measurement of changes in body tissues, such as extent of narrowing of carotid arteries, can be related to the development of atherosclerosis. Markers need to be sensitive and specific to the disease condition.

ACTIONS OF FUNCTIONAL FOODS AND THEIR COMPONENTS

Probiotics. Probiotics are bacteria established in the intestinal tract that exert a beneficial effect. The term "probiotics" was coined to contrast with antibiotics, which destroy harmful bacteria. Probiotics are normally added to dairy products as lactobacilli and bifidobacteria. These bacteria promote improved intestinal microbial balance with a reduction in harmful microbes. Probiotics are beneficial in preventing infection and enhancing the immune system. They aid in preventing pathogens from entering the bloodstream through the mucosal epithelial cells by increasing mucin production and reducing permeability.

Probiotics also enhance antibacterial and anti-inflammatory activities of the intestinal epithelium by stimulating synthesis of specialized protective proteins. Clinical studies have shown that probiotics can reduce the symptoms of irritable bowel syndrome and can be beneficial in maintaining remission in cases of ulcerative colitis and pouchitis (inflammation of the intestinal wall). Other studies have shown that probiotics can help prevent necrotizing enterocolitis in infants.

Prebiotics. Prebiotics are indigestible oligosaccharide carbohydrates that can be fermented by lactobacilli and bifidobacteria. Prebiotics, along with probiotics, act in concert to produce the same beneficial results. Prebiotics can serve as fermenting media for probiotic bacteria already in the intestinal tract or in combination with introduced probiotics. Studies are ongoing to determine appropriate conditions for the use of intact cereals as media for the growth of probiotic strains and to develop processing methods to isolate sources of water-soluble fiber that can serve as prebiotics.

Plant sterols. A review article indicated that plant sterols and tree nuts were beneficial for the prevention of coronary heart disease in most clinical trials, while flavonoids in dark chocolate may protect LDL cholesterol from undergoing oxidative modification. Plant sterols are believed to interfere with the absorption of cholesterol from the small intestine by preventing it from dissolving in the micellular structure. Plant sterols are added to margarine products as a cholesterol-lowering agent, but some consumers have concerns about weight gain. A meta-analysis of fifty-nine randomized clinical trials found that plant sterols that were added to milk, orange juice, or yogurt lowered total cholesterol and LDL cholesterol, but did not do so when added to breads or meats.

Nuts. Many clinical studies have shown that the consumption of walnuts, almonds, pecans, pistachio nuts, and macadamia nuts result in lowered total cholesterol and LDL cholesterol. Epidemiological studies found an inverse relationship between nut consumption and the risk of coronary heart disease. Scientists believe that the beneficial effect of nuts comes from their high content of polyunsaturated fatty acids. Nuts may improve endothelial (blood-vessel wall) function too, resulting in better vasodilation. Nuts also may act as antioxidants, reducing LDL oxidation, one of the steps leading to plaque formation.

Polyphenols. Polyphenols, also known as flavonoids, are widespread in commonly consumed foods. Several hundred have been identified in fruits, vegetables, legumes, whole grains, and nuts, and in beverages such as tea, coffee, and wine. Many studies have examined polyphenols; however, many of these studies have been in vitro (in a laboratory) and at high doses. Epidemiological studies with humans have shown a protective effect of polyphenols on reducing fatal or nonfatal coronary artery disease. Epidemiological studies also have shown a protective effect against lung and colorectal cancers.

Procyanidins and isoflavones. Intervention (controlled) studies have shown that procyanidins found in red wine, grapes, cocoa, cranberries, and apples have pronounced beneficial effects on the vascular system, effects including antioxidant activity, decreased platelet aggregation, decreased LDL concentration, and increased HDL concentration. Isoflavones may have effects on bone mineral density and bone mineral content in women who are postmenopausal.

David A. Olle, M.S.

FURTHER READING

American Dietetic Association. "Functional Foods." Available at http://www.eatright.org/public.

Institute of Food Technologists. "Functional Foods Expert Report: Opportunities and Challenges." Describes in detail FDA regulations governing health-related claims on food labels. Available at http://www.ift.orgknowledge-center.

Milner, John. "Functional Foods: The U.S. Perspective." *American Journal of Clinical Nutrition* 71 (2000): 1654-1659. An overview of functional foods. Includes discussion of public interest and the means of evaluation.

Roberfroid, Marcel. "Concepts and Strategy of Functional Food Science: The European Perspective." *American Journal of Clinical Nutrition* 71 (2000): 1660-1664. Provides an introduction to the science of functional foods and their applications.

Saulnier, Delphine, et al. "Mechanisms of Probiosis and Prebiosis: Considerations for Enhanced Functional Foods." *Current Opinion in Biotechnology* 20, no. 2 (2009): 135-141. Discusses the mechanisms and applications of probiotics and prebiotics.

Vita, Joseph. "Polyphenols and Cardiovascular Disease: Effects on Endothelial and Platelet Function." *American Journal of Clinical Nutrition* 81 (2005): 292-297. A review of epidemiologic studies that support a relationship between higher intakes of polyphenolic flavonoids and reduced risk of cardiovascular disease.

See also: Carotenoids; Diet-based therapies; Food allergies and sensitivities; Functional foods: Introduction; Low-carbohydrate diet; Low-glycemic-index diet; Macrobiotic diet; Probiotics; Raw foods diet; Stanols and sterols; Supplements: Introduction; Vegan diet; Vegetarian diet.

G

GABA

CATEGORY: Herbs and supplements
RELATED TERM: Gamma-aminobutyric acid
DEFINITION: Natural substance of the human body used as a supplement to treat specific health conditions.
PRINCIPAL PROPOSED USE: Hypertension
OTHER PROPOSED USES: Anxiety, insomnia, stress

OVERVIEW

The substance gamma-aminobutyric acid (GABA) is a neurotransmitter, a chemical used by the human nervous system to send messages and modulate its own function. GABA acts in an inhibitory manner, tending to calm the nerves. Drugs in the benzodiazepine-receptor-agonist (BzRA) family (a family that includes true benzodiazepines such as Valium, as well as related drugs such as Ambien and Lunesta) exert their effect by facilitating the ability of GABA to bind to receptor sites in the brain. In turn, this leads to relaxation, relief from anxiety, induction of sleep, and suppression of seizure activity.

When GABA is taken orally, GABA levels in the brain do not increase, presumably because the substance itself cannot pass the blood-brain barrier and enter the central nervous system. For this reason, oral GABA supplements cannot replicate the effect of tranquilizing drugs, even though they work through a GABA-related mechanism. GABA supplements can affect the peripheral nervous system, however, as well as any other part of the body not protected by the blood-brain barrier. Some evidence suggests that orally ingested GABA might cause physiological changes that lead to benefit for hypertension.

REQUIREMENTS AND SOURCES

GABA is not a required nutrient, and it is not found to any extent in food. However, certain probiotics in the *Lactobacillus* family can be induced to produce GABA as they ferment milk and soy products. GABA supplements can also be created entirely synthetically.

THERAPEUTIC DOSAGES

In the best-designed study of GABA for reducing blood pressure, the dosage used was 10 milligrams (mg) daily. Much higher dosages are sometimes recommended by alternative practitioners for treating anxiety or insomnia, as high as 1,000 mg daily, in the (probably vain) hope that some tiny amount of this orally ingested GABA might make it into the brain.

THERAPEUTIC USES

As noted above, GABA is still sometimes recommended for treatment of anxiety and insomnia, but it is almost certainly ineffective for these purposes. However, evidence from animal studies and preliminary studies in humans hint that GABA supplements can reduce blood pressure. In the best of the human trials, thirty-nine people with mild hypertension were given either a fermented milk product providing GABA, at a dose of 10 mg daily, or a placebo, for twelve weeks. The results indicated that GABA modestly decreased blood pressure levels. However, this study was small and suffered from significant problems in design. Additional research will be necessary before GABA can be considered an effective treatment for high blood pressure.

SAFETY ISSUES

No serious adverse effects have been associated with the use of GABA. Nonetheless, comprehensive safety studies have not been performed. Maximum safe doses in young children, pregnant or nursing women, and people with severe liver or kidney disease have not been established.

FURTHER READING

Hirata, H., et al. "Hypotensive Effect of Fermented Milk Containing Gamma-Aminobutyric Acid (GABA) in Subjects with High Normal Blood Pressure." *Journal of the Japanese Society for Food Science and Technology* 51 (2004): 79-86.

Inoue, K., et al. "Blood-Pressure-Lowering Effect of a Novel Fermented Milk Containing Gamma-

Aminobutyric Acid (GABA) in Mild Hypertensives." *European Journal of Clinical Nutrition* 57 (2003): 490-495.

Park, K. B., and S. H. Oh. "Production of Yogurt with Enhanced Levels of Gamma-Aminobutyric Acid and Valuable Nutrients Using Lactic Acid Bacteria and Germinated Soybean Extract." *Bioresource Technology* 98 (2007): 1675-1679.

See also: Anxiety and panic attacks; Hypertension; Insomnia; Stress.

Gallstones

CATEGORY: Condition
RELATED TERM: Gallbladder pain
DEFINITION: Treatment of the sludge, lumps, and hard deposits that form in the bile.
PRINCIPAL PROPOSED NATURAL TREATMENTS: None
OTHER PROPOSED NATURAL TREATMENTS: Artichoke leaf, betaine hydrochloride, boldo, dandelion root, fumitory, greater celandine, milk thistle, peppermint, turmeric, vitamin C

INTRODUCTION

The function of the gallbladder is to store the bile produced by the liver and to release it on an as-needed basis for digestive purposes. However, it is not easy to keep this complex mixture of chemicals in liquid form. The various elements of bile have a natural tendency to form sludge, lumps, and hard deposits called gallstones. The body uses several biochemical methods to prevent such condensation from occurring, but this natural chemistry does not always succeed. More than 20 percent of women and 8 percent of men develop gallstones at some time in their lives.

A person could have gallstones for many years without experiencing any problems. However, sooner or later, a gallstone will likely plug the duct that leads out of the gallbladder, causing pain, often severe.

Generally, gallbladder pain starts in the form of occasional minor attacks that subside rapidly, separated by weeks without discomfort. During this phase, the stones block the duct temporarily and then move on. Eventually, continuous obstruction may develop, causing the gallbladder to become inflamed and perhaps infected. This condition is called cholecystitis, a

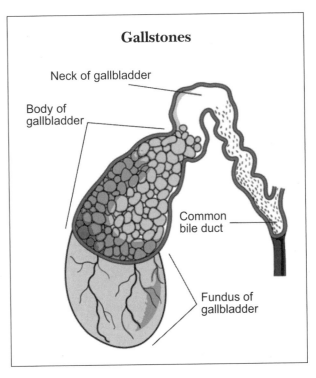

Gallstones

Neck of gallbladder

Body of gallbladder

Common bile duct

Fundus of gallbladder

potentially life-threatening situation because an inflamed, blocked gallbladder can rupture. Another risk is that a stone may escape the gallbladder's own duct and move along to the duct that carries away secretions from both the liver and the gallbladder (the common bile duct). When this happens, the liver cannot unload the bile it produces, putting it at risk of permanent injury and creating a surgical emergency.

The most reliable symptom of cholecystitis is intense pain beneath the right lower rib cage, often occurring from midnight to 3 A.M. Typically, pain radiates to the right shoulder and is accompanied by a loss of appetite and sometimes nausea. Removal of the gallbladder immediately solves the problem. Gallbladder surgery can usually be carried out laparoscopically, resulting in a quick and easy procedure that requires little recovery time.

Living without a gallbladder does not seem to bring any long-term consequences. However, many people are opposed on general principle to removing an organ that is naturally part of the body. Medications that dissolve gallstones may be another option.

PROPOSED NATURAL TREATMENTS

The only time it is appropriate to use alternative treatments for gallstones is during the interval before cholecystitis develops. Once the gallbladder has become completely blocked, surgical treatment is urgent.

However, during the initial period in which pain is only occasional or intermittent, the risks incurred by postponing surgery are slight. If a doctor feels that a trial of stone-dissolving medications might be appropriate, some of the agents described here could present alternative possibilities. None, though, are well established as effective. Medical supervision is essential.

Preliminary clinical trials suggest that formulas containing peppermint and related terpenes (fragrant substances found in plants) can dissolve gallstones. The herb milk thistle, standardized to its silymarin content, has been shown to improve the liquidity of bile, although its actual effects on gallstones are unknown.

Several herbs are prescribed in Germany for gallbladder pain, including artichoke leaf, boldo, dandelion root, fumitory, greater celandine, and turmeric. These herbs are thought to work by causing the gallbladder to contract and thereby expel its stones. However, such an effect is not always positive: Expelled stones might become lodged in the duct of the gallbladder or, worse, the common bile duct. Furthermore, if the duct is already blocked, gallbladder contraction will lead to increased pain and perhaps rupture. Finally, some of these herbs are potentially toxic to the liver. One should consult a qualified physician before trying these treatments.

There is some evidence that regular coffee drinking can reduce the risk of developing gallstones–in men between forty and seventy-five years of age. In an observational study that tracked about 46,000 male physicians for ten years, those who drank two to three cups of caffeinated coffee daily had a 40 percent reduced risk of developing gallstone disease. Those who drank more coffee had an even greater reduction of risk.

It may be that the caffeine in coffee helps, as other sources of caffeine were also associated with reduced risk of gallstones, while decaffeinated coffee did not seem to help. Caffeine is known to increase the flow of bile, so this connection makes sense. However, it is also possible that people who drink more coffee have other unknown characteristics that make them more likely to have gallstones, and that caffeine itself has no effect. Observational studies, in other words, do not show cause and effect. Similarly weak evidence suggests that the regular use of vitamin C supplements might help prevent gallstones in women.

EBSCO CAM Review Board

Further Reading

Clavien, Pierre-Alain, ed. *Diseases of the Gallbladder and Bile Ducts.* 2d ed. Hoboken, N.J.: Wiley-Blackwell, 2006.

Leitzmann, M. F., et al. "A Prospective Study of Coffee Consumption and the Risk of Symptomatic Gallstone Disease in Men." *Journal of the American Medical Association* 281 (1999): 2106-2112.

Simon, J. A., and E. S. Hudes. "Serum Ascorbic Acid and Gallbladder Disease Prevalence Among U.S. Adults." *Archives of Internal Medicine* 160 (2000): 931-936.

See also: Bile acid sequestrant drugs; Cholesterol, high; Gastrointestinal health; Kidney stones; Liver disease; Pancreatitis; Surgery support.

Gamma-linolenic acid

Category: Herbs and supplements

Related terms: Omega-6 fatty acids, omega-6 oils, sources of gamma-linolenic acid, including black currant seed oil, borage oil, and evening primrose oil

Definition: Natural substance essential for health and promoted as a dietary supplement for specific health benefits.

Principal proposed use: Diabetic neuropathy

Other proposed uses:

- *Gamma-linolenic acid:* Attention deficit disorder, cyclic mastalgia, dry eyes (in contact lens wearers), kidney stones, premenstrual syndrome, Raynaud's phenomenon, rheumatoid arthritis, ulcerative colitis, weight loss
- *In combination with fish oil:* Attention deficit and hyperactivity disorder, Huntington's disease, osteoporosis

Probably not effective use: Eczema

Overview

Gamma-linolenic acid (GLA) is one of the two main types of essential fatty acids. These are good fats that are as necessary as vitamins for health. Specifically, GLA is an omega-6 fatty acid. The body uses essential fatty acids to make various prostaglandins and leukotrienes. These substances influence inflammation and pain; some of them increase symptoms, while others decrease them. Taking GLA may swing the balance to the more favorable prostaglandins and leukotrienes, making it helpful for diseases that involve inflammation.

There is some evidence that GLA may be helpful for diabetic neuropathy. The supplement is widely used in the United Kingdom and other parts of Europe to treat eczema and cyclic mastalgia (a condition marked by breast pain associated with the menstrual cycle). Evidence, however, suggests that it may not help. There are many other proposed uses of GLA based on fairly weak evidence.

REQUIREMENTS AND SOURCES

The body ordinarily makes all the GLA it needs from linolenic acid, an omega-6 essential fatty acid found in many foods. In certain circumstances, however, the body may not be able to convert linolenic acid to make GLA efficiently. These circumstances include advanced age, diabetes, high alcohol intake, eczema, cyclic mastitis, viral infections, excessive saturated fat intake, elevated cholesterol levels, and deficiencies of vitamin B_6, zinc, magnesium, biotin, or calcium. In such cases, taking GLA supplements may make up for a genuine deficiency.

Evening Primrose Oil as a Source of GLA

Evening primrose (*Oenothera biennis*) is a plant native to North America, but it grows in Europe and parts of the Southern Hemisphere as well. It has yellow flowers that bloom in the evening. Evening primrose oil contains gamma-linolenic acid (GLA), an essential fatty acid. Essential fatty acids are required by the body for growth and development, and they must be obtained from the diet.

Evening primrose oil is extracted from the seeds of the evening primrose. The oil is usually put into capsules for use, and it is well tolerated by most people. Mild side effects include gastrointestinal upset and headache.

The oil has been used since the 1930s for eczema, a condition in which the skin becomes inflamed, itchy, or scaly because of allergies or other irritation. The oil also has been used for other conditions involving inflammation, such as rheumatoid arthritis; for conditions affecting women, such as breast pain associated with the menstrual cycle, menopausal symptoms, and premenstrual syndrome (PMS); and for cancer and diabetes.

A small amount of GLA is found in the diet. Borage oil is the richest supplemental source (17 to 25 percent GLA), followed by black currant oil (15 to 20 percent) and evening primrose oil (7 to 10 percent). Borage and evening primrose are the most common sources used in studies.

It is commonly stated that people require a certain optimum ratio of omega-3 to omega-6 fatty acids in the diet; however, there is no real evidence that this is true, and some evidence that it is false.

THERAPEUTIC DOSAGES

The typical dosage of GLA when it is used in hopes of alleviating cyclic mastalgia or eczema is about 200 to 400 milligrams (mg) daily (about 2 to 4 grams [g] of evening primrose oil or 1 to 2 g of borage oil). Diabetic neuropathy is typically treated with about 400 to 600 mg daily (about 4 to 6 g of evening primrose or 2 to 3 g of borage oil). In rheumatoid arthritis, doses as high as 2,000 to 3,000 mg have been tried. (Doses this high can only be obtained from purified GLA, as one would need impractically high doses of evening primrose oil or borage oil to get enough.)

GLA should be taken with food. Full benefits (if there are any) may take more than six months to develop.

THERAPEUTIC USES

GLA has shown some promise for the treatment of diabetic neuropathy, a complication of diabetes. This condition consists of pain and numbness caused by progressive nerve damage. However, supporting evidence that GLA is effective for this use is quite limited.

Perhaps the most common use of GLA has been as a treatment for eczema. It was once widely dispensed for this purpose by the British health-care system, but the balance of the evidence indicates that for eczema, GLA is just a placebo treatment.

GLA is also a popular treatment for cyclic mastalgia, but the evidence regarding its effectiveness is more negative than positive. GLA is additionally said to be useful for general premenstrual syndrome (PMS) symptoms, but the supporting evidence for this use is very weak.

Despite many positive anecdotes, GLA has failed to prove effective for attention deficit disorder (ADD). One study that used GLA plus fish oil did find weak evidence of benefits. Extremely weak evidence hints that evening primrose oil might be more effective for

ADD if combined with zinc, but this is more of an untested hypothesis than a conclusion.

GLA has been studied for numerous other conditions, such as rheumatoid arthritis, Raynaud's phenomenon (a condition in which the fingers and toes react to cold in an exaggerated way), weight loss, ulcerative colitis, kidney stones, and multiple sclerosis, and for increasing the effectiveness of the drug tamoxifen in the treatment of breast cancer. Persons undergoing treatment for cancer should not take GLA (or any other supplement) except under physician supervision.

Other studies have investigated the potential benefits of combination treatment using GLA and fish oil. Conditions studied include osteoporosis, chronic fatigue syndrome, periodontitis (gum disease), and Huntington's disease. In these trials, some promising (but far from definitive) results have been seen. However, this combination therapy has failed to prove effective for cyclic mastalgia.

GLA is sometimes suggested as a treatment for tardive dyskinesia, but two double-blind studies have failed to find it helpful for this disorder. GLA has also failed to prove effective for the itching caused by kidney dialysis.

There is some evidence that GLA may benefit persons with eye problems. One randomized trial indicated that orally administered evening primrose oil was more effective than olive oil (placebo) at reducing dry eye symptoms and improving comfort in users of soft contact lenses. In addition, Sjögren's syndrome, an autoimmune condition in which the immune system destroys moisture-producing glands, often causes dry eyes because of a lack of tears. One small double-blind study found that a combination of GLA and the omega-6 fatty acid linolenic acid (found in many vegetable oils) may improve dry eye symptoms in Sjögren's. Finally, persons who undergo laser surgery for vision correction (photorefractive keratectomy) are sometimes left with a hazy appearance to their cornea. Another small randomized trial found some potential benefit of a supplement containing omega-6 fatty acids in preventing this complication.

Thus far, only a fraction of the conditions for which GLA has been proposed as a treatment have been discussed here. Other conditions include asthma, allergies, bursitis, endometriosis, heart disease, irritable bowel syndrome, prostate cancer, benign prostatic hyperplasia, and Sjögren's disease. However, none of these potential uses has been scientifically evaluated to any significant extent.

SCIENTIFIC EVIDENCE

Diabetic neuropathy. Diabetic neuropathy is a gradual degeneration of nerves caused by diabetes. There is some evidence that GLA can be helpful, if it is given time to work. In one double-blind, placebo-controlled study, 111 people with mild diabetic neuropathy received 480 mg daily of either GLA or placebo. After twelve months, the group taking GLA was doing significantly better than the placebo group. Good results were seen in a smaller study too. However, these promising findings lack further research validation. There is some preliminary evidence that GLA may be more effective for diabetic neuropathy when it is combined with lipoic acid.

Eczema. Despite GLA (usually as evening primrose oil) being widely used in Europe to treat eczema, it appears most likely that the treatment is not truly effective. The anecdotes of cure that abound are probably just testimonials to the placebo effect (and to a strong marketing campaign by one evening primrose oil supplier).

A 1989 review of the literature found significant benefit in the nine double-blind controlled studies performed to that date, all involving evening primrose oil. This study led to widespread sales of one evening primrose oil product. However, this review has been sharply criticized for including poorly designed studies and for possibly misinterpreting study results.

Improvements in symptoms were also seen in a later double-blind study of forty-eight children with eczema. However, more recent and better-conducted research has failed to find any benefit. For example, a sixteen-week, double-blind study involving fifty-eight children with eczema found no difference between the effects of evening primrose oil and placebo (substantial improvements were seen, but to the same extent for placebo and evening primrose oil). Lack of specific benefit was also seen with evening primrose oil or evening primrose oil plus fish oil in a sixteen-week, double-blind, placebo-controlled study of 102 persons with eczema. Finally, a double-blind trial followed thirty-nine people with hand dermatitis for twenty-four weeks; it again found no greater benefits than those produced by placebo.

GLA taken orally from borage oil has also failed to prove effective. In a twenty-four-week, double-blind study of 160 adults with eczema, the treatment provided no greater benefits than placebo. The same was seen in a twelve-week, double-blind, placebo-controlled study of 151 adults and children with eczema. Finally, in a double-blind, placebo-controlled study of 118 infants at high risk for developing eczema, a GLA supplement made from borage oil failed to provide a significant protective effect.

However, a double-blind study tested the use of undershirts coated with borage oil for the treatment of eczema. In this two-week study of thirty-two children aged one to ten years, the use of these coated undershirts appeared to reduce eczema symptoms. However, additional, higher-quality research studies need to be undertaken to establish whether or not this method of delivery really works.

Cyclic mastalgia. Cyclic mastalgia, also known as fibrocystic breast disease, cyclic mastitis, and mastodynia, is a condition in which a woman's breasts become painful during the week or two before her menstrual period. The discomfort is accompanied by swelling, inflammation, and sometimes actual cysts that form in the breasts. It is often associated with other PMS symptoms.

The cause of cyclic mastalgia is not known, but some researchers believe that it is associated with an imbalance of fatty acids in the body. On this basis, evening primrose oil became a popular treatment for cyclic mastalgia. However, there are considerable doubts regarding whether it is actually effective.

The main supporting evidence comes from three controlled studies that appeared to find benefit. All of these studies had significant limitations in design and reporting and cannot be taken as reliable. A better-quality study found that evening primrose oil, by itself or with fish oil, is not more effective than placebo for cyclic breast pain. A randomized trial involving eighty-five women also did not support the effectiveness of evening primrose (alone or with vitamin E) for treating breast pain. Other studies have found evening primrose oil ineffective for established breast cysts.

Other premenstrual symptoms. Although several small studies suggest that GLA as evening primrose oil is helpful in reducing overall PMS symptoms, all of these studies had serious flaws that make the results difficult to trust.

Rheumatoid arthritis. According to many studies, fish oil, a source of omega-3 essential fatty acids, improves symptoms of rheumatoid arthritis. A few studies suggest that GLA may also help. One six-month double-blind study followed fifty-six people with rheumatoid arthritis. Participants received either 2.8 g daily of purified GLA or placebo. The group taking GLA experienced significantly fewer symptoms than the placebo group, and the improvements grew over time.

Other small studies have found similar results. The overall conclusion appears to be that purified GLA might offer some benefit for rheumatoid arthritis, especially when used with standard treatment for rheumatoid arthritis, but the evidence is weak.

Raynaud's phenomenon. High dosages of evening primrose oil may be useful for Raynaud's phenomenon, a condition in which a person's hands and feet show abnormal sensitivity to cold temperatures. A small double-blind study found that GLA produced significantly better results than placebo. Similar results have been obtained with the omega-3 fatty acids found in fish oil. However, larger studies would be necessary to actually establish effectiveness.

Osteoporosis. There is some evidence that essential fatty acids may enhance the effectiveness of calcium for the treatment or prevention of osteoporosis. In one study, sixty-five postmenopausal women were given calcium with either placebo or a combination of omega-6 fatty acids (from evening primrose oil) and omega-3 fatty acids (from fish oil) for eighteen months. At the end of the study period, the group receiving essential fatty acids had higher bone density and fewer fractures than the placebo group. However, a twelve-month, double-blind trial of forty-two postmenopausal women found no benefit.

The explanation for the discrepancy may lie in the differences between the women studied. The first study involved women living in nursing homes, while the second studied healthier women living on their own. The latter group of women may have been better nourished and might already have been receiving enough essential fatty acids in their diet.

Attention deficit disorder. Based on evidence that essential fatty acids are necessary for the proper development of brain function in growing children, essential fatty acids have been tried for the treatment of ADD and related conditions. A preliminary double-blind, placebo-controlled trial found some evidence that a supplement containing fish oil and evening primrose oil might improve ADD symptoms. However, a high rate of dropouts makes the results of this study less than reliable. A repeat study found this combination no better than placebo.

Evening primrose oil by itself was found no better than placebo in a double-blind, placebo-controlled trial. In another small placebo-controlled, comparative trial, evening primrose oil proved less effective than standard medical treatment.

Weight loss. A twelve-week, double-blind study that enrolled one hundred significantly overweight women compared the effectiveness of evening primrose oil to placebo. No difference was seen between the groups. However, there was a high dropout rate in this trial (more than 25 percent), which somewhat decreases the meaningfulness of the results. In addition, many participants were known to have "refractory obesity," meaning that they had already failed to respond to other forms of treatment.

Another double-blind trial, involving forty-seven people, tested the unusual hypothesis that evening primrose might only work in persons with a family history of obesity. The results showed that the use of evening primrose oil produced a small but significant loss of weight. Participants whose parents were obese showed even better response. Considering the contradictory nature of this evidence, more research is necessary to determine whether evening primrose oil is really useful for weight loss.

SAFETY ISSUES

Most of the safety information on GLA comes from experience with evening primrose oil. Animal studies suggest that evening primrose oil is completely nontoxic and noncarcinogenic. More than four thousand people have taken GLA or evening primrose oil in scientific studies, and no significant adverse effects have ever been noted.

Early reports suggested that GLA might worsen temporal lobe epilepsy, but there has been no later confirmation. The maximum safe dosage of GLA for young children, pregnant or nursing women, or those with severe liver or kidney disease has not been established.

EBSCO CAM Review Board

FURTHER READING

Aragona, P., et al. "Systemic Omega-6 Essential Fatty Acid Treatment and PGE1 Tear Content in Sjögren's Syndrome Patients." *Investigative Ophthalmology and Visual Science* 46 (2005): 4474-4479.

Harris, W. S. "The Omega-6/Omega-3 Ratio and Cardiovascular Disease Risk: Uses and Abuses." *Current Atherosclerosis Reports* 8 (2006): 453-459.

Kanehara, S., et al. "Clinical Effects of Undershirts Coated with Borage Oil on Children with Atopic Dermatitis." *Journal of Dermatology* 34 (2007): 811-815.

Kokke, K. H., J. A. Morris, and J. G. Lawrenson. "Oral Omega-6 Essential Fatty Acid Treatment in Contact Lens Associated Dry Eye." *Contact Lens and Anterior Eye* 31 (2008): 141-146.

Pruthi, S., et al. "Vitamin E and Evening Primrose Oil for Management of Cyclical Mastalgia." *Alternative Medicine Review* 15 (2010): 59-67.

Stevens, L., et al. "EFA Supplementation in Children with Inattention, Hyperactivity, and Other Disruptive Behaviors." *Lipids* 38 (2003): 1007-1021.

Van Gool, C. J., et al. "Gamma-Linolenic Acid Supplementation for Prophylaxis of Atopic Dermatitis: A Randomized Controlled Trial in Infants at High Familial Risk." *American Journal of Clinical Nutrition* 77 (2003): 943-951.

See also: Diabetes, complications of; Fish oil.

Gamma oryzanol

CATEGORY: Herbs and supplements

DEFINITION: Natural plant product used to treat specific health conditions.

PRINCIPAL PROPOSED USE: High cholesterol

OTHER PROPOSED USES: Heart disease prevention, menopausal symptoms, sports performance and bodybuilding, ulcer prevention

OVERVIEW

Gamma oryzanol is a mixture of substances derived from rice bran oil, including sterols and ferulic acid. It has been approved in Japan for several conditions, including menopausal symptoms, mild anxiety, stomach upset, and high cholesterol. In the United States, it is widely used as a sports supplement, as well as for reducing cholesterol. However, there is no meaningful evidence supporting the use of gamma oryzanol for any of these purposes.

REQUIREMENTS AND SOURCES

There is no daily requirement for gamma oryzanol. Rice bran oil is the principal source of gamma oryzanol, but it is also found in the bran of wheat and other grains, as well as in various fruits, vegetables, and herbs. However, to get enough gamma oryzanol to reach typical therapeutic dosages, one needs to take supplements.

THERAPEUTIC DOSAGES

A typical dosage of gamma oryzanol is 500 milligrams (mg) daily.

THERAPEUTIC USES

Like many other vegetable oils, rice bran oil appears to improve cholesterol profile. Preliminary evidence, including small double-blind, placebo-controlled trials, suggests that the gamma oryzanol portion of rice bran oil may contribute an additional cholesterol-lowering benefit beyond the effects of the fatty acids. Gamma oryzanol is thought to work by impairing cholesterol absorption in the digestive tract.

Additionally, gamma oryzanol has antioxidant properties. It has been hypothesized that antioxidants can help protect against heart disease, cancer, and other illnesses; however, it must be kept in mind that gigantic studies looking for such benefits with the antioxidants vitamin E and beta-carotene have returned negative results.

Gamma oryzanol is used by some athletes based on early reports that suggested gamma oryzanol enhances muscle growth and sports performance. According to numerous Web sites, gamma oryzanol produces these benefits by increasing levels of testosterone, growth hormone, and other anabolic (muscle-building) hormones. However, there is no real evidence that gamma oryzanol either affects these hormones or enhances performance, and some evidence that it does not. For example, a double-blind, placebo-controlled study found that nine weeks' consumption of gamma oryzanol at a dose of 500 mg daily affected neither anabolic hormone levels nor performance. Evidence from animal studies suggests that gamma oryzanol may help prevent ulcers, but meaningful human trials are lacking.

Gamma oryzanol also has been advocated as a treatment for menopausal symptoms, but the basis of this potential use consists of evidence far too weak to be relied upon. In one study, gamma oryzanol injected into rats altered levels of circulating luteinizing hormone (LH). This, in turn, might conceivably help menopausal symptoms, but it is a long way from theoretical benefits in rats to proof of effectiveness in humans. One open study, sometimes touted as direct evidence for benefit in menopause, lacked a control group and therefore means nothing.

SAFETY ISSUES

In the late 1970s, a batch of rice bran oil was contaminated by polychlorobiphenyls (PCBs), resulting in the poisoning of more than two thousand people. This led to studies on the safety of gamma oryzanol products. On balance, the results of these investigations suggest that gamma oryzanol, when taken at normal doses, is nontoxic and noncarcinogenic. However, the maximum safe dosages for young children, pregnant or nursing women, and those with severe liver or kidney disease have not been established.

FURTHER READING

Berger, A., et al. "Similar Cholesterol-Lowering Properties of Rice Bran Oil, with Varied Gamma-Oryzanol, in Mildly Hypercholesterolemic Men." *European Journal of Nutrition* 44, no. 3 (2005): 163-173.

Cicero, A. F., and A. Gaddi. "Rice Bran Oil and Gamma-Oryzanol in the Treatment of Hyperlipoproteinaemias and Other Conditions." *Phytotherapy Research* 15 (2001): 277-289.

Most, M. M., et al. "Rice Bran Oil, Not Fiber, Lowers Cholesterol in Humans." *American Journal of Clinical Nutrition* 81 (2005): 64-68.

See also: Cholesterol, high; Herbal medicine; Menopause; Sports and fitness: Performance enhancement; Ulcers.

Garlic

CATEGORY: Herbs and supplements
RELATED TERM: *Allium sativum*
DEFINITION: Herbal product promoted as a dietary supplement for specific health benefits.
PRINCIPAL PROPOSED USES: Common cold prevention, heart disease prevention, insect repellent
OTHER PROPOSED USES: Athlete's foot, blood thinning, cancer prevention, candida, diabetes, hyper-

tension, immune support, middle ear infection (reducing pain), topical antibiotic, vaginal infection, yeast hypersensitivity

PROBABLY NOT EFFECTIVE USES: High cholesterol, oral antibiotic, ulcers

OVERVIEW

The story of garlic's role in human history could fill a book, as indeed it has, many times. Its species name, *sativum*, means "cultivated," indicating that garlic does not grow in the wild. So fond have humans been of this herb that garlic can be found almost everywhere in the world, from Polynesia to Siberia.

From Roman antiquity through World War I, garlic poultices were used to prevent wound infections. The famous microbiologist Louis Pasteur performed some of the original work showing that garlic could kill bacteria. In 1916, the British government issued a general plea for the public to supply it with garlic to meet wartime needs. Garlic was called Russian penicillin during World War II because, after running out of antibiotics, the Russian government turned to this ancient treatment for its soldiers. After World War II, Sandoz Pharmaceuticals manufactured a garlic

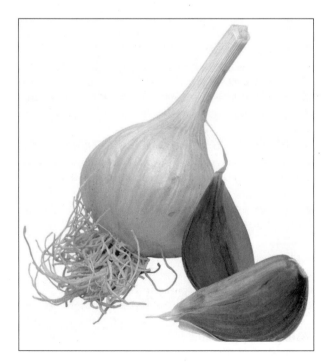

Garlic has been studied for cancer prevention and treatment. (Object Gear)

compound for intestinal spasms, and the Van Patten Company produced another for lowering blood pressure.

USES AND APPLICATIONS

Garlic is widely used as an all-around treatment for preventing or slowing the progression of atherosclerosis (the cause of most heart attacks and strokes). However, there is actually relatively little in the way of meaningful evidence that it works for this purpose. The balance of the evidence suggests that garlic is not effective for treating high cholesterol; there is only minimal evidence that it offers any benefits for people with high blood pressure. According to some studies, garlic might have blood-thinning effects, but whether this translates into any medical benefit remains unclear.

One study found preliminary evidence that the use of garlic could enhance blood sugar control in diabetes. Also, garlic has a long folkloric history as a treatment for colds and is commonly stated to strengthen the immune system. However, not until 2001 was there supporting evidence for this use. A well-designed double-blind study suggested that the regular use of garlic extract can help prevent colds.

In addition, folklore suggesting that garlic ingestion can ward off insect bites may have some truth to it, at least when garlic is taken regularly for several weeks. When applied topically, garlic can kill fungi, and there is preliminary evidence suggesting that ajoene, a compound derived from garlic, might help treat athlete's foot. Topical garlic can also kill bacteria on contact; however, if taken by mouth, garlic will not work like an antibiotic (that is, throughout the body). Furthermore, oral garlic has failed to prove effective for killing *Helicobacter pylori*, the stomach bacteria implicated as a major cause of ulcers.

Traditionally, garlic was often combined with the herb mullein in oil products designed to reduce the pain of middle ear infections (otitis media) but not of external ear infections (known commonly as swimmer's ear). Two double-blind studies support this use. While these products may reduce pain, it is very unlikely that they have any actual effect on the infection because the eardrum prevents them from reaching the site of infection.

Preliminary evidence, including one small double-blind trial, suggests that regular intake of garlic as food or as aged garlic supplements may reduce the risk of various forms of cancer. Based on extremely weak evidence, garlic has been proposed as a treatment for problems related to the yeast *Candida albicans*, problems such as vaginal yeast infection, oral yeast infection (thrush), and the purported condition discussed in some alternative medicine circles as yeast hypersensitivity syndrome.

SCIENTIFIC EVIDENCE

Atherosclerosis. Scant evidence hints that garlic might help prevent atherosclerosis, the most common cause of heart attacks and strokes. Garlic preparations have been found to slow hardening of the arteries in animal studies.

In a double-blind, placebo-controlled study that followed 152 people for four years, standardized garlic powder at a dosage of 900 milligrams (mg) daily significantly slowed the development of atherosclerosis as measured by ultrasound. However, this study had some statistical problems that make its results less than fully reliable.

An observational study of two hundred people measured the flexibility of the aorta, the main artery exiting the heart. Participants who took garlic showed more flexibility, indicating less atherosclerosis. However, because this was not a double-blind trial, its results prove little.

Heart attack prevention. In one study, 432 people who had experienced a heart attack were given either garlic oil extract or no treatment for a period of three years. The results showed a significant reduction of second heart attacks and about a 50 percent reduction in death rate among those taking garlic.

High cholesterol. A number of studies published in the 1980s and early 1990s found evidence that garlic preparations can reduce high cholesterol. However, virtually all subsequent studies have failed to find any significant benefit. One carefully designed study failed to find benefits with raw garlic, garlic powder, or aged garlic. The accumulating impact of these repeated negative results indicates that garlic is not effective for improving cholesterol profile.

Hypertension. Numerous studies have found weak evidence that garlic lowers blood pressure slightly, perhaps in the neighborhood of 5 to 10 percent more than placebo. It remains unclear whether garlic supplements can help persons with high blood pressure safely eliminate or avoid antihypertensive medications.

One study followed forty-seven persons with an average starting blood pressure of 171/101. In a period of twelve weeks, one-half were treated with 600 mg of garlic powder daily standardized to 1.3 percent alliin, while the other one-half were given placebo. The results showed a statistically significant drop of 11 percent in the systolic blood pressure and 13 percent in the diastolic pressure. In comparison, blood pressure fell in the placebo group by 5 and 4 percent, respectively. However, this study had a significant problem: The average starting blood pressures of the placebo and the treated groups were quite different, making comparisons unreliable.

Prevention of colds. The herb garlic has a long history of use for treating or preventing colds. An American study reported in 2001 provides meaningful preliminary evidence that garlic might possess cold-fighting powers. In this twelve-week, double-blind, placebo-controlled trial, 146 people received either placebo or a garlic extract between the months of November and February.

The results showed that participants receiving garlic were almost two-thirds less likely to catch cold than those receiving placebo. Furthermore, participants who did catch cold recovered about one day faster in the garlic group compared with the placebo group. Thus, the regular use of garlic might help prevent colds. However, there is no evidence that taking garlic at the onset of a cold will help a person recover more quickly.

Insect repellent. A twenty-week, double-blind, placebo-controlled crossover trial followed eighty Swedish soldiers and measured the number of tick bites they received while undergoing the garlic and the placebo treatments. The results showed a modest but statistically significant reduction in tick bites when soldiers consumed 1,200 mg of garlic daily for eight to ten weeks. However, the type of garlic used in this study was not stated. Another study failed to find one-time use of garlic helpful for repelling mosquitoes.

Cancer prevention. Evidence from observational studies suggests that garlic may help prevent cancer, particularly cancer of the stomach and colon. In one of the best of these trials, the Iowa Women's Study, 41,837 women were questioned as to their lifestyle habits (beginning in 1986) and then followed in subsequent years. At the four-year follow-up, questionnaires showed that women whose diets included significant quantities of garlic were approximately 30 percent less likely to develop colon cancer.

The interpretations of studies like this one are always a bit controversial. For example, it is possible that the women who ate a lot of garlic also made other healthful lifestyle choices. While researchers looked at this possibility carefully and concluded that garlic was a common factor, it is not clear that the researchers are right. What is really needed to settle the question is an intervention trial, in which some people are given garlic and others are given placebo. However, no studies have been performed to evaluate garlic for cancer prevention.

Antimicrobial. There is no question that raw garlic can kill a wide variety of microorganisms, including fungi, bacteria, viruses, and protozoa, by direct contact. A double-blind study reported in 1999 found that a cream made from the garlic constituent ajoene was just as effective for fungal skin infections as the standard drug terbinafine. These findings may explain why garlic was traditionally applied directly to wounds to prevent infection (but it also can burn the skin). Nevertheless, there is no real evidence that taking garlic orally can kill organisms throughout the body. Thus, it is not an antibiotic in the usual sense; it is more of an antiseptic.

Oral garlic could theoretically offer benefits against organisms in the stomach or intestines because it can come into direct contact with them. However, there is only the slightest evidence that it works for any specific infection of this type. For example, despite test-tube evidence that garlic can kill *H. pylori*, studies in people have not been promising.

Dosage

A typical dosage of garlic is 900 mg daily of a garlic powder extract standardized to contain 1.3 percent alliin, providing about 12,000 micrograms of alliin daily, or 4 to 5 mg of "allicin potential." Alliin-free aged garlic is taken at a dose of 1 to 7.2 grams daily.

Alliin is a relatively odorless substance found in garlic. When garlic is crushed or cut, an enzyme called allinase is brought in contact with alliin, turning it into allicin. Allicin is responsible for much of the typical odor of garlic. It is very active chemically and probably helps the garlic bulb defend itself from attack by insects and other threats. However, allicin is unstable, and it soon breaks down into a variety of other substances. When garlic is ground up and encapsulated, the effect is similar to cutting the bulb: Alliin contacts allinase, yielding allicin, which then breaks down.

Unless something is done to prevent this process, garlic powder will not have any alliin or allicin left by the time it is purchased.

Some garlic producers believe that alliin and allicin are not essential for garlic's effectiveness and do not worry about this breakdown. Aged garlic, for example, has very little of either compound, but other manufacturers believe that allicin is the primary active ingredient in garlic. Because allicin is an unstable chemical, these manufacturers are faced with a challenge.

One solution might be to chemically stabilize allicin so that it does not break down. However, allicin has a strong garlic smell, and a relatively odorless product is preferable. Many manufacturers of garlic powder products seek to stabilize the alliin in the product, and to do so in such a way that the alliin converts to allicin after it is consumed. How well their methods work remains a matter of controversy.

One should not confuse essential oil of garlic with garlic oils. The term "garlic oil" refers to garlic extracted by means of oil. Garlic essential oil is the pure oily component of the herb, and, like other essential oils, it is potentially toxic.

Safety Issues

As a commonly used food, garlic is on the GRAS (Generally Recognized As Safe) list of the U.S. Food and Drug Administration. Test rats have been fed gigantic doses of aged garlic (2,000 mg per kilogram of body weight) for six months without any signs of negative effects. Long-term treatment with standardized garlic powder at a dose equivalent to three times the usual dose, along with fish oil, produced no toxic effects in rats.

The only common side effect of garlic is unpleasant breath odor. Even "odorless garlic" produces an offensive smell in up to 50 percent of those who use it. Other side effects occur only rarely. For example, a study that followed 1,997 people who were given a normal dose of deodorized garlic daily for sixteen weeks showed a 6 percent incidence of nausea, a 1.3 percent incidence of dizziness on standing (perhaps a sign of low blood pressure), and a 1.1 percent incidence of allergic reactions. There were also a few reports of bloating, headaches, sweating, and dizziness.

When raw garlic is taken in excessive doses, it can cause numerous symptoms, such as stomach upset, heartburn, nausea, vomiting, diarrhea, flatulence, facial flushing, rapid pulse, and insomnia. Topical garlic can cause skin irritation, blistering, and even third-degree burns.

Because garlic might "thin" the blood, it is probably imprudent to take garlic pills immediately before or after surgery or labor and delivery because of the risk of excessive bleeding. Similarly, garlic should not be combined with blood-thinning drugs such as warfarin (Coumadin), heparin, aspirin, clopidogrel (Plavix), ticlopidine (Ticlid), or pentoxifylline (Trental). In addition, garlic could conceivably interact with natural products with blood-thinning properties, such as ginkgo, policosanol, or high-dose vitamin E. However, a placebo-controlled study found that actual raw garlic consumed in food at the fairly high dose of 4.2 mg once daily did not impair platelet function. In addition, volunteers who continued to consume the dietary garlic for one week did not show any changes in their normal platelet function.

Garlic may also combine poorly with certain medications for human immunodeficiency virus (HIV) infection. Two HIV-positive persons experienced severe gastrointestinal toxicity from the HIV drug ritonavir after taking garlic supplements. Garlic might also reduce the effectiveness of some drugs used for HIV infection. Garlic is presumed to be safe for pregnant women (except just before and immediately after delivery) and nursing mothers, although this has not been proven.

IMPORTANT INTERACTIONS

Persons should not use garlic except on medical advice if also taking blood-thinning drugs. Taking garlic at the same time as ginkgo, policosanol, or high-dose vitamin E might conceivably cause a risk of bleeding problems. Finally, one should not use garlic if also taking medications for HIV infection.

EBSCO CAM Review Board

FURTHER READING

Gardner, C. D., et al. "Effect of Raw Garlic vs Commercial Garlic Supplements on Plasma Lipid Concentrations in Adults with Moderate Hypercholesterolemia." *Archives of Internal Medicine* 167 (2007): 346-353.

Khoo, Y. S., and Z. Aziz. "Garlic Supplementation and Serum Cholesterol." *Journal of Clinical Pharmacy and Therapeutics* 34 (2009): 133-145.

Ngo, S. N., et al. "Does Garlic Reduce Risk of Colorectal Cancer?" *Journal of Nutrition* 137 (2007): 2264-2269.

Rajan, T. V., et al. "A Double-Blinded, Placebo-Controlled Trial of Garlic as a Mosquito Repellant." *Medical and Veterinary Entomology* 19 (2005): 84-89.

Ried, K., O. R. Frank, and N. P. Stocks. "Aged Garlic Extract Lowers Blood Pressure in Patients with Treated but Uncontrolled Hypertension." *Maturitas* 67 (2010): 144-150.

Sabitha, P., et al. "Efficacy of Garlic Paste in Oral Candidiasis." *Tropical Doctor* 35 (2005): 99-100.

Sobenin, I. A., et al. "Metabolic Effects of Time-Released Garlic Powder Tablets in Type 2 Diabetes Mellitus." *Acta Diabetologica* 45 (2008): 1-6.

See also: Colds and flu; Heart attack; Insect bites and stings.

Gas, intestinal

CATEGORY: Condition
RELATED TERMS: Bloating, intestinal, dyspepsia, flatulence
DEFINITION: Treatment of excess intestinal gas.
PRINCIPAL PROPOSED NATURAL TREATMENTS: None
OTHER PROPOSED NATURAL TREATMENTS: Activated charcoal, artichoke leaf, beta-galactosidase, boldo, carminative herbs (such as chamomile, coriander, caraway, cumin, dill, fennel, garlic, ginger, parsley, and spearmint), peppermint oil, probiotics, turmeric, yucca, zinc

INTRODUCTION

The passing of intestinal gas is a normal process, but it can become unpleasant, uncomfortable, or embarrassing. Intestinal gas has two primary sources: bacteria in the intestines and air swallowed by mouth (aerophagia). Certain foods greatly increase the production of gas in the intestines by providing nutrients to gas-producing bacteria. Common gas-increasing foods include beans, beer, broccoli, cabbage, cauliflower, fructose, onions, prunes, red wine, and sorbitol. In general, high-fiber foods cause more gas than low-fiber ones, and for this reason, people who switch to a whole-foods diet frequently experience more gas.

Certain medical conditions can also increase gas-related symptoms, including celiac sprue, colon cancer, Crohn's disease, fat malabsorption, irritable bowel syndrome (IBS), lactose intolerance, and ulcerative colitis. Finally, some people may experience significant gas discomfort without actually producing more gas than other people.

Treatment of excess gas begins with treating the underlying disease, if there is one. Beyond that, general steps include avoiding gas-producing foods and minimizing habits that cause aerophagia (such as gulping of beverages). Medications such as simethicone, metoclopramide, and antibiotics may also help, although the supporting evidence to indicate that they are effective remains incomplete.

PROPOSED NATURAL TREATMENTS

There has been little meaningful scientific investigation of natural treatments to reduce gas in people who are otherwise healthy. However, some evidence supports the use of natural treatments for reducing gas production among those with IBS (a cluster of nonspecific intestinal complaints) or dyspepsia (a cluster of nonspecific stomach-related complaints). It is likely, although not guaranteed, that the benefits seen in these studies would carry over to people without these conditions.

For example, a four-week, double-blind, placebo-controlled study of sixty people with IBS found that the use of probiotics (friendly bacteria) reduced gas-related discomfort. Probiotics are presumed to work by replacing gas-producing bacteria with others that are less likely to create gas. The initial use of probiotics reportedly can increase gas production for a short time. Other treatments for IBS, such as peppermint oil and flaxseed, also may be helpful.

The herbs turmeric, artichoke leaf, and boldo have shown promise for reducing gas in people with dyspepsia.

Beano, a product containing the enzyme beta-galactosidase, is widely available for reducing gas caused by consuming beans. This enzyme breaks down some of the gas-producing carbohydrates in beans. However, a study designed to test this substance found only weak evidence of its effectiveness.

Activated charcoal taken by mouth may reduce the amount of flatulence, although not all studies agree on this claim. Certain herbs called carminatives are traditionally believed to aid the movement of gas. These herbs include anise, caraway, cardamom, chamomile, coriander, cumin, dill, fennel, garlic, ginger, parsley, and spearmint.

In addition, numerous alternative therapies are said to help improve digestion and reduce gas, including Chinese herbal medicine, intestinal cleansing, and food allergen identification and avoidance. However, there is little supporting evidence for these approaches.

One study in dogs indicates that a combination of charcoal, yucca, and zinc acetate significantly reduced the smell of intestinal gas, although not the amount that was released. Taken separately, charcoal was the most effective of these treatments. Garments containing activated charcoal have also shown promise for reducing the odor of flatulence.

EBSCO CAM Review Board

FURTHER READING

Fink, R. N., and A. J. Lembo. "Intestinal Gas." *Current Treatment Options in Gastroenterology* 4 (2001): 333-337.

Ganiats, T. G., et al. "Does Beano Prevent Gas? A Double-Blind Crossover Study of Oral Alpha-Galactosidase to Treat Dietary Oligosaccharide Intolerance." *Journal of Family Practice* 39 (1994): 441-445.

Hall, R. G., Jr., H. Thompson, and A. Strother. "Effects of Orally Administered Activated Charcoal on Intestinal Gas." *American Journal of Gastroenterology* 75 (1981): 192-196.

Nobaek, S., et al. "Alteration of Intestinal Microflora Is Associated with Reduction in Abdominal Bloating and Pain in Patients with Irritable Bowel Syndrome." *American Journal of Gastroenterology* 95 (2000): 1231-1238.

Suarez, F. L., et al. "Failure of Activated Charcoal to Reduce the Release of Gases Produced by the Colonic Flora." *American Journal of Gastroenterology* 94 (1999): 208-212.

See also: Cetylated fatty acid; Crohn's disease; Diarrhea; Dyspepsia; Gastritis; Gastrointestinal health; Irritable bowel syndrome (IBS); Lactose intolerance; Nondairy milk; Parasites, intestinal; Probiotics.

Gastritis

CATEGORY: Condition

DEFINITION: Treatment of the inflammation of the lining of the stomach.

PRINCIPAL PROPOSED NATURAL TREATMENTS: None

OTHER PROPOSED NATURAL TREATMENTS: Aloe vera,

beeswax extract, betaine hydrochloride, bioflavo-noids, butterbur, cat's claw, cayenne, cinnamon, colostrum, cranberry, cysteine, fish oil, gamma ory-zanol, garlic, glutamine, licorice, marshmallow, methyl sulfonyl methane, probiotics, reishi, seleni-um, slippery elm, suma, vitamin A, vitamin C, wood betony, zinc

HERBS AND SUPPLEMENTS TO USE ONLY WITH CAU-TION: Arginine, cola nut, feverfew, turmeric, white willow

INTRODUCTION

Gastritis is a condition in which the lining of the stomach becomes inflamed, leading to discomfort. If the inflammation is prolonged, either atrophic gas-tritis (a condition in which the glands of the stomach lining disappear) or an ulcer may develop. Under-lying causes of gastritis include infection with the bac-terium *Helicobacter pylori*, excessive stomach acid secre-tion, autoimmune processes (conditions in which the body attacks itself), and damage to the stomach lining caused by alcohol, nonsteroidal anti-inflammatory drugs, corticosteroids, or severe stress.

Gastritis typically causes pain in the upper ab-domen (just below the sternum), but it also may occur without pain. A burning sensation (heartburn) higher up in the chest generally indicates esophageal reflux. Stomach distress may also occur without in-flammation of the stomach wall; in this case, the dis-tress is called dyspepsia.

Conventional treatment for gastritis includes anti-biotics to eliminate *H. pylori*; reducing stomach acidity with medications in the antacid, H_2 blocker, or proton pump inhibitor families; and possibly using medica-tions to protect the stomach lining. One should also reduce alcohol consumption and change (or, if pos-sible, stop taking) medications that damage the stomach. Vitamin B_{12} supplements may be necessary in some cases of atrophic gastritis.

Newer anti-inflammatory drugs in the COX-2 in-hibitor family, such as Celebrex (celecoxib) and Vioxx (rofecoxib), were designed to cause less harm to the stomach than the older drugs in that category (such as aspirin and ibuprofen). However, evidence remains mixed on how much better these drugs really are compared to the old ones. More sophisticated forms of inhibitors may better fulfill the promise of these medications.

Probiotics for Gastritis

Health experts have debated how to define the term "probiotics." One widely used definition, developed by the World Health Organization and the Food and Agriculture Organization of the United Nations, defines "probiotics" as "live microorganisms, which, when administered in adequate amounts, confer a health benefit on the host." (Microorganisms are tiny living organisms—such as bacteria, viruses, and yeasts—that can be seen only under a microscope.)

Probiotics are available in foods and dietary supple-ments (for example, capsules, tablets, and powders) and in some other forms. Examples of foods con-taining probiotics are yogurt, fermented and unfer-mented milk, miso, tempeh, and some juices and soy beverages. In probiotic foods and supplements, the bacteria may have been present originally or added during preparation.

Most probiotics are bacteria similar to those natu-rally found in a person's gut, especially in those of breast-fed infants (who have natural protection against many diseases). Most often, the bacteria come from two groups, *Lactobacillus* or *Bifidobacterium*. Within each group, there are different species (for example, *L. acidophilus* and *B. bifidus*), and within each species, different strains (or varieties). A few common probiotics, such as *Saccharomyces boulardii*, are yeasts, which are different from bacteria.

PROPOSED NATURAL TREATMENTS

No herbs or supplements (other than alkaline substances with direct antacid properties, such as calcium carbonate or hydrotalcite) have been proven effective for gastritis. The treatments mentioned here have merely shown some promise in prelimi-nary studies.

Natural therapies that may affect H. pylori. *H. pylori* is thought to contribute to many cases of gastritis. A number of treatments have been evaluated to see whether they inhibit the growth of *H. pylori*. For ex-ample, evidence suggests that various probiotics (friendly bacteria) in the *Lactobacillus* family can in-hibit the growth of *H. pylori*. While this effect does not appear to be strong enough for probiotic treatment to eradicate *H. pylori* on its own, preliminary studies (one of which was double-blind) suggest that probi-otics may help standard antibiotic therapy work better, improving the rate of eradication and reducing side effects.

Preliminary studies suggest that various bioflavonoids also can inhibit the growth of *H. pylori*. All fruits and vegetables provide bioflavonoids, but these substances can also be taken as supplements. Vitamin C has also shown some ability to act against *H. pylori*.

Despite early reports that garlic inhibits or kills *H. pylori*, studies in people have not been promising. Fish oil in combination with antibiotic therapy has been tried as a treatment for eradicating *H. pylori*, but it did not prove particularly helpful.

The herb cranberry is thought to help prevent bladder infections by preventing adhesion of bacteria to the bladder. Preliminary evidence suggests that it might also help prevent the adhesion of *H. pylori* to the stomach wall. Theoretically, this could help treat gastritis, but there is no direct evidence regarding this potential benefit.

Cayenne does not appear to be helpful against *H. pylori*. However, some evidence suggests that cayenne can protect the stomach against damage caused by anti-inflammatory drugs. Other natural supplements that have shown promise for protecting against the side effects of these drugs include the amino acid cysteine, a special form of licorice known as deglycyrrhizinated licorice, and the breast milk constituent known as colostrum.

Other natural therapies that may protect the stomach lining. A collection of substances extracted from beeswax has been studied as a treatment for preventing and treating ulcers of various kinds, with promising results. Known as D-002, this product is chemically related to policosanol; however, policosanol itself is not thought to have this effect. (A similar beeswax extract is sold in the United States as policosanol.)

Weak evidence also suggests that butterbur and cinnamon might help protect the stomach lining. Other natural substances have also been suggested as aids to stomach health, but there is little to no scientific evidence that they are effective for gastritis. These natural substances include aloe vera, cat's claw, gamma oryzanol, glutamine, marshmallow, methyl sulfonyl methane, reishi, selenium, slippery elm, suma, vitamin A, vitamin C, wood betony, and zinc.

Many naturopathic physicians believe that the supplement betaine hydrochloride can aid gastritis by increasing stomach acid. This sounds paradoxical, because conventional treatment for this condition involves reducing stomach acid. However, according to one theory, lack of stomach acid leads to incomplete digestion of proteins, and these proteins cause allergic reactions and other responses that lead to an increase in ulcer pain. Again, scientific evidence is lacking.

HERBS AND SUPPLEMENTS TO USE ONLY WITH CAUTION

A number of herbs and supplements, including arginine, cola nut, feverfew, turmeric, and white willow, might tend to increase stomach inflammation. In addition, various supplements may interact with drugs used to treat gastritis.

EBSCO CAM Review Board

FURTHER READING

Armuzzi, A., et al. "Effect of *Lactobacillus* GG Supplementation on Antibiotic-Associated Gastrointestinal Side Effects During *Helicobacter pylori* Eradication Therapy." *Digestion* 63 (2001): 1-7.

Burger, O., et al. "A High Molecular Mass Constituent of Cranberry Juice Inhibits *Helicobacter pylori* Adhesion to Human Gastric Mucus." *FEMS Immunology and Medical Microbiology* 29 (2000): 295-301.

Cremonini, F., et al. "Effect of Different Probiotic Preparations on Anti-*Helicobacter pylori* Therapy-Related Side Effects." *American Journal of Gastroenterology* 97 (2002): 2744-2749.

Gawronska, A., et al. "A Randomized Double-Blind Placebo-Controlled Trial of *Lactobacillus* GG for Abdominal Pain Disorders in Children." *Alimentary Pharmacology and Therapeutics* 25 (2007): 177-184.

Shmuely, H., et al. "Effect of Cranberry Juice on Eradication of *Helicobacter pylori* in Patients Treated with Antibiotics and a Proton Pump Inhibitor." *Molecular Nutrition and Food Research* 51 (2007): 746-751.

Wendakoon, C. N., A. B. Thomson, and L. Ozimek. "Lack of Therapeutic Effect of a Specially Designed Yogurt for the Eradication of *Helicobacter pylori* Infection." *Digestion* 65 (2002): 16-20.

See also: Diarrhea; Dyspepsia; Gas, intestinal; Gastritis: Homeopathic remedies; Gastroesophageal reflux disease; Gastrointestinal health; Peptic ulcer disease: Homeopathic remedies; Probiotics; Ulcers.

Gastritis: Homeopathic remedies

CATEGORY: Homeopathy

RELATED TERMS: Irritable stomach, nervous stomach, upset stomach

DEFINITION: Homeopathic treatment of the inflammation of the lining of the stomach.

STUDIED HOMEOPATHIC REMEDIES: *Lycopodium, Nux vomica, Pulsatilla*

SCIENTIFIC EVALUATIONS OF HOMEOPATHIC REMEDIES

Three studies, two of which were randomized, double-blind, placebo-controlled trials, examined the effectiveness of treating mild gastritis with the homeopathic remedy *Nux vomica*. Overall, however, the results were not promising.

The first trial was a double-blind study enrolling 147 participants, each of whom received either *Nux vomica* D4 or placebo. The treatment group did not show a statistically significant improvement in symptoms compared with the control group.

Two other double-blind studies included sixty-nine persons in total; one study tested *Nux vomica* at a strength of D4 and the other used a D30 potency. In both studies, the persons who were treated with the homeopathic remedy did not demonstrate a statistically significant improvement in symptoms compared with the control group. These reasonable-size studies of homeopathic *Nux vomica* suggest that it is probably not effective for treating gastritis.

TRADITIONAL HOMEOPATHIC TREATMENTS

Classical homeopathy offers many possible homeopathic treatments for gastritis. These therapies are chosen based on various specific details of the person seeking treatment.

Homeopathic practitioners have traditionally used *Nux vomica* in the treatment of gastritis. *Nux vomica* is said to be indicated for those who experience heartburn or stomach pain after eating; who wake at night with stomach discomfort, including pain or bloating; and who often have constipation or diarrhea. Symptoms are worsened by rich or spicy foods and relieved by warmth. Irritability and impatience are also prominent parts of the classical symptom picture of this remedy.

Lycopodium may be traditionally indicated when belching, bloating, and easy fullness are prominent

parts of the symptom picture, along with indigestion related to social stress. *Pulsatilla* is frequently recommended for emotional, "clingy" people, who have rapidly changing symptoms, including heartburn and bloating, particularly after eating rich foods.

EBSCO CAM Review Board

FURTHER READING

Diamond, J. A., and W. J. Diamond. "Common Functional Bowel Problems: What Do Homeopathy, Chinese Medicine, and Nutrition Have to Offer?" *Advance for Nurse Practitioners* 15 (2005): 31-34, 72.

Hofbauer, R., at al. "Heparin-Binding Epidermal Growth Factor Expression in KATO-III Cells After *Helicobacter pylori* Stimulation Under the Influence of Strychnos *Nux vomica* and *Calendula officinalis*." *Homeopathy* 99 (2010): 177-182.

Koretz, R. L., and M. Rotblatt. "Complementary and Alternative Medicine in Gastroenterology: The Good, the Bad, and the Ugly." *Clinical Gastroenterology and Hepatology* 2 (2004): 957-967.

See also: Dyspepsia; Irritable bowel syndrome (IBS); Gas, intestinal; Homeopathy.

Gastroesophageal reflux disease

CATEGORY: Condition

RELATED TERMS: Esophageal reflux, GERD, heartburn

DEFINITION: Treatment of the condition that causes stomach acid to enter the esophagus.

PRINCIPAL PROPOSED NATURAL TREATMENTS: None

OTHER PROPOSED NATURAL TREATMENTS: Aloe vera, betaine hydrochloride, bladderwrack, carob, calcium carbonate, folate, hydrotalcite, licorice, marshmallow, multivitamin-multimineral supplements, vitamin B_{12}

INTRODUCTION

In gastroesophageal reflux disease (GERD), acid from the stomach splashes upward, or refluxes, and burns the esophagus (the tube connecting the mouth and throat to the stomach). Normally, a type of sphincter muscle keeps the upper part of the stomach closed, but various factors may loosen it, allowing acid to rise more easily. The result is pain in the chest, commonly known as heartburn. GERD is generally made worse by lying down because gravity no longer restrains the upward movement of stomach contents. In infants, the major issue with GERD is not pain but the spitting up (vomiting) of food or milk.

Certain foods may worsen GERD, and these include alcohol, carbonated beverages, caffeine, chocolate, citrus juices, milk, and peppermint. Cigarette smoking may also increase symptoms. Contrary to earlier beliefs, it does not appear that people with GERD need to cut down on fat intake to help control the disease.

Pregnant women frequently develop GERD because of changes in muscle tone. Also, the connection between obesity and GERD remains unclear.

Treatment for GERD involves elevating the head of one's bed and using medications that reduce the acidity of the stomach. In general, more powerful antacid medications are required for GERD than for ulcers or gastritis. Drugs in the proton pump category are most effective. Surgery may be recommended in certain cases.

If left untreated, GERD causes precancerous alterations in the lower part of the esophagus (a condition called Barrett's esophagus), which can develop into esophageal cancer. Thus, people with GERD are often tested to evaluate the condition of the esophagus.

PROPOSED NATURAL TREATMENTS

Natural antacids, such as calcium carbonate (Tums) or hydrotalcite, may provide short-term relief from GERD. Drugs used to treat GERD tend to deplete the body of certain nutrients, especially vitamin B_{12} but also folate and various minerals. The use of a multivitamin-multimineral supplement should correct this problem.

Deglycyrrhizinated licorice, a special form of the herb licorice, has shown some promise for the treatment of ulcers. A drug (carbenoxolone) that is similar to ingredients in licorice has been studied for the treatment of GERD, with good results.

However, in these studies carbenoxolone was combined with other ingredients, including antacids and alginic acid. It is not clear that carbenoxolone alone will help GERD, and it is even less clear that licorice itself offers any benefit.

A popular over-the-counter drug for GERD, Gaviscon, contains a substance called alginic acid. Alginic acid is thought to form a kind of protective seal at the top of the stomach, reducing reflux. The seaweed bladderwrack is high in alginic acid. However, there is no evidence that whole bladderwrack can reduce heartburn symptoms.

Several other natural supplements are often recommended for the treatment of GERD, including aloe vera, antioxidants, artemesia, fresh garlic, marshmallow, and slippery elm, but there is no scientific evidence to support their use. Milk allergy is thought to contribute to GERD in infants. Whether food allergies play a significant role in adult cases remains unclear. The herb carob may be helpful for infant GERD.

Many naturopathic physicians believe that the supplement betaine hydrochloride can aid GERD by increasing stomach acid. This sounds paradoxical, because conventional treatment involves reducing stomach acid. However, according to one theory, lack of stomach acid leads to incomplete digestion of proteins; these proteins cause allergic reactions and other responses that lead to an increase in reflux. Again, scientific evidence is lacking.

EBSCO CAM Review Board

FURTHER READING

Holtmeier, W., et al. "On-Demand Treatment of Acute Heartburn with the Antacid Hydrotalcite Compared with Famotidine and Placebo." *Journal of Clinical Gastroenterology* 41 (2007): 564-570.

Pehl, C., et al. "Effect of Low- and High-Fat Meals on Lower Esophageal Sphincter Motility and Gastroesophageal Reflux in Healthy Subjects." *American Journal of Gastroenterology* 94 (1999): 1192-1196.

Salvatore, S., and Y. Vandenplas. "Gastroesophageal Reflux and Cow Milk Allergy: Is There a Link?" *Pediatrics* 110 (2002): 972-984.

Wenzl, T. G., et al. "Effects of Thickened Feeding on Gastroesophageal Reflux in Infants: A Placebo-Controlled Crossover Study Using Intraluminal Impedance." *Pediatrics* 111 (2003): e355-e359.

See also: Antacids; Dyspepsia; Gas, intestinal; Gastritis; Gastrointestinal health; Proton pump inhibitors.

Gastrointestinal health

CATEGORY: Issues and overviews

DEFINITION: Complementary and alternative therapies considered for use in gastrointestinal health.

OVERVIEW

The gastrointestinal (GI) system includes the esophagus, stomach, intestines, colon, rectum, and anus. Many other organs assist in the digestive process of the GI system; they include the gallbladder, pancreas, and liver.

GI conditions are often chronic, can cause various degrees of discomfort, and can affect a person's quality of life. Millions of people look to complementary and alternative medicine (CAM) as an adjunct to or a substitute for traditional medical therapy. While many CAM therapies do relieve symptoms, one should use them with caution because some therapies and dietary supplements can affect other modes of care and can lead to adverse reactions.

A National Health Interview Survey showed that 3.7 percent of Americans use CAM for GI care. Many persons with GI problems do not disclose their use of CAM to their doctor, which may also impact optimal care.

GI disorders may be functional (the system appears normal but does not "work" properly) or structural (the system includes swelling, obstruction, or other visual symptom). Constipation and irritable bowel are common functional disorders, and hemorrhoids and cancer are examples of structural disorders.

COMMON CAM THERAPIES

The National Center for Complementary and Alternative Medicine (NCCAM), part of the National Institutes of Health, categorizes CAM into four major categories: biologically based (supplementing the diet with nutrients, herbs, particular foods, or extracts), manipulative and body-based (using touch and manipulation such as chiropractic or massage), mind/body (connecting the mind to the body and spirit with practices such as yoga and meditation), and energy therapies (aiming to restore balance to the body's energy with therapies such as qigong and Reiki). Other whole, ancient medical systems include traditional Chinese medicine, Ayurveda, homeopathic medicine, and naturopathic medicine.

COMMON GASTROINTESTINAL CONDITIONS

The most common GI health issues addressed by CAM include nausea and vomiting, dyspepsia, irritable bowel syndrome (IBS), inflammatory bowel disease (IBD), diarrhea and constipation, liver disease (hepatitis B and C and alcohol-related disease), and cancer.

Nausea and vomiting. Nausea and vomiting can be quite unsettling. They often arise in pregnancy, with an infection, or during medical treatment. Certain CAM therapies have been used for the relief of symptoms, including relaxation for chemotherapy-induced nausea and vomiting and the herb ginger, the most commonly employed supplement to relieve nausea and vomiting. Some studies have demonstrated that ginger improves GI motility and acts as an antiemetic (blocks serotonin receptors in the GI tract and in the central nervous system). Ginger also has been used with some success for morning sickness, motion sickness, chemotherapy, and postoperative nausea.

Acupuncture and acupressure have been shown to reduce symptoms of nausea and vomiting, and their use has been supported by much research on their effectiveness. Many hospitals have acupuncturists on staff.

Dyspepsia. Mild dyspepsia is often self-managed with CAM therapeutic agents, including bananas, red pepper, peppermint, caraway, and turmeric. Most have shown efficacy over placebo in randomized-control trials and are common in the average home. Other lesser-known herbs also have shown promise. These include celandine, liu-jun-zi-tang, shenxiahewining, and STW 5.

Irritable bowel syndrome. IBS affects about 5 to 10 percent of Americans, mostly women. Many CAM therapies have been investigated to relieve the discomfort. Bulking agents such as psyllium have been most studied and prescribed. Psyllium, a first-line of treatment for many, has been shown to speed up bowel movements. Allergic reactions to psyllium are possible, but rare.

Many other CAM therapies have been used for IBS, including acupuncture, Ayurvedic medicine, Chinese herbal medicine, homeopathy, hypnotherapy, peppermint oil, probiotic therapy, and STW 5. Randomized-control trials have shown positive results for many of these therapies.

Diarrhea and constipation. Several herbal supplements are commonly used to improve colonic health.

The Organs of the Gastrointestinal System

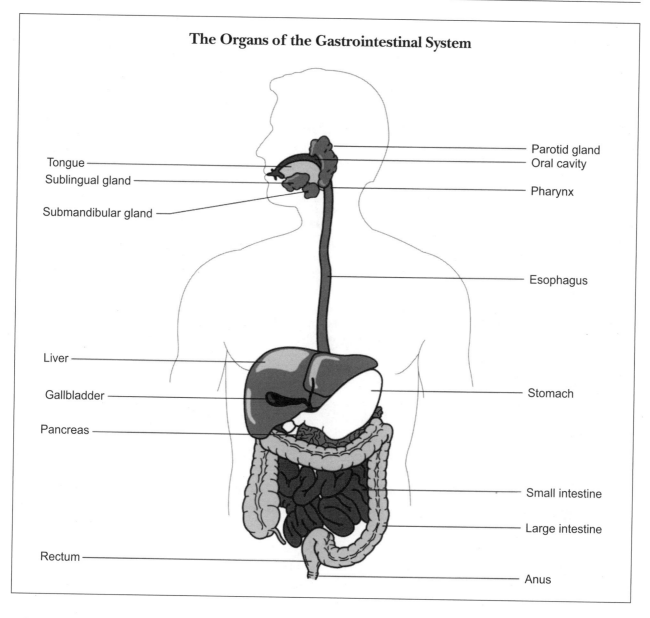

Tongue
Sublingual gland
Submandibular gland
Liver
Gallbladder
Pancreas
Rectum

Parotid gland
Oral cavity
Pharynx
Esophagus
Stomach
Small intestine
Large intestine
Anus

These supplements include aloe, apple pectin, cascara sagrada, chamomile, clove, echinacea, fennel, fenugreek, ginger, hibiscus, magnesium citrate, marshmallow, oat bran, Oregon grape, papaya, psyllium, raspberry, rhubarb, senna, spirulina, valerian, and yellow dock. Nearly all of these herbs stimulate action and have a laxative effect. Few adverse reactions have been reported. Some of these herbs, however, may interfere with other blood-thinning medications and should be discussed with a doctor before use.

Probiotics, good bacteria found in a healthy gut, are also used to prevent diarrhea and constipation. They are essential to overall gut health. Infection, the use of antibiotics, and even modern-day stress can lower healthy amounts of good bacteria in the gut. Antibiotics can disturb the balance of the gut's ecosystem by killing friendly bacteria. It appears that the regular use of probiotics can generally improve the health of the GI system by stocking the gut with healthy bacteria and making less room for harmful bacteria and yeasts.

Commonly Used CAM Therapies for Gastrointestinal Health

Acupuncture	A Chinese medicine technique that utilizes needles at defined locations to move *qi*, or energy. It aims to restore balance and energy to the body's organs.
Ayurveda	An ancient whole-body system from India rooted in diet and lifestyle recommendations to improve overall health.
Colonic irrigation therapy	Cleansing of the colon through various oral and enema solutions to improve digestive health.
Herbal medicine	The use of a variety of herbal therapies, supplements, vitamins, and probiotics to improve the function of the digestive system.
Homeopathy	Based on the principle "like cured with like," homeopathy uses diluted formulas to reduce sensitivity and increase tolerance to help the body adjust and cure itself.
Hypnosis	Inducing a deeply relaxed state and making helpful suggestions to alter a person's behavior and response.
Meditation and relaxation	A regular practice of relaxation, reflection, and contemplation to bring about a sense of calm and well-being.
Reflexology	Massage and pressure applied to areas of the feet that are said to coincide with organs of the body.

Certain strains of *Lactobacillus* were shown to help restore colonic health after a course of antibiotics. *L. casei* Shirota and *L. rhamnosus* are helpful bacteria for treating chronic constipation. Also, a mixture of *Bifidobacteria* and *Lactobacilli* was shown to improve symptoms. In another study, a combination of *B. lactis* and *B. longus* showed promise for improving bowel regularity in persons in nursing homes. In a six-week double-blind, placebo-controlled trial of 274 people with constipation-predominant IBS, the use of a probiotic formula containing *B. animalis* significantly improved stool frequency.

Cultured dairy products such as yogurt and kefir are good sources of acidophilus and other probiotic bacteria. Supplements are widely available in powder,

liquid, capsule, or tablet form. Grocery stores and natural-food stores both carry milk that contains live acidophilus.

In addition to probiotics, related substances known as prebiotics may enhance the colonization of healthy bacteria in the intestinal tract. It is important to note that many products sold on the market may not contain viable cultures at the time of purchase. A study reported in 1990 found that most acidophilus capsules on the market contained no living acidophilus. The situation has improved in subsequent evaluations, but some products still have no living organisms and therefore will provide no benefit. Some container labels guarantee the units of living organisms at the time of purchase, not just at the time of manufacture.

Other CAM therapies that have been used to treat IBS include biofeedback, abdominal massage, homeopathy, and colonic irrigation.

MIND/BODY THERAPIES

The power of the mind to heal and bring about well-being has been demonstrated in self-reported quality-of-life measures. Strong evidence in the form of randomized-control trials is lacking, in part because of the difficulty in devising placebo/sham therapies and because of funding obstacles. Many practices, such as yoga, meditation, and Tai Chi, are said to help reduce abdominal symptoms and bring about a sense of relaxation.

Deep breathing and yoga are often used by persons with IBS. Stress can exacerbate symptoms, so any sort of practice that reduces stress and helps one cope with stress can reduce symptoms. Yoga focuses on a healthy spine for a healthy body and incorporates deep-breathing exercises. Different poses and movements involving twist and balance are said to stimulate the nerves along the spine and promote circulation and the flow of energy.

Many professional athletes practice some form of yoga for increased flexibility. It is often incorporated into cross-training exercise routines. Some adolescents are embracing mind/body forms of CAM. One study showed that adolescents between the ages of twelve and nineteen with IBS were likely to engage in or consider meditation or prayer, or both, for symptom management.

ENERGY THERAPIES

Acupuncture is commonly employed to reduce GI symptoms. While acupuncture may be helpful for some people and for certain conditions, the evidence for its effectiveness is unclear. Studies have shown no difference in acupuncture versus sham acupuncture. Several well-designed studies have shown both sham and treatment groups improving at the same rate. Modern science is still not clear how or if acupuncture works.

Chinese medicine has outlined hundreds of meridians, or channels, along the body that are thought to stimulate certain organs or systems. According to Chinese medicine, these channels conduct the flow of energy, or *qi*, a vital force that flows through the body. It is thought that blockages along the vital channels can result in pain or illness. Acupuncture is thought to remove blockages from the system and restore the normal circulation of *qi*. There is no scientific evidence, however, for the existence of the meridians or of *qi*. These channels have never been seen under a microscope or mapped, and they do not correspond to major nerve pathways.

Deanna M. Neff, M.P.H.

FURTHER READING

Feldman, Mark, Lawrence S. Friedman, and Lawrence J. Brandt, eds. *Sleisenger and Fordtran's Gastrointestinal and Liver Disease: Pathophysiology, Diagnosis, Management.* 8th ed. 2 vols. Philadelphia: Saunders/Elsevier, 2006. A comprehensive textbook of gastrointestinal diseases and physiology. Contains excellent chapters and endoscopic photographs.

Micozzi, Marc S., ed. *Fundamentals of Complementary and Integrative Medicine.* 3d ed. St. Louis, Mo.: Saunders/Elsevier, 2006. A good overview of complementary, alternative, and integrative medicine basics.

National Center for Complementary and Alternative Medicine. http://nccam.nih.gov. A comprehensive U.S. government resource for articles, scientific studies, and general consumer information about complementary and alternative medicine.

See also: Compulsive overeating; Dyspepsia; Eating disorders; Gas, intestinal; Gastritis; Gastroesophageal reflux disease; Obesity and excessive weight; Peptic ulcer disease: Homeopathic treatment; Probiotics; Weight loss, undesired; Ulcers.

Gattefossé, René-Maurice

CATEGORY: Biography
IDENTIFICATION: French chemist who is a founder of contemporary aromatherapy
BORN: 1881; Montchat, near Lyon, France
DIED: 1950; Casablanca, Morocco

OVERVIEW

René-Maurice Gattefossé was a French chemist and a founder of contemporary aromatherapy. He also is credited with coining the term "aromatherapy."

Gattefossé's family developed perfume and other aromatics. His father founded a group called Etablissements Gattefossé in southern France in 1880 (it remains in business today), which produced various oils, perfume components, ointments, and related products. Gattefossé studied chemical engineering at the University of Lyon, subsequently worked with his family business, and eventually went on to join other research groups to investigate the potential roles of aromatics and essential oils for cosmetology, dermatology, psychology, and general clinical use. In 1907, Gattefossé formally joined a research group that investigated the scientific properties of various aromatics and oils, although he later parted ways with the group to conduct his own research studies.

Sources suggest that Gattefossé first discovered aromatherapy when he was working in a laboratory, after he burned his hand and doused it with the nearest liquid: lavender oil. Many historians suggest that this "self-experimentation" was no accident. After this experience, Gattefossé found that his hand healed more quickly than expected, which led him to investigate the therapeutic properties of other, similar aromatic oils. Gattefossé went on to provide both preventive treatment and post injury treatment to several persons during the 1918 influenza epidemic.

Many researchers before the time of Gattefossé speculated that various aromatic derivatives had antimicrobial and therapeutic capacities, but Gattefossé's research and publications clearly articulated these effects and went beyond the conclusions of many previous studies. In 1937, he first used the term "aromatherapy" in print, in a book on the subject, *Aromathérapie: Les Huiles Essentielles, Hormones Végétales* (*Gattefossé's Aromatherapy*, 1993). Thus he is recognized as a key figure in clinical aromatherapy.

During his career, Gattefossé claimed that various essential oils had antiseptic, bactericidal, antiviral, and antitoxic properties. In particular, he claimed in his writings that he had used oils to cure skin cancer, skin ulcers, gangrene, and poisonous spider bites, in addition to many other ailments. Gattefossé also speculated that essential oils had various psychological and calming effects, and he suggested that different aromatics and oil combinations could produce intentional effects in exposed persons. Many modern-day aromatherapists credit Gattefossé with launching this ever-growing field.

Brandy Weidow, M.S.

FURTHER READING

Gattefossé, René-Maurice. *Gattefossé's Aromatherapy*. 2d ed. Edited by Robert B. Tisserand. New York: Random House, 2004.

Schnaubelt, Kurt. *Medical Aromatherapy: Healing with Essential Oils*. Berkeley, Calif.: Frog Books, 1999.

Valnet, Jean. *The Practice of Aromatherapy: A Classic Compendium of Plant Medicines and Their Healing Properties*. Edited by Robert B. Tisserand. Rochester, Vt.: Healing Arts Press, 1990.

See also: Aromatherapy.

Genistein

CATEGORY: Herbs and supplements
DEFINITION: Natural plant product used to treat specific health conditions.
PRINCIPAL PROPOSED USES: None
OTHER PROPOSED USES: Amyotrophic lateral sclerosis, blood sugar control (prediabetes), cancer prevention, high cholesterol, menopausal symptoms, osteoporosis

OVERVIEW

Genistein, a naturally occurring chemical present in soy, has attracted scientific interest for its possible benefits in cancer and heart disease prevention. Genistein is a type of chemical called a phytoestrogen, an estrogen-like substance present in some plants. There are two main types of phytoestrogens: isoflavones and lignans. Soy is the most abundant source of isoflavones, with genistein the most abundant isoflavone in soy. Red clover is also a good sourse of genistein.

Like other phytoestrogens, genistein can work in two ways: by either increasing or decreasing the effects of estrogen. This happens because genistein binds to special sites on cells called estrogen receptors. Genistein stimulates these receptors, but not as strongly as real estrogen; at the same time, it blocks estrogen itself from attaching. The net result is that when there is a lot of estrogen in the body, such as before menopause, genistein may partly block its effects. Since estrogen appears to increase the risk of various forms of cancer, regular use of genistein by premenopausal women might help reduce this risk. On the other hand, if there is little human estrogen present, such as after menopause, genistein can partly make up for it. This is one rationale for using genistein to treat menopausal symptoms and to prevent osteoporosis. Genistein might also be helpful for reducing heart disease risk.

REQUIREMENTS AND SOURCES

Genistein is found in high quantities in soy and in negligible quantities in a few other foods. Most soy foods contain about 1 to 2 milligrams (mg) of genistein per gram of protein.

THERAPEUTIC DOSAGES

The optimum dosage of genistein is unknown. In Asia, population groups who daily eat soy foods containing 20 to 80 mg of genistein have lower rates of breast and prostate cancer than do groups in the West with less genistein in their diets. However, it is not known if genistein or even soy isoflavones generally are responsible for this effect.

THERAPEUTIC USES

Double-blind, placebo-controlled studies have found that genistein may be helpful for preventing heart disease and preventing or treating osteoporosis. Genistein may additionally improve blood sugar control in people with prediabetes. Weaker evidence suggests potential benefits in cancer prevention, cancer treatment, and amyotrophic lateral sclerosis (ALS).

Isoflavone mixtures containing genistein have undergone considerably more study than genistein

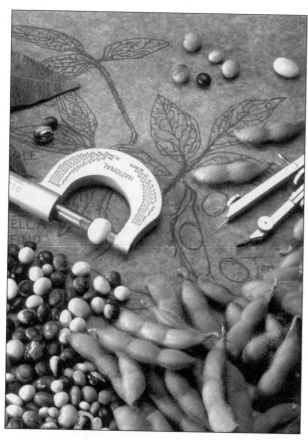

Genistein, the main isoflavone in soybeans, is classified as a key anticancer agent by the National Cancer Institute. (U.S. Department of Agriculture)

alone. Mixed isoflavones have shown promise for most of the conditions just mentioned, as well as for menopausal symptoms and cyclic mastalgia.

SCIENTIFIC EVIDENCE

Osteoporosis. Estrogen has a powerful protective effect on bone. In women, osteoporosis most often occurs after menopause, when the ovaries stop producing estrogen. Animal studies, as well as double-blind, placebo-controlled trials in humans, suggest that genistein can help restore bone protection.

For example, in a twenty-four-month double-blind, placebo-controlled study of 389 postmenopausal women with mild bone loss, use of genistein at a dose of 54 mg daily significantly improved bone density, compared with a placebo. (All participants were additionally given calcium and vitamin D.)

In a previous twelve-month study, ninety women aged forty-seven to fifty-seven were given genistein, standard hormone replacement therapy (HRT), or a placebo. The results showed that genistein increased bone density to approximately the same extent as HRT. No adverse effects on the uterus or breast were seen. Evidence suggests that unlike estrogen, which primarily helps prevent the destruction of bone, genistein may also assist in creating new bone.

However, in one animal study, while a small dose of genistein helped protect the rats' bones, a larger dose of genistein seemed to have the opposite effect: causing increasing bone destruction. Studies in humans are needed to determine whether genistein is truly effective and to find the optimum dose. Other studies have evaluated the effects of soy products containing other constituents besides genistein.

Menopausal symptoms (hot flashes). A double-blind study of 247 women suffering from menopausal hot flashes compared the effects of a placebo and genistein over a period of one year. Genistein was taken at a dose of 54 mg per day. The results indicated that use of genistein significantly reduced hot flashes, compared with placebo. No adverse effects were seen.

Cancer. Genistein may help reduce risk of various forms of cancer. In one study, newborn female rats treated with genistein had less breast cancer later in life than those treated with a placebo. However, other studies suggest that genistein or other isoflavones could promote breast cancer under certain conditions.

In the test tube, genistein has been found to suppress the growth of a wide range of cancer cells, including forms of cancer that are not affected by estrogen. For example, genistein has been found to inhibit skin cancer when it was applied to the skin of mice or fed to rats. Furthermore, in test-tube studies, genistein has been found to enhance the effects of chemotherapy drugs.

Heart disease. One double-blind, placebo-controlled study found that use of genistein helped relax the artery wall (the endothelium), an effect that would be expected to help prevent heart disease. In addition, test-tube studies suggest that genistein may help keep cholesterol in the blood from being deposited in blood vessel walls. Finally, very early test-tube research suggests that genistein may also inhibit the formation of blood clots, which are a major cause of heart attacks.

Genistein for Menopausal Hot Flashes

Genistein is an isoflavone, a plant-source substance with estrogen-like qualities (a phytoestrogen). Soy is the most abundant common source of isoflavones, and genistein is the most abundant isoflavone in soy. Red clover is also a good source of genistein.

Like other phytoestrogens, genistein can have two opposite effects, depending on the circumstances in which it is taken. In some circumstances, it acts as an antagonist to estrogen, decreasing the hormone's effects in the body. In other situations, it acts as an estrogen substitute, producing estrogenic effects where the hormone is failing to do so. It can have these opposite effects because it binds to special sites on cells called estrogen receptors and mildly stimulates them. This stimulation is not as strong as that produced by estrogen itself; however, genistein effectively occupies these sites and keeps estrogen from having any effect on them. The net result is that when women with high levels of estrogen take genistein, estrogenic activity in the body decreases. Conversely, in women with relatively little natural estrogen, genistein can partly make up for what is lacking.

This second effect is the rationale for using genistein as a treatment for problems associated with menopause. Estrogen reduces many symptoms of menopause, such as hot flashes. Estrogen, however, is somewhat dangerous, increasing the risk of heart disease and cancer. It has been hypothesized that genistein and other isoflavones could "split the difference," providing some of estrogen's benefits without the risks.

Numerous studies have looked at genistein for this purpose. Most have evaluated possible beneficial effects regarding osteoporosis. In 2007, a study was published that looked at genistein's effects on hot flashes. This was a double-blind study that included 247 women who had problematic hot flashes caused by menopause. Participants were given either placebo or genistein at a dose of 54 milligrams per day. The results indicated that the use of genistein significantly reduced the rate and severity of hot flashes, compared with placebo. No adverse effects were seen in this study. Importantly, genistein did not have any harmful effects on the uterus. Estrogen, taken by itself, causes precancerous changes in the uterus, so this is a distinct advantage.

Estrogen is also thought to increase breast cancer and heart disease risk. Genistein most likely does not present the same issues, but this has not been conclusively proven.

Steven Bratman, M.D.

SAFETY ISSUES

Most safety studies that have implications for genistein involved mixed isoflavones from soy or red clover. Regarding genistein alone, one large study reported that genistein caused significant gastrointestinal side effects in almost 20 percent of participants.

Additionally, some evidence suggests that the genistein in particular might impair immunity. One study in mice found that injected genistein has negative effects on the thymus gland (an organ that is important for immunity) and also causes changes in the prevalence of various white blood cells consistent with impaired immunity. Although the genistein was injected rather than administered orally, the blood levels of genistein that these injections produced were not excessively high; they were comparable to (or even lower than) what occurs in children fed soy milk formula. In addition, there are several reports of impaired immune responses in infants fed soy formula. While it is too early to conclude that genistein impairs immunity, these findings are a potential cause for concern.

FURTHER READING

Allred, C. D., et al. "Soy Diets Containing Varying Amounts of Genistein Stimulate Growth of Estrogen-Dependent (Mcf-7) Tumors in a Dose-Dependent Manner." *Cancer Research* 61 (2001): 5045-5050.

Atteritano, M., et al. "Effects of the Phytoestrogen Genistein on Some Predictors of Cardiovascular Risk in Osteopenic, Postmenopausal Women." *Journal of Clinical Endocrinology and Metabolism* 92, no. 8 (2007): 3068-3075.

D'Anna, R., et al. "Effects of the Phytoestrogen Genistein on Hot Flushes, Endometrium, and Vaginal Epithelium in Postmenopausal Women." *Menopause* 16, no. 2 (2009): 301-306.

Marini, H., et al. "Effects of the Phytoestrogen Genistein on Bone Metabolism in Osteopenic Postmenopausal Women." *Annals of Internal Medicine* 146 (2007): 839-847.

Messina, M., C. Gardner, and S. Barnes. "Gaining Insight into the Health Effects of Soy, but a Long Way Still to Go: Commentary on the Fourth International

Symposium on the Role of Soy in Preventing and Treating Chronic Disease." *Journal of Nutrition* 132 (2002): 547S-551S.

Morabito, N., et al. "Effects of Genistein and Hormone-Replacement Therapy on Bone Loss in Early Postmenopausal Women." *Journal of Bone and Mineral Research* 17 (2002): 1904-1912.

Persky, V. W., et al. "Effect of Soy Protein on Endogenous Hormones in Postmenopausal Women." *American Journal of Clinical Nutrition* 75 (2002): 145-153.

Squadrito, F., et al. "Effect of Genistein on Endothelial Function in Postmenopausal Women." *American Journal of Medicine* 114 (2003): 470-476.

Yellayi, S., et al. "The Phytoestrogen Genistein Induces Thymic and Immune Changes: A Human Health Concern?" *Proceedings of the National Academy of Sciences* 99 (2002): 7616-7621.

See also: Amyotrophic lateral sclerosis; Cancer risk reduction; Cholesterol, high; Diabetes; Estrogen; Isoflavone; Lignans; Menopause; Osteoporosis; Soy.

Gentian

CATEGORY: Herbs and supplements
RELATED TERM: *Gentiana lutea*
DEFINITION: Natural plant product used to treat specific health conditions.
PRINCIPAL PROPOSED USES: Appetite, digestive aid

OVERVIEW

For reasons that are not entirely clear, bitter plants have the capacity to stimulate appetite, and gentian ranks high on the scale of bitterness. Two of its constituents, gentiopicrin and amarogentin, taste bitter even when diluted by a factor of fifty thousand.

In traditional European herbology, gentian and other bitter herbs are believed to strengthen the digestive system when taken over a period of time. However, in Chinese medicine, gentian is regarded as a rather intense herb that should seldom be taken over the long term. Experts are not sure which view is right, although most lean toward the Chinese viewpoint and recommend gentian only for short-term use.

THERAPEUTIC DOSAGES

A typical dosage of gentian is twenty drops of tincture fifteen minutes before meals. To make the intensely bitter taste more tolerable, one can mix the tincture in juice or water.

THERAPEUTIC USES

Gentian extracts are widely sold in liquor stores under the name "bitters," for the purpose of increasing appetite. Tinctures are also sold medicinally for the same purpose.

SAFETY ISSUES

Gentian is somewhat mutagenic, meaning that it can cause changes in the DNA of bacteria. For this reason, gentian should not be taken during pregnancy. Safety in young children, nursing women, or those with severe liver or kidney disease is also not established. In the short term, gentian rarely causes any side effects, except for occasional worsening of ulcer pain and heartburn. (For some people, it relieves stomach problems.)

EBSCO CAM Review Board

FURTHER READING

Lininger, S. W., et al. *The Natural Pharmacy.* Rocklin, Calif.: Prima, 1998.

Morimoto, I., et al. "Mutagenic Activities of Gentisin and Isogentisin from *Gentianae Radix* (Gentianaceae)." *Mutation Research* 116 (1983): 103-117.

See also: Dyspepsia; Herbal medicine; Weight loss, unintended.

Germander

CATEGORY: Herbs and supplements
RELATED TERM: *Teucrium chamaedrys*
DEFINITION: Toxic plant product claimed to be a treatment for specific health conditions.

OVERVIEW

The herb germander is a dramatic counterexample to the widely held belief that if a treatment has been used for thousands of years, it must be safe.

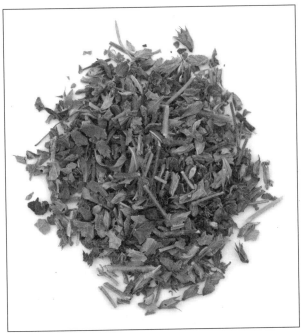

The herb germander is a dramatic counterexample to the widely held belief that if a treatment has been used for thousands of years, it must be safe. (Geoff Kidd/Photo Researchers, Inc.)

Germander grows wild in the Mediterranean region, especially in Greece and Syria. It has a long tradition of use for gout, as well as for febrile illnesses, asthma, coughs, depression, and congestive heart failure. It was also said to improve digestion and increase appetite. What traditional herbalists appear to have missed is that germander is toxic to the liver.

In the 1980s, germander became a popular treatment for weight control in France. A small epidemic of hepatitis was the result. Subsequent research demonstrated conclusively that the herb is toxic to the liver, but this same research has not precisely identified the constituents at fault. Problems also have occurred when products labeled as containing skullcap have turned out to contain germander instead. Germander was subsequently banned in France and many other countries. Numerous Web sites continue to promote the use of this herb.

EBSCO CAM Review Board

FURTHER READING

De Berardinis, V., et al. "Human Microsomal Epoxide Hydrolase Is the Target of Germander-Induced Autoantibodies on the Surface of Human Hepatocytes." *Molecular Pharmacology* 58 (2000): 542-551.

Loeper, J., et al. "Human Epoxide Hydrolase Is the Target of Germander Autoantibodies on the Surface of Human Hepatocytes: Enzymatic Implications." *Advances in Experimental Medicine and Biology* 500 (2001): 121-124.

Polymeros, D., et al. "Acute Cholestatic Hepatitis Caused by *Teucrium polium* (Golden Germander) with Transient Appearance of Antimitochondrial Antibody." *Journal of Clinical Gastroenterology* 34 (2002): 100-101.

Stickel, F., et al. "Hepatotoxicity of Botanicals." *Public Health Nutrition* 3 (2000): 113-124.

See also: Herbal medicine; The Internet and CAM; Scientific evidence.

Gerson, Max

CATEGORY: Biography
IDENTIFICATION: German physician and scientist who developed a specialized dietary system to treat disease
BORN: October 18, 1881; Wongrowitz, Germany
DIED: March 8, 1959; New York, New York

OVERVIEW

Max Gerson was a German physician and orthomolecularist who developed Gerson therapy, an alternative dietary system to cure cancer and various chronic and degenerative diseases. Gerson described his approach in the book *A Cancer Therapy: Results of Fifty Cases* (1958). However, the American Medical Association and the National Cancer Institute have found this method to be ineffective and unsupported.

Gerson was born to a Jewish family in Germany and was said to have decided to study medicine because of anti-Semitism and because the medical field was open to Jewish persons. Gerson was said to suffer from migraine headaches as a young man and thus decided to alter his diet; he found that, with this new diet, his headaches disappeared.

After entering private practice, Gerson prescribed the diet to patients to overcome health problems, including migraine headaches. Gerson also reported that skin lesions related to tuberculosis were remedied by his diet. In 1928, he conducted a clinical study that included a woman with serious cancer, and he claimed that his diet cured her. He suggested that artificial fertilizers and pesticides might be causing a number of diseases, and he spoke of a need for regulating agricultural practices.

After fleeing Nazi Germany, he settled in the United States in 1936. Here, he reportedly treated several persons with cancer with success, although most people in the scientific community found his results unconvincing.

Current proponents of Gerson's diet think it was effective because it helped one avoid eating foods with contaminants, such as fertilizers. In addition, the Gerson diet included the consumption of raw plants, drinking an eight-ounce glass of organic juice every waking hour, and supplementing one's diet with various vitamins and other similar agents. The diet also restricted intake of water, berries, nuts, animal products, various oils, and other harmful substances, such as tobacco and alcohol. The diet often was coupled with enemas, including those using coffee, which have since been exposed as dangerous and ineffective by independent investigators and regulatory agencies.

Gerson's daughter, Charlotte Gerson, promoted the therapy and founded the Gerson Institute in 1977. Since this time, a number of retrospective studies have been performed—by both proponents and opponents of Gerson therapy—to investigate the usefulness of the approach. In summary, the results of such studies have been mixed, although it is worth noting that proponents typically concluded the therapy extended patient life and reduced side effects, whereas the opponents typically concluded the therapy had no clinical benefits. Also of note, no clinical trials have found the therapy to be useful in treating cancer, although some researchers have indicated the therapy may have psychological benefits to its users.

Brandy Weidow, M.S.

FURTHER READING

Gerson, Charlotte, and Beata Bishop. *Healing the Gerson Way: Defeating Cancer and Other Chronic Diseases.* New ed. Carmel, Calif.: Gerson Health Media, 2010.
_____, and Morton Walker. *The Gerson Therapy: The Proven Nutritional Program for Cancer and Other Illnesses.* Rev. ed. New York: Kensington Books, 2006.
Straus, Howard, and Barbara Marinacci. *Dr. Max Gerson: Healing the Hopeless.* 2d ed. Carmel, Calif.: Totality Books, 2009.

See also: Cancer risk reduction; Diet-based therapies.

Ginger

CATEGORY: Herbs and supplements
RELATED TERM: *Zingiber officinale*
DEFINITION: Herbal product promoted as a dietary supplement for specific health benefits.
PRINCIPAL PROPOSED USES: Morning sickness in pregnancy, motion sickness, postsurgical nausea
OTHER PROPOSED USES: Atherosclerosis, high cholesterol, migraine headaches, osteoarthritis, rheumatoid arthritis

OVERVIEW

Native to southern Asia, ginger is a perennial that is two to four feet in length and produces grasslike leaves up to one foot long and almost one inch wide. Although it is called ginger root in the grocery store, the part of the herb used is actually the rhizome, the underground stem of the plant, with its outer covering (similar to bark) scraped off.

Ginger has been used as food and medicine for millennia. Arabian traders carried ginger root from China and India to be used as a food spice in ancient Greece and Rome, and tax records from the second century show that ginger was a source of revenue for the Roman treasury.

Chinese medical texts from the fourth century B.C.E. suggest that ginger is effective in treating nausea, diarrhea, stomachache, cholera, toothaches, bleeding, and rheumatism. Ginger was later used by Chinese herbalists to treat a variety of respiratory conditions, including coughs and the early stages of colds.

Ginger's modern use dates to the early 1980s, when a scientist named D. Mowrey noticed that ginger-filled capsules reduced his nausea during an episode of flu. Inspired by this, he performed the first double-blind study of ginger. Germany's Commission E subsequently approved ginger as a treatment for indigestion and motion sickness.

One of the most prevalent ingredients in fresh ginger is the pungent substance gingerol. However, when ginger is dried and stored, its gingerol rapidly converts to the substances shogaol and zingerone. It remains unknown if any of these substances has medicinal effects.

USES AND APPLICATIONS

Some evidence suggests that ginger may be slightly helpful for the prevention and treatment of various forms of nausea, including motion sickness, the nausea and vomiting of pregnancy (morning sickness), and postsurgical nausea. (Women who are pregnant and persons undergoing surgery should not self-treat with ginger except under physician supervision.)

Scant preliminary evidence suggests that ginger might be helpful for osteoarthritis. One small study suggests that it may be beneficial for high cholesterol. Ginger has been suggested as a treatment for numerous other conditions, including atherosclerosis, migraine headaches, rheumatoid arthritis, ulcers, depression, and impotence. However, there is negligible evidence for these uses.

In traditional Chinese medicine, hot ginger tea taken at the first sign of a cold is believed to offer the possibility of averting the infection. However, there is no scientific evidence for this use.

SCIENTIFIC EVIDENCE

Nausea. The evidence for ginger's effectiveness in various forms of nausea remains mixed. It has been suggested that in some negative studies, poor-quality ginger powder might have been used. In general, while most antinausea drugs influence the brain and the inner ear, ginger appears to act directly on the stomach.

Motion sickness. Ginger has shown inconsistent promise for the treatment of motion sickness. A double-blind, placebo-controlled study of seventy-nine Swedish naval cadets at sea found that 1 gram (g) of ginger could decrease vomiting and cold sweating, but without significantly decreasing nausea and vertigo. Benefits were also seen in a double-blind study of thirty-six persons given ginger, dimenhydrinate, or placebo.

However, a 1984 study funded by the National Aeronautics and Space Administration using intentionally stimulated motion sickness found that ginger was not any more effective than placebo. Two other small studies have also failed to find any benefit. The reason for the discrepancy may lie in the type of ginger used or in the severity of the stimulant used to bring on motion sickness.

Nausea and vomiting during pregnancy. Four double-blind, placebo-controlled studies enrolling 246 women found ginger more effective than placebo for the treatment of morning sickness. For example, a double-blind, placebo-controlled trial of seventy pregnant women evaluated the effectiveness of ginger for morning sickness. Participants received either placebo or 250 milligrams of powdered ginger three times daily

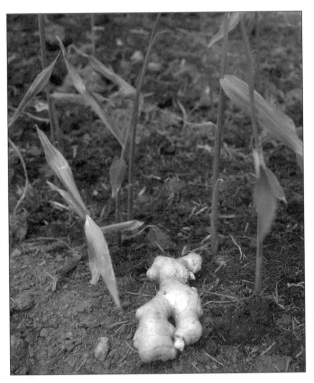

The root and shoots of the ginger plant. (Hans Reinhard/ Okapia/Photo Researchers, Inc.)

for four days. The results showed that ginger significantly reduced nausea and vomiting. No significant side effects occurred.

A minimum of three studies compared ginger to vitamin B_6, a commonly recommended treatment for morning sickness. Two studies found them to be equally beneficial, while the third found ginger to be somewhat better. However, because the effectiveness of vitamin B_6 for morning sickness is not solidly established (the evidence rests largely on one fairly old study), these findings are of questionable value. Despite its use in these studies, ginger has not been proven safe for pregnant women.

Postsurgical nausea. Although there have been some positive studies, on balance, the evidence regarding ginger for reducing nausea and vomiting following surgery is discouraging. A double-blind British study compared the effects of ginger, placebo, and metoclopramide (Reglan) in the treatment of nausea following gynecological surgery. The results in sixty women indicated that both treatments produced similar benefits compared with placebo.

A similar British study followed 120 women receiving elective laparoscopic gynecological surgery. Whereas nausea and vomiting developed in 41 percent of the participants given placebo, in the groups treated with ginger or metoclopramide, these symptoms developed in only 21 and 27 percent, respectively. Benefits were also seen in a double-blind study of eighty people. A study of sixty people found marginally positive results. However, a double-blind study of 108 people undergoing similar surgery found no benefit with ginger compared with placebo. If ginger is effective for postsurgical nausea, the effect is very slight.

Other forms of nausea. One study failed to find ginger helpful for reducing nausea caused by the cancer chemotherapy drug cisplatin. In a second study, ginger did not add to the effectiveness of standard medications to treat chemotherapy-induced nausea and vomiting.

Osteoarthritis. A large double-blind study (more than 250 participants) found that a combination of ginger and another Asian spice called galanga (*Alpinia galanga*) can significantly improve arthritis symptoms. This study was widely publicized as proving that ginger is effective for osteoarthritis. However, the study design makes it impossible to draw any conclusions on the effectiveness of the ginger component of the mixture. Ginger alone has been tested only in two small double-blind studies, and they had contradictory results.

DOSAGE

For most purposes, the standard dosage of powdered ginger is 1 to 4 g daily, divided into two to four doses per day. To prevent motion sickness, one should begin treatment one or two days before a trip and continue it throughout the period of travel.

SAFETY ISSUES

Ginger is on the GRAS (Generally Recognized As Safe) list of the U.S. Food and Drug Administration as a food, and the treatment dosages of ginger are comparable to dietary usages. No significant side effects have been observed.

Like onions and garlic, extracts of ginger inhibit blood coagulation in test-tube experiments. European studies with actual oral ginger taken alone in normal quantities have not found any significant effect on blood coagulation, but it is still theoretically possible that a weak anticoagulant could amplify the effects of drugs that have a similar effect, such as warfarin (Coumadin), heparin, clopidogrel (Plavix), ticlopidine (Ti-

clid), pentoxifylline (Trental), and aspirin. One fairly solid case report appears to substantiate these theoretical concerns: The use of a ginger product markedly (and dangerously) increased the effect of an anticoagulant drug closely related to Coumadin. However, a double-blind study failed to find any interaction between ginger and Coumadin, leaving the truth regarding this potential risk unclear. Finally, the maximum safe doses of ginger for pregnant or nursing women, young children, or persons with severe liver or kidney disease has not been established.

IMPORTANT INTERACTIONS

Ginger could amplify the effects of strong blood-thinning drugs such as Coumadin, heparin, clopidogrel, ticlopidine, pentoxifylline, and aspirin. Also, ginger might increase the risk of bleeding problems.

EBSCO CAM Review Board

FURTHER READING

Alizadeh-Navaei, R., et al. "Investigation of the Effect of Ginger on the Lipid Levels." *Saudi Medical Journal* 29 (2008): 1280-1284.

Ensiyeh, J., and M. A. Sakineh. "Comparing Ginger and Vitamin B6 for the Treatment of Nausea and Vomiting in Pregnancy." *Midwifery* 25 (2009): 649-653.

Takahashi, M., et al. "Clinical Effectiveness of KSS Formula, a Traditional Folk Remedy for Alcohol Hangover Symptoms." *Journal of Natural Medicines* 64 (2010): 487-491.

Wu, K. L., et al. "Effects of Ginger on Gastric Emptying and Motility in Healthy Humans." *European Journal of Gastroenterology and Hepatology* 20 (2008): 436-440.

Zick, S. M., et al. "Phase II Trial of Encapsulated Ginger as a Treatment for Chemotherapy-Induced Nausea and Vomiting." *Supportive Care in Cancer* 17 (2009): 563-572.

See also: Morning sickness; Nausea; Pregnancy support; Vertigo.

Ginkgo

CATEGORY: Herbs and supplements
RELATED TERM: *Ginkgo biloba*
DEFINITION: Natural plant product used to treat specific health conditions.

PRINCIPAL PROPOSED USES: Alzheimer's disease, enhancing memory and mental function in healthy people, intermittent claudication, non-Alzheimer's dementia

OTHER PROPOSED USES: Anxiety, complications of diabetes, depression, glaucoma, increasing efficacy and reducing side effects of phenothiazines and atypical antipsychotics, macular degeneration, multiple sclerosis, premenstrual syndrome, Raynaud's phenomenon, vertigo, vitiligo

OVERVIEW

Traceable to three hundred million years ago, the ginkgo is the oldest surviving species of tree. Although it died out in Europe during the Ice Age, ginkgo survived in China, Japan, and other parts of East Asia. It has been cultivated extensively for both ceremonial and medical purposes, and some particularly revered trees have been tended for more than one thousand years.

In traditional Chinese herbology, tea made from ginkgo seeds has been used for numerous problems, most particularly asthma and other respiratory illnesses. The leaf was not used. In the 1950s, however, German researchers started to investigate the medical possibilities of ginkgo leaf extracts rather than remedies using the seeds. Thus, modern ginkgo preparations are not the same as the traditional Chinese herb, and the comparisons often drawn are incorrect.

THERAPEUTIC DOSAGES

The standard dosage of ginkgo is 40 milligrams (mg) to 80 mg three times daily of a 50:1 extract standardized to contain 24 percent ginkgo-flavone glycosides. Levels of toxic ginkgolic acid and related alkylphenol constituents should be kept under five parts per million. In an analysis performed in 2006 by a respected testing organization, some tested ginkgo products were found to be contaminated with lead.

THERAPEUTIC USES

Fairly good evidence indicates that ginkgo is effective for Alzheimer's disease and other severe forms of memory and mental function decline. When used for this purpose, ginkgo appears to be as effective as standard drugs.

Inconsistent evidence hints that ginkgo might also be helpful for enhancing memory and mental function in seniors without severe memory loss. Weak evidence hints that ginkgo, alone or in combination with ginseng or vinpocetine, may be helpful for enhancing memory or alertness in younger people. Combining phosphatidylserine, another substance used to enhance mental function, with ginkgo might increase its efficacy.

In addition, ginkgo may be effective for the treatment of restricted circulation in the legs due to hardening of the arteries, known as intermittent claudication. One substantial, well-designed double-blind, placebo-controlled study found evidence that ginkgo extract taken at a dose of 240 mg or 480 mg daily may be helpful for anxiety. Weak, and in some cases inconsistent, evidence from preliminary double-blind trials hints that ginkgo might be helpful for glaucoma, macular degeneration, conjunctivitis, premenstrual syndrome (PMS), Raynaud's disease, sudden hearing loss, vertigo, and vitiligo. Although study results conflict, on balance the evidence suggests that ginkgo is not helpful for tinnitus (ringing in the ear).

Three small, double-blind trials enrolling a total of about one hundred people found preliminary evidence that use of the herb *Ginkgo biloba* can help prevent altitude sickness. However, a large-scale, double-blind study enrolling 614 people failed to find benefit. (The drug acetazolamide, however, did provide significant benefits compared to placebo.) A similarly designed smaller study enrolling fifty-seven people also failed to find ginkgo effective. Overall, the balance of evidence suggests that ginkgo is not effective for this purpose.

Numerous case reports and uncontrolled studies raised hope that ginkgo might be an effective treatment for sexual dysfunction in men or women, particularly in those cases related to certain antidepressant medications. However, the results of a number of double-blind studies indicate that ginkgo is no more effective than placebo, whether or not subjects are taking antidepressants.

One small study failed to find ginkgo helpful for the treatment of cocaine dependence. Two studies failed to find ginkgo helpful in multiple sclerosis.

Chinese research suggests that ginkgo might enhance the effects of drugs used for schizophrenia, both phenothiazines as well as atypical antipsychotic drugs. Antipsychotic drugs can cause a neurological condition called tardive dyskinesia, which involves troubling, uncontrollable body movements. One randomized study found that ginkgo (240 mg/day for twelve weeks) was more helpful than placebo in reducing tardive dyskinesia symptoms in people with schizophrenia.

An open study evaluated combination therapy with ginkgo extract and the chemotherapy drug 5FU for the treatment of pancreatic cancer, on the theory that ginkgo might enhance blood flow to the tumor and thereby help 5FU penetrate better. The results were promising, but much better research must be performed before ginkgo can be recommended for this use. Similarly inadequate evidence hints at benefits in dyslexia. Ginkgo has also been proposed as a treatment for depression and diabetic retinopathy, but there is little evidence that it is effective for these conditions.

SCIENTIFIC EVIDENCE

Alzheimer's disease and non-Alzheimer's dementia. In the past, European physicians believed that the cause of mental deterioration with age (senile dementia) was reduced circulation in the brain due to atherosclerosis. Since ginkgo is thought to improve circulation, they assumed that ginkgo was simply getting more blood to brain cells and thereby making them work better.

However, the contemporary understanding of age-related memory loss and mental impairment no longer considers chronically restricted circulation the primary issue. Ginkgo (and other drugs used for dementia) may instead function by directly stimulating nerve cell activity and protecting nerve cells from further injury, although improvement in circulatory capacity may also play a role.

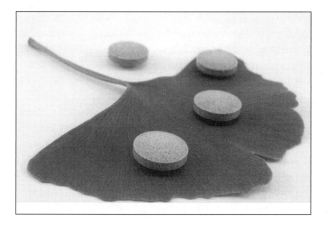

Ginkgo leaf and pills. (©Truembie/Dreamstime.com)

Numerous double-blind, placebo-controlled studies have found ginkgo extract effective for dementia; among these, studies rated as "high-quality" by accepted scientific norms enrolled a total of more than two thousand people. For example, one major trial in the United States published in 1997 enrolled more than three hundred people with Alzheimer's disease or non-Alzheimer's dementia. Participants were given either 40 mg of *Ginkgo biloba* extract or placebo three times daily for a period of fifty-two weeks. The results showed significant but not entirely consistent improvements in the treated group.

Another study, published in 2007, followed four hundred people for twenty-two weeks and used twice the dose of ginkgo. The results of this trial indicated that ginkgo was significantly superior to placebo. (Technically, it was superior in the primary outcome measure, the SKT cognitive test battery, as well as on all secondary outcome measures.) The areas in which ginkgo showed the most marked superiority, compared with placebo, included "apathy/indifference, anxiety, irritability/lability, depression/dysphoria and sleep/nighttime behaviour." In addition, a six-month study found ginkgo just as effective as the drug donepezil (taken at a dose of 5 mg daily).

On the other hand, one fairly large study drew headlines for finding ginkgo extract ineffective. This twenty-four-week, double-blind, placebo-controlled study of 214 people with either mild to moderate dementia or ordinary age-associated memory loss found no effect with ginkgo extract at a dose of 160 mg or 240 mg daily. This study has been sharply criticized for a number of serious flaws in its design. However, in another community-based study among 176 elderly subjects with early-stage dementia, researchers found no beneficial effect for 120 mg of ginkgo extract given daily for six months.

A 2011 systematic review of nine placebo-controlled, randomized trials found more promising evidence for ginkgo. The trials, which involved 2,372 people with Alzheimer's disease or another form of dementia, ranged from twelve to fifty-two weeks. Those in the ginkgo group did have improvements in their cognition scores. A subgroup of people with Alzheimer's disease also showed improvements in their activities of daily living.

The ability of ginkgo to prevent or delay a decline in cognitive function is less clear. In a placebo-controlled trial of 118 cognitively intact adults eighty-five years or older, ginkgo extract seemed to effectively slow the decline in memory function in a forty-two-month period. The researchers also reported a higher incidence of stroke in the group that took ginkgo, a finding that requires more investigation.

In a 2009 review of thirty-six randomized trials involving 4,423 persons with declining mental function, including dementia, researchers concluded that ginkgo appears to be safe. However, there is inconsistent evidence regarding whether it works.

Enhancing mental function in healthy people. Ginkgo has shown less consistent promise for enhancing mental function in people who experience the relatively slight decline in cognitive function that typically accompanies increased age. For example, in a double-blind, placebo-controlled trial, 241 elderly persons with mildly impaired memory were given either placebo or ginkgo for twenty-four weeks. The results showed that ginkgo produced modest improvements in certain types of memory.

Another double-blind, placebo-controlled trial examined the effects of ginkgo extract in forty men and women, aged fifty-five to eighty-six, who did not have any mental impairment. In a six-week period, the results showed improvements in measurements of mental function. Possible benefits were also seen in six other trials involving a total of about 250 people.

Set against these positive findings is the twenty-four-week study mentioned above, which found no benefit in ordinary age-related memory loss. The reason for this negative outcome may be flaws in this trial's design. However, three other studies enrolling a total of about four hundred elderly persons also failed to find significant benefit with daily use of ginkgo. Another double-blind, placebo-controlled study used a one-time dose of ginkgo and again found no benefits.

Besides these negative trials, there is another weakness in the evidence: inconsistency even among positive trials. There are numerous measurable aspects of memory and mental function, and studies of ginkgo have examined a great many of these, but the exact areas of benefits seen vary widely.

For example, in one positive study, ginkgo may speed the ability to memorize letters but not expand the number of letters that can be retained while in another positive study, the reverse may be true. This type of inconsistency tends to decrease the confidence one can place in these apparently positive studies, because

if ginkgo were really working, one would expect its effects to be more reproducible.

A total of about fifteen controlled trials have examined the effects of ginkgo on memory and mental function in younger people. However, results are again inconsistent, with many negative results and the positive ones failing to indicate a consistent pattern of benefit.

Several small double-blind, placebo-controlled studies have evaluated combined treatment with ginseng or vinpocetine for enhancing mental function in young people. The results, overall, are unconvincing. Weak evidence suggests that combining phosphatidyl-serine with ginkgo might increase its efficacy. In two studies, ginkgo combined with the Ayurvedic herb brahmi failed to improve mental function.

It remains unclear whether ginkgo actually enhances memory and mental function in healthy seniors or healthy younger people. Benefits, if they do exist, are probably slight.

Intermittent claudication. In intermittent claudication, impaired circulation can cause a severe, cramplike pain in one's legs after walking only a short distance. According to nine double-blind, placebo-controlled trials, ginkgo can significantly increase pain-free walking distance.

One double-blind study enrolled 111 people for twenty-four weeks. Subjects were measured for pain-free walking distance by walking up a 12 percent slope on a treadmill at 3 kilometers per hour (about 2 miles per hour). At the beginning of treatment, both the placebo and ginkgo (120 mg daily) groups were able to walk about 350 feet without pain. By the end of the trial, both groups had improved, although the ginkgo group had improved significantly more. Participants taking ginkgo showed about a 40 percent increase in pain-free walking distance, compared with only a 20 percent improvement in the placebo group. Similar improvements were also seen in a double-blind, placebo-controlled trial of sixty people who had achieved maximum benefit from physical therapy.

A twenty-four-week, double-blind, placebo-controlled study of seventy-four people with intermittent claudication found that ginkgo was more effective at a dose of 240 mg per day than at 120 mg per day. A 2009 review of eleven trials with 477 participants suggested that those who took *Ginkgo biloba* were able to walk farther than control patients, although the results were limited by differences among the trials. However, not all studies have been positive. In a randomized trail involving sixty-two persons averaging seventy years of age, 300 mg of ginkgo per day was no better than placebo at improving pain-free walking distance over four months of treatment.

PMS symptoms. One double-blind, placebo-controlled study evaluated the benefits of ginkgo extract for women with PMS symptoms. This trial enrolled 143 women, eighteen to forty-five years of age, and followed them for two menstrual cycles. Each woman received either the ginkgo extract (80 mg twice daily) or placebo beginning on day sixteen of the first cycle. Treatment was continued until day five of the next cycle and resumed on day sixteen of that cycle. Compared with placebo, ginkgo significantly relieved major symptoms of PMS, especially breast pain and emotional disturbance. In another, similarly designed trial involving eighty-five university students, *Ginkgo biloba* L. significantly reduced PMS symptom severity compared to placebo.

Anxiety. In a double-blind, placebo-controlled study of 107 people with various forms of anxiety (specifically, generalized anxiety disorder or adjustment disorder with anxious mood), ginkgo extract taken at a dose of 240 mg or 480 mg daily proved significantly more effective than placebo.

Macular degeneration. Macular degeneration, one of the most common causes of vision loss in seniors, may respond to ginkgo. In a six-month, double-blind, placebo-controlled study of twenty people with macular degeneration, use of ginkgo at a dose of 160 mg daily resulted in improved visual acuity.

A twenty-four-week, double-blind study of ninety-nine people with macular degeneration compared ginkgo extract at a dose of 240 mg per day with ginkgo at a dose of 60 mg daily. The results showed that vision improved in both groups, but to a greater extent with the higher dose.

Vertigo. A three-month, double-blind trial of seventy people with a variety of vertigo conditions found that ginkgo extract given at a dose of 160 mg twice daily produced results superior to placebo. By the end of the trial, 47 percent of the people given ginkgo had significantly recovered, versus only 18 percent in the placebo group.

Glaucoma. A small double-blind, placebo-controlled trial found that use of ginkgo extract at a dose of 120 mg daily for eight weeks significantly improved the visual field in people with glaucoma.

Tinnitus. Studies of *Ginkgo biloba* extract for treating tinnitus have yielded conflicting results. While some small studies found benefit, the largest and best-designed of these trials failed to find ginkgo effective. In a twelve-week, double-blind trial, 1,121 people with tinnitus were given either placebo or standardized ginkgo at a dose of 50 mg three times daily. The results showed no difference between the treated and the placebo groups.

SAFETY ISSUES

Ginkgo appears to be relatively safe. Extremely high doses have been given to animals for long periods of time without serious consequences, and results from human trials are also generally reassuring. Safety in young children, pregnant or nursing women, or those with severe liver or kidney disease, however, has not been established.

In all the clinical trials of ginkgo up through 1991 combined, involving a total of almost ten thousand participants, the incidence of side effects produced by ginkgo extract was extremely small. There were twenty-one cases of gastrointestinal discomfort and even fewer cases of headaches, dizziness, and allergic skin reactions.

However, there are some potential problems. Perhaps the most serious have been the numerous case reports of internal bleeding associated with use of ginkgo (spontaneous as well as following surgery). Based on these reports, as well as previous evidence that ginkgo inhibits platelet function, studies have been performed to determine whether ginkgo significantly affects bleeding time or other measures of blood coagulation, with somewhat inconsistent results. Prudence suggests that ginkgo should not be used by anyone during the periods before or after surgery or labor and delivery, or by those with bleeding problems such as hemophilia. It also seems reasonable to hypothesize that ginkgo might interact with blood-thinning drugs, amplifying their effects on coagulation. However, two studies found no interaction between ginkgo and warfarin (Coumadin), and another found no interaction with clopidogrel. (Although, it did find a slight interaction with the related drug cilostazol.) While these findings are reassuring, prudence indicates physician supervision before combining ginkgo with blood-thinning drugs.

One study found that when high concentrations of ginkgo were placed in a test tube with hamster sperm and ova, the sperm were less able to penetrate the ova. However, since researchers have no idea whether this much ginkgo can actually come into contact with sperm and ova when they are in the body rather than a test tube, these results may not be meaningful in real life.

The ginkgo extracts approved for use in Germany are processed to remove alkylphenols, including ginkgolic acids, which have been found to be toxic. The same ginkgo extracts are available in the United States. However, other ginkgo extracts and whole ginkgo leaf might contain appreciable levels of these dangerous constituents.

Seizures have also been reported with the use of ginkgo leaf extract in people with previously well-controlled epilepsy; in one case, the seizures were fatal. It has been suggested that ginkgo might interfere with the effectiveness of some antiseizure medications, specifically phenytoin and valproic acid. Another possible explanation is contamination of ginkgo-leaf products with ginkgo seeds; the seeds of the ginkgo plant contain a neurotoxic substance called 4-methoxypyridoxine (MPN). Finally, the drug tacrine (also used to improve memory) has been associated with seizures, and ginkgo may affect the brain in ways similar to tacrine. Regardless of the explanation, prudence suggests that people with epilepsy should avoid ginkgo.

According to a study in rats, ginkgo extract may cause the body to metabolize the drug nicardipine (a calcium channel blocker) more rapidly, thereby decreasing its effects. In addition, this finding also suggests potential interactions with numerous other drugs, although more research is needed to determine which ones might be affected.

Antibiotics in the aminoglycoside family can cause hearing loss by damaging the nerve carrying hearing sensation from the ear. One animal study evaluated the potential benefits of ginkgo for preventing hearing loss but found instead that the herb increased damage to the nerve. Based on this finding, individuals using aminoglycosides should avoid ginkgo.

It has been suggested that ginkgo might cause problems for people with type 2 diabetes by altering blood levels of medications, as well as by directly affecting the blood-sugar-regulating system of the body. However, the most recent and best-designed studies have failed to find any such actions. Nonetheless, until this situation is clarified, people with diabetes should use ginkgo only under physician supervision.

IMPORTANT INTERACTIONS

Taking blood-thinning drugs–such as aspirin and other nonsteroidal anti-inflammatory drugs (ibuprofen), cilostazol, clopidogrel (Plavix), heparin, pentoxifylline (Trental), ticlopidine (Ticlid), and warfarin (Coumadin)–while simultaneously using ginkgo could theoretically cause bleeding problems and should not be undertaken without physician supervision. Ginkgo might also reduce the effectiveness of channel blockers.

Using ginkgo while also taking antipsychotic medications in the phenothiazine family, as well as atypical antipsychotic drugs, such as clozapine and olanzapene, might help these drugs work better with fewer side effects. Use of ginkgo simultaneously with ainoglycoside antibiotics might increase risk of hearing loss. Finally, ginkgo might interfere with the effectiveness of medications to prevent seizures.

EBSCO CAM Review Board

FURTHER READING

Dodge, H. H., et al. "A Randomized Placebo-Controlled Trial of *Ginkgo biloba* for the Prevention of Cognitive Decline." *Neurology* 6, no. 70 (2008): 1809-1817.

Gardner, C. D., et al. "Effect of *Ginkgo biloba* (EGB 761) on Treadmill Walking Time Among Adults with Peripheral Artery Disease." *Journal of Cardiopulmonary Rehabilitation and Prevention* 28 (2008): 258-265.

McCarney, R., et al. "*Ginkgo biloba* for Mild to Moderate Dementia in a Community Setting." *International Journal of Geriatric Psychiatry* 23, no. 12 (2008): 1222-1230.

Meston, C. M., et al. "Short- and Long-Term Effects of *Ginkgo biloba* Extract on Sexual Dysfunction in Women." *Archives of Sexual Behavior* 37, no. 4 (2008): 530-547.

Ozgoli, G., et al. "A Randomized, Placebo-Controlled Trial of *Ginkgo biloba* L. in Treatment of Premenstrual Syndrome." *Journal of Alternative and Complementary Medicine* 15 (2009): 845-851.

Russo, V., et al. "Clinical Efficacy of a *Ginkgo biloba* Extract in the Topical Treatment of Allergic Conjunctivitis." *European Journal of Ophthalmology* 19 (2009): 331-336.

Weinmann, S., et al. "Effects of *Ginkgo biloba* in Dementia." *BMC Geriatrics* 10 (2010): 14.

See also: Alzheimer's disease and non-Alzheimer's dementia; Herbal medicine; Intermittent claudication; Memory and mental function impairment; Mental health.

Ginseng

CATEGORY: Herbs and supplements
RELATED TERMS: *Panax ginseng, P. quinquefolius*
DEFINITION: Natural plant product used as a dietary supplement for specific health benefits.
PRINCIPAL PROPOSED USES: Colds and flu, diabetes, general well-being, immune support, mental function enhancement, stress
OTHER PROPOSED USES: Cancer prevention, male sexual function, sports performance
PROBABLY INEFFECTIVE USE: Menopause

OVERVIEW

Three different herbs are commonly called ginseng: Asian or Korean ginseng (*Panax ginseng*), American ginseng (*P. quinquefolius*), and Siberian ginseng (*Eleutherococcus senticosus*). The latter herb, however, is actually not ginseng.

Asian ginseng is a perennial herb with a taproot resembling the shape of the human body. It grows in northern China, Korea, and Russia; its close relative, *P. quinquefolius*, is cultivated in the United States. Because ginseng must be grown for five years before it is harvested, it commands a high price, with top-quality roots easily selling for more than ten thousand U.S. dollars. Dried, unprocessed ginseng root is called white ginseng, and steamed, heat-dried root is red ginseng. Chinese herbalists believe that each form has its own particular benefits.

Ginseng is commonly regarded as a stimulant. According to persons who use it seriously, however, this description is inadequate. In traditional Chinese herbology, *P. ginseng* was used to strengthen the digestion and the lungs, to calm the spirit, and to increase overall energy. Before World War II, a Russian scientist named Israel I. Brekhman became interested in the herb and came up with a new way to describe it: as an adaptogen.

An adaptogen is part of a hypothetical treatment that helps the body adapt to stresses of various kinds, whether heat, cold, exertion, trauma, sleep deprivation, toxic exposure, radiation, infection, or psychological stress. Furthermore, an adaptogen, by definition, should cause no side effects, should be effective in treating a wide variety of illnesses, and should help return an organism toward balance.

Perhaps the only indisputable example of an adaptogen is a healthful lifestyle. By eating right, exercising regularly, and generally living a life of balance and moderation, a person can increase physical fitness and the ability to resist illnesses of all types. Whether there are any substances that can do as much remains unclear. Brekhman believed that ginseng produced similarly universal benefits.

Traditional Chinese medicine does not align with Brekhman's idea. There is no one-size-fits-all in Chinese medical theory. Like any other herb, ginseng is said to be helpful for those people who need its particular effects and to be neutral or harmful for others. In Europe, Brekhman's concept took hold, and ginseng is now widely believed to be a universal adaptogen.

THERAPEUTIC DOSAGES

The typical recommended daily dosage of *P. ginseng* is 1 to 2 grams (g) of raw herb or 200 mg daily of an extract standardized to contain 4 to 7 percent ginsenosides. In one study of American ginseng for diabetes, the dose used was 3 g daily.

There are dozens of ginsenosides in ginseng. Because different ginsenosides have different effects, two different ginseng products with similar total ginsenoside content will not necessarily have similar efficacy. Scientific knowledge does not allow experts to make informed recommendations on which specific ginsenosides are useful for which conditions.

Ordinarily, a two- to three-week period of using ginseng is recommended, followed by a one- to two-week "rest" period. Russian tradition suggests that ginseng should not be used by those persons younger than age forty years. However, there is no scientific evidence to support these recommendations.

THERAPEUTIC USES

If Brekhman was right, ginseng should be the right treatment for the stresses of modern life. Ginseng is widely used for this purpose in Russia and Eastern Europe. However, the scientific basis for this use is largely limited to animal studies and human trials of unacceptably low quality.

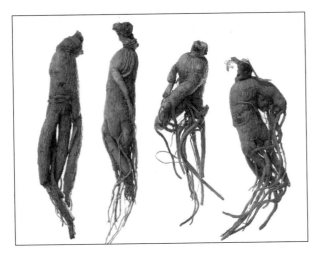

Ginseng roots. (©Antaratma Images/Dreamstime.com)

There have been a few better-quality studies of various forms of ginseng for certain more specific purposes, such as strengthening immunity against colds and flu and other infections (including herpes), helping to control diabetes, stimulating the mind, increasing a general sense of well-being, and improving physical performance capacity. Some of these studies have found positive results with the use of ginseng.

The active ingredients in ginseng are believed to be substances called ginsenosides. Ginseng low in ginsenosides may not be effective. However, different ginsenosides appear to have differing actions, and the exact mixture of the ginsenosides in a given ginseng product may play a large role in its efficacy.

Two preliminary studies suggest that Korean red ginseng may have some benefits for impotence (erectile dysfunction). A poorly designed study using an untreated control group found indications that *P. ginseng* might improve sperm count and motility, thereby enhancing male fertility.

Highly preliminary evidence suggests that *P. quinquefolius* might improve the effectiveness of breast cancer chemotherapy drugs. *P. ginseng* also is said to help prevent cancer and to fight chemical dependency, but the scientific evidence for these uses is minimal at best. Another study failed to find ginseng helpful for menopausal symptoms.

SCIENTIFIC EVIDENCE

Adaptogenic effects. Numerous studies have evaluated the effects of oral *P. ginseng* on animals under condi-
tions of extreme stress. The results suggest that ginseng increases physical endurance and causes physiological changes that may help the body adapt to adverse conditions. In addition, studies in mice found that consuming *P. ginseng* before exposure to a virus significantly increased the survival rate and the number of antibodies produced. However, most of these studies fall far beneath modern scientific standards.

Colds and flu. A double-blind, placebo-controlled study of 323 people found meaningful evidence that an extract of American ginseng taken at 400 milligrams (mg) daily may help prevent the common cold. Participants who used the extract for four months had a reduced number of colds compared with those taking the placebo. Comparative benefits also were seen in the percentage of participants who developed two or more colds and in the severity and duration of cold symptoms that did develop. Similar benefits were seen in a study of forty-three people.

In addition, two double-blind, placebo-controlled studies indicate that *P. quinquefolius* may be able to prevent flulike illness in the elderly.

A double-blind, placebo-controlled study suggests that ginseng can also help prevent flulike illnesses. This trial enrolled 227 participants at three medical offices in Milan, Italy. One-half were given ginseng at a dosage of 100 mg daily, the other one-half placebo. Four weeks into the study, all participants received influenza vaccine. The results showed a significant decline in the frequency of colds and flu in the treated group compared with the placebo group (fifteen versus forty-two cases, respectively). Also, antibody measurements in response to the vaccination rose higher in the treated group than in the placebo group.

On a much more theoretical level, two other studies found evidence that ginseng increases the number of immune cells in the blood, while a third study did not find this effect. (In any case, measuring changes in the number of immune cells is not a reliable method of demonstrating immune-system enhancement.) Also, a nonblinded pilot study provides weak evidence that ginseng might be helpful in chronic bronchitis.

Diabetes. In preliminary double-blind studies performed by a single research group, the use of American ginseng (*P. quinquefolius*) appeared to improve blood sugar control. In some studies, the same researchers reported potential benefit with Korean red ginseng.

A different research group tested ordinary ginseng and claimed to find it effective. However, this study was somewhat substandard in both its design and its reporting. In other studies, ordinary ginseng seemed to worsen blood sugar control rather than improve it, while yet another group found benefits. It appears possible that certain ginsenosides (found in high concentrations in some American ginseng products) may lower blood sugar, while others (found in high concentration in some *P. ginseng* products) may raise it. It has been suggested that because the actions of these various constituents are not well defined, ginseng should not be used to treat diabetes until more is known.

Mental function. Several studies have found indications that *P. ginseng* might enhance mental function. However, the specific benefits seen have varied considerably from trial to trial, tending to make the actual cognitive effects of ginseng (if there are any) difficult to discern. A double-blind, placebo-controlled study found that *P. ginseng* can improve some aspects of mental function. For two months, 112 healthy, middle-aged adults took either ginseng or placebo. The results showed that ginseng improved abstract thinking ability. However, there was no significant difference between the two groups in reaction time, memory, concentration, or overall subjective experience.

Another double-blind, placebo-controlled study of fifty men found that an eight-week treatment with a *P. ginseng* extract improved ability in completion of a detail-oriented editing task. Also, a double-blind trial of sixteen healthy males found favorable changes in ability to perform mental arithmetic in those given *P. ginseng* for twelve weeks.

A double-blind, placebo-controlled trial of sixty elderly people found that fifty or one hundred days of treatment with *P. ginseng* produced improvements in numerous measures of mental function, including memory, attention, concentration, and ability to cope. Benefits were still evident at the fifty-day follow-up. However, virtually no improvement was seen in the placebo group, a result that is highly unusual and raises doubts about the accuracy of the study. In addition, three double-blind, placebo-controlled studies evaluated combined treatment with *P. ginseng* and ginkgo and found some evidence of improved mental function.

Sports performance. The evidence for *P. ginseng* as a sports supplement is mixed at best. An eight-week, double-blind, placebo-controlled trial evaluated the effects of *P. ginseng* with and without exercise in forty-one persons. The participants were given either ginseng or placebo, and then they underwent exercise training or remained untrained throughout the study. The results showed that ginseng improved aerobic capacity in persons who did not exercise but offered no benefit in those who did exercise. In a nine-week, double-blind, placebo-controlled trial of thirty highly trained athletes, treatment with *P. ginseng* alone or in combination with vitamin E produced significant improvements in aerobic capacity. Another double-blind, placebo-controlled trial of thirty-seven persons also found some benefit.

A double-blind, placebo-controlled study of 120 people found that *P. ginseng* gradually improved reaction time and lung function in a twelve-week treatment period among those persons forty to sixty years old. No benefits were seen in younger persons.

However, numerous studies have failed to find *P. ginseng* effective. For example, an eight-week double-blind trial that followed sixty healthy men in their twenties found no evidence of ergogenic benefit. Many other small trials of *P. ginseng* also failed to find evidence of benefit.

General well-being. A double-blind study compared the effects of a nutritional supplement with and without *P. ginseng* extract on the feeling of well-being in 625 people whose average age was just under forty years. Quality of life was measured by a set of eleven questions. People taking the ginseng-containing supplement reported significant improvement compared with those taking the supplement without ginseng (the control group). Similar findings were reported in a double-blind, placebo-controlled study of thirty-six people newly diagnosed with diabetes. After eight weeks, participants who had been taking 200 mg of ginseng daily reported improvements in mood, well-being, vigor, and psychophysical performance that were significant compared with the reports of control participants.

A twelve-week, double-blind, placebo-controlled study of 120 people found improvement in general well-being among women aged thirty to sixty years and men aged forty to sixty years, but not among men aged thirty to thirty-nine years.

However, a double-blind, placebo-controlled trial of thirty young people found marginal benefits at four weeks and no significant benefits at eight weeks. Similarly, a sixty-day, double-blind, placebo-controlled trial of eighty-three adults in their mid-twenties found no effect on mood or psychological well-being.

A double-blind study of fifty-three people undergoing cancer treatment found equivocal evidence of benefit with a special form of ginseng modified to contain higher levels of certain constituents.

Impotence (erectile dysfunction). Two double-blind, placebo-controlled trials, involving a total of about 135 people, have found evidence that Korean red ginseng may improve erectile function. In the better of the two trials, 45 participants received either placebo or Korean red ginseng at a dose of 900 mg three times daily for eight weeks. The results indicate that while using Korean red ginseng, men experienced significantly better sexual function than while they were taking placebo.

In an analysis combining the results of six controlled trials, researchers found some evidence for the benefits of Korean red ginseng. However, the small size and generally low quality of the studies left some doubts about this conclusion.

Preventing cancer. An observational study on ginseng and cancer prevention has been widely publicized, but a close look at the data arouses serious suspicions. This study was performed in South Korea and followed a total of 4,587 men and women aged thirty-nine years and older from 1987 to 1991. People who regularly consumed *P. ginseng* were compared with otherwise similar people (matched in gender, age, alcohol use, smoking, education, and economic status) who did not.

The reported results were impressive. Those who used ginseng showed a 60 percent decrease in risk of death from cancer. Lung cancer and gastric cancer were particularly reduced. The more ginseng consumed, the greater the effect.

However, there is something not right about this study. The use of ginseng fewer than three times per year reportedly led to a 54 percent reduction in risk. It is difficult to believe that so occasional a use of ginseng could reduce cancer mortality by more than one-half.

Menopause. A double-blind, placebo-controlled study of 384 women experiencing menopausal symptoms found no significant benefit with *P. ginseng* and no evidence of hormonal effects.

SAFETY ISSUES

Ginseng appears to be nontoxic, both in the short term and the long term, according to the results of studies in mice, rats, chickens, and dwarf pigs.

Reported side effects in humans are rare. There are a few case reports of breast tenderness, postmenopausal vaginal bleeding, and menstrual abnormalities associated with *P. ginseng* use. Such side effects suggest that it has estrogenic properties. However, a large double-blind trial of *P. ginseng* found no estrogen-like effects. Another double-blind trial found no effects on estrogen or testosterone, and a carefully designed test-tube study showed that ginseng is not estrogenic. Therefore, it is possible that these apparent side effects were coincidental; another possibility is that adulterants in the ginseng product used caused the problem. Ginseng and other Asian herbal products have often been found to contain unlisted herbs and pharmaceuticals.

Estrogen itself stimulates the growth of breast cancer cells. In a test-tube study, *P. ginseng* was again found to be nonestrogenic, and yet, it nonetheless stimulated the growth of breast cancer cells. Although the mechanism of this effect is not known, the results suggest that women who have had breast cancer should avoid using ginseng.

Unconfirmed reports suggest that highly excessive doses of *P. ginseng* can cause insomnia, can raise blood pressure, can increase heart rate, and can cause other significant effects. Whether some of these cases were actually caused by caffeine mixed in with ginseng remains unclear. One double-blind study failed to find any effect on blood pressure.

One case report and one double-blind trial suggest that *P. ginseng* can reduce the anticoagulant effects of Coumadin (warfarin), but another trial failed to find such an interaction. The reason for this discrepancy is not clear, so one should not combine ginseng and warfarin.

Two reports indicate that combination treatment with *P. ginseng* and antidepressant drugs may result in a manic episode. There are also theoretical concerns regarding the use of ginseng by people with diabetes. If it is true, as the foregoing preliminary studies suggest, that ginseng can reduce blood sugar levels, people with diabetes who take ginseng might need to reduce their dose of medication. On the other hand, if certain types of ginseng have the opposite effect (as researchers hypothesize), this could necessitate an increase in medication. People with diabetes should use ginseng only under physician supervision.

In 1979, an article in the *Journal of the American Medical Association* claimed that people can become addicted to *P. ginseng* and can develop blood pressure elevations, nervousness, sleeplessness, diarrhea, and hypersexuality. However, this report has since been thoroughly discredited and should no longer be taken seriously.

Chinese tradition suggests that *P. ginseng* should not be used by pregnant or nursing women, and one animal study hints that ginseng use by a pregnant woman could cause birth defects. Safety in young children or in persons with severe liver or kidney disease has not been established.

IMPORTANT INTERACTIONS

In persons taking antidepressants, *P. ginseng* might cause manic episodes. For persons using insulin or oral hypoglycemics, various forms of ginseng may unpredictably alter the dosage need. For persons taking Coumadin, *P. ginseng* might possibly decrease its effect. However, *P. ginseng* might increase the effectiveness of the influenza vaccine.

EBSCO CAM Review Board

FURTHER READING

Ellis, J. M., and P. Reddy. "Effects of *Panax ginseng* on Quality of Life." *Annals of Pharmacotherapy* 36 (2002): 375-379.

Hartz, A. J., et al. "Randomized Controlled Trial of Siberian Ginseng for Chronic Fatigue." *Psychological Medicine* 34 (2004): 51-61.

Jang, D. J., et al. "Red Ginseng for Treating Erectile Dysfunction." *British Journal of Clinical Pharmacology* 66 (2008): 444-450.

Kim, J. H., C. Y. Park, and S. J. Lee. "Effects of Sun Ginseng on Subjective Quality of Life in Cancer Patients." *Journal of Clinical Pharmacy and Therapeutics* 31 (2006): 331-334.

Predy, G. N., et al. "Efficacy of an Extract of North American Ginseng Containing Poly-Furanosyl-Pyranosyl-Saccharides for Preventing Upper Respiratory Tract Infections." *CMAJ* 173 (2005): 1043-1048.

Reay, J. L., D. O. Kennedy, and A. B. Scholey. "The Glycaemic Effects of Single Doses of *Panax ginseng* in Young Healthy Volunteers." *British Journal of Nutrition* 96 (2006): 639-642.

Vuksan, V., and J. L. Sievenpiper. "Herbal Remedies in the Management of Diabetes: Lessons Learned from the Study of Ginseng." *Nutrition, Metabolism, and Cardiovascular Diseases* 15 (2005): 149-160.

See also: Cancer risk reduction; Colds and flu; Diabetes; Herbal medicine; Immune support; Sexual dysfunction in men; Sports and fitness support: Enhancing performance; Stress; Traditional Chinese herbal medicine.

Glaucoma

CATEGORY: Condition
DEFINITION: Treatment of damage to the eye's optic nerve that leads to impaired vision or blindness.
PRINCIPAL PROPOSED NATURAL TREATMENTS: None
OTHER PROPOSED NATURAL TREATMENTS: Forskolin (from *Coleus forskohlii*), ginkgo, lipoic acid, magnesium, melatonin, omega-3 fatty acids, vitamin C

INTRODUCTION

Glaucoma is a group of related diseases that cause damage to the eye's optic nerve and result in visual impairment or blindness. Most often, glaucoma occurs in the presence of increased intraocular pressure (pressure inside the eye). However, glaucoma can also occur when intraocular pressure is normal (although treatment that reduces the pressure appears to benefit this kind of glaucoma too).

Glaucoma is the second leading cause of legal blindness in the United States and is the leading cause of blindness in African Americans. Most of the time, glaucoma presents no symptoms until permanent damage has been done. It is estimated that 2.5 million Americans have glaucoma, and one-half do not know they have it. For this reason, regular checkups are advisable for people at high risk for glaucoma. Risk factors include African American descent, being sixty years of age and older, a family history of glaucoma, and the use of corticosteroid drugs (including steroid inhalers for asthma).

Physicians diagnose glaucoma by measuring intraocular pressure, by examining the optic nerve, and by special vision tests. Eye drops that reduce intraocular pressure are safe and highly effective for most cases of glaucoma.

PROPOSED NATURAL TREATMENTS

A small, double-blind, placebo-controlled trial found that the use of ginkgo extract at a dose of 120 milligrams daily for eight weeks significantly improved vision in people with glaucoma. Ginkgo is thought to work by enhancing circulation.

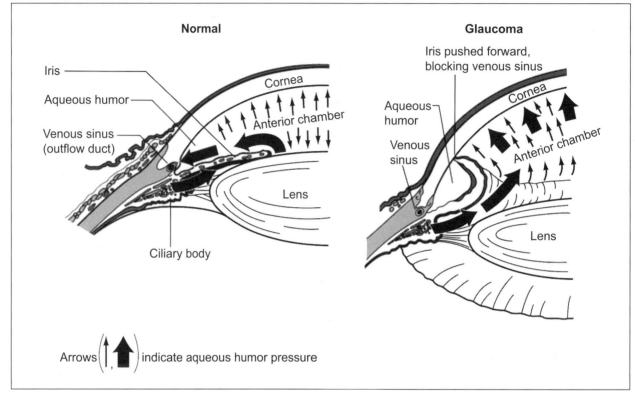

A normal eye versus an eye affected by glaucoma.

Small, double-blind, placebo-controlled trials suggest that eye drops containing the chemical forskolin, a constituent of the herb *Coleus forskohlii*, reduce intraocular pressure in people without glaucoma. However there is no evidence that forskolin is an effective treatment. In any case, forskolin is not available except for research, and using ordinary preparations of the herb directly in the eye is not recommended. (There is no reason to believe that the oral use of *C. forskohlii* will benefit glaucoma.)

Preliminary evidence suggests that certain dietary supplements, including high-dose vitamin C, melatonin, and omega-3 fatty acids, may also reduce intraocular pressure. However, there is no reliable evidence that any of these supplements enhances the effect of standard treatment, and they definitely cannot be used as substitutes for it. Weak evidence suggests that the supplement lipoic acid could improve vision in people with glaucoma. Magnesium has been suggested for the same purpose, but in one preliminary study, the use of magnesium failed to produce statistically significant benefits. The herbs bilberry, ginkgo, oregano, and pilocarpus, and the supplements citrus bioflavonoids and oligomeric proanthocyanidin complexes are sometimes recommended for preventing or treating glaucoma, but there is no meaningful evidence to indicate that they work.

EBSCO CAM Review Board

FURTHER READING

Gaby, A. R. "Nutritional Therapies for Ocular Disorders." *Alternative Medicine Review* 13 (2008): 191-204.

Gaspar, A. Z., P. Gasser, and J. Flammer. "The Influence of Magnesium on Visual Field and Peripheral Vasospasm in Glaucoma." *Ophthalmologica* 209 (1995): 11-13.

Quaranta, L., et al. "Effect of *Ginkgo biloba* Extract on Preexisting Visual Field Damage in Normal Tension Glaucoma." *Ophthalmology* 110 (2003): 359-362.

See also: Aging; Blepharitis; Cataracts; Corticosteroids; Conjunctivitis; Elder health; Macular degeneration; Night vision, impaired; Retinitis pigmentosa; Uveitis.

Glucomannan

CATEGORY: Herbs and supplements
RELATED TERM: *Amorphophallus konjac*
DEFINITION: Natural plant product used to treat specific health conditions.
PRINCIPAL PROPOSED USE: High cholesterol
OTHER PROPOSED USES: Constipation, diabetes, high blood pressure, hyperthyroidism, weight loss

OVERVIEW

Glucomannan is a dietary fiber derived from the tubers of *Amorphophallus konjac.* Konjac flour (made from these tubers) is used to make a jelly called konyaku, a common food product in Japan.

Fiber-containing foods, such as oats, are known to help reduce cholesterol and improve constipation and may also help regulate blood sugar and assist in weight reduction by creating a feeling of fullness. However, many people have a hard time consuming enough fiber from food, so they turn to fiber supplements, such as guar gum and pectin, to help meet their daily requirements. Glucomannan offers one advantage over these forms of fiber: much smaller doses are necessary. When glucomannan is placed in water, it can swell up to seventeen times its original volume. These qualities make it potentially quite convenient as a fiber supplement.

REQUIREMENTS AND SOURCES

Although glucomannan can be derived from other sources, such as yeast, most studies have used glucomannan purified from the konjac root.

THERAPEUTIC DOSAGES

Most of the studies described here used 3 to 5 grams (g) per day in divided doses before meals. However, there are concerns regarding the form of glucomannan used.

THERAPEUTIC USES

Several small controlled studies have found glucomannan to be effective for improving the cholesterol profile. Glucomannan appears to reduce LDL (bad) cholesterol and, according to some studies, increase HDL (good) cholesterol. In addition, it may improve blood pressure.

By expanding in the stomach, glucomannan might be useful for people trying to lose weight. Many people report a feeling of fullness after taking glucomannan, and some studies found a significant weight loss among those taking glucomannan compared to those on a placebo. However, not all studies of glucomannan for weight loss have had positive results.

Glucomannan may also help the body to regulate blood sugar levels and therefore could be helpful in treating diabetes. Additionally, glucomannan might be helpful for individuals who experience episodes of low blood sugar following stomach surgery. Like other dietary fibers, glucomannan may help treat constipation.

Hyperthyroidism is a state in which levels of thyroid hormone are too high. A preliminary trial found some evidence that when glucomannan is added to standard treatment, normal thyroid hormone levels are restored more rapidly.

SCIENTIFIC EVIDENCE

High cholesterol and high blood pressure. In a double-blind study, sixty-three people were given either 3.9 g per day of glucomannan or a placebo for four weeks and then switched to the other treatment. While taking glucomannan, participants showed significant reductions in total cholesterol, LDL cholesterol, and triglycerides, compared with the placebo. In addition, their systolic blood pressure (the upper number in the blood pressure reading) was also reduced. However, there was no significant increase in HDL cholesterol and no improvement in the ratio of LDL to HDL cholesterol.

Participants in another study were given either 3 g per day of glucomannan or a placebo over an eight-week period. The glucomannan group showed improvements in total and HDL cholesterol, as well as a reduction in systolic blood pressure. Those taking glucomannan also lost weight, whereas the placebo group gained weight over the length of the trial.

Several other controlled studies have found similar results. In addition, in a mathematical review combining the results of fourteen studies, glucomannan significantly reduced total and LDL cholesterol levels.

Weight loss. A few small double-blind studies suggest that glucomannan may be helpful for people trying to lose weight; however, in other studies, no such benefit was seen. One double-blind, placebo-controlled trial of twenty women who were more than 20 percent over their ideal weight found glucomannan to be more effective than placebo at promoting weight loss. All participants were instructed not to change their eating or exercise habits while on the treatment. Those in the treatment group took 1 g of glucomannan three times a day for eight weeks and lost an average of 5.5 pounds during that period; in comparison, those in the placebo group gained an average of 1.5 pounds, a significant difference. The glucomannan group also had a reduction of total and LDL cholesterol, as well as triglyceride levels. Benefits were also seen in a double-blind, placebo-controlled trial of twenty-eight overweight people who had just experienced a heart attack.

However, another double-blind trial of sixty obese children did not find a significant difference in weight loss between the glucomannan and the placebo groups. In this study, the children received either 1 g of glucomannan or 1 g of placebo twice a day for eight weeks.

Diabetes. A study of individuals with diabetes tested the effectiveness of glucomannan fiber-enriched biscuits against wheat bran biscuits for blood sugar control. While using the glucomannan biscuits, people experienced a significant improvement in glucose control, compared with those using the wheat bran biscuits. Other studies have also found evidence that glucomannan can improve blood sugar control.

SAFETY ISSUES

In Japan, food products containing glucomannan have a long history of use and are believed to be safe. However, there are some concerns about taking glucomannan as a supplement. Some people taking glucomannan complain of excess gas, stomach distension, or mild diarrhea. These symptoms usually abate within a couple of days of treatment or with a reduction of the dosage.

In a few cases, glucomannan tablets have caused obstruction of the esophagus when they expanded before reaching the stomach. In response to these reports, tablets of this type have been banned. Capsules, however, do not seem to pose the same risk because their casing prevents the glucomannan from contacting water until it reaches the stomach. The dramatic expansion of glucomannan has also raised some concerns that it could cause an obstruction in the intestines; nonetheless, there have been no reports of this actually happening. One option to offset all expansion risk is to mix glucomannan powder in water so that it expands before it is ingested; however, this strategy reduces the convenience of this form of fiber.

EBSCO CAM Review Board

FURTHER READING

Azezli, A. D., et al. "The Use of Konjac Glucomannan to Lower Serum Thyroid Hormones in Hyperthyroidism." *Journal of the American College of Nutrition* 26 (2007): 663-668.

Chen, H. L., et al. "Supplementation of Konjac Glucomannan into a Low-Fiber Chinese Diet Promoted Bowel Movement and Improved Colonic Ecology in Constipated Adults." *Journal of the American College of Nutrition* 27 (2008): 102-108.

Sood, N., et al. "Effect of Glucomannan on Plasma Lipid and Glucose Concentrations, Body Weight, and Blood Pressure." *American Journal of Clinical Nutrition* 88 (2008): 1167-1175.

Vasques, C. A., et al. "Evaluation of the Pharmacotherapeutic Efficacy of *Garcinia cambogia* Plus *Amorphophallus konjac* for the Treatment of Obesity." *Phytotherapy Research* 22 (2008): 1135-1140.

Vuksan, V., et al. "Konjac-Mannan (Glucomannan) Improves Glycemia and Other Associated Risk Factors for Coronary Heart Disease in Type 2 Diabetes." *Diabetes Care* 22 (1999): 913-919.

See also: Cholesterol, high; Constipation; Diabetes; Herbal medicine; Hypertension; Hyperthyroidism; Obesity and excess weight.

Glucosamine

CATEGORY: Herbs and supplements

RELATED TERMS: Glucosamine hydrochloride, glucosamine sulfate, N-acetyl glucosamine

DEFINITION: Natural substance of the human body used as a supplement to treat specific health conditions.

PRINCIPAL PROPOSED USE: Osteoarthritis

OTHER PROPOSED USES: Muscle injury prevention, osteochondritis, rheumatoid arthritis, tendonitis

OVERVIEW

Glucosamine, most commonly used in the form glucosamine sulfate, is a simple molecule derived from glucose, the principal sugar found in blood. In glucosamine, one oxygen atom in glucose is replaced by a nitrogen atom. The chemical term for this modified form of glucose is amino sugar. Glucosamine is produced naturally in the body, where it is a key building block for making cartilage.

REQUIREMENTS AND SOURCES

There is no U.S. Dietary Reference Intake for glucosamine. One's body makes all the glucosamine it needs from building blocks found in foods. Glucosamine is not usually obtained directly from food. Glucosamine supplements are derived from chitin, a substance found in the shells of shrimp, lobsters, and crabs.

THERAPEUTIC DOSAGES

Osteoarthritis is a disease in which cartilage in joints becomes stiffer and may wear away. Glucosamine is used to treat this condition. A typical dosage of glucosamine is 500 milligrams (mg) three times daily. A 1,500-mg dose taken once daily is another option.

Glucosamine is available in three forms: glucosamine sulfate, glucosamine hydrochloride, and N-acetyl glucosamine. All three forms are sold as tablets or capsules. There is some dispute over which form is best. One study provides some evidence that glucosamine hydrochloride and glucosamine sulfate are equally effective. Glucosamine is often sold in combination with chondroitin. It is not known whether this combination treatment is better than glucosamine alone, although animal studies suggest that this may be the case.

THERAPEUTIC USES

Glucosamine is widely accepted as a treatment for osteoarthritis. However, the current evidence from double-blind studies is highly inconsistent, with many of the most recent and best-designed studies failing to find significant benefit. According to the positive studies, glucosamine acts more slowly than

---

Long-term Glucosamine Study

New data from a long-term study of the dietary supplements glucosamine and chondroitin for treating knee osteoarthritis pain reveal that persons who took the supplements (alone or in combination) had outcomes similar to those experienced by persons who took celecoxib (Celebrex) or placebo pills. Earlier studies examined the effects of glucosamine and chondroitin on pain associated with osteoarthritis of the knee over a short duration—twenty-four weeks. This study, part of the Glucosamine/Chondroitin Arthritis Intervention Trial (GAIT), funded by the National Center for Complementary and Alternative Medicine and the National Institute of Arthritis and Musculoskeletal and Skin Diseases, was the first to assess the safety and effectiveness of the supplements over two years.

The study enrolled 662 GAIT participants with moderate-to-severe knee osteoarthritis, who received either glucosamine (500 milligrams [mg] three times daily), chondroitin sulfate (400 mg three times daily), glucosamine and chondroitin sulfate combined (same doses), Celebrex (200 mg once daily), or placebo. The study's primary outcome measure was a 20 percent reduction in pain scores (using the WOMAC pain scale).

All treatment groups experienced improvement in pain and function over the two-year study period, with clinically detectable improvements seen as early as twenty-four weeks in all groups. However, none of the treatments was significantly better than placebo. The odds of obtaining a 20 percent decline on the WOMAC scale when taking Celebrex were 1.2 times greater than the odds of obtaining this decline when taking placebo. Likewise, the odds of obtaining a 20 percent decline for glucosamine alone, glucosamine and chondroitin sulfate combined, and chondroitin sulfate alone were 1.16, 0.83, and 0.69 times that for placebo, respectively. There were no statistically significant differences among the four treatment groups. Adverse reactions were mild and occurred among all treatment groups, and serious adverse events were rare.

The researchers noted that findings from their study provide important longer-term safety information on the use of glucosamine and chondroitin and on the use of Celebrex, adding to the existing scientific literature on treatments people use for pain associated with osteoarthritis of the knee. Researchers also pointed out that their study data were obtained with dosages typically used to treat osteoarthritis of the knee.

conventional treatments, such as ibuprofen, but eventually produces approximately equivalent benefits. In addition, unlike conventional treatments, glucosamine might also help prevent progressive joint damage, thereby slowing the course of the disease. However, both these potential benefits remain controversial in light of the most recent trials. Glucosamine has also shown some promise for osteochondritis of the knee, a cartilage disease related to osteoarthritis.

Some athletes use glucosamine, in the (unproven) belief that it can prevent muscle and tendon injuries. It has also been suggested as a treatment for tendonitis. However, there is no meaningful scientific evidence to support these potential uses. Exercise can also produce short-term muscle soreness. In one study, use of glucosamine not only failed to prove effective for reducing this type of pain but also increased it. However, one study found somewhat inconsistent evidence hinting that glucosamine might aid recovery from acute knee injuries experienced by competitive athletes.

Glucosamine might also be helpful for rheumatoid arthritis, according to a double-blind, placebo-controlled study of fifty-one people. In this study, use of glucosamine at a dose of 1,500 mg daily significantly improved symptoms. It did not, however, alter measures of inflammation as determined through blood tests.

SCIENTIFIC EVIDENCE

Relieving osteoarthritis symptoms. Inconsistent evidence suggests that glucosamine supplements might relieve pain and other symptoms of osteoarthritis. Two types of studies have been performed, those that compared glucosamine against placebo and those that compared it against standard medications.

In the placebo-controlled category, one of the best trials was a three-year, double-blind study of 212 people with osteoarthritis of the knee. Participants receiving glucosamine showed reduced symptoms, compared with those receiving placebo. Benefits were also seen in other double-blind, placebo-controlled studies, enrolling a total of more than a thousand people and ranging in length from four weeks to three years.

Other double-blind studies, enrolling a total of more than four hundred people, compared glucosamine against ibuprofen. These studies found glucosamine and the drug equally effective. Furthermore,

one of the placebo-controlled trials noted above (only reported in abstract form) also included people given the drug piroxicam and again found equivalent benefits.

However, most recent studies have been less promising. In four studies involving a total of about five hundred people, use of glucosamine failed to provide any meaningful improvement in symptoms. The list goes on. In a study involving 222 participants with hip osteoarthritis, two years of treatment with glucosamine was no better than a placebo for pain, function, or X-ray findings. Another trial involving 147 women with osteoarthritis found glucosamine to be no more effective than home exercises over an eighteen-month period.

In a double-blind trial, researchers evaluated the effects of stopping glucosamine after taking it for six months. Involving 137 people with osteoarthritis of the knee, the study found that participants who stopped using glucosamine (and, unbeknownst to them, took a placebo instead) did no worse than people who stayed on glucosamine.

In another, very large (1,583-participant) study, neither glucosamine (as glucosamine hydrochloride) nor glucosamine plus chondroitin was more effective than a placebo. Another trial failed to find benefit with glucosamine plus chondroitin. Finally, in a systematic review including ten randomized trials involving 3,803 patients with osteoarthritis of hip or knee, researchers found that glucosamine alone or with chondroitin did not improve pain. It appears that most of the positive studies were funded by manufacturers of glucosamine products, and most of the studies performed by neutral researchers failed to find benefit.

Many popular glucosamine products combine this supplement with methylsulfonylmethane (MSM). One study published in India reported that both MSM and glucosamine improved arthritis symptoms, compared with a placebo, but that the combination of MSM and glucosamine was even more effective than either supplement separately. However, India has not achieved a reputation for conducting reliable medical trials.

Slowing the course of osteoarthritis. Conventional treatments for osteoarthritis reduce the symptoms but do not slow the progress of the disease. In fact, nonsteroidal anti-inflammatory drugs, such as indomethacin, might actually speed the progression of osteoarthritis by interfering with cartilage repair and promoting cartilage destruction (though the evidence for this is weak). In contrast, two studies reported that glucosamine can slow the progression of osteoarthritis.

A three-year, double-blind, placebo-controlled study of 212 people found indications that glucosamine may protect joints from further damage. Over the course of the study, individuals given glucosamine showed some actual improvement in pain and mobility, while those given placebo worsened steadily. Perhaps even more important, X-rays showed that glucosamine treatment prevented progressive damage to the knee joint. Another large, three-year study enrolling 202 people found similar results. Furthermore, a follow-up analysis, done five years after the conclusion of these two studies, found suggestive evidence that use of glucosamine reduced the need for knee-replacement surgery.

Like the positive studies of glucosamine for reducing symptoms, all of these studies were funded by a major glucosamine manufacturer.

Relieving knee pain due to osteochondritis. A twelve-week, double-blind, placebo-controlled study examined the effectiveness of glucosamine at 2,000 mg daily in fifty people with continuing knee pain, mostly caused by osteochondritis (damage to the articular cartilage of the knee) rather than osteoarthritis. The results were somewhat equivocal but appeared to indicate that glucosamine could improve symptoms. Some participants may have also had osteoarthritis, so the results of this study are a bit difficult to interpret.

SAFETY ISSUES

Glucosamine appears to be a generally safe treatment and has not been associated with significant side effects. A few case reports and animal studies raised concerns that glucosamine might raise blood sugar in people with diabetes, but subsequent studies have tended to lay these concerns to rest. Glucosamine does not appear to affect cholesterol levels either. There is one case report of an allergic reaction to a glucosamine/chondroitin product, causing exacerbation of asthma.

EBSCO CAM Review Board

FURTHER READING

Arendt-Nielsen, L., et al. "A Double-Blind Randomized Placebo-Controlled Parallel Group Study Evaluating the Effects of Ibuprofen and Glucosamine Sulfate on Exercise-Induced Muscle Soreness." *Journal of Musculoskeletal Pain* 15 (2007): 21-28.

Herrero-Beaumont, G., et al. "Glucosamine Sulfate in the Treatment of Knee Osteoarthritis Symptoms: A Randomized, Double-Blind, Placebo-Controlled Study Using Acetaminophen as a Side Comparator." *Arthritis and Rheumatism* 56, no. 2 (2007): 555-567.

Kawasaki, T., et al. "Additive Effects of Glucosamine or Risedronate for the Treatment of Osteoarthritis of the Knee Combined with Home Exercise." *Journal of Bone and Mineral Metabolism* 26 (2008): 279-287.

Ostojic, S. M., et al. "Glucosamine Administration in Athletes: Effects on Recovery of Acute Knee Injury." *Research in Sports Medicine* 15 (2007): 113-124.

Rozendaal, R. M., et al. "Effect of Glucosamine Sulfate on Hip Osteoarthritis." *Annals of Internal Medicine* 148 (2008): 268-277.

Usha, P. R., and M. U. Naidu. "Randomised, Double-Blind, Parallel, Placebo-Controlled Study of Oral Glucosamine, Methylsulfonylmethane, and Their Combination in Osteoarthritis." *Clinical Drug Investigation* 24 (2004): 353-363.

See also: Osteoarthritis; Rheumatoid arthritis; Tendonitis.

Glutamine

CATEGORY: Herbs and supplements
RELATED TERMS: Glutamic acid, L-glutamine
DEFINITION: Natural substance of the human body used as a supplement to treat specific health conditions.
PRINCIPAL PROPOSED USES: None
OTHER PROPOSED USES: Angina, attention deficit disorder, Crohn's disease, enhancing mental function, food allergies, human immunodeficiency virus infection support, irritable bowel syndrome, overtraining syndrome, post-exercise colds, ulcerative colitis, ulcers, undesired weight loss

OVERVIEW

Glutamine, or L-glutamine, is an amino acid derived from another amino acid, glutamic acid. Glutamine plays a role in the health of the immune system, digestive tract, and muscle cells, as well as of other bodily functions. It appears to serve as a fuel for the cells that line the intestines. Heavy exercise, infection,

Glutamine and Athletic Training

Glutamine may be theorized to be ergogenic (performance-enhancing) in various ways. Glutamine is an important fuel for some cells of the immune system, such as lymphocytes and macrophages, which may be decreased with prolonged intense exercise, such as that related to overtraining. Glutamine may also promote muscle glycogen synthesis, and it has been studied for potential enhancement of muscular strength.

Several investigators theorize that athletes who overtrain may experience decreased plasma glutamine levels, which may impair functions of the immune system and predispose the athlete to various illnesses. Illness may impair training and eventual performance. Research findings are equivocal, with some studies reporting lower incidence rates of infection among athletes who consumed a glutamine-supplement drink following intense training. However, others reported that although glutamine supplementation helped maintain plasma glutamine levels following intense exercise, it had no effect on various tests of the immune response. Recent reviews indicate that there is little support from controlled studies to recommend glutamine ingestion for enhanced immune function.

Although glutamine may simulate muscle glycogen synthesis, reviewers recently concluded that there is no advantage over ingestion of adequate carbohydrates alone. Moreover, several recent studies indicate that neither short-term nor long-term glutamine supplementation has an ergogenic effect on muscle mass or strength performance. Glutamine supplementation one hour before testing had no effect on resistance exercise to fatigue, nor did six weeks of glutamine supplementation during resistance training increase lean muscle mass or strength more than the placebo treatment.

Source: Adapted from Melvin Williams. "Dietary Supplements and Sports Performance: Amino Acids." *Journal of the International Society of Sports Nutrition* 2 (2005): 63-67. The electronic version of this open-access article is available at http://www.jissn.com/content/2/2/63.

surgery, and trauma can deplete the body's glutamine reserves, particularly in muscle cells.

The fact that glutamine does so many good things in the body has led people to try glutamine supplements as a treatment for various conditions, including preventing the infections that often follow endurance exercise, reducing symptoms of overtraining syndrome, improving nutrition in critical illness, alleviating allergies, and treating digestive problems.

REQUIREMENTS AND SOURCES

There is no daily requirement for glutamine because the body can make its own supply. As mentioned earlier, various severe stresses may result in a temporary glutamine deficiency. High-protein foods such as meat, fish, beans, and dairy products are excellent sources of glutamine. Typical daily intake from food ranges from approximately 1 to 6 grams (g).

THERAPEUTIC DOSAGES

Typical therapeutic dosages of glutamine used in studies ranged from 3 to 30 g daily, divided into several separate doses.

THERAPEUTIC USES

Endurance athletes frequently catch cold after completing a marathon or similar forms of exercise. Preliminary evidence, including one small double-blind, placebo-controlled trial, suggests that glutamine supplements might help prevent such infections.

Another small double-blind, placebo-controlled trial suggests that glutamine might support standard therapy for angina. Angina is too dangerous a disease for self-treatment. A person who has angina should not take glutamine (or any other supplement) except on the advice of a physician.

Because, as noted above, cells of the intestine use glutamine for fuel, the supplement has been tried as a supportive treatment for various digestive conditions, with mixed results. Tested uses include reducing diarrhea caused by the drug nelfinavir (used for treatment of human immunodeficiency virus, or HIV), digestive distress caused by cancer chemotherapy, and symptoms of inflammatory bowel disease.

Glutamine appears to help reduce leakage through the intestinal wall. On this basis, glutamine has also been suggested as a treatment for food allergies, according to the idea that in some people, whole proteins leak through the wall of the digestive tract and enter the blood, causing allergic reactions (so-called leaky gut syndrome). However, there is no reliable evidence that glutamine actually provides any benefits for food allergies.

Preliminary evidence suggests that glutamine combined with antioxidants or other nutrients may help people with HIV to gain weight. Glutamine (often combined with other nutrients) also appears to be useful as a nutritional supplement for people undergoing recovery from major surgery or critical illness.

Glutamine has been tried as an ergogenic aid for bodybuilders, but two small trials failed to find any evidence of benefit. Based on glutamine's role in muscle, it has been suggested that glutamine might be useful for athletes experiencing overtraining syndrome. As the name suggests, this syndrome is the cumulative effect of a training regimen that allows too little rest and recovery between workouts. Symptoms include depression, fatigue, reduced performance, and physiological signs of stress. Glutamine supplements have additionally been proposed as treatment for attention deficit disorder and ulcers, and as a " brain booster." However, there is little to no scientific evidence for any of these uses.

SCIENTIFIC EVIDENCE

Infections in athletes. Endurance exercise temporarily reduces immunity to infection. This effect may be due in part to reduction of glutamine in the body, although not all studies agree.

A double-blind, placebo-controlled study evaluated the benefits of supplemental glutamine (5 g) taken at the end of exercise in 151 endurance athletes. The results showed a significant decrease in infections among treated athletes. Only 19 percent of the athletes taking glutamine got sick, compared with 51 percent of those on a placebo.

Recovery from critical illness. One small double-blind study found that glutamine supplements might have significant nutritional benefits for seriously ill people. In this study, eighty-four critically ill hospital patients were divided into two groups. All the patients were being fed through a feeding tube. One group received a normal feeding-tube diet, whereas the other group received this diet plus supplemental glutamine. After six months, fourteen of the forty-two patients re-

ceiving glutamine had died, compared with twenty-four of the control group. The glutamine group also left both the intensive care ward and the hospital significantly sooner than the patients who did not receive glutamine. Benefits have been seen in other controlled trials as well.

HIV support. One double-blind, placebo-controlled study of twenty-five people found that use of glutamine at 30 g daily for seven days reduced diarrhea caused by the protease inhibitor nelfinavir. In addition, combination supplements containing glutamine may help reverse HIV-related weight loss. For example, a double-blind, placebo-controlled study found that a combination of glutamine and antioxidants (vitamins C and E, beta-carotene, selenium, and N-acetyl cysteine) led to significant weight gain in people with HIV who had lost weight. Another small double-blind trial found that combination treatment with glutamine, arginine, and beta-hydroxy beta-methylbutyrate (HMB) could increase muscle mass and possibly improve immune status.

Cancer chemotherapy. There is mixed evidence regarding whether glutamine can reduce the side effects of cancer chemotherapy. A double-blind, placebo-controlled trial of seventy people undergoing chemotherapy with the drug 5-FU for colorectal cancer found that glutamine at a dose of 18 g daily improved intestinal function and structure and reduced the need for antidiarrheal drugs. However, a double-blind trial of sixty-five women undergoing various forms of chemotherapy for advanced breast cancer failed to find glutamine at 30 g per day helpful for reducing diarrhea. Based on a review of several studies, there is some preliminary evidence that glutamine may help relieve the pain associated with nerve damage (peripheral neuropathy) caused by some chemotherapy drugs.

Angina. Researchers conducted investigations in rats and found that glutamine could protect the heart from damage caused by loss of oxygen. Based on these findings, they went on to evaluate the effects of glutamine in ten people with chronic angina who were also taking standard medication. In this double-blind, placebo-controlled trial, each participant received a single oral dose of glutamine (80 mg per kg of body weight) or placebo forty minutes before a treadmill test. A week later, each participant received the opposite treatment. The results showed that use of glutamine significantly enhanced the ability of participants to exercise without showing signs of heart stress. Based on the results in rats, researchers suggest that a higher dose of glutamine would be worth trying.

Crohn's disease. Because glutamine is the major fuel source for cells of the small intestine, glutamine has been proposed as a treatment for Crohn's disease, a disease of the small intestine. However, two double-blind trials enrolling a total of thirty people found no benefit.

Sports performance. A double-blind, placebo-controlled trial of thirty-one people ranging from eighteen to twenty-four years of age evaluated the potential benefits of glutamine as a sports supplement for improving response to resistance training (weight lifting). Participants received either a placebo or glutamine at a dose of 0.9 g per kg of lean tissue mass. After six weeks of resistance training, participants taking glutamine showed no relative improvement in performance, composition, or muscle protein degradation. Similarly, negative results were seen in a small double-blind, placebo-controlled trial of weightlifters using a dose of 0.3 g per kg of total body weight.

SAFETY ISSUES

As a naturally occurring amino acid, glutamine is thought to be a safe supplement when taken at recommended dosages. There is strong evidence that glutamine is safe at levels up to 14 g per day, although higher dosages have been tested without apparent adverse effects.

Nevertheless, those who are hypersensitive to monosodium glutamate (MSG) should use glutamine with caution, as the body metabolizes glutamine into glutamate. In addition, because many antiepilepsy drugs work by blocking glutamate stimulation in the brain, high dosages of glutamine might conceivably overwhelm these drugs and pose a risk to people with epilepsy. In one case report, high doses of the supplement L-glutamine (more than 2 g per day) may have triggered episodes of mania in two people not previously known to have bipolar disorder. In a small randomized trial including thirty older people, L-glutamine did not cause any clinically significant changes in lab tests. The researchers did urge caution, though, since there were some statistically significant changes for certain kidney levels. Maximum safe dosages for young children, pregnant or nursing women, and those with severe liver or kidney disease have not been determined.

IMPORTANT INTERACTIONS

Persons taking antiseizure medications, including carbamazepine, phenobarbital, phenytoin (Dilantin), primidone (Mysoline), and valproic acid (Depakene), should use glutamine only under medical supervision. Persons taking nelfinavir or other protease inhibitors for HIV, or cancer chemotherapy drugs should note that concurrent glutamine may reduce intestinal side effects.

EBSCO CAM Review Board

FURTHER READING

Amara, S. "Oral Glutamine for the Prevention of Chemotherapy-Induced Peripheral Neuropathy." *Annals of Pharmacotherapy* 42, no. 10 (2008): 1481-1485.

Antonio, J., et al. "The Effects of High-Dose Glutamine Ingestion on Weightlifting Performance." *Journal of Strength and Conditioning Research* 16 (2002): 157-160.

Candow, D. G., et al. "Effect of Glutamine Supplementation Combined with Resistance Training in Young Adults." *European Journal of Applied Physiology* 86 (2001): 142-149.

Clark, R. H., et al. "Nutritional Treatment for Acquired Immunodeficiency Virus-Associated Wasting Using Beta-Hydroxy Beta-Methylbutyrate, Glutamine, and Arginine." *JPEN: Journal of Parenteral and Enteral Nutrition* 24 (2000): 133-139.

Daniele, B., et al. "Oral Glutamine in the Prevention of Fluorouracil-Induced Intestinal Toxicity." *Gut* 48 (2001): 28-33.

Galera, S. C., et al. "The Safety of Oral Use of L-Glutamine in Middle-Aged and Elderly Individuals." *Nutrition* 26, no. 4 (2010): 375-381.

Khogali, S. E., et al. "Is Glutamine Beneficial in Ischemic Heart Disease?" *Nutrition* 18 (2002): 123-126.

Quan, Z. F., et al. "Effect of Glutamine on Change in Early Postoperative Intestinal Permeability and Its Relation to Systemic Inflammatory Response." *World Journal of Gastroenterology* 10 (2004): 1992-1994.

Shao, A., and J. N. Hathcock. "Risk Assessment for the Amino Acids Taurine, L-Glutamine, and L-Arginine." *Regulatory Toxicology and Pharmacology* 50, no. 3 (2008): 376-399.

See also: Angina; Attention deficit disorder; Allergies; Colds and flu; HIV support; Irritable bowel syndrome (IBS); Ulcers; Weight loss, undesired.

Glutathione

CATEGORY: Herbs and supplements
DEFINITION: Natural substance of the human body used as a supplement to treat specific health conditions.
PRINCIPAL PROPOSED USES: None
OTHER PROPOSED USE: Antioxidant

OVERVIEW

Dangerous naturally occurring substances in the body called free radicals pose a risk to many tissues. The body deploys an antioxidant defense system to hold free radicals in check. Glutathione, a protein made from the amino acids cysteine, glutamic acid, and glycine, is one of the most important elements of this system.

Glutathione does much of its work in the liver, although it is also found elsewhere in the body. Besides fighting free radicals, it helps keep various essential biological molecules in a chemical state called reduced (as opposed to oxidized). In addition, glutathione can act on toxins such as pesticides, lead, and dry cleaning solvents, transforming them in such a way that the body can excrete them more easily.

Nutrients such as vitamin C and vitamin E also help neutralize free radicals. In the 1990s, such antioxidant supplements were widely promoted for preventing a variety of diseases, including cancer and heart disease. During this period, oral glutathione became popular as an additional antioxidant supplement. Glutathione is not absorbed when taken by mouth, so such supplements are almost certainly useless. It may be possible, however, to raise glutathione levels in the body by taking other supplements, such as vitamin C, cysteine, lipoic acid, and N-acetylcysteine. Whether doing so would offer any health benefits remains unclear.

REQUIREMENTS AND SOURCES

There is no dietary requirement for glutathione. The body makes it from scratch, utilizing vitamins and common amino acids found in food. Glutathione levels in the body are reduced by cigarette smoking. Various diseases are associated with reduced levels of glutathione, including cancer, cataracts, diabetes, and human immunodeficiency virus (HIV) infection.

THERAPEUTIC DOSAGES

A typical recommended dose of oral glutathione is 50 milligrams twice daily. However, as noted above,

---

Glutathione as an Antioxidant

Antioxidants are substances that may prevent potentially disease-producing cell damage that can result from natural bodily processes and from exposure to certain chemicals. There are a number of different antioxidants found in foods and available as dietary supplements, including glutathione.

Oxidation, one of the body's natural chemical processes, can produce free radicals, which are highly unstable molecules that can damage cells. For example, free radicals are produced when the body breaks down foods for use or storage. They are also produced when the body is exposed to tobacco smoke, radiation, and environmental contaminants. Free radicals can cause damage, known as oxidative stress, which is thought to play a role in the development of many diseases, including Alzheimer's disease, cancer, eye disease, heart disease, Parkinson's disease, and rheumatoid arthritis. In laboratory experiments, antioxidant molecules counter oxidative stress and its associated damage.

---

when glutathione is taken by mouth it is destroyed. Therefore, no matter what the dose, it will not make any difference. It is possible that some glutathione may be absorbed if it is held in the mouth and allowed to dissolve, but this has not been well studied.

A more promising method for raising glutathione levels in the body involves taking supplemental cysteine or antioxidant supplements. Evidence suggests that cysteine (often supplied in the form of whey protein, which is high in cysteine) can raise glutathione levels in people with cancer, hepatitis, or HIV.

In addition, because vitamin C has overlapping functions with glutathione, vitamin C supplements may spare some of the body's glutathione from being used up, thereby increasing its levels in the body. The antioxidant supplement lipoic acid appears to raise glutathione levels as well. Other supplements that might raise glutathione levels include N-acetylcysteine, glutamine, methionine, and S-adenosyl methionine (SAMe).

THERAPEUTIC USES

Various Web sites promote glutathione for a wide variety of health problems, from preventing aging to enhancing sports performance. However, oral glutathione supplements are almost certainly use-less for any condition, since they are not absorbed.

There is a bit of evidence that injected glutathione might offer a few health benefits, such as preventing blood clots during surgery, reducing the side effects and increasing the effectiveness of cancer chemo-therapy drugs such as cisplatin, treating male infer-tility, and alleviating symptoms of early Parkinson's disease. Although oral glutathione is not likely to provide the same benefits, it is at least theoretically possible that taking the nutrients described in the previous section (and thereby raising glutathione levels indirectly) could offer similar benefits. How-ever, there is no direct evidence to indicate that this hypothesis is true.

SAFETY ISSUES

Oral glutathione should be entirely safe, since it is not absorbed.

FURTHER READING

Bharath, S., et al. "Glutathione, Iron, and Parkinson's Disease." *Biochemical Pharmacology* 64 (2002): 1037-1048.

Bounous, G. "Whey Protein Concentrate (WPC) and Glutathione Modulation in Cancer Treatment." *Anticancer Research* 20 (2000): 4785-4792.

De Rosa, S. C., et al. "N-Acetylcysteine Replenishes Glutathione in HIV Infection." *European Journal of Clinical Investigation* 30 (2000): 915-929.

Droge, W., and R. Breitkreutz. "Glutathione and Im-mune Function." *Proceedings of the Nutrition Society* 59 (2000): 595-600.

Hultberg, B., et al. "Lipoic Acid Increases Gluta-thione Production and Enhances the Effect of Mercury in Human Cell Lines." *Toxicology* 175 (2002): 103-110.

Lenzi, A., et al. "Lipoperoxidation Damage of Sper-matozoa Polyunsaturated Fatty Acids (PUFA): Scavenger Mechanisms and Possible Scavenger Therapies." *Frontiers in Bioscience* 5 (January, 2000): E1-E15.

Packer, L., et al. "Molecular Aspects of Lipoic Acid in the Prevention of Diabetes Complications." *Nutri-tion* 17 (2001): 888-895.

See also: Antioxidants; Smoking addiction.

Glycine

CATEGORY: Herbs and supplements
DEFINITION: Natural substance of the human body used as a supplement to treat specific health con-ditions.
PRINCIPAL PROPOSED USE: Schizophrenia
OTHER PROPOSED USES: Cancer prevention, diabe-tes, enhancing memory and mental function, epi-lepsy, immune support, kidney protection, liver protection, prostate enlargement, sports perfor-mance, strokes

OVERVIEW

Glycine is the simplest of the twenty different amino acids used as building blocks to make proteins for the body. It works in concert with glutamine, a sub-stance that plays a major role in brain function. Gly-cine has shown some promise as an aid in the treat-ment of schizophrenia and may have other uses related to the brain as well, such as enhancing mental function.

REQUIREMENTS AND SOURCES

The body makes glycine using another amino acid, serine. Because one can manufacture glycine, one does not have to consume any, so it is called a nones-sential amino acid. Most people get about 2 grams (g) of glycine a day from the foods eaten regularly. This dietary glycine comes mostly from high-protein foods, such as meat, fish, dairy products, and legumes. For treating certain disease conditions, however, much larger amounts than are normally consumed have been advocated; such high doses can be obtained only by taking supplements.

THERAPEUTIC DOSAGES

Dosages of oral glycine used in clinical trials for therapeutic purposes range from 2 to 60 g daily.

THERAPEUTIC USES

Several studies have evaluated glycine as a sup-portive treatment for schizophrenia. According to some of these studies, high doses of glycine (15 to 60 g daily) might augment the effectiveness of medi-cations used for this condition. The notable excep-tion is clozapine (Clozaril); one study suggests that gly-cine may decrease the effectiveness of this drug.

One large double-blind study suggests that low doses of glycine may be helpful for limiting the spreading brain damage that occurs during stroke. However, there are also theoretical concerns that glycine could increase such damage, so one should not try this treatment except under physician supervision.

A small double-blind study found evidence that glycine may help improve long-term blood sugar control in people with type 2 diabetes. One small study weakly suggests that glycine may enhance memory and mental function. Glycine alone and in combination with other amino acids has shown a bit of promise for enhancing wound healing.

Animal studies suggest that dietary glycine may protect against chemically induced damage to the liver or kidneys. Other studies in laboratory animals suggest that dietary glycine may prevent tumor formation and growth in the livers of mice and rats. However, it is too early to say whether glycine has cancer-preventive effects in humans.

Manufacturers advertising glycine supplements have made a number of additional claims for it, including prevention of epileptic seizures, reducing acid in the stomach, multiple sclerosis, boosting the immune system, and calming the mind. It is also proposed as a sports supplement, said to work in this capacity by increasing release of human growth hormone (HGH). There is no real scientific evidence that glycine works for any of these purposes. Because it has a sweet taste, glycine has also been recommended as a sugar substitute for people with diabetes.

SCIENTIFIC EVIDENCE

Schizophrenia. Glycine might enhance the effectiveness of drugs used for schizophrenia, especially those in the older phenothiazine category. It has also shown equivocal promise for enhancing the effectiveness of the drugs risperidone and olanzapine. However, it may not be helpful for people using clozapine.

Phenothiazine drugs are most effective for the "positive" symptoms of schizophrenia, such as hallucinations and delusions. (Such symptoms are called positive because they indicate the presence of abnormal mental functions rather than the absence of normal mental functions.) In general, however, these medications are less helpful for the "negative" symptoms of schizophrenia, such as apathy, depression, and social withdrawal. Glycine might be of benefit here.

A double-blind, placebo-controlled trial enrolled twenty-two participants who continued to experience negative symptoms of schizophrenia despite standard therapy. The results showed that the use of glycine significantly improved negative symptoms. In addition, glycine also appeared to reduce some of the side effects caused by the prescription drugs. No changes were seen in positive symptoms (for instance, hallucinations), but it is not possible to tell whether that is because these symptoms were already being controlled by prescription medications or if glycine simply has no effect on those particular symptoms of schizophrenia.

Three earlier double-blind, placebo-controlled clinical trials of glycine together with standard drugs for schizophrenia also found it to be helpful for negative symptoms. All of these studies used very small groups (from twelve to eighteen people), so much larger trials are still needed to verify glycine's effectiveness. The trials just discussed were conducted before atypical antipsychotics were widely available. These drugs cause fewer side effects and also provide benefits for the negative symptoms of schizophrenia along with the positive. One study found that glycine augmented the effectiveness of two of these drugs: olanzapine and risperidone. However, another study suggests that adding glycine to the atypical antipsychotic clozapine may not be a good idea. In this study, glycine was found to reduce the benefits of clozapine. Two other double-blind, placebo-controlled trials of glycine and clozapine simply failed to find benefit. Another recent study, not specifically limited to clozapine, also failed to find benefit with glycine.

Stroke. Glycine's potential usefulness for treating individuals who have undergone strokes was investigated in a double-blind, placebo-controlled study with two hundred participants. The results suggest that glycine can protect against the spreading damage to the brain that usually follows a stroke. Participants were given either 1 to 2 g of glycine sublingually (dissolved under the tongue) or a placebo treatment for a period of five days. The results suggest that glycine can prevent neural damage. This appears to be an impressive result, but further research is necessary.

Although other researchers using glycine for brain disorders have reported that such small doses of glycine would not be sufficient to cross the blood-brain barrier, measurements of amino acids in the cerebrospinal fluid during the above study suggest that it did enter the brain. However, there are potential concerns that high-dose glycine could increase stroke damage.

SAFETY ISSUES

No serious adverse effects from using glycine have been reported, even at doses as high as 60 g per day. One participant in the twenty-two-person trial described above developed stomach upset and vomiting, but it ceased when the glycine was discontinued.

In contradiction to the study on strokes mentioned above, theoretical concerns have been raised that suggest glycine might increase brain injury in strokes. In fact, drugs that block glycine have been investigated as treatments to limit stroke damage. However, the authors of the study on strokes described above make an argument that suggests the overall effect of glycine is protective. Until this controversy is settled, prudence suggests not using glycine following a stroke, except on the advice of a physician.

In addition, as noted above, it is possible that use of glycine could reduce the benefits of clozapine. Maximum safe doses for young children, pregnant or nursing women, or people with liver or kidney disease are not known. Persons taking clozapine should not take glycine except under the supervision of a physician.

FURTHER READING

Buchanan, R. W., et al. "The Cognitive and Negative Symptoms in Schizophrenia Trial (CONSIST): The Efficacy of Glutamatergic Agents for Negative Symptoms and Cognitive Impairments." *American Journal of Psychiatry* 64 (2007): 1593-1602.

Diaz, P., et al. "Double-Blind, Placebo-Controlled, Crossover Trial of Clozapine Plus Glycine in Refractory Schizophrenia Negative Results." *Journal of Clinical Psychopharmacology* 25 (2005): 277-278.

Heresco-Levy, U., et al. "High-Dose Glycine Added to Olanzapine and Risperidone for the Treatment of Schizophrenia." *Biological Psychiatry* 55 (2004): 165-171.

Javitt, D. C., et al. "Reversal of Phencyclidine-Induced Effects by Glycine and Glycine Transport Inhibitors." *Biological Psychiatry* 45 (1999): 668-679.

See also: Cancer risk reduction; Diabetes; Immune support; Liver disease; Sports and fitness support: Enhancing performance; Schizophrenia; Strokes.

Goldenrod

CATEGORY: Herbs and supplements
RELATED TERM: *Solidago* species
DEFINITION: Natural plant product used to treat specific health conditions.
PRINCIPAL PROPOSED USES: Bladder and kidney stones, bladder infections

OVERVIEW

Goldenrod often is falsely considered an intensely allergenic plant, because of its tendency to bloom brightly at the same time and often in locations quite near to the truly allergenic ragweed. However, actual allergic reactions to this gorgeous herb are unusual.

There are numerous species of goldenrod (twenty-seven have been collected in Indiana alone), but all seem to possess similar medicinal properties, and various species are used interchangeably in Europe.

THERAPEUTIC DOSAGES

A typical dosage is 3 to 4 grams (g) of dried herb two to three times daily. Make sure to drink plenty of water while taking goldenrod, to help it do its job.

THERAPEUTIC USES

In Germany, goldenrod is used as a supportive treatment for bladder infections, irritation of the urinary tract, and bladder/kidney stones. Goldenrod is said to wash out bacteria and kidney stones by increasing the flow of urine and also to soothe inflamed tissues and calm muscle spasms in the urinary tract. It is not used as a cure but rather as an adjunct to other, more definitive treatments, such as (in the case of bladder infections) antibiotics.

However, it is not known if goldenrod helps. Several studies have found that goldenrod does increase urine flow, but there is no direct evidence that this leads to any other medical benefits. Urinary conditions such as kidney stones are potentially serious. For this reason, medical advice is recommended.

SAFETY ISSUES

The safety of goldenrod has not been fully evaluated. However, no significant reactions or side effects have been reported. Safety in young children, pregnant and nursing women, or those with severe liver or kidney disease has not been established. Individuals

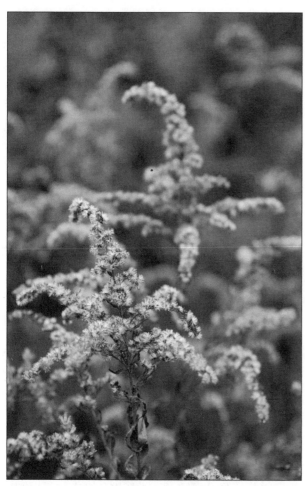

Goldenrod is said to wash out bacteria and kidney stones by increasing the flow of urine and also to soothe inflamed tissues and calm muscle spasms in the urinary tract. (Joshua Sheldon/Getty Images)

taking the medication lithium should use herbal diuretics such as goldenrod only under the supervision of a physician, as dehydration can be dangerous with this medication.

FURTHER READING

Pyevich, D., and M. P. Bogenschutz. "Herbal Diuretics and Lithium Toxicity." *American Journal of Psychiatry* 158 (2001): 1329.

See also: Bladder infection; Bladder infection: Homeopathic remedies; Kidney stones.

Goldenseal

CATEGORY: Herbs and supplements
RELATED TERM: *Hydrastis canadensis*
DEFINITION: Natural plant product used to treat specific health conditions.
PRINCIPAL PROPOSED USES: None
OTHER PROPOSED USES: Athlete's foot, congestive heart failure, dyspepsia, heart arrhythmia, high blood pressure, high cholesterol, infectious diarrhea, irritable bowel syndrome, minor wounds, vaginal yeast infection, urinary tract infections

OVERVIEW

Although goldenseal root is one of the most popular herbs sold, it is taken almost entirely for the wrong reasons. Originally, it was used by Native Americans both as a dye and as a treatment for skin disorders, digestive problems, liver disease, diarrhea, and eye irritations. European settlers learned of the herb from the Iroquois and other tribes and quickly adopted goldenseal as a part of early colonial medical care.

In the early nineteenth century, herbalist Samuel Thompson created a wildly popular system of medicine that swept the country. Thompson spoke of goldenseal as a nearly magical cure for many conditions. His evangelism led to a dramatic upsurge in demand, followed by overcollection and decimation of the wild plant. Prices skyrocketed but then collapsed when Thompsonianism faded away.

Goldenseal has passed through several more booms and busts. Again in great demand, it is under intentional cultivation.

THERAPEUTIC DOSAGES

When goldenseal is used as a topical treatment for minor skin wounds, a sufficient quantity of goldenseal cream, ointment, or powder should be applied to cover the wound. It is important to be sure to clean the wound at least once a day to prevent goldenseal particles from becoming trapped in the healing tissues.

For mouth sores and sore throats, goldenseal tincture is swished or gargled. Goldenseal may also be used as strong tea for this purpose, made by boiling 0.5 to 1 gram in a cup of water. The herb has a bitter taste. Goldenseal tea is also used as a douche for vaginal yeast infections.

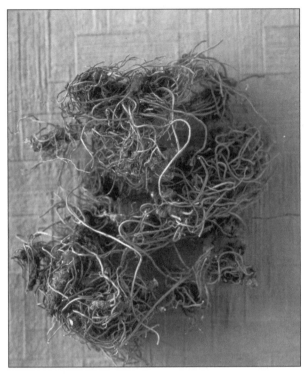

Goldenseal contains a substance called berberine that has been found to inhibit or kill many microorganisms, including fungi, protozoa, and bacteria. (Time & Life Pictures/ Getty Images)

THERAPEUTIC USES

Goldenseal contains a substance called berberine that has been found to inhibit or kill many microorganisms, including fungi, protozoa, and bacteria. On this basis, contemporary herbalists often use goldenseal as a topical antibiotic for skin wounds, as well as to treat viral mouth sores and superficial fungal infections, such as athlete's foot. However, there is no direct scientific evidence that goldenseal is effective for any of these purposes.

Goldenseal is not likely to work as an oral antibiotic, because the blood levels of berberine that can be achieved by taking goldenseal orally are far too low to matter. However, goldenseal could theoretically be beneficial in treating sore throats and diseases of the digestive tract (such as infectious diarrhea) because it can contact the affected area directly. Since berberine is concentrated in the bladder, goldenseal could be useful for bladder infections. Nonetheless, there is no direct evidence that goldenseal is effective for these uses.

Extremely weak evidence (far too weak to rely upon) suggests that goldenseal or berberine may be helpful for various heart-related conditions, including arrhythmias, congestive heart failure, high cholesterol, diabetes, and high blood pressure. Similarly, infinitesimal evidence hints that goldenseal could be helpful for conditions in which spasms of smooth muscle play a role, such as dyspepsia (nonspecific stomach distress) and irritable bowel syndrome, as well as various forms of pain caused by inflammation.

Ironically, goldenseal's most common uses are entirely inappropriate. Goldenseal is frequently combined with the herb echinacea to be taken as a "traditional immune booster" and "antibiotic" for the prevention and treatment of colds. However, as the noted herbalist Paul Bergner has pointed out, there are three things wrong with this packaging. First, there is no credible evidence that goldenseal increases immunity. Only one study weakly hints at an immune-strengthening effect. Second, colds are caused by viruses and do not respond to antibiotics, even if goldenseal were an effective systemic (whole-body) antibiotic, which it almost certainly is not. Third, goldenseal was never used traditionally for the common cold.

The other myth that has helped drive the sales of goldenseal is the widespread belief that it can block a positive drug screen. The origin of this false idea dates back to a work of fiction published in 1900 by a pharmacist and author named John Uri Lloyd. In *Stringtown on the Pike*, a dead man is found to have traces of goldenseal in his stomach. In fact, he had taken goldenseal regularly as a digestive aid, but a toxicology expert mistakes the goldenseal for strychnine and deduces intentional murder.

This work of fiction sufficed to create a folkloric connection between goldenseal and drug testing. Although the goldenseal in the story actually made a drug test come out falsely positive, this has been turned around to become a belief that goldenseal can make urine drug screens come out negative. A word to the wise: It does not work.

SAFETY ISSUES

Although there are no reports of severe adverse effects attributed to use of goldenseal, this herb has not undergone much safety testing. One study suggests that topical use of goldenseal could cause photosensitivity (an increased tendency to react to sun exposure).

Goldenseal should not be used by pregnant women because the herb has been reported to cause uterine contractions. In addition, berberine may increase levels of bilirubin and cause genetic damage. The last of these effects indicates that individuals with elevated bilirubin levels (jaundice) also should avoid use of goldenseal. Safety in young children, nursing women, or those with severe liver or kidney disease is also not established.

Just as there are incorrect rumors regarding the benefits of goldenseal, there are popular but incorrect beliefs regarding its health risks. For example, it is often said that goldenseal can disrupt the normal bacteria of the intestines. However, there is no scientific evidence that this occurs. Another fallacy is that small overdoses of goldenseal are toxic, causing ulcerations of the stomach and other mucous membranes. This idea is based on a misunderstanding of old literature.

Some evidence suggests that goldenseal might interact with various medications by altering the way they are metabolized in the liver. One study found that berberine impairs metabolism of the drug cyclosporine, thereby raising its levels. This could potentially cause toxicity. It is important, therefore, to speak with a physician before taking goldenseal with other medications.

FURTHER READING

Hubbard, M. A., et al. "Clinical Assessment of Cyp2d6-Mediated Herb-Drug Interactions in Humans: Effects of Milk Thistle, Black Cohosh, Goldenseal, Kava Kava, St. John's Wort, and Echinacea." *Molecular Nutrition and Food Research* 52, no. 7 (2008): 755-763.

Inbaraj, J. J., et al. "Photochemistry and Photocytotoxicity of Alkaloids from Goldenseal (*Hydrastis canadensis* L.)." *Chemical Research in Toxicology* 14 (2001): 1529-1534.

Scazzocchio, F., et al. "Antibacterial Activity of *Hydrastis canadensis* Extract and Its Major Isolated Alkaloids." *Planta Medica* 67 (2001): 561-564.

Wu, X., et al. "Effects of Berberine on the Blood Concentration of Cyclosporin A in Renal-Transplanted Recipients: Clinical and Pharmacokinetic Study." *European Journal of Clinical Pharmacology* 61, no. 8 (2005): 567-572.

Zhang, Y., et al. "Treatment of Type 2 Diabetes and Dyslipidemia with the Natural Plant Alkaloid Berberine." *Journal of Clinical Endocrinology and Metabolism* 93, no. 7 (2008): 2559-2565.

See also: Arrhythmia; Athlete's foot; Cholesterol, high; Congestive heart failure; Diarrhea; Dyspepsia; Hypertension; Irritable bowel syndrome (IBS); Immune support; Vaginal infection.

Gotu kola

CATEGORY: Herbs and supplements
RELATED TERM: *Centella asiatica*
DEFINITION: Natural plant product used to treat specific health conditions.
PRINCIPAL PROPOSED USE: Venous insufficiency/varicose veins
OTHER PROPOSED USES: Anal fissures, anxiety, burn healing, cellulite, hemorrhoids, improving mental performance, keloid scars, liver cirrhosis, periodontal disease, scleroderma, wound healing

OVERVIEW

Gotu kola is a creeping plant native to subtropical and tropical climates. Gotu kola has a long history of use in Ayurvedic medicine (the traditional medicine of India) to promote wound healing and slow the progress of leprosy. It was also reputed to prolong life, increase energy, and enhance sexual potency. Other uses of gotu kola included treating skin diseases, anxiety, diarrhea, menstrual disorders, vaginal discharge, and sexually transmitted diseases.

Based on these many traditional indications, gotu kola was accepted as a drug in France in the 1880s. British physicians in Africa used a special extract to treat leprosy.

THERAPEUTIC DOSAGES

The usual dosage of gotu kola is 20 to 60 milligrams (mg) three times daily of an extract standardized to contain 40 percent asiaticoside, 29 to 30 percent asiatic acid, 29 to 30 percent madecassic acid, and 1 to 2 percent madecassoside. When using it for venous insufficiency, give gotu kola at least four weeks to work. For the prevention of keloid scars (a purpose for which gotu kola has not been proven effective), the herb is typically taken for three months prior to surgery and for another three months afterward.

THERAPEUTIC USES

The best-documented use of gotu kola is to treat chronic venous insufficiency, a condition closely related to varicose veins. In these conditions, blood pools in the legs, causing aching, pain, heaviness, swelling, fatigue, and unsightly visible veins. Preliminary double-blind, placebo-controlled studies indicate that gotu kola extract provides improvement in major venous insufficiency symptoms, reducing swelling, pain, fatigue, sensation of heaviness, and fluid leakage from the veins. However, no studies have evaluated whether regular use of gotu kola can make visible varicose veins disappear or prevent new ones from developing. Gotu kola has also been suggested as a treatment for hemorrhoids because they are a type of varicose vein, but there is no direct evidence that it is helpful for this purpose.

Like other herbs used for the treatment of varicose veins, gotu kola is thought to work by strengthening connective tissues. This has led to trials of gotu kola extracts for preventing or treating keloid scars and treating anal fissures, bladder ulcers, burns, cellulite, dermatitis, liver cirrhosis, periodontal disease, scleroderma, and wounds. However, again, there is no real evidence that gotu kola is effective for any of these conditions.

One study provides weak evidence that gotu kola might be helpful for anxiety. Gotu kola has a reputation for improving memory, and the positive results from a study in rats performed in 1992 produced a temporary rush of public interest in gotu kola as a brain booster. However, benefits in humans have not been demonstrated. Gotu kola should not be confused with the caffeine-containing kola nut used in original recipes for Coca-Cola.

SCIENTIFIC EVIDENCE

Venous insufficiency/varicose veins. There is significant, but not definitive, scientific evidence for the effectiveness of gotu kola for the treatment of varicose veins/venous insufficiency. For example, a two-month double-blind, placebo-controlled study of ninety-four people with venous insufficiency of the lower limb compared the benefits of gotu kola extract at 120 mg daily and 60 mg daily against a placebo. The results showed a significant dose-related improvement in the treated groups in symptoms such as subjective heaviness, discomfort, and edema.

Another two-month study of double-blind design enrolled ninety people with varicose veins and compared the benefits of gotu kola at 60 mg and 30 mg daily against a placebo. Again, the results showed improvements in both treated groups, but greater improvement at the higher dose. In one study of people with venous insufficiency, two weeks of treatment with gotu kola extracts was shown to reduce the time necessary for the swelling to disappear.

Another study of double-blind design followed eighty-seven people with varicose veins and compared the benefits of gotu kola at 60 mg and 30 mg daily against a placebo. Again, the results showed improvements in both treated groups, but greater improvement at the higher dose.

Anxiety. Gotu kola has been used in traditional Ayurvedic medicine to treat anxiety. Because evidence suggests that easy startling is related to anxiety, researchers have attempted to test this use by measuring the acoustic startle response. In this double-blind, placebo-controlled trial, forty study participants were given either gotu kola or a placebo and then subjected to sudden loud noises. Researchers measured eye blinks and found a significantly reduced startle response in those treated with gotu kola. This suggests, but does not prove, that gotu kola may be helpful for anxiety.

SAFETY ISSUES

When taken orally, gotu kola seldom causes any side effects other than the occasional allergic skin rash, and safety studies suggest that it is essentially nontoxic. However, one animal study hints that gotu kola might have carcinogenic effects if applied topically to the skin.

Although gotu kola has not been proven safe for pregnant or nursing women, studies in rabbits suggest that it does not harm fetal development, and Italian physicians have given it to pregnant women. Safety in young children and those with severe liver or kidney disease has not been established.

EBSCO CAM Review Board

FURTHER READING

Bradwejn, J., et al. "A Double-Blind, Placebo-Controlled Study on the Effects of Gotu Kola (*Centella asiatica*) on Acoustic Startle Response in Healthy Subjects." *Journal of Clinical Psychopharmacology* 20 (2000): 680-684.

Klovekorn, W., et al. "A Randomized, Double-Blind, Vehicle-Controlled, Half-Side Comparison with a

Herbal Ointment Containing *Mahonia aquifolium, Viola tricolor,* and *Centella asiatica* for the Treatment of Mild-to-Moderate Atopic Dermatitis." *International Journal of Clinical Pharmacology and Therapeutics* 45 (2007): 583-591.

Shukla, A., et al. "In Vitro and In Vivo Wound Healing Activity of Asiaticoside Isolated from *Centella asiatica.*" *Journal of Ethnopharmacology* 65 (1999): 1-11.

See also: Anxiety and panic attacks; Burns, minor; Cirrhosis; Hemorrhoids; Periodontal disease; Scar tissue; Scleroderma; Varicose veins; Venous insufficiency.

Gout

CATEGORY: Condition
DEFINITION: Treatment of inflammation caused by the deposit of uric acid crystals in joints and tissues.
PRINCIPAL PROPOSED NATURAL TREATMENTS: None
OTHER PROPOSED NATURAL TREATMENTS: Aspartic acid, bromelain, celery juice, cherry juice, devil's claw, fish oil, folate, olive leaf, selenium, vitamin A, vitamin C, vitamin E

INTRODUCTION

Gout is an inflammatory condition that is caused by the deposit of uric acid crystals in joints (primarily the big toe) and tissues. Typically, attacks of fierce pain, redness, swelling, and heat punctuate pain-free intervals. Conventional medical treatment consists of anti-inflammatory drugs for acute attacks and of uric acid-lowering drugs for prevention.

PROPOSED TREATMENTS

The following herbs and supplements are widely recommended for gout, but they have no reliable scientific support:

- *Vitamin C.* In a double-blind, placebo-controlled study of 184 people without gout, the use of vitamin C at a daily dose of 500 milligrams significantly reduced uric acid levels. This suggests, but falls far short of proving, that vitamin C might be helpful for preventing or treating gout.
- *Folate.* Folate has been recommended as a preventive treatment for gout since the last decades of the twentieth century. Some clinicians report

that it can be highly effective. Scientific evidence on the method is contradictory. It has been suggested that a contaminant found in folate, pterin-6-aldehyde, may actually be responsible for the positive effects observed by some clinicians.

- *Devil's claw.* The herb devil's claw is sometimes recommended as a pain-relieving treatment for gout based on evidence for its effectiveness in various forms of arthritis. However, it has not been tested in gout.
- *Other supplements.* On the basis of certain reasoning but no concrete evidence of effectiveness, fish oil, olive leaf, vitamin E, selenium, bromelain, vitamin A, and aspartic acid have also been recommended for both prevention and treatment of gout.
- *Folk remedies.* A traditional remedy for gout (with negligible scientific evidence) calls for the consumption of one-half to one pound of cherries per day. Over-the-counter tablets containing concentrated cherry juice are available too. Celery juice is another folk remedy for gout that is said to be widely used in Australia.

HERBS AND SUPPLEMENTS TO USE WITH CAUTION

Various herbs and supplements may interact adversely with drugs used to treat gout, so persons should

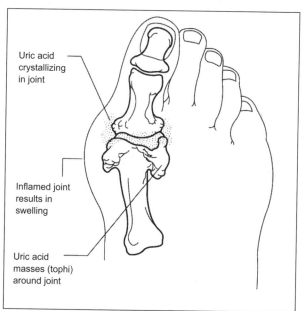

The big toe is a common site for gout.

What Is Gout?

Gout is an ancient and common form of inflammatory arthritis, and is the most common inflammatory arthritis among men. Gout may remit for long periods, followed by flare-ups for days or weeks, or the condition can become chronic.

Gout is caused by an uncontrolled metabolic disorder, hyperuricemia, which leads to the deposition of monosodium urate crystals in tissue, causing joint pain. Hyperuricemia means too much uric acid in the blood. Uric acid is a metabolic product resulting from the metabolism of purines, which are found in many foods and in human tissue.

Hyperuricemia is caused by an imbalance in the production and excretion of urate, that is, in urate's overproduction, underexcretion, or both. Underexcretion is the most common cause, thought to account for 80 to 90 percent of hyperuricemia. Hyperuricemia is not the same as gout. Asymptomatic hyperuricemia does not need to be treated.

Risk factors for gout include being overweight or obese, having hypertension, drinking alcohol (beer and spirits more than wine), using diuretics, and eating a rich diet of meat and seafood. Weight loss lowers the risk for gout.

---

be cautious when considering the use of herbs and supplements.

EBSCO CAM Review Board

FURTHER READING

Huang, H. Y., et al. "The Effects of Vitamin C Supplementation on Serum Concentrations of Uric Acid." *Arthritis and Rheumatism* 52 (2005): 1843-1847.

Lewis, A. S., et al. "Inhibition of Mammalian Xanthine Oxidase by Folate Compounds and Amethopterin." *Journal of Biological Chemistry* 259 (1984): 12-15.

Parker, James N., and Philip M. Parker, eds. *The 2002 Official Patient's Sourcebook on Gout.* San Diego, Calif.: Icon Health, 2002.

See also: Bone and joint health; Bursitis; Herbal medicine; Osteoarthritis; Soft tissue pain.

Grass pollen extract

CATEGORY: Herbs and supplements
DEFINITION: Natural plant product used to treat specific health conditions.
PRINCIPAL PROPOSED USE: Prostate enlargement
OTHER PROPOSED USES: High cholesterol, menopausal symptoms, premenstrual syndrome, prostate cancer, prostatitis

OVERVIEW

Like the more famous saw palmetto, extracts of grass pollen are used to treat prostate enlargement. The grass mixture utilized to make this preparation consists of 92 percent rye, 5 percent timothy, and 3 percent corn. Grass pollen also has been investigated for its potential to treat prostatitis, prostate cancer, and symptoms of menopause and premenstrual syndrome (PMS), as well as to reduce cholesterol.

Related grass pollen extracts are used for allergy shots. The grass pollen extracts described have their allergenic component removed, so they cannot possibly work to treat hay fever. Grass pollen is also an entirely different product from bee pollen.

REQUIREMENTS AND SOURCES

Grass pollen extract tablets for prostate disease are available in pharmacies and health food stores or can be ordered from a number of sources on the Internet.

THERAPEUTIC DOSAGES

The recommended dosage for grass pollen extract tablets is between 80 and 120 milligrams (mg) per day.

THERAPEUTIC USES

Two double-blind, placebo-controlled studies have found that grass pollen extract can help reduce symptoms of benign prostate enlargement (technically called benign prostatic hyperplasia, or BPH). One small double-blind study found evidence that a product containing grass pollen, the pistils (seed-bearing parts) of grass, and royal jelly (a product made by bees) may be helpful for PMS. Another small double-blind study found benefit with the same combination for treatment of menopausal symptoms.

Grass pollen extract has also shown promise for treating prostatitis. In a six-month, double-blind study of sixty men with nonbacterial prostatitis, use of the grass pollen extract was more effective than placebo in relieving symptoms.

Grass pollen has additionally been investigated for its usefulness in treating inflammation or infection of the prostate, prostate cancer, and high cholesterol. Animal studies also suggest that it may protect the liver from damage by some types of poisons. However, the scientific evidence for all of these remains very weak.

Scientific Evidence

Two double-blind, placebo-controlled studies have found that grass pollen extract can improve symptoms of BPH. In the first double-blind, placebo-controlled study, 103 people with BPH were assigned to take either a placebo or two capsules of a standardized grass pollen extract three times daily for a period of twelve weeks. At the end of the study, 69 percent of the participants who had been taking the grass pollen had reduced the number of trips they had to make to the bathroom at night. In the placebo group, only 37 percent reported improvement in this symptom. The amount of urine remaining in the bladder following urination was reduced in the treatment group by 24 milliliters (ml) and in the placebo group by 4 ml. Both of these were statistically significant improvements for those taking grass pollen.

The second double-blind, placebo-controlled study lasted longer but enrolled fewer participants. Fifty-seven men with prostate enlargement were enrolled in the study, with thirty-one taking 92 mg of the grass pollen extract daily for six months and the remaining twenty-six taking a placebo. As with the previous study, statistically significant improvements in nighttime frequency of urination and emptying of the bladder were found with use of grass pollen extract. Additionally, 69 percent of the participants receiving treatment reported overall improvement, while only 29 percent of the group taking the placebo felt they had improved, another statistically significant difference.

An important finding in this study was that, according to ultrasound measurements, prostate size decreased in men taking grass pollen. Not all treatments for BPH can reduce prostate size. It may be that treatments that shrink the prostate can reduce the need for surgery; such is the case, at least, with the prescription

drug finasteride. Whether grass pollen offers this same potential benefit is not known.

Two additional studies compared grass pollen to other alternative treatments for prostate enlargement rather than to a placebo. An open study pitted grass pollen against pygeum. Although pygeum is considered a more established treatment for prostate enlargement, grass pollen appeared to work better. The pollen extract was found to be significantly more effective in improving the flow of urine, emptying of the bladder, and the participants' perceptions of relief. Those in the grass pollen group also had a significant reduction in prostate size, while there was no reduction of size in the pygeum group. It appears from this that grass pollen is a more effective treatment than pygeum, but since the study was not blinded, the results are somewhat questionable.

A double-blind comparative study pitted grass pollen against an amino acid preparation and found no significant difference between the two. Because it is not known how well the amino acid medication works, the result has little meaning.

No one is certain how the grass pollen extract might cause the beneficial results seen in the studies. One theory is that it inhibits the body's manufacturing of prostaglandins and leukotrienes, which might relieve congestion and act as an anti-inflammatory. This, however, probably would not explain the reduction in prostate size, meaning that there may be more than one mechanism at work.

Safety Issues

No serious side effects have been reported with the use of grass pollen extract. No adverse reactions were observed in any of the clinical trials discussed above, although one review author mentioned rare reports of stomach upset and skin rash.

Although many people are allergic to grass pollen, the grass pollen products discussed in this article are processed to remove allergenic proteins. For this reason, it is unlikely that grass-allergic individuals will have an allergic reaction. Maximum safe doses for young children, pregnant or nursing women, or those with liver or kidney disease are not known.

EBSCO CAM Review Board

Further Reading

Elist, J. "Effects of Pollen Extract Preparation Prostat/ Poltit on Lower Urinary Tract Symptoms in Patients with Chronic Nonbacterial Prostatitis/Chronic Pelvic Pain Syndrome." *Urology* 67 (2006): 60-63.

Winther, K., et al. "Femal, a Herbal Remedy Made from Pollen Extracts, Reduces Hot Flushes and Improves Quality of Life in Menopausal Women." *Climacteric* 8 (2005): 162-170.

See also: Cholesterol, high; Menopause; Premenstrual syndrome (PMS); Prostatitis.

Greater celandine

CATEGORY: Herbs and supplements
RELATED TERM: *Chelidonium majus*
DEFINITION: Natural plant product used to treat specific health conditions.
PRINCIPAL PROPOSED USES: None
OTHER PROPOSED USES: Dyspepsia, warts

OVERVIEW

The herb greater celandine (*Chelidonium majus*), a relative of the poppy, contains an orange-colored juice that has been used medicinally for thousands of years. It has been applied topically for eye and skin problems and taken internally for bronchitis, jaundice, indigestion, cancer, and whooping cough. However, traditional herbalists appear to have missed one major problem with this herb: It can damage the liver. Greater celandine contains toxic constituents, and it is not recommended for use.

THERAPEUTIC DOSAGES

A typical dosage of greater celandine extract is standardized to supply 4 milligrams of the substance chelidonine three times daily. However, experts advise against its use. For the treatment of warts, greater celandine is applied directly to the wart and allowed to dry there.

THERAPEUTIC USES

Test-tube and animal studies provide weak evidence that greater celandine may both stimulate and relax the gallbladder. In Europe, it is commonly believed that minor gallbladder problems are a cause of indigestion. On this basis, celandine was approved in 1985 by Germany's Commission E, which has evaluated the usefulness of three hundred herbs, as a treatment for dyspepsia, or nonspecific digestive distress. While there is some supporting evidence for this use, in view of the safety risks associated with celandine, using it for this purpose (or any other) is not recommended.

Preliminary evidence hints suggests that constituents of celandine may also have cancer-preventive and antimicrobial properties. Celandine has traditionally been advocated as a topical treatment for warts. However, there is no reliable evidence that it is effective for this purpose.

SAFETY ISSUES

Numerous case reports indicate that use of celandine can lead to severe, potentially fatal liver injury. It should be noted that most people who use greater celandine do not develop liver problems. It may be that certain individuals have an especially high level of susceptibility. However, since it is not possible to determine in advance who would be at risk, experts recommend that the internal use of greater celandine should be avoided entirely.

EBSCO CAM Review Board

FURTHER READING

Benninger, J., et al. "Acute Hepatitis Induced by Greater Celandine (*Chelidonium majus*)." *Gastroenterology* 117 (1999): 1234-1237.

Song, J. Y., et al. "Immunomodulatory Activity of Protein-Bound Polysaccharide Extracted from *Chelidonium majus*." *Archives of Pharmacal Research* 25 (2002): 158-164.

Stickel, F., et al. "Acute Hepatitis Induced by Greater Celandine (*Chelidonium majus*)." *Scandinavian Journal of Gastroenterology* 38 (2003): 565-568.

See also: Dyspepsia; Warts.

Green coffee bean extract

CATEGORY: Herbs and supplements
RELATED TERM: Chlorogenic acid
DEFINITION: Natural plant product used to treat specific health conditions.
PRINCIPAL PROPOSED USE: Hypertension
OTHER PROPOSED USES: Diabetes prevention, weight loss

OVERVIEW

Just as black tea is made by processing green tea leaves from their original state, ordinary coffee is made by roasting green coffee beans. This processing alters the chemical makeup of the plant product. In an analogy to the medicinal study of green tea, an extract made from green coffee beans is undergoing increasing investigation as a possible health-promoting supplement.

Like green tea, green coffee bean extract (GCBE) contains strong antioxidants in the polyphenol family. The primary polyphenol antioxidants in green coffee bean extract are in a family known as chlorogenic acids (CGA). Meaningful, if still preliminary, evidence hints that CGA may help reduce blood pressure. Other proposed uses of GCBE are based primarily on its caffeine content, as well as observational studies of ordinary coffee consumption and the possible health benefits of antioxidants in general.

THERAPEUTIC DOSAGES

In a large human trial of GCBE for hypertension, the extract was most effective when taken at a dose of 185 milligrams (mg) daily.

THERAPEUTIC USES

Animal studies have found evidence that chlorogenic acids from GCBE can reduce blood pressure. Based on this, researchers have conducted human trials.

In a double-blind, placebo-controlled study of 117 males with mild hypertension, GCBE was given for one month at 46 mg, 93 mg, or 185 mg daily. After twenty-eight days, the results showed a significant improvement in blood pressure, compared with placebo, in the 93-mg and 185-mg groups. The results seen were dose-related, meaning that the greater the dose, the greater the improvement. The finding of dose-relatedness tends to increase the likelihood that a studied treatment is actually effective. Antihypertensive benefits were also seen in a much smaller study using purified chlorogenic acids.

GCBE has also shown a bit of promise for aiding weight loss, perhaps in part due to its chlorogenic acid content. The caffeine in GCBE might also provide a slight weight-loss benefit.

GCBE products are sometimes said to help prevent diabetes. However, this claim derives only from weak evidence involving consumption of ordinary coffee and cannot be relied upon.

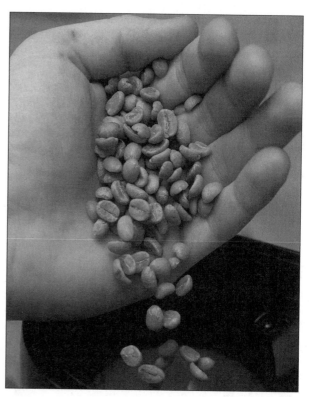

Like green tea, green coffee bean extract (GCBE) contains strong antioxidants in the polyphenol family. (AP Photo)

Roasted (as opposed to green) coffee beans contain the substances kahweol and cafestol, which appear to increase levels of low-density lipoprotein (LDL, or bad cholesterol). The fact that GCBE does not contain these substances is used as an argument in its favor. However, these substances remain in the coffee grounds, and they are also not present in standard beverage coffee, so this is probably not a significant point. (Unfiltered or boiled coffee, with the grounds left in, however, may present a risk.)

Since green coffee bean extract typically contains about 30 percent chlorogenic acids, this works out to a dose of about 60 mg of chlorogenic acids daily. Another study used 140 mg of purified chlorogenic acids daily.

SAFETY ISSUES

GCBE is thought to be a safe substance. In human trials, no significant adverse effects have been seen.

In theory, the caffeine content of GCBE could potentially cause problems for some people. However, since GCBE contains only about 10 percent caffeine by weight, a high daily dose contains no more than about 20 percent of the caffeine content that is in a strong cup of coffee. Maximum safe doses in pregnant or nursing women, young children, and people with liver or kidney disease have not yet been established.

EBSCO CAM Review Board

FURTHER READING

Kozuma, K., et al. "Antihypertensive Effect of Green Coffee Bean Extract on Mildly Hypertensive Subjects." *Hypertension Research* 28 (2006): 711-718.

Ranheim, T., and B. Halvorsen. "Coffee Consumption and Human Health: Beneficial or Detrimental? Mechanisms for Effects of Coffee Consumption on Different Risk Factors for Cardiovascular Disease and Type 2 Diabetes Mellitus." *Molecular Nutrition and Food Research* 49 (2005): 274-284.

Van Dam, R. M., and E. J. Feskens. "Coffee Consumption and Risk of Type 2 Diabetes Mellitus." *The Lancet* 360 (2002): 1477-1478.

Watanabe, T., et al. "The Blood Pressure-Lowering Effect and Safety of Chlorogenic Acid from Green Coffee Bean Extract in Essential Hypertension." *Clinical and Experimental Hypertension* 28 (2006): 439-449.

See also: Diabetes; Herbal medicine; Hypertension; Obesity and excess weight.

Green-lipped mussel

CATEGORY: Herbs and supplements
RELATED TERM: *Perna canaliculus*
DEFINITION: Natural seafood product used to treat specific health conditions.
PRINCIPAL PROPOSED USE: Osteoarthritis
OTHER PROPOSED USES: Asthma, rheumatoid arthritis

OVERVIEW

The green-lipped mussel, a common appetizer in sushi restaurants, contains healthy fats in the omega-3 family. Like fish oil, another source of omega-3 fatty acids, green-lipped mussel has shown some promise for reducing inflammation. Inflammation is the cause of symptoms in numerous illnesses, ranging from arthritis to asthma. On this basis, green-lipped mussel has been promoted as a treatment for these conditions. However, the evidence that it provides any meaningful benefits remains highly preliminary.

THERAPEUTIC DOSAGES

A typical dose of green-lipped mussel is about 200 milligrams (mg) per day of the lipid extract or 1,000 mg per day of the freeze-dried powder.

THERAPEUTIC USES

There are two major forms of arthritis: osteoarthritis and rheumatoid arthritis. Rheumatoid arthritis is primarily a disease of inflammation, and the anti-inflammatory omega-3 fatty acids found in fish oil have been successfully used to treat it. Inflammation plays a relatively less important role in osteoarthritis. However, green-lipped mussel has been tried for both conditions, with, at present, inconclusive results.

Unlike standard nonsteroidal anti-inflammatory drugs (NSAIDs), which harm the stomach wall, green-lipped mussel might help prevent ulcers. Green-lipped mussel has also been shown to ease asthma.

SCIENTIFIC EVIDENCE

Arthritis. The evidence regarding use of green-lipped mussel for arthritis remains weak and inconsistent. Several animal studies performed by a single research group have reported that green-lipped mussel reduces symptoms of osteoarthritis. However, the results from human studies remain inconsistent. Of five reported controlled studies of green-lipped mussel for osteoarthritis, two found benefit.

Asthma. In an eight-week, double-blind, placebo-controlled trial of 46 people with allergic asthma, those who received a green-lipped mussel extract showed some improvement in wheezing and peak flow of air.

SAFETY ISSUES

In studies, green-lipped mussel has not caused much in the way of side effects, other than occasional mild digestive distress. People with shellfish allergies, however, should avoid green-lipped mussel. Unlike oysters, green-lipped mussel does not appear to contain heavy metals.

EBSCO CAM Review Board

FURTHER READING

Cho, S. H., et al. "Clinical Efficacy and Safety of Lyprinol, a Patented Extract from New Zealand

Green-Lipped Mussel (*Perna canaliculus*) in Patients with Osteoarthritis of the Hip and Knee." *Allergie et Immunologie* 35 (2003): 212-216.

Cobb, C. S., and E. Ernst. "Systematic Review of a Marine Nutriceutical Supplement in Clinical Trials for Arthritis: The Effectiveness of the New Zealand Green-Lipped Mussel *Perna canaliculus.*" *Clinical Rheumatology* 25, no. 3 (2006): 275-284.

Emelyanov, A., et al. "Treatment of Asthma with Lipid Extract of New Zealand Green-Lipped Mussel." *European Respiratory Journal* 20 (2002): 596-600.

Halpern, G. M. "Anti-Inflammatory Effects of a Stabilized Lipid Extract of *Perna canaliculus* (Lyprinol)." *Allergie et Immunologie* 32 (2000): 272-278.

Rojas de Astudillo, L., et al. "Heavy Metals in Green Mussel (*Perna viridis*) and Oysters (*Crassostrea*) from Trinidad and Venezuela." *Archives of Environmental Contamination and Toxicology* 42 (2002): 410-415.

See also: Asthma; Herbal medicine; Osteoarthritis; Rheumatoid arthritis.

Green tea

CATEGORY: Functional foods
RELATED TERM: *Camellia sinensis*
DEFINITION: Natural plant product consumed for specific health benefits.
PRINCIPAL PROPOSED USES: Cancer prevention, gingivitis
OTHER PROPOSED USES: Diabetes, heart disease prevention, high cholesterol, influenza prevention, liver disease prevention, rosacea, sun damage protection, weight loss

OVERVIEW

People have been drinking tea for thousands of years, and more recently, a number of potential health benefits have been attributed to this ancient beverage. Black tea and green tea are made from the same plant, but a higher level of the original substances endure in the less-processed green form.

USES AND APPLICATIONS

Green tea contains high levels of substances called catechin polyphenols, known to possess strong antioxidant, anticarcinogenic, antitumorigenic, and even antibiotic properties. Based on these findings and on observational studies, green tea has become popular as a daily drink for preventing cancer and heart disease. However, some observational trials failed to find indications of benefit with green tea. Furthermore, only double-blind, placebo-controlled studies can prove a treatment effective, and there is little direct evidence of this type of study regarding green tea and cancer or heart disease prevention.

One such study found that green teas produced short-term improvements in cholesterol profile, with the benefits disappearing after four weeks. More positive results were seen in a study that evaluated a form of green tea enriched with the substance theaflavin, which is found in black tea. In this fairly large (more than two hundred participants), three-month study, the use of the tea product resulted in significant, ongoing reductions in LDL (bad) cholesterol compared with placebo. A green tea extract enhanced with catechins has also shown promise for reducing LDL levels, according to one somewhat flawed double-blind study. However, a study involving catechin-enhanced green tea in Japanese children was less convincing.

Preliminary studies suggest that certain green tea polyphenols may help prevent skin cancer if they are applied directly to the skin. In addition, there is some evidence that green tea constituents might help protect the skin from sun damage. Unlike normal sunscreen preparations, green tea does not physically block ultraviolet light. Rather, it seems to protect cells from some of the damage caused by ultraviolet light. Because it works by such a different mechanism of action, green tea might offer synergistic benefits if combined with standard sunscreens. However, in an eight-week double-blind, placebo-controlled study of forty women who already had symptoms of aging skin, the combined use of oral green tea and a topical green tea cream failed to prove more effective than placebo. Some possible benefits were seen in the microscopic evaluation of the skin condition.

Topical green tea extracts have also shown some promise for the treatment of cervical dysplasia, while oral green tea extracts might reduce the risk of prostate cancer, according to a small pilot study. Combining the results of thirteen observational studies, researchers found conflicting evidence for green tea's effect on the risk of stomach cancer. In a Japanese pilot study, green tea extract supplements lowered the risk of recurrent colorectal polyps. In a review of nine observational studies involving more

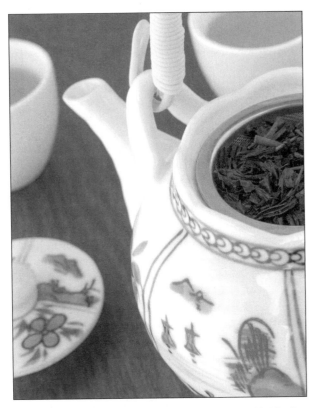

Green tea is being studied as a cancer preventive. (© Monkey Business Images/Dreamstime.com)

than 5,600 cases of breast cancer, researchers failed to find reliable evidence for a reduction in the incidence of breast cancer. However, they did find weak evidence for a decrease in breast cancer recurrence among women who consumed more than three cups of green tea daily

On a completely different note, one study tested the effectiveness of gargling with green tea catechins as a means of preventing influenza. In this double-blind, placebo-controlled study, 124 residents of a Japanese nursing home gargled with green tea catechins or placebo for three months. All participants received standard influenza vaccine. The results showed that residents who gargled with the tea extract were less likely to develop influenza than those using the placebo. In addition, another double-blind study found preliminary evidence that oral consumption of a green tea extract might help prevent colds and flu.

A small double-blind, placebo-controlled trial found weak evidence that green tea chew candy might reduce gum inflammation in persons with periodontal disease

(gingivitis). Green tea extract has shown some promise for treating borderline diabetes. However, one double-blind study failed to find that a combined extract of black and green tea was helpful for controlling blood sugar levels in people with type 2 diabetes. Green tea also has been proposed as a means of preventing liver disease, but the evidence remains unconvincing.

Green tea is sometimes recommended for weight loss on the basis of rather theoretical evidence that it speeds up metabolism. However, there is little direct scientific backing for this use. If green tea does increase metabolism, the effect is extremely small. One study conducted in Thailand reported weight-loss benefits with green tea, as did a second study of oolong tea enriched with green tea extracts. However, a Dutch study failed to find green tea helpful for preventing weight regain after weight loss. In another study, the use of green tea failed to produce significant weight loss in overweight women with polycystic ovary syndrome. Green tea extract enriched with catechins has done somewhat better, enhancing weight loss in one substantial but flawed trial. However, a study in overweight Japanese children did not support the effectiveness of green tea catechins for weight reduction. Similar results were obtained in another placebo-controlled trial involving seventy-eight overweight women after twelve weeks of treatment.

One preliminary study found some evidence that green tea cream may be helpful for the skin condition rosacea. The results of another study weakly hint that green tea extracts taken orally might reduce symptoms of benign prostatic hyperplasia. One study found that inhaled tea catechins could reduce levels of resistant staph carried in the sputum of disabled elderly persons. One should not, however, attempt to inhale green tea products.

DOSAGE

Studies weakly suggest that three cups of green tea daily might provide protection from cancer. However, because not everyone wants to take the time to drink green tea, manufacturers have offered extracts that can be taken in pill form. A typical dosage is 100 milligrams (mg) to 150 mg three times daily of a green tea extract standardized to contain 80 percent total polyphenols and 50 percent epigallocatechin gallate. Whether these extracts offer any benefit remains unknown. Furthermore, there are growing concerns about liver toxicity with the use of green tea extracts.

In an analysis performed in 2006, some tested green tea products were found to be contaminated with lead.

SAFETY ISSUES

As a widely consumed beverage, green tea is generally regarded as safe. It does contain caffeine, at perhaps a slightly lower level than black tea, and can therefore cause insomnia, nervousness, and the other well-known symptoms of excess caffeine intake.

Green tea extracts, however, may not be safe. There are a growing number of case reports in which the use of a concentrated green tea extract was associated with liver inflammation. In most cases, liver problems disappeared after the extract was discontinued, but in two cases, permanent liver failure ensued, requiring liver transplantation. While it is not certain that the green tea extract caused the liver problems, or how it might do so, these reports do raise significant concerns about the use of green tea extracts, especially by those with liver disease or those who are prone to it.

Green tea should not be given to infants and young children. There are theoretical concerns that high dosages of epigallocatechin gallate might be unsafe for pregnant women.

Dried green tea leaf contains significant levels of vitamin K on a per-weight basis. On this basis, it has been stated that people using blood thinners in the warfarin (Coumadin) family should avoid green tea, because vitamin K antagonizes the effect of those drugs. However, green tea taken as a beverage provides such small amounts of the vitamin that the risk seems minimal for normal consumption. There is one case report of problems that developed in a person on warfarin who consumed as much as 1 gallon of green tea daily.

Important interactions. The caffeine in green tea could cause serious problems in persons who are taking monoamine oxidase inhibitors. One should avoid drinking large quantities of green tea if also taking warfarin. Finally, green tea may decrease the absorption of folic acid into the bloodstream.

EBSCO CAM Review Board

FURTHER READING

Boehm, K., et al. "Green Tea (*Camellia sinensis*) for the Prevention of Cancer." *Cochrane Database of Systematic Reviews* (2009): CD005004. Available through *EBSCO DynaMed Systematic Literature Surveillance* at http://www.ebscohost.com/dynamed.

Hsu, C. H., et al. "Effect of Green Tea Extract on Obese Women." *Clinical Nutrition* 27 (2008): 363-370.

Katiyar, S. K., N. Ahmad, and H. Mukhtar. "Green Tea and Skin." *Archives of Dermatology* 136 (2000): 989-994.

Liu, J., J. Xing, and Y. Fei. "Green Tea (*Camellia sinensis*) and Cancer Prevention." *Chinese Medicine* 3 (2008): 12.

Mackenzie, T., L. Leary, and W. B. Brooks. "The Effect of an Extract of Green and Black Tea on Glucose Control in Adults with Type 2 Diabetes Mellitus." *Metabolism* 56 (2007): 1340-1344.

Matsuyama, T., et al. "Catechin Safely Improved Higher Levels of Fatness, Blood Pressure, and Cholesterol in Children." *Obesity* 16 (2008): 1338-1348.

Myung, S. K., et al. "Green Tea Consumption and Risk of Stomach Cancer." *International Journal of Cancer* 124 (2009): 670-677.

Ogunleye, A. A., F. Xue, and K. B. Michels. "Green Tea Consumption and Breast Cancer Risk or Recurrence." *Breast Cancer Research and Treatment* 119 (2010): 477-484.

Rowe, C. A., et al. "Specific Formulation of *Camellia sinensis* Prevents Cold and Flu Symptoms and Enhances T Cell Function." *Journal of the American College of Nutrition* 26 (2007): 445-452.

Sarma, D. N., et al. "Safety of Green Tea Extracts: A Systematic Review by the U.S. Pharmacopeia." *Drug Safety* 31 (2008): 469-484.

See also: Black tea; Cancer risk reduction; Folk medicine; Functional beverages; Herbal medicine; Hypertension; Kombucha tea; Red tea.

Guarana

CATEGORY: Herbs and supplements

RELATED TERM: *Paullinia cupana*

DEFINITION: Natural plant product used to treat specific health conditions.

PRINCIPAL PROPOSED USES: Enhancing mental function, fatigue

OTHER PROPOSED USES: Sports performance enhancement, weight loss

OVERVIEW

Guarana, an herb from the Amazon rainforest, has a long history of use as a stimulant beverage. It has

also been used to treat arthritis, diarrhea, and headaches.

THERAPEUTIC DOSAGES

A typical dose of guarana supplies 50 milligrams
(mg) of caffeine, which is about half the amount in a
cup of strong coffee. However, a 1998 analysis of products on the market indicated that many guarana products contain less than the advertised amount of guarana.

THERAPEUTIC USES

Like tea, coffee, and chocolate, guarana contains
alkaloids in the caffeine family, such as theobromine
and theophylline. Caffeine is known to reduce pain,
treat migraine headaches, and fight fatigue. In addition, it may, under certain circumstances, enhance
sports performance, improve mental function, and
modestly aid weight loss.

Most of the proposed uses of guarana fall into line
with these effects of caffeine. For example, in a
double-blind, placebo-controlled study of 129 healthy
young adults, the one-time use of guarana plus vitamins and minerals improved mental function and
reduced mental fatigue among those undergoing a
battery of cognitive tests. In another double-blind,
placebo-controlled study, use of guarana alone or
guarana plus ginseng appeared to improve mental
function (though the study suffered from some design problems). In two other studies, no benefits
were seen.

Another double-blind, placebo-controlled study
tested the effects of guarana plus ephedra for weight
loss. In this trial, a total of sixty-seven overweight
people were given either placebo or a combination of
guarana and ephedra for a period of eight weeks. The
results showed significantly greater weight loss in the
treated group than in the placebo group. However,
ephedra is an unsafe substance.

SAFETY ISSUES

The side effects of guarana would be expected to
be similar to those of tea or coffee, such as heartburn,
gastritis, insomnia, anxiety, and heart arrythmias (benign palpitations or more serious disturbances of
heart rhythm). Combination products containing
guarana and ephedra would be expected to present
additional risk. Finally, all drug interactions that can
occur with caffeine would be expected to occur with
guarana as well. Young children, pregnant or nursing

women, and people with heart disease should not use
guarana.

IMPORTANT INTERACTIONS

For people taking monoamine oxidase (MAO) inhibitors while simultaneously using guarana, the caffeine in guarana could cause dangerous drug interactions. The stimulant effects of guarana might be
amplified if one used it while simultaneously taking
stimulant drugs, such as Ritalin. Guarana might also
interfere with the action of drugs taken to prevent
heart arrythmias or to treat insomnia or anxiety.

EBSCO CAM Review Board

FURTHER READING

Boozer, C. N., et al. "An Herbal Supplement Containing Ma Huang-Guarana for Weight Loss." *International Journal of Obesity and Related Metabolic Disorders* 25 (2001): 316-324.

Cannon, M. E., et al. "Caffeine-Induced Cardiac Arrhythmia: An Unrecognised Danger of Healthfood
Products." *Medical Journal of Australia* 174 (2001):
520-521.

Kennedy, D. O., et al. "Improved Cognitive Performance and Mental Fatigue Following a Multi-vi-
tamin and Mineral Supplement with Added Guarana (*Paullinia cupana*)." *Appetite* 50, nos. 2/3
(2008): 506-13.

See also: Fatigue; Obesity and excess weight; Sports
and fitness support: Enhancing performance.

Guggul

CATEGORY: Herbs and supplements
RELATED TERM: *Commiphora mukul*
DEFINITION: Natural plant product used to treat spe-
cific health conditions.
PRINCIPAL PROPOSED USE: High cholesterol
OTHER PROPOSED USES: Acne, diabetes, weight loss

OVERVIEW

Guggul, the sticky gum resin from the mukul
myrrh tree, plays a major role in Ayurveda, the traditional herbal medicine of India. It was traditionally
combined with other herbs for the treatment of arthritis, skin diseases, pains in the nervous system,

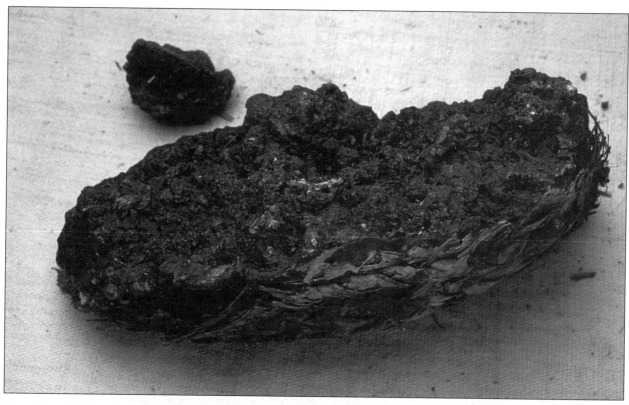

Guggul, a resin from the mukul myrrh tree. (Jerry Mason/Photo Researchers, Inc.)

obesity, digestive problems, infections in the mouth, and menstrual problems.

THERAPEUTIC DOSAGES

Guggul is manufactured in a standardized form that provides a fixed amount of guggulsterones, the presumed active ingredients in guggul. The typical daily dose should provide 100 milligrams (mg) of guggulsterones.

THERAPEUTIC USES

Based on preliminary studies, guggul has become a popular herbal treatment for high cholesterol. However, the best-designed trial failed to find benefit.

Other potential uses of guggul have no more than minimal supporting evidence. One small study hints that guggul might be helpful for acne. In addition, a study in mice found potential antidiabetic effects.

Recently, guggul has been promoted as a weight-loss agent. Supposedly, it works by enhancing thyroid function. However, there is little evidence that guggul actually affects the thyroid, and one small double-blind, placebo-controlled trial failed to find it effective for weight loss.

SCIENTIFIC EVIDENCE

High cholesterol. Three double-blind studies performed in India found evidence that guggul can reduce cholesterol levels. However, the largest placebo-controlled study failed to find benefit.

One of the positive placebo-controlled studies enrolled sixty-one individuals and followed them for twenty-four weeks. After twelve weeks of following a healthy diet, half the participants received placebo and the other half received guggul at a dose providing 100 mg of guggulsterones daily. The results after twenty-four weeks of treatment showed that the treated group experienced an 11.7 percent decrease in total cholesterol, along with a 12.7 percent decrease in low-density lipoprotein (LDL, or bad cholesterol), a 12 percent decrease in triglycerides, and an 11.1 percent decrease in the total cholesterol/high-density lipoprotein (HDL, or good cholesterol) ratio. These improvements were significantly greater than what was seen in the placebo group. Similar results were seen in a double-blind, placebo-controlled trial of forty individuals.

A double-blind study of 228 individuals given either guggul or the standard drug clofibrate found approximately equal efficacy between the two treatments. However, the absence of a placebo group makes these results less than reliable.

In contrast to these results, a double-blind, placebo-controlled study of 103 people failed to find guggul effective at a dose of 75 mg or 150 mg of guggulsterones daily. In fact, the herb seemed to worsen levels of LDL (bad) cholesterol. The reason for this discrepancy is not clear.

Acne. A small controlled trial compared oral gugulipid (50 mg of guggulsterones twice daily) against tetracycline for the treatment of acne and reported equivalent results. However, the study report does not state whether this trial was double-blind, and it also lacked a placebo group.

SAFETY ISSUES

In clinical trials of standardized guggul extract, no significant side effects other than occasional mild gastrointestinal distress or allergic skin rashes have been seen. Laboratory tests done in the course of these trials did not reveal any alterations in liver or kidney function, blood cell numbers and appearance, heart function, or blood chemistry.

Drugs in the statin family used to reduce cholesterol can cause a potentially serious condition called rhabdomyolysis, in which muscle fibers break down. One case report hints that this could also occur with guggul. Safety in young children, pregnant or nursing women, and those with severe liver or kidney disease has not been established.

EBSCO CAM Review Board

FURTHER READING

Antonio, J., et al. "Effects of a Standardized Guggulsterone Phosphate Supplement on Body Composition in Overweight Adults." *Current Therapeutic Research* 60 (1999): 220-227.

Bianchi, A., et al. "Rhabdomyolysis Caused by Commiphora Mukul, a Natural Lipid-Lowering Agent." *Annals of Pharmacotherapy* 38 (2004): 1222-1225.

Singh, R. B., et al. "Hypolipidemic and Antioxidant Effects of Commiphora Mukul as an Adjunct to Dietary Therapy in Patients with Hypercholesterolemia." *Cardiovascular Drugs and Therapy* 8 (1994): 659-664.

Szapary, P. O., et al. "Guggulipid for the Treatment of Hypercholesterolemia." *Journal of the American Medical Association* 290 (2003): 765-772.

See also: Acne; Ayurveda; Cholesterol, high; Diabetes; Obesity and excess weight.

Guided imagery

CATEGORY: Therapies and techniques
RELATED TERMS: Affirmations, mental imagery, visualization
DEFINITION: A therapy involving the use of imagined scenes and activities to influence the body.
PRINCIPAL PROPOSED USES: Promote healing, relaxation, stress reduction
OTHER PROPOSED USES: Asthma, athletics, blood pressure, blood sugar control in diabetes, boost the immune cells, breast milk production, chemotherapy side effects, depression and anxiety, headaches, immune system, insomnia, pain, premenstrual syndrome, promote healing, surgery preparation, weight loss

OVERVIEW

Guided imagery has been used since ancient times by the Greeks and Egyptians. Normally, a person uses imagery many times each day when anticipating events or activities. Some of the imagery is negative and causes worrying. A person develops thoughts about who he or she is through mental imagery. Guided imagery channels this use of the mind to affect the body.

When initiating guided imagery, it helps to relax, because doing so makes the body more receptive to mental images. Some persons use guided imagery when they wake up in the morning and before they go to sleep at night. Guided imagery can be effective when practiced regularly, but it takes time to learn and to see its effects. Guided imagery should be practiced a minimum of twice per day.

Guided imagery is sometimes referred to as visualization or affirmations. Both visualization and affirmations apply the same principles as guided imagery.

MECHANISM OF ACTION

Guided imagery uses the mind/body connection

to change the body or its functioning. The mind already has a great deal of control over the body, and this control can be increased by using guided imagery.

The brain does not "understand" words; rather it understands only pictures or images, and these mental images must be repeatedly reviewed. With enough repetition, the brain and unconscious mind will attempt to make these images real. Positive imagery can trigger the release of brain chemicals, such as serotonin and endorphins, which are natural tranquilizers.

Guided imagery is more effective if all of the senses are used in forming the images. For example, a runner imaging his or her performance in a race should imagine the smell of perspiration, feel the pain in the legs and chest, imagine the dryness of the mouth, see competitors through peripheral vision, see the finish line, feel sweat running down the neck, and hear feet beating the ground as he or she pulls ahead and crosses the finish line first. One can then imagine the joy of winning the race and receiving a trophy or medal.

USES AND APPLICATIONS

Guided imagery assists in relaxing the body, controlling some body functions, and increasing the effectiveness of performance. It can be used to treat depression, anxiety, cancer, the side effects of chemotherapy, pain, high blood pressure, obesity, diabetes, insomnia, headaches, wounds, premenstrual syndrome, asthma, spastic colon, and low white-blood-cell counts.

SCIENTIFIC EVIDENCE

Much research has been conducted to determine the effectiveness of guided imagery. Many of the studies examined guided imagery as a CAM therapy for healing, reducing the side effects of drugs, or initiating personal change. In general, however, the effectiveness of guided imagery depends on the efforts of the individual person and cannot be controlled or measured accurately.

One study of women with breast cancer demonstrated such questionable results. The study, performed by the Oregon Health and Science University in 2002, looked at twenty-five women with either stage one or stage two breast cancer. They were taught guided imagery to see the natural killer cells of their immune system destroying the cancer cells. The initial session was taped; participants were asked to practice at home with the tape three times per week for eight weeks. Their immune function and emotional

state were measured three times: before the study began, at the end of eight weeks, and three months after the study ended. Participants reported being less depressed. The measure of their immune system demonstrated higher levels of natural killer cells but no change in the physical effects of the killer cells.

CHOOSING A PRACTITIONER

Guided imagery can be done without a practitioner. Audiotapes and CDs are available to provide guided imagery coaching. Good books describe the process and include scripts for guided imagery. A mental health counselor or a physician can provide coaching in guided imagery, and trained guided imagery counselors can be consulted.

SAFETY ISSUES

There are no known safety issues with guided imagery. However, intense worrying can have negative physical and emotional effects.

Christine M. Carroll, R.N., B.S.N.

FURTHER READING

"Guided Imagery: Using Your Imagination." In *Stress Management for Life: A Research-Based Experiential Approach*, edited by Michael Olpin and Margie Hesson. Belmont, Calif.: Wadsworth/Cengage Learning, 2010.

Naparstek, Belleruth. *Staying Well with Guided Imagery*. New York: Grand Central, 1995.

Rossman, Martin L. *Guided Imagery for Self-Healing*. 2d ed. Tiburon, Calif.: H. J. Kramer/New World Library, 2000.

See also: Art therapy; Biofeedback; Color therapy; Depression, mild to moderate; Faith healing; Humor and healing; Hypnosis; Meditation; Mental health; Mind/body medicine; Music therapy; Pet ownership; Self-care; Spirituality; Stress; Transcendental Meditation.

Gymnema

CATEGORY: Herbs and supplements

RELATED TERMS: Gumar, *Gymnema sylvestre*

DEFINITION: Natural plant product used to treat specific health conditions.

PRINCIPAL PROPOSED USE: Diabetes

OVERVIEW

Native to the forests of India, *Gymnema sylvestre* (also called gumar) has a coincidental double relationship to sugar: When placed on the tongue, it blocks the sensation of sweetness, and when taken internally, it might help control blood sugar levels in people with diabetes. (There does not seem to be any connection between these two uses.)

Practitioners of Ayurveda, the traditional medicine of India, first used gymnema to treat diabetes almost two thousand years ago. In the 1920s, preliminary scientific studies found some evidence that gymnema leaves can reduce blood sugar levels, but nothing much came of this observation for decades. Research in India picked up again in the 1980s and 1990s, leading to the publication of promising preliminary studies in people.

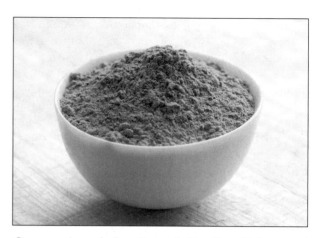

Gymnema is an herb native to India. (Lew Robertson/ Getty Images)

THERAPEUTIC DOSAGES

Gymnema is usually taken at a dosage of 400 to 600 milligrams daily of an extract standardized to contain 24 percent gymnemic acid.

THERAPEUTIC USES

Gymnema has become increasingly popular in the United States as a supportive treatment for diabetes. However, the evidence that it works remains weak. Only double-blind, placebo-controlled studies can prove a treatment effective, and none have been reported for gymnema. Current evidence is limited to a few animal studies and human open trials.

Gymnema is advocated as a support to standard treatment, not as a replacement for it. This herb definitely cannot be used as a substitute for insulin treatment, and it has not been proven strong enough for use in lieu of oral diabetes medications. There are also potential risks involved in adding gymnema to an existing treatment regimen.

SAFETY ISSUES

When used in appropriate dosages, gymnema appears to be fairly safe, although extensive studies have not been performed. One obvious risk is that if gymnema is successful, it may lower blood sugar levels too much, causing a dangerous hypoglycemic reaction. For this reason, medical supervision is essential. Safety in young children, pregnant or nursing women, and those with severe kidney or liver disease has not been established.

IMPORTANT INTERACTIONS

For people who are taking insulin or oral medications to reduce blood sugar levels, gymnema might cause these medications to work even better, potentially causing hypoglycemia. Therefore, individuals may need to reduce their doses of medication.

EBSCO CAM Review Board

FURTHER READING

Joffe, D. J., and S. H. Freed. "Effect of Extended Release *Gymnema sylvestre* Leaf Extract Alone or in Combination with Oral Hypoglycemics or Insulin Regimens for Type 1 and Type 2 Diabetes." *Diabetes Control Newsletter* 76, no. 1 (2001): 1-4.

See also: Ayurveda; Diabetes; Herbal medicine.

H

H$_2$ blockers

CATEGORY: Drug interactions
DEFINITION: Medications used to decrease the production of stomach acid.
INTERACTIONS: Folate, magnesium, minerals, vitamin B$_{12}$, vitamin D
DRUGS IN THIS FAMILY: Cimetidine (Tagamet), famotidine (Pepcid), nizatidine (Axid), ranitidine hydrochloride (Zantac)

VITAMIN B$_{12}$
Effect: Probable Need for Supplementation

H$_2$-receptor blockers appear to impair the absorption of vitamin B$_{12}$ from food. This is thought to occur because the vitamin B$_{12}$ in food is attached to proteins. Stomach acid separates them and allows the B$_{12}$ to be absorbed.

Persons who regularly use H$_2$ blockers should take vitamin B$_{12}$ supplements. These supplements can be absorbed easily because they are not attached to proteins.

FOLATE
Effect: Supplementation Possibly Helpful

There is some evidence that H$_2$ blockers may slightly reduce the absorption of folate. Folate is an important nutrient and one that is commonly deficient in the diet. Experts recommend that persons taking H$_2$ blockers should also take folate supplements.

MINERALS
Effect: Supplementation Possibly Helpful

By reducing stomach acid levels, H$_2$ blockers might interfere with the absorption of iron, zinc, and perhaps other minerals. Taking mineral supplements that provide the U.S. Dietary Reference Intake (formerly known as the Recommended Dietary Allowance) of these substances should help.

MAGNESIUM
Effect: Take at a Different Time of Day

Magnesium supplements may interfere with the absorption of H$_2$ blockers. However, the interference may be too minor to cause a real problem. Persons who think that their magnesium supplements are interfering with their medication should take these minerals a minimum of two hours before or after taking an H$_2$-blocking medication.

VITAMIN D
Effect: Possible Inhibition by Cimetidine

Cimetidine may interfere with vitamin D metabolism. Other H$_2$ blockers may not interact. It is not known whether taking more vitamin D is useful.

EBSCO CAM Review Board

FURTHER READING
Bachmann, K. A., et al. "Drug Interactions of H2-Receptor Antagonists." *Scandinavian Journal of Gastroenterology* 206, suppl. (1994): S14-S19.

DeVault, K. R., and N. J. Talley. "Insights into the Future of Gastric Acid Suppression." *Nature Reviews: Gastroenterology and Hepatology* 6, no. 9 (2009): 524-532.

Odes, H. S. "Effect of Cimetidine on Hepatic Vitamin D Metabolism in Humans." *Digestion* 46, no. 2 (1990): 61-64.

See also: Antacids; Folate; Food and Drug Administration; Magnesium; Proton pump inhibitors; Vitamin B$_{12}$; Vitamin D; Vitamins and minerals. Supplements: Overview.

Hackett, George S.

CATEGORY: Biography
IDENTIFICATION: American physician who developed prolotherapy
FLOURISHED: 1940s

OVERVIEW
George S. Hackett was an American physician often considered the founder of prolotherapy, an al-

ternative method that involves injecting an otherwise nonpharmacological solution into the body to strengthen weakened connective tissues and to alleviate musculoskeletal pain. Hackett reportedly used the term "prolotherapy" as a shortened form of the words "fibroproliferative therapy" (or "proliferant injection therapy"). Accordingly, this technique is still sometimes referred to as proliferation therapy or regenerative injection therapy. Most proponents of prolotherapy claim that it works by reinitiating an inflammatory response in an affected area, which leads to the strengthening of the area to overcome pain signals.

Hackett earned his medical degree from Cornell Medical College around 1916. He was trained as a general surgeon and was said to have a particular interest in cases of trauma, including follow-up surgery and rehabilitation. He noted his trauma patients' regular comments about their chronic postsurgical pain and disabilities. Based on his interactions with patients, he came to believe that their pain was caused not by bone-related issues but by the "soft tendons" (tendons and ligaments) that failed to heal after surgery. At this time, there was no diagnostic method for detecting such issues (beyond a thorough physical examination). Also, no therapies existed for treating these patients.

Hackett likely was aware of nineteenth-century practices, whereby various materials were injected into the body to form scar tissue or to heal topical wounds. In line with this knowledge, he formally developed the field of prolotherapy in the 1940s. He experimented with many different preparations and techniques to optimize results. He is said to have carried out in vivo experiments using rabbits to test different materials and doses. He also relied on microscopy to observe the results of treatments at the cellular level.

Hackett was reportedly the first modern clinician to rigorously investigate and document the use of prolotherapy, both in experimental systems and in humans. In particular, he was known to treat joint pain and hernias. He published his study results in popular medical journals of his time. In 1958, he also published the book *Ligament and Tendon Relaxation: Treated by Prolotherapy*.

By the 1950s, Hackett began teaching prolotherapy. One of his primary students, Gustav Hemwall, expanded on Hackett's methods from the 1950s to the 1990s.

Based on his own clinical experiences, Hackett reported that more than 80 percent of the thousands of persons he had treated with prolotherapy had indicated that the treatment relieved their chronic pain. Prolotherapy is still used today.

Brandy Weidow, M.S.

FURTHER READING

Darrow, Marc. *Prolotherapy: Living Pain Free*. Los Angeles: Protex Press, 2004.

Hackett, George Stuart, et al. *Ligament and Tendon Relaxation: Treated by Prolotherapy*. Oak Brook, Ill.: Institute in Basic Life Principles, 1993.

Hauser, Ross A., and Marion A. Hauser. *Prolo Your Pain Away! Curing Chronic Pain with Prolotherapy*. 3d ed. Oak Park, Ill.: Beulah Land Press, 2007.

Rabago, D., A. Slattengren, and A. Zgierska. "Prolotherapy in Primary Care Practice." *Primary Care* 37, no. 1 (2010): 65-80.

See also: Pain management; Prolotherapy.

Hahnemann, Samuel

CATEGORY: Biography

IDENTIFICATION: German physician who first proposed homeopathy

BORN: April 10, 1755; Meissen, Saxony (now in Germany)

DIED: July 2, 1843; Paris, France

OVERVIEW

Samuel Hahnemann, a German physician, introduced the alternative form of medicine called homeopathy, or the use of highly diluted preparations. Some also consider him to be the founder of experimental pharmacology, because he was the first physician known to prepare medicines in a purposeful, specialized way.

Before Hahnemann's time, most medical preparations were administered to ailing persons based primarily on the speculative (or sometimes superstitious) properties of the agents, rather than on experimental verification of the agent's effects. Hahnemann wrote critically of several of the practices of his time; he thought many of the methods were nonspecific (did more harm than good) and that some were altogether irrational.

Hahnemann is credited for experimentally investigating and ultimately discovering the potentialities of

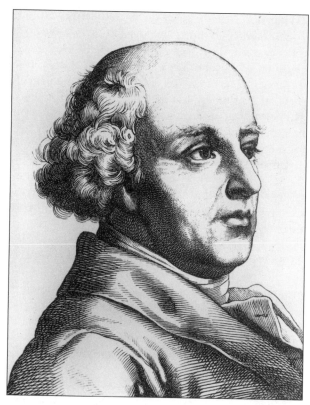

Samuel Hahnemann. (Hulton Archive/Getty Images)

a variety of natural substances (such as silica and vegetable charcoal). In addition, Hahnemann is considered the first person to describe the different disease states as either "acute" (transitory or temporary) or "chronic" (lifelong). He posited that some acute ailments could progress to the chronic state if they were left untreated or treated inappropriately.

Hahnemann was born in Meissen, Saxony. At a young age, he became proficient in many languages, including English, Italian, and French. He worked as a translator and language teacher, while further expanding his own knowledge of additional languages, including Arabic and Hebrew. He attended medical school in both Leipzig and Vienna, before transferring to the University of Erlangen, where he obtained his medical degree in 1779.

Hahnemann worked as a family physician for a few years and as a curator to supplement his income for his expanding family (he would have eleven children). However, becoming increasingly disenchanted with existing medical practices, he stopped practicing medicine in 1784 and worked full-time as a writer and translator of scientific and medical texts. He practiced this profession for a number of years and used it as an opportunity to further explore the shortcomings of medicine and to consider potential solutions. In 1790, while translating *A Treatise on the Materia Medica*, a well-known book by William Cullen, he read about Cullen's belief that the bark (called cinchona) of a Peruvian tree could treat malaria because of its astringency and its ability to strengthen a person's stomach. Equipped with his background in medicine, Hahnemann questioned the reason for the bark's utility and speculated that the bark worked by another mechanism of action.

Hahnemann went on to investigate the antimalaria effect of other astringents, including experiments that involved self-application. (He apparently also included some family members and friends in his various experiments.) After ingesting bark for multiple days, he found that it had caused him to experience malaria-like symptoms (despite the absence of these symptoms before eating the bark).

As a result of this experiment and many others over the course of several years, Hahnemann developed a practical healing system based on what he called the law of similars (or the natural law of "like cured by like"). This system was based on the idea that an item that can produce symptoms in a healthy person can be used to treat a sick person who displays the same symptoms. Hahnemann eventually named this approach homeopathy, a term that was first used in an article he published in 1807. Hahnemann studied many potential homeopathic substances for much of his career, meticulously recording his experimental methods and results, and ultimately cataloguing those agents useful for medicinal purposes. He also is known for introducing the so-called coffee theory, which posited that many diseases are caused by coffee; he later abandoned this theory.

Hahnemann had three major publications on homeopathy during his lifetime: the first, the *Organon der rationellen Heilkunde* (1810; *Organon of the Art of Healing*, 1833; best known as *Organon of Medicine*), describes the fundamentals of homeopathy; the second, *Materia Medica Pura* (1811; English translation, 1846) details the precise symptoms of certain diseases and the effects of the curative agents used to treat them; and the third, *Die chronischen Krankheiten, ihre eigenthümliche Natur und homöopathische Heilung* (1837; *The Chronic Diseases, Their Specific Nature and*

Their Homeopathic Treatment: Antipsoric Remedies, 1845) describes how certain diseases progress to the chronic state when they fail to be properly treated. These books, especially the first of the three, continue to be used today to educate students of homeopathy.

Throughout his life, Hahnemann practiced and researched homeopathy, taught, and published many articles on the topic. He died of bronchitis in Paris in 1843. A medical center, Hahnemann University Hospital, which is located in Philadelphia, is named in his honor.

Brandy Weidow, M.S.

FURTHER READING

Haehl, Richard. *Life and Work of Samuel Hahnemann.* Translated by Marie L. Wheeler and W. H. R. Grundy. New Delhi, India: B. Jain, 2003. This reference book describes Hahnemann's life, his therapeutic developments, the development of his potencies, and the arguments he had with traditional medical professionals.

Hahnemann, Samuel. *The Chronic Diseases: Their Peculiar Nature and Their Homeopathic Cure.* Charleston, S.C.: BiblioBazaar, 2009. This book is a pre-1923 historical reproduction that has been updated to improve the readability of the original.

_____. *Organon of the Medical Art.* Edited by Wenda Brewster O'Reilly and Jeremy Sherr. Palo Alto, Calif.: Birdcage Books, 1996. A new translation of one of Hahnemann's first books, with annotations and updated editing. The original book, published in 1810, is considered to be a cornerstone of homeopathy. This updated version preserves Hahnemann's voice but contains updated language for modern general readers.

See also: Homeopathy: Overview.

Hawthorn

CATEGORY: Herbs and supplements

RELATED TERM: *Crataegus oxyacantha*

DEFINITION: Natural plant product used to treat specific health conditions.

PRINCIPAL PROPOSED USE: Congestive heart failure

OTHER PROPOSED USES: Benign heart palpitations, high blood pressure, orthostatic hypotension

OVERVIEW

The name "hawthorn" is derived from "hedgethorn," reflecting this spiny tree's use as a type of living fence in much of Europe. Besides protecting estates from trespassers, hawthorn has also been used medicinally since ancient times. Roman physicians used hawthorn as a heart drug in the first century C.E., but most of the literature from that period focuses on its symbolic use for religious rites and political ceremonies.

During the Middle Ages, hawthorn was used for the treatment of dropsy, a condition now called congestive heart failure (CHF). It was also used for treating other heart ailments and for treating sore throat.

THERAPEUTIC DOSAGES

The usual dosage of hawthorn is 300 to 600 milligrams (mg) three times daily of an extract standardized to contain about 2 to 3 percent flavonoids or 18 to 20 percent procyanidins. Studies indicate that full effects may take up to six months to develop, although some improvement should be apparent much sooner.

THERAPEUTIC USES

Meaningful evidence indicates that hawthorn is a safe and effective treatment for CHF. Like other treatments used for CHF, hawthorn improves the heart's pumping ability. It also may offer some important advantages over certain conventional drugs used for this condition.

Digoxin, as well as other medications that increase the power of the heart, also make the heart more susceptible to dangerous irregularities of rhythm (arrhythmias). In contrast, preliminary evidence indicates that hawthorn may have the unusual property of both strengthening the heart and stabilizing it against arrhythmias.

It is thought to do so by lengthening what is called the refractory period: the short period following a heartbeat during which the heart cannot beat again. Many irregularities of heart rhythm begin with an early beat. Digoxin shortens the refractory period, making such a premature beat more likely, while hawthorn protects against such potentially dangerous breaks in the heart's even rhythm.

Another advantage of hawthorn is its lower toxicity. With digoxin, the difference between the proper dosage and the toxic dosage is dangerously small. Hawthorn has an enormous range of safe dosing.

However, keep in mind that digoxin is itself an outdated drug. There are a great many newer drugs for CHF, such as angiotensin-converting enzyme (ACE) inhibitors, that are much more effective than digoxin. Many of these have been proven to prolong life in people with advanced CHF. There is no reliable evidence that hawthorn offers the same benefit, although one large study found tantalizing hints that it might. One small study concluded that it may be safe to combine hawthorn and digoxin, but whether hawthorn interacts safely with other heart drugs remains to be determined.

Finally, CHF is simply too dangerous a condition to rely solely on self-treatment. People who have CHF should not use hawthorn except under close physician supervision.

In addition to CHF, hawthorn is sometimes used as a treatment for annoying heart palpitations that have been thoroughly evaluated and found to be harmless. Common symptoms include occasional thumping, as well as episodes of racing heartbeat. These may occur without any identifiable cause and may not require any medical treatment, except for purposes of comfort. However, there is no evidence that hawthorn is effective for this purpose. Furthermore, because there are many dangerous kinds of heart palpitations, it is absolutely necessary for individuals to get a thorough checkup first. It is only worth considering hawthorn as a treatment for palpitations if a doctor tells a patient that he or she has no medically significant heart problems.

Hawthorn is sometimes recommended for the treatment of high blood pressure, but its effects appear to be marginal at best. Furthermore, there is some evidence that a combination herbal treatment made from hawthorn and camphor can help prevent the sudden fall in blood pressure that may occur on standing up from a sitting or lying position (orthosatic hypotension). In these studies, the mixture acted to increase blood pressure.

Hawthorn has also been tried for other heart-related conditions, such as angina and atherosclerosis in general. However, there is no reliable evidence to support these uses.

SCIENTIFIC EVIDENCE

Several reasonable-quality, double-blind, placebo-controlled trials, involving a total of more than 750 participants, have found hawthorn effective for the

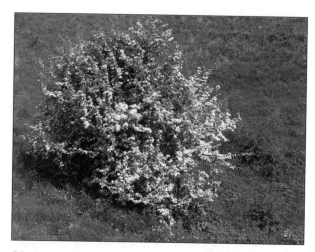

Meaningful evidence indicates that hawthorn is a safe and effective treatment for congestive heart failure (CHF). (Adrian Bicker/Photo Researchers, Inc.)

treatment of mild to moderate congestive heart failure. In one of the best of these studies, 209 people with relatively advanced congestive heart failure (technically, New York Heart Association [NYHA] class III) were given either 900 mg or 1,800 mg of standardized hawthorn extract or matching placebo. The results after sixteen weeks of therapy showed significant improvements in the hawthorn groups, compared with the placebo groups. Benefits in the high-dose hawthorn group included a reduction in subjective symptoms, as well as an increase in exercise capacity. Subjective symptoms improved to a similar degree in the lower-dose hawthorn group, but there was no improvement in exercise capacity.

In an analysis that mathematically combined the results of ten controlled trials involving 855 patients, hawthorn extract was found to be significantly better than placebo for improving exercise tolerance, decreasing shortness of breath and fatigue, and enhancing the physiologic function of an ailing heart in mild to moderate CHF. In another study, however, researchers found that persons with mild-to-moderate CHF taking a special extract of hawthorn, 900 mg daily, were more likely to experience an initial worsening of their condition compared to those taking a placebo. By the end of six months, however, there was no difference in the two groups. In light of numerous other studies supporting the safety and effectiveness of hawthorn in CHF, the results of this special extract study need to be repeated before drawing any firm conclusions.

A comparative study suggests that hawthorn extract (900 mg) is about as effective as a low dose of the conventional drug captopril. However, while captopril and other standard drugs in the same family have been shown to help reduce hospitalizations and mortality associated with CHF, there is no similar evidence for hawthorn.

SAFETY ISSUES

Hawthorn appears to be generally safe. Germany's Commission E lists no known risks, contraindications, or drug interactions with hawthorn, and mice and rats have been given very large doses without showing significant toxicity. In clinical trials, reported side effects were relatively rare and nonspecific, consisting primarily of mild dizziness, stomach upset, headache, and occasional allergic reactions (skin rash).

Perhaps the biggest risk with hawthorn is that using it instead of conventional treatment might increase risk of death or other complications of CHF. In addition, it is not known whether hawthorn can be safely combined with other drugs that affect the heart. Therefore, individuals should not self-treat CHF with hawthorn; a physician's supervision is essential.

Safety in young children, pregnant or nursing women, or those with severe liver, heart, or kidney disease has not been established. Taking hawthorn could cause problems for people who are simultaneously using any medications that affect the heart.

EBSCO CAM Review Board

FURTHER READING

Daniele, C., et al. "Adverse-Event Profile of *Crataegus* SPP." *Drug Safety* 29 (2006): 523-535.

Degenring, F. H., et al. "A Randomised Double-Blind. Placebo-Controlled Clinical Trial of a Standardised Extract of Fresh Crataegus Berries (Crataegisan) in the Treatment of Patients with Congestive Heart Failure." *Phytomedicine* 10 (2003): 363-369.

Tankanow, R., et al. "Interaction Study Between Digoxin and a Preparation of Hawthorn (*Crataegus oxyacantha*)." *Journal of Clinical Pharmacology* 43 (2003): 637-642.

Walker, A. F., et al. "Hypotensive Effects of Hawthorn for Patients with Diabetes Taking Prescription Drugs." *British Journal of General Practice* 56 (2006): 437-443.

Zick, S. M., et al. "The Effect of *Crataegus oxyantha* Special Extract WS 1442 on Clinical Progression in Patients with Mild to Moderate Symptoms of Heart Failure." *European Journal of Heart Failure* 10, no. 6 (2008): 587-593.

See also: Arrhythmia; Congestive heart failure; Digoxin; Hypertension.

Headache, cluster

CATEGORY: Condition
DEFINITION: Treatment of severe headaches that strike suddenly after a long time without an episode.
PRINCIPAL PROPOSED NATURAL TREATMENTS: None
OTHER PROPOSED NATURAL TREATMENTS: Hyperbaric oxygen therapy, magnesium, melatonin

INTRODUCTION

First recognized in 1867, cluster headaches remain one of the most painful and frustrating headache syndromes. Their cause is unclear, and no treatment is fully effective. People with cluster headaches may go for more than one year without any attacks and then suddenly have headaches that strike several times a day. Each headache lasts from thirty minutes to two hours and consists of severe pain on one side of the head, generally in the region of the eye. These daily headaches continue for four to eight weeks and then disappear for another year or more. A more chronic, continuous form of cluster headaches can also occur.

Cluster headaches are different from migraine headaches (although they may possess some underlying similarities) and are much more difficult to treat. During cluster headache episodes, rapid-acting treatments are usually used to ease pain and stop the headache. Treatments include aerosolized ergotamine, pure oxygen, lidocaine nasal spray, and anesthetic inhalation. For prevention, drugs such as ergotamine, prednisone, methysergide, and lithium may reduce the severity and frequency of attacks.

PROPOSED NATURAL TREATMENTS

Some evidence suggests that people with cluster headaches have lower than average levels of the hormone melatonin. In a double-blind, placebo-controlled study of twenty people with cluster headaches, the use of melatonin (10 milligrams daily) for fourteen days significantly reduced headache severity or frequency (or both) compared with placebo. About one-half the participants given melatonin responded well to the treatment.

The inhalation of 100 percent oxygen is sometimes used to treat cluster headache attacks. In preliminary controlled trials, the use of hyperbaric oxygen (oxygen under pressure) not only treated the headaches but also helped prevent further attacks. The intravenous use of magnesium has shown promise for cluster headache relief. However, the use of oral magnesium has not been evaluated.

EBSCO CAM Review Board

FURTHER READING

Di Sabato, F., and M. Giacovazzo et al. "Effect of Hyperbaric Oxygen on the Immunoreactivity to Substance P in the Nasal Mucosa of Cluster Headache Patients." *Headache* 36 (1996): 221-223.

Di Sabato, F., and M. Rocco et al. "Hyperbaric Oxygen in Chronic Cluster Headaches: Influence on Serotonergic Pathways." *Undersea Hyperbaric Medicine* 24 (1997): 117-122.

Jena, S., et al. "Acupuncture in Patients with Headache." *Cephalalgia* 28 (2008): 969-979.

Leone, M., et al. "Melatonin Versus Placebo in the Prophylaxis of Cluster Headache." *Cephalalgia* 16 (1996): 494-496.

Mauskop, A., et al. "Intravenous Magnesium Sulfate Rapidly Alleviates Headaches of Various Types." *Headache* 36 (1996): 154-160.

Nestoriuc, Y., et al. "Biofeedback Treatment for Headache Disorders." *Applied Psychophysiology and Biofeedback* 33 (2008): 125-140.

See also: Acupressure; Acupuncture; Headache, tension; Magnesium; Melatonin; Migraines; Pain management; Premenstrual syndrome (PMS); Stress.

Headache, tension

CATEGORY: Condition

DEFINITION: Treatment of aching, dull, and throbbing pain most commonly felt in the forehead, temples, and base of the skull.

PRINCIPAL PROPOSED NATURAL TREATMENTS: Acupuncture, chiropractic

OTHER PROPOSED NATURAL TREATMENTS: Aromatherapy; body-mind therapies such as biofeedback, hypnosis, relaxation therapies, and therapeutic touch; butterbur; 5-hydroxytryptophan; massage; osteopathic manipulation; prolotherapy

HERBS AND SUPPLEMENTS TO AVOID: Kava

INTRODUCTION

Modern life is stressful, and tension headaches are one result of that stress. People with such headaches often describe a sensation like a tight band around the head; this band may in fact exist as a contracted muscle. Other characteristics of tension headache include aching, dull, or throbbing pain, usually concentrated in the forehead, temples, or base of the skull. Symptoms may overlap those of migraine, cluster, or sinus headaches, and medical advice may be necessary to distinguish among them.

Medical treatment for tension headaches generally involves the use of nonsteroidal anti-inflammatory drugs and sometimes muscle relaxants. Physicians may also recommend physical therapy techniques in hopes of addressing the causes of tension headaches, such as muscle tension in the neck or jaw.

PRINCIPAL PROPOSED NATURAL TREATMENTS

Both acupuncture and chiropractic have undergone significant evaluation as treatments for tension headaches.

Acupuncture. Placebo-controlled studies of acupuncture for tension headaches have yielded mixed results. One study compared six sessions of traditional acupuncture with sham acupuncture in eighteen people with chronic tension headache. The real treatment caused a 31 percent reduction in pain and was found to be significantly more effective than placebo. A study of twenty-nine students with various types of headaches found that a single acupuncture treatment decreased the number of days during which headaches occurred and the total use of medications. A statistically insignificant reduction in the number of days of attacks was seen in the placebo group.

Another study enrolled forty-three children with headaches (migraine or tension) and compared laser acupuncture with placebo laser acupuncture. An individualized treatment approach based on the principles of traditional Chinese medicine was used. The results indicated that the use of real laser acupuncture was statistically more effective than placebo acupuncture. In a large randomized trial involving 3,182 headache patients, the group that received fifteen individualized acupuncture sessions in three months experienced significantly fewer headache days and less pain compared to the group receiving usual care. However, despite its large size and positive results, this study did not include a placebo group.

On the negative side, a study of thirty-nine participants with a tension headache found no convincing evidence that acupuncture was helpful. In addition, a single-blind study of fifty participants with tension headache found that a special brief-acupuncture style given once a week for six weeks did not reduce headache frequency. Several other trials also failed to find evidence of benefit with various forms of acupuncture.

In a 2008 analysis of five randomized controlled trials that were considered highest in quality, researchers determined that real acupuncture has limited effectiveness over sham acupuncture for tension headache. While it is clear that many headache patients benefit from acupuncture, at present it is unclear whether or not this represents more than a placebo effect.

Chiropractic spinal manipulation. Neck tension can cause tension and pain in the head. Such cervicogenic headaches overlap closely with tension headaches. Chiropractic spinal manipulation has shown some promise for these conditions, but the evidence is incomplete and somewhat contradictory.

In a controlled trial of 150 participants, investigators compared spinal manipulation to the drug amitriptyline for the treatment of chronic tension-type headaches. By the end of the six-week treatment period, participants in both groups had improved similarly. However, four weeks after treatment was stopped, people who had received spinal manipulation showed statistically better reduction in headache intensity and frequency and used fewer over-the-counter medications than those who had used the amitriptyline.

In another positive trial, fifty-three participants with cervicogenic headaches received chiropractic spinal manipulation or laser acupuncture plus massage. Chiropractic manipulation was more effective. However, a similar study of seventy-five participants with recurrent tension headaches found no difference between the two groups. Other, smaller studies of spinal manipulation have been reported too, with mixed results.

In a later controlled trial, two hundred people with cervicogenic headaches were randomly assigned to

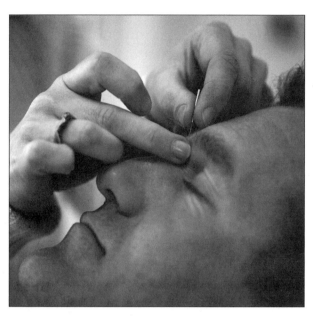

Acupuncture is being used here to treat a tension headache. (Chris Knapton/Photo Researchers, Inc.)

receive one of four therapies: manipulation, a special exercise technique, exercise plus manipulation, or no therapy. Each participant received a minimum of eight to twelve treatments in a six-week period. All three treatment approaches produced better results than no treatment, and all had approximately the same effect. While these results may sound promising, in fact they prove nothing, since any treatment will generally produce better results than no treatment because of the power of suggestion. Ordinarily, researchers get around this problem by using double-blind, placebo-controlled trials. While it is not possible to do a truly double-blind trial of chiropractic, the better foregoing trials used a form of placebo treatment, making them more reliable than this one.

OTHER PROPOSED NATURAL TREATMENTS

A number of other alternative treatments have undergone some evaluation for their usefulness in the treatment of tension headaches.

Several techniques in the category of body-mind medicine have shown promise. These techniques include hypnosis, biofeedback, and relaxation techniques, often used with each other. In a careful review of multiple controlled studies, researchers concluded that biofeedback is useful for tension

Using Acupuncture for Pain

Acupuncture, among the oldest healing practices in the world, is a form of traditional Chinese medicine. Acupuncture practitioners stimulate specific points on the body, most often by inserting thin needles through the skin. In traditional Chinese medicine theory, this stimulation regulates the flow of qi (vital energy) along pathways known as meridians.

According to the 2007 U.S. National Health Interview Survey (NHIS), which included a comprehensive survey of complementary and alternative medicine use by Americans, 1.4 percent of respondents (an estimated 3.1 million persons) said they had used acupuncture in the year preceding the study. A special analysis of acupuncture data from an earlier NHIS found that pain or musculoskeletal complaints accounted for seven of the top ten conditions for which people use acupuncture. Back pain was the most common, followed by joint pain, neck pain, severe headache, migraine headache, and recurring pain.

headaches, particularly when combined with other relaxation therapies. Another review of twenty control trials found psychological interventions, such as cognitive behavioral therapy, biofeedback, relaxation, and coping strategies, to be associated with reduced chronic headache or migraine pain in 589 children. These treatments were compared with placebo, standard treatment, waiting list control, or other active treatments.

A topical ointment known as Tiger Balm is a popular remedy for headaches, muscle pain, and other conditions. Tiger Balm contains the aromatic substances camphor, menthol, cajuput, and clove oil, making it a form of aromatherapy. A double-blind study enrolling fifty-seven people with acute tension headache compared Tiger Balm (applied to the forehead) with placebo ointment and with the drug acetaminophen (Tylenol). The placebo ointment contained mint essence to make it smell like Tiger Balm. Real Tiger Balm proved more effective than placebo. In addition, it was just as effective as acetaminophen and acted more rapidly. Another form of aromatherapy, peppermint oil applied to the forehead, has also shown promise, but studies remain highly preliminary.

Therapeutic touch is a form of energy healing popular in the American nursing community. In a blinded study, sixty participants with tension headaches were randomly assigned to receive either therapeutic touch or a placebo form of the therapy. The true therapy proved to be more effective than placebo.

A study of twenty-eight people with tension headaches compared one session of osteopathic manipulation to two forms of sham treatment and found evidence that the real treatment provided a greater improvement in headache pain. Prolotherapy, massage, and reflexology (a special form of massage) have all been recommended for the treatment of tension headaches, but there is little evidence to support their use.

The herb butterbur is thought to have antispasmodic and anti-inflammatory properties, making it potentially useful for tension headaches. The supplement 5-hydroxytryptophan (5-HTP) has shown some promise for migraine headaches. However, an eight-week, double-blind, placebo-controlled trial of sixty-five people with tension headaches found that 5-HTP did not significantly reduce the number of headaches experienced. It did, however, reduce participants' need to use other pain-relieving medications.

HERBS AND SUPPLEMENTS TO AVOID

The herb kava is sometimes suggested as a muscle relaxant and stress reducer. However, there is no meaningful evidence that kava is effective for tension headaches (or any form of muscle tension), and it has been taken off the market in many countries for safety reasons: Its use has been linked with severe liver damage. Finally, numerous herbs and supplements may interact adversely with prescription drugs used to treat tension headaches.

EBSCO CAM Review Board

FURTHER READING

Astin, J., and E. Ernst. "The Effectiveness of Spinal Manipulation for the Treatment of Headache Disorders." *Cephalalgia* 22 (2002): 617-623.

Davis, M. A., et al. "Acupuncture for Tension-Type Headache." *Journal of Pain* 9 (2008): 667-677.

Eccleston, C., et al. "Psychological Therapies for the Management of Chronic and Recurrent Pain in Children and Adolescents." *Cochrane Database of Systematic Reviews* (2009): CD003968. Available through *EBSCO DynaMed Systematic Literature Surveillance* at http://www.ebscohost.com/dynamed.

Gottschling, S., et al. "Laser Acupuncture in Children with Headache." *Pain* 137 (2008): 405-412.

Jena, S., et al. "Acupuncture in Patients with Head-ache." *Cephalalgia* 28 (2008): 969-979.

Nestoriuc, Y., W. Rief, and A. Martin. "Meta-analysis of Biofeedback for Tension-Type Headache: Efficacy, Specificity, and Treatment Moderators." *Journal of Consulting and Clinical Psychology* 76 (2008): 379-396.

See also: Acupuncture; Chiropractic.

Head injury: Homeopathic remedies

CATEGORY: Homeopathy

DEFINITION: Homeopathic treatment of injuries to the head, including the brain.

STUDIED HOMEOPATHIC REMEDIES: *Arnica, Natrum sulph*

INTRODUCTION

Injury to the head is one of the most feared complications of vehicle and bicycle accidents and other forms of trauma, primarily because it can lead to temporary or permanent impairment of brain function. In many cases, complete recovery does occur, but only after many months or even years of care and therapy. In other cases, mental and physical deficits continue for the rest of the injured person's life, despite intensive therapy and medical care. One should never rely on homeopathic remedies as the sole treatment for head injury. A physician evaluation is essential to treat this type of emergency.

SCIENTIFIC EVALUATIONS OF HOMEOPATHIC REMEDIES

A four-month, double-blind, placebo-controlled pilot study of fifty people evaluated the effects of a constitutional, or classical, homeopathic remedy in the treatment of mild head injury. The results, however, were not impressive.

The investigators recruited the participants from a clinic that specializes in the treatment of head injuries. All participants were evaluated according to classical homeopathic principles and assigned an individualized remedy at 200c (centesimal) potency. Then, one-half of the participants were randomly assigned to received placebo instead of the prescribed

remedy. However, after four months of treatment, most of the assessment techniques used to evaluate rate of recovery failed to indicate any benefits in the treated group compared with the placebo group.

TRADITIONAL HOMEOPATHIC TREATMENTS

Classical homeopathy offers other homeopathic treatments for head injury. These therapies are chosen based on specific details of the person seeking treatment. The homeopathic remedy *Arnica* is commonly utilized for any form of trauma, including concussion and head injury. *Natrum sulph* may be used when head injury is accompanied by difficulty breathing.

EBSCO CAM Review Board

FURTHER READING

Chapman, E. H., et al. "Homeopathic Treatment of Mild Traumatic Brain Injury." *Journal of Head Trauma Rehabilitation* 14 (1999): 521-542.

Ludtke, R., and D. Hacke. "On the Effectiveness of the Homeopathic Remedy *Arnica montana*." *Wiener Medizinische Wochenschrift* 155 (2006): 482-490.

Oberbaum, M., et al. "Homeopathy in Emergency Medicine." *Wiener Medizinische Wochenschrift* 155 (2005): 491-497.

Zuzak, T. J., et al. "Medicinal Systems of Complementary and Alternative Medicine: A Cross-Sectional Survey at a Pediatric Emergency Department." *Journal of Alternative and Complementary Medicine* 16 (2010): 473-479.

See also: Homeopathy; Injuries, minor; Sports and fitness support: Enhancing recovery; Sports-related injuries: Homeopathic remedies.

Health freedom movement

CATEGORY: Issues and overviews

RELATED TERMS: Antiaging medicine, Codex Alimentarius, Dietary Supplement Health and Education Act, European Union Food Supplements Directive, megavitamin therapy, naturopathic medicine, orthomolecular medicine

DEFINITION: A collective of organizations, consumers, activists, product manufacturers, and medical practitioners campaigning worldwide for unregulated access to health care.

OVERVIEW

The term "health freedom movement" gained currency in the United States during the 1990s amid public debate about proposed legislation concerning dietary supplements. The Dietary Supplement Health and Education Act (DSHEA) was signed into law in 1994 by U.S. president Bill Clinton, who welcomed the act as a victory for consumers. DSHEA did represent a significant step forward for freedom of choice in health care. Putting the onus on the U.S. Federal Drug Administration (FDA) to prove a given supplement's potential danger, rather than obliging supplement manufacturers to provide proof of their products' safety and efficacy, the legislation largely exempted dietary supplements from federal regulation.

As always, the health freedom movement made for strange bedfellows. DSHEA had been supported by both Democratic senator Tom Harkin and conservative Republican senator Orrin Hatch. More recently, the health freedom movement has been embraced in the United States by the Texas free market libertarian representative and presidential candidate Ron Paul and in Great Britain by the heir to the throne, Prince Charles.

One reason the movement remains so decentralized is that its primary goal is opposition to regulation, which is by definition site-specific. Another is that the movement is adamantly opposed to centralization, which is viewed as inimical to the very notion of choice. Trade blocs, it is argued, tend to promote the interests of business, particularly those of agribusiness and the pharmaceutical industry, over those of individual countries and their citizens. Of particular concern is the Codex Alimentarius Commission, a body established in 1963 by the United Nations. The stated goals of the commission are protecting consumer health and ensuring fair trade practices in international food trade. In 2005, the commission adopted the Codex Alimentarius, guidelines for standardization of dietary supplements that quickly raised the suspicions of the health freedom movement, suspicions that were fueled by the European Union's (EU) adoption of the Food Supplements Directive (2002), aimed at tightening rules concerning sales of vitamins and other dietary supplements.

KEY OBJECTIVES

The movement strives for freedom of choice in every area of health care, including mainstream and conventional medical treatments. Nonetheless, activists driving the movement tend to favor medical alternatives such as orthomolecular therapy and naturopathic medicine. Unfettered access to all manner of vitamins, minerals, herbs, and other supplements unites them, as does their general mistrust of pharmaceutical manufacturers. Like advocates of antiaging medicine, health freedom activists argue for the nutritional prevention and treatment of chronic diseases, advocating the use of, for example, high dosages of vitamins C and E, despite a dearth of research supporting such therapies. Any restrictions on supplements are viewed as favoring the pharmaceutical industry, which many believe has a vested interest not in promoting public health but in perpetuating disease.

A corollary to the movement's demands for freedom of choice in nutrition is its belief that persons should be free to opt out of overarching government health programs, such as water fluoridation, mandatory childhood vaccination, national electronic health records, and the sharing of genetic information without patient consent. In March 2007, then Virginia governor Tim Kaine signed legislation allowing state citizens over the age of fourteen to refuse medical treatment for ailments such as cancer, heralding a victory for health freedom. In 2010, the states of Idaho and Tennessee passed legislation challenging a new federal mandate requiring uninsured citizens to purchase health insurance; these laws, too, are by-products of the health freedom movement. Skeptics claim, however, that such victories are hollow and pernicious.

Because the movement cannot legitimately pursue its goals in what would otherwise be the proper forum (science), health freedom turns to the political arena. Laws like the foregoing, critics argue, succeed only in further disenfranchising sick, poor, frightened, and desperate persons who pursue unproven medical treatments not because they wish to exercise their freedom of choice but because they have, or have been led to believe they have, no other options.

Lisa Paddock, Ph.D.

FURTHER READING

Alliance for Natural Health International. http://www.anhinternational.org. An organization based in the United Kingdom that was originally founded to challenge the European Union's Food Supplements Directive.

Institute for Health Freedom. http://www.forhealth-freedom.org. A think tank established in 1996 and dedicated to promoting public policies supporting personal choice in health care in the United States.

Miller, Kevin P. *We Become Silent: The Last Days of Health Freedom* (2005). A short documentary film about health freedom directed by Kevin Miller, a longtime movement activist whose 1994 film *Let Truth Be the Bias* helped to marshal public support for the DSHEA Act in the United States. Available at http://video.google.com/videoplay?docid=451097355502728465#.

Walker, Martin J. "A Bibliographic History of the Health Freedom Movement." Available at http://www.laleva.org/eng/2005/08/martin_walker_a_bibliographic_history_of_the_health_freedom_movement.html. This Web-based bibliographic essay is a rare extended written narrative about the health freedom movement.

See also: American Academy of Anti-Aging Medicine; Codex Alimentarius Commission; Dietary Supplement Health and Education Act of 1994; Insurance coverage; National Health Federation; Naturopathy; Orthomolecular medicine; Popular Health movement; Vitamins and minerals.

Hearing loss

CATEGORY: Condition

RELATED TERMS: Age-related hearing loss, idiopathic sudden hearing loss, noise-induced hearing loss, presbycusis, sudden hearing loss, unilateral idiopathic sudden hearing loss

DEFINITION: Prevention of hearing loss and treatment of the inability to hear.

PRINCIPAL PROPOSED NATURAL TREATMENTS

- *Prevention of noise-induced hearing loss:* Magnesium
- *Treatment of sudden hearing loss:* Ginkgo

OTHER PROPOSED NATURAL TREATMENT: Lipoic acid

INTRODUCTION

There are many possible causes of hearing loss, ranging from wax in the ear canal to problems with the nerves that receive sound and transmit it to the brain. Two of the most common causes are age-related hearing loss (presbycusis) and noise-induced hearing loss. The treatment for hearing loss depends on its cause, and for this reason, one should consult a doctor. This article discusses a few herbs and supplements that have shown promise for various forms of hearing loss.

PRINCIPAL PROPOSED NATURAL TREATMENTS

Two natural treatments have been evaluated in double-blind, placebo-controlled trials for the prevention or treatment of hearing loss: magnesium and *Ginkgo biloba*.

Magnesium for preventing noise-induced hearing loss. Long-term exposure to loud sounds, such as gunfire or rock music, can cause permanent hearing loss. A two-month, double-blind, placebo-controlled study of three hundred military recruits found daily supplementation with magnesium helped protect the ear from noise-induced damage. The dosage used in this study was quite small–only 167 milligrams (mg) of magnesium daily–but tests showed that even this amount was sufficient to raise magnesium levels inside cells and apparently protect the ear from damage. Soldiers who received the magnesium were less likely to experience permanent hearing damage than those in the placebo group, and when they did experience hearing damage, it was less severe.

It is not clear how magnesium might protect hearing. Studies in animals suggest that magnesium deficiency can increase the stress on cells involved with hearing and thereby make them more susceptible to damage caused by intense noise. However, human magnesium deficiency is believed to be rare, so it is possible that supplemental magnesium acts in some entirely different way.

Only the use of noise-reduction devices (such as headsets that block sound) has been proven effective for preventing noise-induced hearing loss, and the forgoing study does not indicate that magnesium supplements can replace this effective approach. However, the study suggests that a safe, low dose of magnesium may add an additional level of protection.

Ginkgo for treating sudden hearing loss. Some people develop hearing loss suddenly, usually in one ear. This condition is called unilateral idiopathic sudden hearing loss. Its cause is unknown, but problems with circulation may play a role in some cases. The herb *Ginkgo biloba* is thought to increase circulation, and for this reason it has been tried as a treatment for this condition.

In a double-blind, placebo-controlled trial, 106 participants with a carefully defined form of sudden

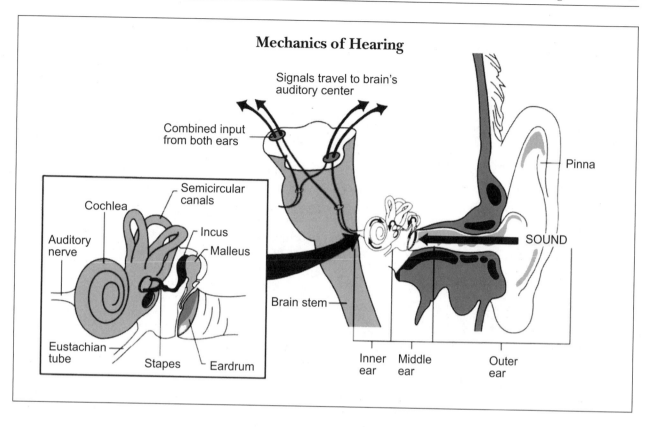

Mechanics of Hearing

hearing loss were given either a full dose of ginkgo extract (120 milligrams [mg] twice daily) or a low dose of the herb (12 mg twice daily). The lower dose was chosen in the belief that it could not possibly offer any benefit and would therefore serve as placebo. However, researchers were surprised to find that most participants in each group recovered by the end of the eight-week trial. There are two possibilities to explain this: low-dose ginkgo is effective, or many people with sudden hearing loss recover on their own anyway.

Because both groups improved to such a great extent, the overall results of the trial did not prove ginkgo effective. An exploratory look at the data provided some hints that high-dose ginkgo may have helped ensure full recovery, but for statistical reasons these hints cannot be taken as proof.

Another double-blind study compared ginkgo to pentoxifylline, a circulation-enhancing drug used in Germany for the treatment of sudden hearing loss. The results indicate that ginkgo was at least as effective as the medication. However, because pentoxifylline itself is not a proven treatment for this condition, the results prove little. Additional research will be necessary to discover whether ginkgo is actually effective for sudden hearing loss

OTHER PROPOSED NATURAL TREATMENTS

A study in animals suggests that the supplement lipoic acid might help prevent age-related hearing loss. Another animal study suggests that melatonin may help prevent hearing loss induced by noise.

Free radicals are naturally occurring substances that cause damage to many parts of the body, including the ear. Antioxidants are substances that fight free radicals. Antioxidant supplements have shown promise for preventing various forms of hearing loss, including age-related hearing loss and hearing damage caused by medications. Commonly used antioxidants include citrus bioflavonoids, coenzyme Q_{10}, lipoic acid, lutein, lycopene, oligomeric proanthocyanidins, vitamin C, and vitamin E.

Other natural treatments sometimes used for various forms of hearing loss, but which lack meaningful scientific support, include folate, manganese, myrrh, potassium, zinc, and vitamins B_1, B_2, B_6, and B_{12}.

EBSCO CAM Review Board

FURTHER READING

Blakley, B. W., et al. "Strategies for Prevention of Toxicity Caused by Platinum-Based Chemotherapy." *Laryngoscope* 112 (2002): 1997-2001.

Burschka, M. A., et al. "Effect of Treatment with *Ginkgo biloba* Extract EGb 761 (Oral) on Unilateral Idiopathic Sudden Hearing Loss in a Prospective Randomized Double-Blind Study of 106 Outpatients." *European Archives of Oto-Rhino-Laryngology* 258 (2001): 213-219.

Henderson, D., et al. "The Role of Antioxidants in Protection from Impulse Noise." *Annals of the New York Academy of Sciences* 884 (November 28, 1999): 368-380.

Karlidag, T., et al. "The Role of Free Oxygen Radicals in Noise Induced Hearing Loss: Effects of Melatonin and Methylprednisolone." *Auris Nasus Larynx* 29 (2002): 147-152.

Reisser, C. H., and H. Weidauer. "*Ginkgo biloba* Extract EGb 761W or Pentoxifylline for the Treatment of Sudden Deafness." *Acta Otolaryngologica* 121 (2001): 579-584.

Seidman, M. D. "Effects of Dietary Restriction and Antioxidants on Presbyacusis." *Laryngoscope* 110 (2000): 727-738.

_____, et al. "Biologic Activity of Mitochondrial Metabolites on Aging and Age-Related Hearing Loss." *American Journal of Otolaryngology* 21 (2000): 161-167.

See also: Aging; Ear infections; Elder health; Ginkgo; Lipoic acid; Magnesium; Tinnitus.

Heart attack

CATEGORY: Condition
RELATED TERM: Myocardial infarction
DEFINITION: Treatment of the acute condition caused by blocked blood flow to the heart.
PRINCIPAL PROPOSED NATURAL TREATMENTS: Natural treatments for atherosclerosis, high cholesterol, high blood pressure, and high homocysteine
OTHER PROPOSED NATURAL TREATMENTS: Antioxidants (such as vitamin A, vitamin C, vitamin E, and beta-carotene), arginine, coenzyme Q_{10}, fish oil, garlic oil, glycine, hawthorn, inosine, L-carnitine, lifestyle modification, lipoic acid, red yeast rice, selenium

PROBABLY INEFFECTIVE TREATMENTS: Chelation therapy, magnesium

INTRODUCTION

As an active muscle, the heart needs a continuous supply of oxygen. The coronary arteries have the job of carrying oxygen to the heart. These arteries have a difficult job to do because they undergo intense compression every time the heart beats. This job becomes even more difficult when the arteries are damaged by atherosclerosis (commonly, though not quite accurately, called hardening of the arteries) in a condition called coronary artery disease.

In coronary artery disease, the passages inside the coronary arteries become narrowed by plaque deposits, which decreases blood flow. When the blood flow is decreased to a sufficient extent, pain caused by oxygen deprivation occurs. This pain is known as angina pectoris. Angina tends to wax and wane, generally worsening with exercise.

A heart attack may occur after years of angina or with no warning. Most heart attacks occur when a blood clot (thrombus) forms on the roughened wall of an atherosclerotic coronary artery. Such a blood clot may lead to a sudden and complete blockage of the artery. More rarely, a spasm of a coronary artery may cut off blood flow. In either case, the cells of the heart fed by that artery begin to die. The region of dead cells is called an infarct, leading to the technical name for a heart attack: myocardial infarction (MI).

The classic symptom of a heart attack is intense, central chest pressure. Other common symptoms include pain or heaviness in the left arm, nausea, shortness of breath, increased perspiration, and a feeling of impending doom. Many people who have had an MI describe chest discomfort or pain in the jaw, teeth, arm, or abdomen. Women are more likely than men to feel pain in their backs. Often, symptoms appear gradually and are intermittent or vague. One-quarter of persons, more often women and people with diabetes, experience no symptoms.

When a heart attack occurs, emergency treatment at a hospital can minimize the extent of permanent damage to the heart. "Clot busting" drugs, if given soon enough, can open the coronary arteries, allowing blood to flow again. Other methods of restoring blood flow include procedures known as angioplasty, stenting, and bypass surgery. The aim is to save those heart cells that are in danger of dying. Recovery after a

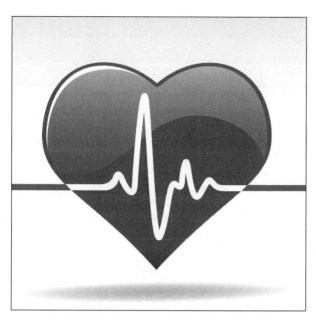

Most heart attacks occur when a blood clot (thrombus) forms on the roughened wall of an atherosclerotic coronary artery. Such a blood clot may lead to a sudden and complete blockage of the artery. (© iStockphoto.com)

heart attack depends on the extent of heart damage. If only a small portion of the heart has died, or if it is in a relatively less important region, symptoms may be slight. More severe damage can cause the heart to pump improperly, leading to congestive heart failure.

During the first several days following a heart attack, the heart has a tendency to lose its normal rhythm and fall into a dysfunctional pattern of beating that does not properly circulate blood. Treatment aimed to prevent or treat this condition, called an arrhythmia, is conducted in a cardiac intensive care unit.

Long-term treatment to reduce the risk of heart attacks generally involves aspirin to prevent blood clots and treatments to slow, stop, or reverse atherosclerosis. The latter is accomplished through the use of medications that keep cholesterol and blood pressure within normal limits and by increasing exercise and improving other aspects of one's lifestyle.

PRINCIPAL PROPOSED NATURAL TREATMENTS

The most important contribution of natural medicine in the realm of heart attacks is prevention, not treatment. Atherosclerosis, which causes most heart attacks, is accelerated by high blood pressure and high cholesterol, and possibly by high levels of homocysteine in the blood. Natural treatments used for these conditions are worth considering. However, natural therapies for high blood pressure and high cholesterol are generally less effective than the conventional approaches. Persons interested in using natural treatments should first consult with a physician to determine how long it is safe to experiment. If natural therapies have not controlled the heart condition within the prescribed time, it may better to use conventional therapies.

OTHER PROPOSED NATURAL TREATMENTS

Several natural treatments have shown promise for use with conventional treatment in the period following a heart attack. Note, however, that people who have recently had a heart attack should not use any herbs or supplements except under the supervision of a physician. Furthermore, none of these treatments can substitute for standard care; at most, they might be helpful if used in addition to it.

Coenzyme Q_{10}. The supplement coenzyme Q_{10} (CoQ_{10}) is thought to improve heart function. In a double-blind trial, 145 people who had recently experienced a heart attack were given either placebo or 120 milligrams (mg) of CoQ_{10} daily for twenty-eight days. The results showed that participants receiving CoQ_{10} experienced significantly fewer heart-related problems, such as episodes of angina pectoris or arrhythmia, or recurrent heart attacks. CoQ_{10} taken with the mineral selenium has also shown promise for people who have survived a heart attack.

L-carnitine. The amino acid L-carnitine has shown potential value during the first few weeks after an MI. A double-blind, placebo-controlled study that followed 101 people for one month after a heart attack found that the use of L-carnitine, in addition to standard care, reduced the size of the infarct (area of dead heart tissue). Other complications of heart attack were reduced too. Similar benefits also were seen in a one-year, controlled study of 160 people who had just experienced a heart attack; however, because this study was not double-blind, its results are not reliable.

In the months following a severe heart attack, the heart often enlarges and loses function. L-carnitine has shown some potential for helping the first of these complications, but not the second. In a twelve-month, double-blind, placebo-controlled study of 472 people

Fish Oil for Heart Health

Medical interest in fish oil began with the observation that heart disease is extremely rare among the Inuit (Eskimo) people, despite the fact that they consume a great deal of fat. Close investigation showed that the Inuit diet includes high amounts of an unusual type of fat found primarily in cold-water fish, seals, and whales.

This finding led to an enormous amount of scientific investigation into the potential health effects of what came to be called fish oil. However, despite decades of research and hundreds of clinical trials, it has proved difficult to conclusively demonstrate that fish oil does in fact prevent heart disease.

The active ingredients in fish oil are two fats in the omega-3 category: eicosapentaenoic acid (EPA) and docosahexaenoic acid (DHA). Fairly solid evidence indicates that EPA and DHA can reduce levels of triglycerides. A triglyceride is a substance that is related to cholesterol and helps to create the artery-clogging plaque.

Much weaker evidence hints that EPA and DHA might raise HDL (good) cholesterol levels, thin the blood, prevent dangerous heart arrhythmias, slow heart rate, improve blood vessel tone, and decrease blood pressure. All of these effects would be expected to help protect against heart attacks and other forms of heart disease. Studies designed to examine the effects of fish, fish oil, or its component omega-3 fatty acids on the incidence of heart disease have failed to produce consistently positive findings. Some have shown benefit; some have shown no effect; one even found evidence that fish oil could, in certain cases, make heart disease worse.

In 2007, however, the results of a gigantic study were published that appeared to settle the question at last. The heart-protective effects of fish oil had been proven. However, this study had severe design flaws, and because of this, it proves little or nothing.

More than eighteen thousand people were enrolled in the trial. All had high cholesterol, and all were using standard drugs in the statin family to lower their LDL (bad) cholesterol. About one-half of the participants were additionally given 1,800 milligrams of purified EPA daily, while the other one-half were given no extra treatment. Researchers then followed the participants for about five years. What they wanted to know was whether the use of EPA with statins further reduced the rate of major cardiac events (broadly defined to include sudden cardiac death, fatal and nonfatal heart attack, unstable angina, angioplasty, stenting, or coronary artery bypass grafting).

The outcome was quite positive. Participants in the group taking EPA plus statins showed a 19 percent reduction of major cardiac events, compared with those taking statins alone. This was positive, but far short of proof. This study was an open trial, meaning that participants knew whether they were taking the treatment or not taking it. Open trials are notoriously unreliable. Only double-blind studies can actually establish the effectiveness of a medical treatment.

In double-blind, placebo-controlled studies, some participants are given the real treatment while others are given an identical-appearing placebo, and both participants and researchers are kept in the dark (are "blind") as to which is which. The following discussion treats only one of the many possible problems that can occur when a study is not double-blind: the so-called halo effect.

As has been established in thousands of studies, when people know they are being given a treatment in a medical trial, they take better care of themselves in general. They may exercise more, eat a better diet, follow their doctor's advice more closely, and seek medical care for symptoms they might otherwise ignore. The net result can be a dramatic improvement in health that has nothing to do with the treatment under study.

This is not a merely theoretical problem; quite to the contrary, the power of the halo effect is known to be substantial. In this particular study, the entire relative benefit could easily have been caused not by the EPA itself but by the "halo" that surrounded the use of EPA.

The doubt always raised by lack of blinding was further worsened by a specific detail in the outcome of this study: No significant difference between the two groups was seen regarding death rate. It was only in the more subjective, elective case of major cardiac events that EPA showed relative benefit, such as in the frequency of angioplasty procedures. These are relatively subjective outcomes, which are inherently susceptible to psychological influence.

Steven Bratman, M.D.

who had just experienced a heart attack, the use of carnitine at a dose of 6 grams per day significantly decreased the rate of heart enlargement. However, heart function was not improved. A three-month, double-blind, placebo-controlled study of sixty people who had just had a heart attack also failed to find improvements in heart function with L-carnitine. (Heart enlargement was not studied.)

Results consistent with those of the foregoing studies were seen in a six-month, double-blind, placebo-controlled study of 2,330 people who had just had a heart attack. Carnitine failed to produce significant reductions in mortality or heart failure (serious decline in heart function) over the six-month period. However, it did find reductions in early death. (For statistical reasons, the meaningfulness of this last finding is questionable: It was a secondary endpoint rather than a primary one.)

Fish oil. Fish oil contains healthy fats in the omega-3 fatty acid category. Incomplete evidence suggests that fish oil supplements may help prevent heart attacks and prevent sudden death after a heart attack. This benefit may come from a number of fish oil's actions, including preventing dangerous heart arrhythmias and reducing heart rate.

Garlic. In one study, 432 people who had had a heart attack were given either garlic oil extract or no treatment for three years. The results showed a significant reduction of second heart attacks and about a 50 percent reduction in death rate among those taking garlic. People who take aspirin to prevent heart attacks should not take garlic supplements, as the combination could lead to excessive bleeding.

Red yeast rice. Because of its purported ability to lower cholesterol, red yeast rice (made by fermenting a type of yeast called *Monascus purpureus* over rice) has been studied in persons with heart disease. A double-blind study in China compared an alcohol extract of red yeast rice (Xuezhikang) with placebo in almost five thousand people with heart disease. In the four-year study period, the use of the supplement reportedly reduced the heart attack rate by about 45 percent compared with placebo, and total mortality was reduced by about 35 percent. At least three other studies, all from this same original population of participants, have found similar results in diabetics with heart disease and in persons with a previous heart attack, with surprisingly large reductions in the rates of coronary events (such as heart attack) and mortality. These levels of reported benefit, however, are so high and so similar as to raise questions about their reliability.

Antioxidants. Antioxidant supplements help neutralize free radicals, which are dangerous, naturally occurring chemicals that may accelerate heart cell death following a heart attack (among their many other harmful effects). In a double-blind trial, people who had just experienced a heart attack were given either placebo or a mixture of antioxidants (vitamin A, vitamin C, vitamin E, and beta-carotene) for twenty-eight days. The results indicated that the use of antioxidants minimized the extent of heart cell damage.

Magnesium. The mineral magnesium is sometimes suggested for stabilizing the heart after a heart attack, but one study actually found a negative effect. In this one-year, double-blind, placebo-controlled trial of 468 people who had just experienced a heart attack, the use of a magnesium supplement at a dose of 360 mg daily failed to prevent heart-related events (defined as heart attack, sudden cardiac death, or need for cardiac bypass) and actually may have increased the risk slightly.

Arginine. The supplement arginine has been proposed for aiding recovery from a heart attack. In one double-blind study, arginine did not cause harm, and it showed potential modest benefit. However, in another study, arginine failed to prove helpful and possibly increased the death rate of those who had a heart attack.

Other herbs and supplements. Other herbs and supplements that are sometimes said to be useful after a heart attack, but that lack reliable substantiation, include glycine, hawthorn, inosine, and lipoic acid.

Lifestyle modifications. Evidence suggests that intensive lifestyle modification, involving an extremely low-fat diet, exercise, and stress reduction, can actually reverse coronary artery disease in people who have had, or are at high risk for, heart attacks. It is not clear whether less ascetic approaches can achieve similar effects. However, there is evidence that less intensive low-fat and Mediterranean-style (low-fat plus high fish oil) diets can decrease the risk of recurrent heart attacks and similar cardiac events in persons who already have experienced a heart attack.

Chelation therapy. Some alternative medicine physicians recommend the use of intravenous infusions of a chemical called ethylenediaminetetraacetic acid to clear out the arteries of the heart, a method called chelation therapy. This method is based on an outmoded understanding of atherosclerosis, and it is most likely ineffective.

HERBS AND SUPPLEMENTS TO USE WITH CAUTION

Numerous herbs and supplements may interact adversely with drugs used to prevent or treat heart attacks.

EBSCO CAM Review Board

FURTHER READING

Calo, L., et al. "N-3 Fatty Acids for the Prevention of Atrial Fibrillation After Coronary Artery Bypass Surgery." *Journal of the American College of Cardiology* 45 (2005): 1723-1728.

Lu, Z., et al. "Effect of Xuezhikang, an Extract from Red Yeast Chinese Rice, on Coronary Events in a Chinese Population with Previous Myocardial Infarction." *American Journal of Cardiology* 101 (2008): 1689-1693.

Mozaffarian, D. "Fish and N-3 Fatty Acids for the Prevention of Fatal Coronary Heart Disease and Sudden Cardiac Death." *American Journal of Clinical Nutrition* 87 (2008): 1991S-1996S.

Raitt, M. H., et al. "Fish Oil Supplementation and Risk of Ventricular Tachycardia and Ventricular Fibrillation in Patients with Implantable Defibrillators." *Journal of the American Medical Association* 293 (2005): 2884-2891.

Schulman, S. P., et al. "L-arginine Therapy in Acute Myocardial Infarction: The Vascular Interaction with Age in Myocardial Infarction (VINTAGE MI) Randomized Clinical Trial." *Journal of the American Medical Association* 295 (2006): 58-64.

Tarantini, G., et al. "Metabolic Treatment with L-carnitine in Acute Anterior ST Segment Elevation Myocardial Infarction." *Cardiology* 106 (2006): 215-223.

Tuttle, K. R., et al. "Comparison of Low-Fat Versus Mediterranean-Style Dietary Intervention After First Myocardial Infarction (from the Heart Institute of Spokane Diet Intervention and Evaluation Trial)." *American Journal of Cardiology* 101 (2008): 1523-1530.

Yokoyama, M., et al. "Effects of Eicosapentaenoic Acid on Major Coronary Events in Hypercholesterolaemic Patients (JELIS)." *The Lancet* 369 (2007): 1090-1098.

See also: Angina; Arrhythmia; Atherosclerosis and heart disease prevention; Cholesterol, high; Congestive heart failure; Hypertension; Strokes.

Heart disease

CATEGORY: Issues and overviews

RELATED TERMS: Angina, atherosclerosis, cardiovascular disease, congestive heart failure, coronary heart disease, hypertension, peripheral vascular disease

DEFINITION: Complementary and alternative medicines and therapies to prevent and treat cardiovascular disease, or diseases of the heart.

OVERVIEW

With the advent of lifesaving antibiotics in the early to mid-twentieth century, conventional or allopathic medicine became the preeminent form of health care in the United States. Although most of the other health-care systems continued to function, they were deemed unscientific. Moreover, as a result of public health interventions, such as better sanitation, the populace enjoyed greater longevity. As the gradual aging of the population began to significantly increase the prevalence of chronic illnesses such as arthritis, diabetes, high blood pressure, and heart disease, mainstream medicine began to address these conditions.

Cardiovascular disease (CVD) is the leading cause of death in the United States. Of note, CVD includes all conditions affecting the heart and the blood vessels. While many risk factors for CVD may be addressed by lifestyle changes such as stopping smoking and by adherence to diets low in saturated fats and trans fatty acids, the aging process and hereditary factors predispose for risk factors that cannot be altered. Until the age of fifty years, men are at greater risk than women of developing CVD, although once a woman enters menopause, her risk increases threefold.

Many people with CVD have low levels of high-density lipoproteins (HDL) or good cholesterol or high levels of low-density lipoproteins (LDL) or bad cholesterol (or both), and the levels of both are more specifically linked to CVD than is total cholesterol. Atherosclerosis (hardening of the arteries) is the most frequent cause of heart attacks, and it usually occurs in persons with high cholesterol. Overweight persons are more likely to have additional risk factors related to heart disease, specifically hypertension, high blood-sugar levels, high cholesterol, high triglycerides, and diabetes. Most often, recommended treatments for cardiovascular diseases by conventional physicians are invasive and include stents and bypass graft surgery. There are, however, instances when complementary and alternative medicine (CAM) or integrative therapies can augment or even preclude invasive measures.

CAM AND HEART HEALTH

The National Center for Complementary and Alternative Medicine (NCCAM), a branch of the National Institutes of Health (NIH), was established in 1998 to ensure that high-quality scientific research is conducted in CAM practices. Complementary medicine is used together with conventional medicine, an example being aromatherapy, and alternative medicine is used in place of conventional medicine, an example being the Zone diet to lower LDL and raise HDL levels. Integrative medicine is a combination of conventional medicine with therapies for which there is evidence of both safety and efficacy, such as relaxation and therapeutic touch in addition to the administration of analgesics for postoperative pain. CAM may be classified into five types of therapy (some systems or therapies may fit into two or more categories) as they pertain to CVD: alternative medicine systems, mind/body medicine, manipulative and body-based systems, energy therapies, and biologically based therapies.

Alternative medicine systems are based upon complete systems of theory and practice, such as homeopathic and naturopathic medicine in Western culture; non-Western systems include traditional Chinese medicine such as acupuncture and ancient Indian medicine such as Ayurveda, which originated in India more than eight thousand years ago. Ayurveda uses an integrated approach combining meditation, exercise, lifestyle changes, diet, and herbs such as guggulipid (guggul) and its extracts, which have been used to lower lipids in persons with ischemic heart disease, hypercholesterolemia, and obesity. Clinical studies conducted in India have shown that guggul is effective in lowering triglycerides and total cholesterol. In the first clinical randomized trial of guggul in 103 healthy adults, no effect was observed on their lipids. Gastrointestinal upset, rash, headache, and nausea were noted. Guggul has been shown to interfere with the prescription heart medications propranolol and diltiazem. The herbal/mineral *abana* formulation may lessen angina symptoms, reduce high blood pressure, and improve cardiac function.

Mind/body medicine uses meditation, prayer, music therapy, and yoga to provide a positive influence upon the mind to improve a person's health; mind/body medicine's clinical correlates to CVD unite both social and biological aspects of CVD. An increasing body of evidence suggests that persons with depression are predisposed to cardiovascular events; persons with depression after a myocardial infarction were shown to have greater mortality rates than their cohorts who were not depressed. Stress is another psychosocial determinant of cardiovascular pathology and disease, such as high blood pressure; in the Framingham study, high blood pressure was linked to more than 80 percent of all cardiovascular deaths and was at least twice as strong a predictor of death as high cholesterol levels or smoking.

Mind/body techniques have been used as adjuncts to traditional therapies in treating heart diseases. For coronary heart disease, these CAM techniques include stress reduction, meditation (yoga), and group support. CAM includes biofeedback, stress reduction, and group support for arrhythmia; guided imagery for presurgery therapy; stress reduction and meditation for elevated cholesterol levels; group support and biofeedback for congestive heart failure; and group support, biofeedback, meditation (yoga), and pet companionship for high blood pressure.

A 2009 study was undertaken to determine whether breathing exercises practiced in yoga meditations would be of benefit to persons with hypertension. Sixty men and women (twenty to sixty years of age) with stage I essential hypertension were equally divided into groups of controls: those who did slow-breathing exercises and those who did fast-breathing exercises. Subjects were assessed using parameters including baseline and postintervention measurements of blood pressure, standing-to-lying ratio, Valsalva ratio, and the hand-grip and cold pressor response; both types of breathing exercises appeared to benefit persons with hypertension. Improvement in both sympathetic and parasympathetic reactivity was associated with those in the slow-breathing group.

Manipulative and body-based systems include massage and therapeutic touch; their clinical correlates to CVD unite both the social and the biological aspects of CVD. The real benefit of energy treatments might be as adjuncts to improve optimism by restoring a sense of peace, serenity, and emotional connection. This approach may be helpful as long as it does not preclude conventional therapy and does no harm.

Therapeutic touch was tested by meta-analysis; of the eleven trials evaluated, seven demonstrated a positive effect, including anxiety reduction in a coronary care unit, reduced need for postsurgical pain medications, and enhanced wound healing. Because many of these techniques are unproven or may result from a placebo effect, it is best to consult a physician before undergoing therapy.

Energy therapies, which use natural energy fields to promote health and healing, include qigong, Reiki, therapeutic touch, and acupuncture. Acupuncture has become increasingly popular among those wanting to treat or prevent CVD. This ancient Chinese medicine employs tiny needles that are carefully and strategically inserted in the body to improve health. The basis for this improvement is the movement, throughout the body, of energy that may have become blocked; it is believed that acupuncture helps to unblock and redirect energy. Studies have shown that acupuncture can be used to reduce high blood pressure and reduce the incidence of angina and blood vessel spasms; those who were treated by acupuncture for angina recovered more quickly from an attack than those who had been taking drugs. Reliable acupuncturists are usually certified by the National Certification Commission for Acupuncture and Oriental Medicine. Acupuncture is covered by some medical insurance; the cost of visits varies widely, so one should consult several practitioners to find out about their fees.

Biologically based therapies use substances found in nature, such as vitamins, herbs, and omega-3 fatty acids, and special diets to lose weight or prevent CVD.

This illustration shows atherosclerotic coronary artery disease. (Monica Schroeder/Science Source/Photo Researchers, Inc.)

Herbal supplements have been used for thousands of years in the East and have had a recent resurgence in popularity among consumers in the West; more than fifteen million people in the United States consume herbal remedies or high-dose vitamins, and the total number of visits to CAM providers far exceeds those to primary physicians, amounting to more than $34 billion in out-of-pocket costs for CAM annually. Multiple factors contribute to the increased use of CAM, including the obesity epidemic, the prevalence of chronic disorders and pain syndromes, anxiety, depression, the general desire for good health and wellness, disease prevention, the increasing cost of conventional medicines, and the often mistaken belief that CAM remedies are safer and more effective.

The use of herbal remedies in the United States is widespread and increasing dramatically. Generally defined as any form of plant or plant product, herbs make up the largest proportion of CAM use in the United States. Because herbs are regarded as food products, they are not subject to the same scrutiny and regulation as traditional medications; manufacturers are exempt from premarket safety and efficacy testing and from any surveillance after marketing. Although herbal remedies are perceived as being natural, and therefore safe, many have adverse effects that can sometimes produce life-threatening consequences. Thus, one should consult a physician or other health-care professional about using herbs. Physicians are often unaware of their patients' use of such products because they do not ask about it; also, patients rarely volunteer such information.

Tetrandine. This vasoactive alkaloid is used in Chinese medicine to treat hypertension and angina. Because its vasodilation effect comes from the inhibition of the L-type calcium channels, there is possible competition with other calcium-channel blockers.

Aconite. Traditional Chinese practitioners use aconite for relief of pain caused by trigeminal and intercostal neuralgia, rheumatism, migraine, and general debilitation. Aconite is also a mild diaphoretic and is used to slow a rapid pulse. Atrial or ventricular fibrillation, however, may result from the direct effect of aconite on the myocardium. Side effects may occur following contact with leaves or sap from *Aconitum* plants and can range from bradycardia and hypotension to fatal ventricular arrhythmia.

Gynura. Widely used in Chinese folk medicine, gynura purportedly improves microcirculation and relieves pain; however, it has been associated with hepatic toxicity and has been shown to inhibit angiotensin-converting enzyme activity, resulting in hypotension in animals.

Ginseng. To determine whether there was a link between ginseng intake and mortality in a Korean population, 6,282 persons age fifty-five years and older were followed from March 1985, to December 2003. After adjusting for age, education, smoking, body mass index, and blood pressure, the all-cause mortality rate for males who used ginseng was lower. This effect was not observed in female cohorts. Mortality caused by cardiovascular disease was not related to ginseng consumption in either females or males.

Ginkgo biloba. This herb has been used to treat intermittent claudication in persons with peripheral artery blockage. A meta-analysis looked at eight randomized, placebo-controlled, double-blind studies of 415 persons. The results from the trials showed that *Ginkgo biloba* significantly increased walking distance in tested persons by 111.54 feet. Ginkgo should not be given with digitalis, warfarin, aspirin, nonsteroidal anti-inflammatory drugs, or thiazide diuretics.

Cinnamon. Two daily doses of a dried water-soluble cinnamon extract seemed to lower the risk factors for heart disease and diabetes in a small study led by a U.S. Department of Agriculture chemist. It was found that the daily doses of the cinnamon extract improved the antioxidant status of the subjects, a group of obese men and women, and also decreased their fasting blood sugar (glucose) levels. For this twelve-week study, the twenty-two participants were randomly divided into two groups; one group received 250 milligrams of cinnamon extract twice per day with their usual diets, and the other group was given placebos. The positive changes seen in the lab values of the cinnamon group suggested a reduction in the risk of both diabetes and cardiac disease.

Hawthorn. A peripheral vasodilator, hawthorn has been used to treat high blood pressure, ischemic

heart disease, arrhythmia, coronary heart disease, cor pulmonale (pulmonary heart disease), and atherosclerosis. Several double-blind studies of persons with heart failure have shown objective improvement in cardiac performance using bicycle ergometry. In some studies of persons with mild heart failure, hawthorn outperformed digitalis. Care should be taken, however, when taking hawthorn with drugs such as digitalis, beta-blockers, and anti-arrhythmics.

Vitamins. Vitamins used to prevent or treat CVD include B_{12}, B_6, and folate. Having elevated blood levels of the amino acid homocysteine (found in high amounts in animal protein) is a strong risk factor for CVD. Studies have also shown that when high homocysteine levels are reduced, the incidence of heart attack is cut by 20 percent, the risk of blood-clot-related strokes by 40 percent, and the risk of venous blood clots elsewhere in the body by 60 percent. Studies have shown that dietary intake of vitamins B_{12}, B_6, and folate can help to lower elevated homocysteine levels, as can lowering the amount of animal-based protein ingested. At least 10 percent of the population, however, has a genetic propensity for elevated levels of homocysteine. Persons should consult their health care providers to determine homocysteine level; if above 7, activated folic acid (L-methyl folate), vitamin B_{12}, and vitamin B_6 should be added to the diet.

Observational data suggest that fruit and vegetable consumption lower the risk of developing CVD. It has been postulated that the antioxidant component of fruits and vegetables accounts for the observed protection. Decreased risk of cardiovascular death has been associated with higher blood levels of vitamin C and coenzyme Q_{10} (CoQ_{10}). In addition, vitamin C, vitamin E, and CoQ_{10} have demonstrated antioxidant effects, including beneficial effects on oxidation of low-density lipoprotein. There is evidence that these vitamins may affect other risk factors for CVD, such as hypertension. Vitamin E may also reduce coronary artery blockage by decreasing blood platelet aggregation. Thus, supplementation with these antioxidants could decrease the risk of developing CVD.

CoQ_{10} is produced in all body tissues, acting like a free-radical scavenger that can stabilize membranes. There have been more than forty clinical trials of CoQ_{10} use in persons with CVD, demonstrating both subjective and objective benefits. Both a recent review and a meta-analysis have shown the benefits of CoQ_{10}, which has also been shown to significantly reduce cardiotoxicity of cancer drugs such as Adriamycin (doxorubicin). Although not serious, side effects have been reported with CoQ_{10} usage, most frequently insomnia, higher levels of liver enzymes, upper abdominal pain, sensitivity to light, irritability, headache, dizziness, heartburn, and extreme fatigue.

HEART HEALTHY DIETS

In 2006, American Heart Association (AHA) dietary guidelines underscored the importance of limiting "bad fats" and stated that less than 7 percent of calories consumed daily should come from saturated fats (and less than 1 percent from trans-fats). A range between 25 to 35 percent for total fat consumption is suggested for most people, not just for those trying to lose weight. Saturated fats are typically found in meat products and in tropical oils, such as coconut and palm oil. Trans-fat, also known as partially hydrogenated fat, is human-made and is found mostly in commercially baked goods.

The AHA promotes two types of dietary guidelines. The first restricts cholesterol consumption to less than 200 milligrams per day and less than 7 percent of calories as saturated fat, and the second recommends eating foods such as margarine, which contains plant sterols. In 2010, a Tufts University study found that eating such margarine with three meals per day lowered LDL. Other suggestions include soy products, soluble fiber, and walnuts and almonds to lower LDL (low-density lipoprotein), or bad cholesterol. Soy-based phytoestrogen foods have been found to reduce oxidation of lipids. Favorable effects of soy phytoestrogens on lipid profiles and thrombosis and vascular reactivity have been reported. Intake of foods containing phytoestrogens have been linked to a favorable cardiovascular risk profile, as demonstrated by 939 postmenopausal women participating in the Framingham Off-Spring Study.

Eating protein-rich foods other than red meat could play an important role in lowering the risk of heart disease. In a recent study, Harvard School of Public Health researchers found that women who consumed higher amounts of red meat had a greater risk of coronary heart disease (CHD). Substituting other foods high in protein, such as fish, poultry, and nuts, in place of red meat was associated with a lower risk of CHD; eating one serving per day of nuts in place of red meat was linked to a 30 percent lower risk of CHD; substituting a serving of fish showed a 24 percent lower risk, poultry a 19 percent lower risk, and low-fat dairy a 13 percent lower risk.

Many previous studies have focused on either the nutrient composition of protein-rich foods (the amount of saturated fat or iron) or dietary patterns (Mediterranean-style diet or Western-style diet) and how they relate to heart disease risk. This study, which appeared in the August 16, 2010, issue of *Circulation*, evaluated the substitution of one protein-rich food for another, which may be easier for a person to do, compared with substituting one nutrient or one dietary pattern for another, to reduce the risk of heart disease. The researchers followed 84,136 women age thirty to fifty-five years in the Nurses' Health Study (based at Brigham and Women's Hospital) over a period of twenty-six years. The participants had no known cancer, diabetes, stroke, angina, or other cardiovascular disease. To assess diets, the participants filled out a questionnaire every four years about the types of food they ate and how often.

A low-carbohydrate diet based on animal products was associated with higher all-cause mortality in both men and women. According to a study published in the September 7, 2010, issue of *Annals of Internal Medicine*, a low-carbohydrate diet may reduce the risk of death from all medical causes in both men and women, whereas a vegetable-based low-carbohydrate diet was associated with lower all-cause mortality and cardiovascular disease mortality. Researchers had followed more than 85,000 women for twenty-six years and 44,000 men for twenty years as a follow-up to earlier studies.

This wide-ranging study gives credence to the Eco-Atkins diet popularized by David Jenkins (*Archives of Internal Medicine*, 2009), who created a diet high in plant proteins, fruits, and vegetables. In the Jenkins study, forty-seven overweight hyperlipidemic men and women consumed one of two diets: a low-carbohydrate (26 percent of total calories), high vegetable protein (31 percent from gluten, soy, nuts, fruit, vegetables, and cereals), and vegetable oil (43 percent) plant-based diet or a high-carbohydrate lacto-ovo (milk and eggs) vegetarian style diet (58 percent carbohydrate, 16 percent protein, and 25 percent fat). The dieting lasted four weeks and had a parallel-study design. The study food was provided at 60 percent of calorie requirements. While the Jenkins study does not suggest that the diet will result in longevity, Eco-Atkins (the low-carbohydrate diet) was shown to improve cholesterol levels and promote weight loss.

The Ornish diet, designed by Dean Ornish, is a low-fat vegetarian diet with less than 10 percent of daily calories derived from fat (an average of 15 to 25 grams per day), 70 to 75 percent from carbohydrates, and 15 to 20 percent from protein. The diet encourages consumption of beans, fruits, vegetables, and whole grains and restricts intake of processed foods, high-fat dairy products, alcohol, and simple sugars. There are two versions of the Ornish diet: the reversal diet, for people with existing heart disease wanting to reduce their risk of heart attack or other coronary event, and the prevention diet, for otherwise healthy persons with levels of LDL cholesterol greater than 150 milligrams per deciliter or for those with a ratio of total cholesterol to high-density lipoprotein (HDL, or good cholesterol) that is less than 3.0.

The Ornish diet is completely vegetarian. Excluded are cholesterol, saturated fat, and animal products, except egg whites and nonfat dairy products. All nuts, seeds, avocados, chocolate, olives, coconuts, and oils are eliminated too, except for a small amount of canola oil for cooking and for oil that supplies omega-3 essential fatty acids. The Ornish diet also prohibits caffeine but allows a moderate intake of alcohol and salt. There is no restriction on calorie intake, but the diet suggests several small meals each day rather than three large meals. Based on available research, the Ornish diet appears to be more successful in lowering the risk of heart disease than other diets, but it also has been described as one of the more difficult diets to follow.

The Zone diet, designed by Barry Sears, determines total daily caloric intake based on daily protein intake. Once the amount of daily protein is established, the next step is to divide this protein into "blocks," each of which contains approximately 7 grams of protein, then divide the protein blocks into five or more meals to be eaten throughout the day. For example, one can consume four blocks at breakfast, three at lunch, two as afternoon snacks, four at dinner, and two as late-night snacks. For each protein block eaten, one carbohydrate block and one fat block should also be consumed. Each carbohydrate block contains 9 grams of carbohydrate, and each fat block has 1.5 grams of fat. Suggested daily protein intake will vary based on daily activity and lean body mass. For the average over-

weight American, total caloric intake might be 1,400 calories per day. For an average marathon runner, the daily intake might be about 1,750 calories per day. Minimum daily protein recommendation is 75 grams for women and 100 grams for men.

After sixteen years of study, the U.S. Centers for Medicare and Medicaid Services announced a proposed decision to provide Medicare coverage for the comprehensive Zone diet program. This is the first time Medicare has decided to provide coverage for an integrative medicine, or CAM, program.

The Pritikin diet is a low-fat diet largely based on vegetables, grains, and fruits. Fat in the diet accounts for 10 percent of daily intake. Nathan Pritikin promoted the concept of wellness through lowering cholesterol and helping diabetics normalize their blood sugar without taking insulin. That people lost weight was a plus. Pritikin's son, Robert, then altered the diet; its staples remained the same plant-based foods of the original diet, and the fat content remained very low. Again altered by Robert, the diet now focuses on caloric density: Not just calories are important, but also how dense these calories are in a given food. For example, one pound of broccoli has fewer calories than one pound of cookies, which is also rich in simple sugars and saturated fat. Since 1976, more than 70,000 people have attended Pritikin Longevity Centers.

An article in the *Journal of the American Medical Association* (2005) reported on a single-center randomized trial at an academic medical institution in Boston of overweight or obese adults age twenty-two to seventy-two years with known hypertension, dyslipidemia, or fasting hyperglycemia. The study compared the Atkins, Ornish, Weight Watchers, and Zone diets for weight loss and heart disease risk reduction. The study set out to assess adherence rates and the effectiveness of the four popular diets for weight loss and cardiac risk factor reduction. A total of 160 people were randomly assigned to four diet groups: Atkins (carbohydrate restriction), Zone (macronutrient balance), Weight Watchers (calorie restriction), and Ornish (fat restriction) diet groups.

Each diet was found to significantly reduce the LDL/HDL-cholesterol ratio by approximately 10 percent, with no significant effects on blood pressure or glucose at one year. The amount of weight loss was associated with self-reported dietary adherence, but not with diet type. For each diet, decreasing levels of total/HDL cholesterol, C-reactive protein, and insulin were significantly associated with weight loss with no significant difference among diets. Each popular diet modestly reduced body weight and several cardiac risk factors at one year. Overall dietary adherence rates were low, although increased adherence was associated with greater weight loss and cardiac risk factor reductions for each diet.

Those persons looking for a CAM practitioner who can address heart health should contact national organizations such as NCCAM, the American Heart Association, and the National Institutes of Health, and also specific therapy organizations such as the American Association of Oriental Medicine. One can also consult his or her health care provider for suggestions.

Cynthia F. Racer, M.A., M.P.H.

FURTHER READING

American Heart Association. http://www.americanheart.org. Provides comprehensive information on heart disease and conditions, healthy lifestyles, and resources, and also provides interactive health tools.

Baum, Seth J. *The Total Guide to a Healthy Heart: Integrative Strategies for Preventing and Reversing Heart Disease.* New York: Kensington, 2000. Brings together the practices of both conventional and alternative approaches to reversing heart disease and maintaining heart health.

Eisenberg, D. M., et al. "Trends in Alternative Medicine Use in the United States, 1990-1997: Results of a Follow-Up National Survey." *Journal of the American Medical Association* 280 (1998): 1569-1575. Discusses the results of a widespread study on the use of CAM among persons in the United States.

National Center for Complementary and Alternative Medicine. http://nccam.nih.gov. A comprehensive U.S. government resource for news articles, scientific studies, and general consumer information about complementary and alternative medicine.

"Top-Selling Medicinal Herbs in the U.S., 1999-2003." In *The World Almanac and Book of Facts*, edited by K. Park. New York: St. Martin's Press, 2005. An informative look at the use of CAM herbal remedies in America.

The U.S. Weight Loss and Diet Control Market. 9th ed.,Tampa, Fla.: Marketdata Enterprises, 2007. Examines from a business and marketing perspective the popular weight-loss and dieting programs in the United States.

See also: Angina; Atherosclerosis and heart disease prevention; Cholesterol, high; Congestive heart failure; Diet-based therapies; Exercise; Guided imagery; Heart attack; Hypertension; Obesity and excess weight; Smoking addiction; Strokes.

Hellerwork

CATEGORY: Therapies and techniques
RELATED TERMS: Bodywork, movement therapy, Rolfing, somatic education, structural integration
DEFINITION: Treatment and therapy involving the use of massage, patient education, and patient-practitioner dialogue.
PRINCIPAL PROPOSED USES: Body alignment, posture, and balance; breathing; chronic pain; mobility; relaxation; stress
OTHER PROPOSED USES: Fasciitis, headaches, musculoskeletal conditions, sciatica, spine pain, sports and repetitive stress injuries, whiplash

OVERVIEW

Hellerwork was developed in 1979 by Joseph Heller, an aerospace engineer and Rolfing practitioner. Hellerwork is a form of structural integration based on the principles of Rolfing, manipulation of the muscles, but it acknowledges the mind/body relationship. It encompasses bodywork (deep tissue massage), movement education, and verbal dialogue to realign the body, improve balance and posture, reduce stress, boost energy, and promote overall health and well-being.

MECHANISM OF ACTION

Hellerwork assumes that bodily muscles and tissues and the brain possess memories and that physical healing affects emotional well-being. Hellerwork seeks to restore health by manipulating the connective tissue known as fascia. It uses hands-on bodywork techniques to release accumulated tension, thereby making the fascia more flexible. Movement education is designed to teach awareness and ease daily activities (sitting, walking, standing), while verbal dialogue completes the mind/body relationship by connecting physical tension to emotions.

USES AND APPLICATIONS

Hellerwork is used to improve posture, balance, alignment, and mobility. It can help relieve anxiety, tension, and stress to promote relaxation and better health. It may be useful in treating physical problems including chronic muscle and joint pain and sports and repetitive stress injuries.

SCIENTIFIC EVIDENCE

As is true of many other complementary and alternative therapies, a lack of quality scientific research documents the effectiveness of Hellerwork. Although Hellerwork has been suggested for various conditions, most evidence supporting its effectiveness is anecdotal.

Some studies suggest that Hellerwork improves posture and reduces muscular tension. However, the safety and effectiveness of Hellerwork have not been validated by Western standards through randomized, double-blind, placebo-controlled clinical trials.

Studying the effectiveness of hands-on mind/body therapies is difficult because of various research challenges, including inadequate study design, blinding procedures, control groups, treatment length, and enrollment.

Hellerwork has become an attractive treatment option because of its stress-relieving and relaxation effects. However, more research is required to properly assess its clinical effectiveness.

CHOOSING A PRACTITIONER

One should chose a certified, licensed Hellerwork practitioner to avoid injury.

SAFETY ISSUES

The safety of Hellerwork has not been extensively examined. A health care professional should be consulted before beginning treatment.

Hellerwork involves deep tissue massage, so it may cause bruising or physical discomfort and may worsen some conditions. It should not be performed on persons with heart or spinal disease, diabetes, respiratory problems, broken bones, skin damage, psychosis, bleeding disorders, or blood clots, or on women who are pregnant.

Rose Ciulla-Bohling, Ph.D.

FURTHER READING

Claire, Thomas. *Body Work: What Kind of Massage to Get and How to Make the Most of It.* 2d ed. Laguna Beach, Calif.: Basic Health, 2006.

Heller, Joseph, and William A. Henkin. *Bodywise: An Introduction to Hellerwork for Regaining Flexibility and Well-Being.* Berkeley, Calif.: North Atlantic Books, 2004.

Hellerwork Structural Integration. "What Is Hellerwork?" Available at http://www.hellerwork.com.

Levine, Andrew S., and Valerie J. Levine. *The Bodywork and Massage Sourcebook.* Los Angeles: Lowell House, 1999.

See also: Aston-Patterning; Back pain; Manipulative and body-based practices; Massage therapy; Neck pain; Osteopathic manipulation; Progressive muscle relaxation; Reflexology; Relaxation therapies; Rolfing; Sciatica; Shiatsu; Soft tissue pain; Sports and fitness support: Enhancing recovery; Walking, mind/body.

Hemorrhoids

CATEGORY: Condition

RELATED TERM: Piles

DEFINITION: Treatment of swollen and inflamed veins in the rectum.

PRINCIPAL PROPOSED NATURAL TREATMENTS: Bioflavonoids such as citrus bioflavonoids, oxerutins, and bilberry

OTHER PROPOSED NATURAL TREATMENTS: Butcher's broom, calendula, *Collinsonia*, gotu kola, horse chestnut, mesoglycan, oak bark, oligomeric proanthocyanidins, slippery elm, witch hazel

INTRODUCTION

Hemorrhoids are swollen, inflamed veins in the rectum that can ache and bleed. They are common and are usually caused by constipation, a low-fiber diet, a sedentary lifestyle, pregnancy, or liver cirrhosis.

The most important interventions for hemorrhoids aim at reversing their causes. Adopting a high-fiber diet, sitting down less, getting plenty of exercise, and maintaining regular bowel habits can make a significant difference. Medical treatment consists mainly of stool softeners and moist heat. In more severe cases, surgical procedures may be used.

Contrary to popular belief, it does not appear that the consumption of foods spiced with hot chili peppers causes any discomfort or harm to people with hemorrhoids; a double-blind study found no difference in symptoms following consumption of hot peppers or placebo.

PRINCIPAL PROPOSED NATURAL TREATMENTS

Bioflavonoids are colorful substances that occur widely in the plant kingdom. Reasonably good, though not indisputable, evidence suggests that the citrus bioflavonoids diosmin and hesperidin (in a special micronized combination preparation) may be helpful for hemorrhoids.

A two-month, double-blind, placebo-controlled trial of 120 persons with recurrent hemorrhoid flare-ups found that treatment with combined diosmin and hesperidin significantly reduced the frequency and severity of hemorrhoid attacks. Another double-blind, placebo-controlled trial of one hundred persons had positive results with the same bioflavonoids in relieving symptoms once a flare-up of hemorrhoid pain had begun. A ninety-day double-blind trial of one hundred persons with bleeding hemorrhoids also found significant benefits for treatment of acute attacks and prevention of new ones. Finally, this bioflavonoid combination was found to compare favorably with surgical treatment of hemorrhoids. However, less impressive results were seen in a double-blind, placebo-controlled study in which all participants were given a fiber laxative with either combined diosmin and hesperidin or placebo.

Other sources of bioflavonoids have been studied too. In a four-week, double-blind, placebo-controlled trial of forty people with hemorrhoids, the use of an extract made from the bioflavonoid-rich herb bilberry significantly reduced hemorrhoid symptoms compared with placebo. In addition, according to some double-blind studies, the semisynthetic bioflavonoids known as oxerutins may also be helpful for hemorrhoids, including the hemorrhoids that occur during pregnancy. Although it is not known precisely how flavonoids work, it is thought that they stabilize the walls of blood vessels, making them less susceptible to injury.

OTHER PROPOSED NATURAL TREATMENTS

Preliminary evidence suggests that an extract made from pig intestines called mesoglycan can improve the symptoms of hemorrhoids. Another study reported benefit for hemorrhoids by using a combination of olive oil, honey, and beeswax. However, because this trial lacked a placebo group, its results mean little.

The natural treatments used for varicose veins are also often recommended for hemorrhoids, because a

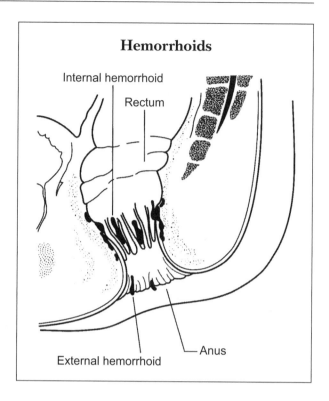

Hemorrhoids

Internal hemorrhoid

Rectum

External hemorrhoid

Anus

hemorrhoid is actually a special kind of varicose vein. Some of the most commonly mentioned treatments include horse chestnut, oligomeric proanthocyanidins, gotu kola, and butcher's broom.

Traditional herbal remedies for hemorrhoids include calendula (applied topically), *Collinsonia* root (oral or topical), oak bark (topical), slippery elm (oral or topical), and witch hazel (topical). However, there has been little to no scientific evaluation of these treatments.

EBSCO CAM Review Board

FURTHER READING

Al-Waili, N. S., et al. "The Safety and Efficacy of a Mixture of Honey, Olive Oil, and Beeswax for the Management of Hemorrhoids and Anal Fissure." *Scientific World Journal* 6 (2006): 1998-2005.

Alonso-Coello, P., et al. "Meta-analysis of Flavonoids for the Treatment of Haemorrhoids." *British Journal of Surgery* 93 (2006): 909-920.

Altomare, D. F., et al. "Red Hot Chili Pepper and Hemorrhoids: The Explosion of a Myth." *Diseases of the Colon and Rectum* 49 (2006): 1018-1023.

Ho, Y. H., M. Tan, and F. Seow-Choen. "Micronized Purified Flavonidic Fraction Compared Favorably with Rubber Band Ligation and Fiber Alone in the Management of Bleeding Hemorrhoids." *Diseases of the Colon and Rectum* 43 (2000): 66-69.

Misra, M. C., and R. Parshad. "Randomized Clinical Trial of Micronized Flavonoids in the Early Control of Bleeding from Acute Internal Haemorrhoids." *British Journal of Surgery* 87 (2000): 868-872.

See also: Bilberry; Citrus bioflavonoids; Oxerutins.

Hemorrhoids: Homeopathic remedies

CATEGORY: Homeopathy
DEFINITION: Homeopathic treatment of swollen and inflamed veins in the rectum caused by constipation, pregnancy, a low-fiber diet, and other factors.
STUDIED HOMEOPATHIC REMEDIES: *Aesculus, Collinsonia, Hamamelis, Nitricum acidum*

INTRODUCTION

Hemorrhoids are swollen, inflamed veins in the rectum that can ache and bleed. They are very common and are usually caused by constipation, a low-fiber diet, a sedentary lifestyle, or pregnancy. They may be accompanied by a tear in the anus called an anal fissure.

SCIENTIFIC EVALUATIONS OF HOMEOPATHIC REMEDIES

One study evaluated the effectiveness of the homeopathic remedy *Nitricum acidum* for the treatment of anal fissures, a possible complication of hemorrhoids. This fifteen-day, double-blind, placebo-controlled trial of thirty-one people tested *N. acidum* 9c (centesimals) given for fifteen days. The results showed that the burning sensation caused by the anal fissure was significantly improved in the homeopathic group compared with the placebo group. However, scores for other symptoms, such as itching, lesions, and pain during and after defecation, were not significantly improved.

TRADITIONAL HOMEOPATHIC TREATMENTS

Classical homeopathy offers many possible homeopathic treatments for hemorrhoids. These therapies are chosen based on various specific details of the person seeking treatment.

The homeopathic remedy *Aesculus* is frequently used for hemorrhoids. Aspects of the symptom picture for this remedy include external hemorrhoids that feel better when they are bleeding, sensations like small poking sticks in the rectum, symptoms made worse by urination or passing stool, and reduction of symptoms in cool, open air.

Collinsonia is often used when hemorrhoidal pain is associated with alternating diarrhea and constipation, and with heart palpitations and swelling of the lips. *Hamamelis* may be indicated when there is a throbbing, raw, aching pain in the anus, made worse for many hours after passing stool and accompanied by significant bleeding. The affected person also may have back pain.

EBSCO CAM Review Board

FURTHER READING

Ernst, E. "Herbal Medicinal Products During Pregnancy: Are They Safe?" *BJOG: An International Journal of Obstetrics and Gynaecology* 109 (2002): 227-235.

Gan, T., et al. "Traditional Chinese Medicine Herbs for Stopping Bleeding from Haemorrhoids." *Cochrane Database of Systematic Reviews* (2010): CD006791. Available through EBSCO DynaMed Systematic Literature Surveillance at http://www.ebscohost.com/dynamed.

Kucukkurt, I., et al. "Beneficial Effects of *Aesculus hippocastanum* L. Seed Extract on the Body's Own Antioxidant Defense System on Subacute Administration." *Journal of Ethnopharmacology* 129 (2010): 18-22.

See also: Constipation; Diarrhea; Pregnancy support.

Heparin

CATEGORY: Drug interactions
DEFINITION: A blood-thinning drug that is delivered by injection.
INTERACTIONS: Chondroitin, garlic, ginkgo, PC-SPES, phosphatidylserine, policosanol, vitamin C, vitamin D, white willow, and other herbs and supplements

CHONDROITIN

Effect: Possible Harmful Interaction

Based on chondroitin's chemical similarity to the anticoagulant drug heparin, it has been suggested that chondroitin might have anticoagulant effects as well. There are no case reports of any problems related to this, and studies suggest that chondroitin has at most a mild anticoagulant effect. Nonetheless, chondroitin should not be combined with heparin except under physician supervision.

GARLIC

Effect: Possible Harmful Interaction

The herb garlic (*Allium sativum*) is taken to lower cholesterol, among many other proposed uses. Because garlic has a blood-thinning effect, it might be dangerous to combine garlic with heparin. Two cases have been reported in which the combination of garlic and the blood thinner warfarin doubled the time it took for blood to clot. Though warfarin thins the blood in a different way than heparin, there are concerns that garlic might interact similarly with heparin.

GINKGO

Effect: Possible Harmful Interaction

The herb ginkgo (*Ginkgo biloba*) has been used to treat Alzheimer's disease and ordinary age-related memory loss, among many other conditions. Ginkgo thins the blood by reducing the ability of blood-clotting cells called platelets to stick together. Because case reports have implicated use of *Ginkgo biloba* in the development of serious bleeding abnormalities, combining ginkgo with heparin might be expected to intensify the danger.

PC-SPES

Effect: Possible Harmful Interaction

PC-SPES is an herbal combination that has shown promise for the treatment of prostate cancer. One case report suggests that PC-SPES might increase risk of bleeding complications if combined with blood-thinning medications.

PHOSPHATIDYLSERINE

Effect: Possible Harmful Interaction

The supplement phosphatidylserine is promoted to treat Alzheimer's disease and ordinary age-related memory loss. A test-tube study suggests that phosphatidylserine might amplify heparin's blood-thinning effects. If this effect were to occur inside the body, it could increase the risk of abnormal bleeding. Persons taking heparin should consult a doctor before taking phosphatidylserine.

POLICOSANOL

Effect: Possible Harmful Interaction

Policosanol, derived from sugarcane, has been taken for hyperlipidemia and intermittent claudication. Human trials suggest that policosanol makes blood platelets more slippery, an action that could potentiate the blood-thinning effects of heparin, possibly causing a risk of abnormal bleeding episodes. A thirty-day double-blind placebo-controlled trial of twenty-seven persons with high cholesterol levels found that policosanol at 10 milligrams (mg) daily markedly reduced the ability of blood platelets to clump together. Another double-blind placebo-controlled study of thirty-seven healthy volunteers found evidence that the blood-thinning effect of policosanol increased as the dose was increased: the larger the policosanol dose, the greater the effect. Another double-blind placebo-controlled study of forty-three healthy volunteers compared the effects of policosanol (20 mg daily), the blood-thinner aspirin (100 mg daily), and policosanol and aspirin combined at these same doses. The results again showed that policosanol substantially reduced the ability of blood platelets to stick together, and that the combined therapy exhibited additive effects. Based on these findings, one should not combine heparin and policosanol except under medical supervision.

VITAMIN C

Effect: Possible Harmful Interaction

Test-tube studies suggest that high amounts of vitamin C may reduce the blood-thinning effect of heparin. However, it is not clear whether the interaction is significant enough to make a practical difference.

WHITE WILLOW

Effect: Possible Harmful Interaction

The herb white willow (*Salix alba*), also known as willow bark, is used to treat pain and fever. White willow contains a substance that is converted by the body into a salicylate similar to aspirin. Since combining aspirin with heparin increases the risk of abnormal bleeding, it would not be advisable to combine white willow with heparin.

OTHER HERBS AND SUPPLEMENTS

Effect: Possible Harmful Interaction

Based on their known effects or constituents, the following herbs and supplements might not be safe to combine with heparin, though this has not been proven: bromelain (in the fruit and stem of pineapple, *Ananas comosus*), papaya (*Carica papaya*), chamomile (*Matricaria recutita*), *Coleus forskohlii*, danshen (*Salvia miltorrhiza*), devil's claw (*Harpogophytum procumbens*), dong quai (*Angelica sinensis*), feverfew (*Tanacetum parthenium*), ginger (*Zingiber officinale*), horse chestnut (*Aesculus hippocastanum*), red clover (*Trifolium pratense*), reishi (*Ganoderma lucidum*), mesoglycan, fish oil, OPCs (oligomeric proantho cyanidins), and vitamin E.

VITAMIN D

Effect: Supplementation Possibly Helpful

High doses or long-term use of heparin may interfere with the proper handling of vitamin D by the body. Because vitamin D is needed for calcium absorption and utilization, this may in turn lead to bone loss and osteoporosis. Additionally, heparin may directly interfere with bone formation. This interaction is of special concern during pregnancy, a period of greater calcium demand and diminished levels of a hormone that pushes calcium into bones. In fact, there have been several reports of fractured and collapsed vertebrae in pregnant women on heparin therapy. Supplementary calcium and vitamin D may help prevent heparin-induced osteoporosis. It might also be advisable to have one's bone density checked during long-term heparin therapy.

EBSCO CAM Review Board

FURTHER READING

Abdel Fattah, W., and T. Hammad. "Chondroitin Sulfate and Glucosamine: A Review of Their Safety Profile." *Journal of the American Nutraceutical Association* 3 (2001): 16-23.

Arruzazabala, M. L., et al. "Effect of Policosanol on Platelet Aggregation in Type II Hypercholesterolemic Patients." *International Journal of Tissue Reactions* 20 (1998): 119-124.

Rosenblatt, M., and J. Mindel. "Spontaneous Hyphema Associated with Ingestion of *Ginkgo biloba* Extract." *New England Journal of Medicine* 336 (1997): 1108.

Rowin, J., and S. L. Lewis. "Spontaneous Bilateral Subdural Hematomas with Chronic *Ginkgo biloba* Ingestion." *Neurology* 46 (1996): 1775-1776.

Vale, S. "Subarachnoid Hemorrhage Associated with *Ginkgo biloba*." *The Lancet* 352 (1998): 36.

See also: Chondroitin; Food and Drug Administration; Garlic; Ginkgo; PC-SPES; Phosphatidylserine; Policosanol; Supplements: Introduction; Vitamin C; Vitamin D; White Willow.

Hepatitis, alcoholic

CATEGORY: Condition

RELATED TERMS: Alcoholic liver disease, cirrhosis

DEFINITION: Treatment of liver disease caused by chronic overconsumption of alcohol.

PRINCIPAL PROPOSED NATURAL TREATMENT: Reduced alcohol consumption

OTHER PROPOSED NATURAL TREATMENTS: General nutritional support, magnesium, milk thistle, omega-3 essential fatty acids, omega-6 essential fatty acids, s-adenosylmethionine, trimethylglycine

HERBS AND SUPPLEMENTS TO AVOID: Beta-carotene (excessive dose), coltsfoot, comfrey, germander, greater celandine, kava, kombucha, pennyroyal, prepackaged Chinese herbal remedies, vitamin A (excessive dose)

INTRODUCTION

The liver is a sophisticated chemical laboratory, capable of carrying out thousands of chemical transformations on which the body depends. The liver produces some important chemicals from scratch and modifies others to allow the body to use them better. In addition, the liver neutralizes an enormous range of toxins.

A number of influences can severely damage the liver, of which alcohol is the most common. This powerful liver toxin harms the liver in three stages: alcoholic fatty liver, alcoholic hepatitis, and cirrhosis. Although the first two stages of injury are usually reversible, cirrhosis is not. Generally, liver cirrhosis is a result of more than ten years of heavy alcohol abuse.

Usually, alcoholic hepatitis is discovered through blood tests that detect levels of enzymes released from the liver. The blood levels of these enzymes, which are known by acronyms such as SGOT, SGPT, ALT, AST, and GGT, rise as damage to the liver (by any cause) progresses.

If blood tests show that a person has alcoholic hepatitis (or any other form of liver disease), it is essential that the person stop drinking. There is little in the way of specific treatment beyond this.

Alcoholic Liver Disease

Because the liver is the chief organ responsible for metabolizing alcohol, it is especially vulnerable to alcohol-related injury. Consuming as few as three drinks at one time may have toxic effects on the liver when combined with certain over-the-counter medications, such as those containing acetaminophen.

Alcoholic liver disease includes three conditions: fatty liver, alcoholic hepatitis, and cirrhosis. Heavy drinking for as little as a few days can lead to "fatty" liver, or steatosis—the earliest stage of alcoholic liver disease and the most common alcohol-induced liver disorder. Steatosis is marked by an excessive buildup of fat inside liver cells. This condition can be reversed, however, when drinking stops.

Drinking heavily for longer periods may lead to a more severe, and potentially fatal, condition called alcoholic hepatitis—an inflammation of the liver. Symptoms include nausea, lack of appetite, vomiting, fever, abdominal pain and tenderness, jaundice, and mental confusion. Scientists believe that if a person with alcoholic hepatitis continues to drink, the inflammation eventually will lead to alcoholic cirrhosis, in which healthy liver cells are replaced by scar tissue (to form fibrosis), leaving the liver unable to perform its vital functions.

The presence of alcoholic hepatitis is a red flag that cirrhosis may soon follow: Up to 70 percent of all persons with alcoholic hepatitis eventually may develop cirrhosis. Persons with alcoholic hepatitis who stop drinking may have a complete recovery from liver disease, or they still may develop cirrhosis.

PRINCIPAL PROPOSED NATURAL TREATMENTS

Several herbs and supplements have shown promise for protecting the liver from alcohol-induced damage. However, none of these has been conclusively proven effective, and cutting down (or eliminating) alcohol consumption is undoubtedly more effective than any other treatment. Following is a discussion of the treatments used specifically to treat early liver damage caused by alcohol.

Milk thistle. Numerous double-blind, placebo-controlled studies enrolling several hundred people have evaluated whether the herb milk thistle can successfully counter alcohol-induced liver damage. However, these studies have yielded inconsistent results. For example, a double-blind, placebo-controlled study performed in 1981 followed 106 Finnish soldiers with alcoholic liver disease over a period of four weeks. The treated group showed a significant decrease in elevated liver enzymes and improvement in liver structure, as evaluated by biopsy in twenty-nine subjects.

Two similar studies enrolling approximately sixty people also found benefits. However, a three-month, double-blind, placebo-controlled study of 116 people showed little to no additional benefit, perhaps because most participants reduced their alcohol consumption and almost one-half of them stopped drinking entirely. Another study found no benefit in seventy-two persons who were followed for fifteen months.

A 2007 review of published and unpublished studies on milk thistle as a treatment for liver disease concluded that benefits were seen only in low-quality trials, and even in those, milk thistle did not show more than a slight benefit. A subsequent 2008 review of nineteen randomized trials drew a similar conclusion for alcoholic liver disease generally, although it did find a modest reduction in mortality for persons with severe liver cirrhosis.

Other proposed natural treatments. The supplement S-adenosylmethionine (SAMe) has also shown some promise for preventing or treating alcoholic hepatitis, but there is no reliable evidence to support its use for this purpose. The supplement trimethylglycine helps the body create its own SAMe and has also shown promise in preliminary studies.

HERBS AND SUPPLEMENTS TO AVOID

High doses of the supplements beta-carotene and vitamin A might cause alcoholic liver disease to develop more rapidly in people who abuse alcohol. Nutritional supplementation at the standard daily requirement level should not cause a problem.

Although one animal study suggests that the herb kava might aid in alcohol withdrawal, the herb can cause liver damage; therefore, it should not be used by people with alcoholic liver disease (and probably not by anyone). Numerous other herbs possess known or suspected liver-toxic properties, including coltsfoot, comfrey, germander, greater celandine, kombucha, pennyroyal, and various prepackaged Chinese herbal remedies. For this reason, people with alcoholic liver disease should use caution before taking any medicinal herbs.

EBSCO CAM Review Board

FURTHER READING

Abittan, C. S., and C. S. Lieber. "Alcoholic Liver Disease." *Current Treatment Options in Gastroenterology* 2 (1999): 72-80.

Leo, M. A., and C. S. Lieber. "Alcohol, Vitamin A, and Beta-carotene: Adverse Interactions, Including Hepatotoxicity and Carcinogenicity." *American Journal of Clinical Nutrition* 69 (1999): 1071-1085.

McClain, C. J., et al. "S-adenosylmethionine, Cytokines, and Alcoholic Liver Disease." *Alcohol* 27 (2002): 185-192.

Ni, R., et al. "Toxicity of Beta-carotene and Its Exacerbation by Acetaldehyde in HepG2 Cells." *Alcohol and Alcoholism* 36 (2001): 281-285.

Rambaldi, A., and C. Gluud. "S-adenosyl-l-methionine for Alcoholic Liver Diseases." *Cochrane Database of Systematic Reviews* (2001): CD002235. Available through *EBSCO DynaMed Systematic Literature Surveillance* at http://www.ebscohost.com/dynamed.

Rambaldi, A., B. Jacobs, and C. Gluud. "Milk Thistle for Alcoholic and/or Hepatitis B or C Virus Liver Diseases." *Cochrane Database of Systematic Reviews* (2007): CD003620. Available through *EBSCO DynaMed Systematic Literature Surveillance* at http://www.ebscohost.com/dynamed.

See also: Alcoholism; Beta-carotene; Cirrhosis; Hepatitis, viral; Liver disease; Milk thistle; Vitamin A.

Hepatitis, viral

CATEGORY: Condition

DEFINITION: Treatment of viral infections of the liver.

PRINCIPAL PROPOSED NATURALS TREATMENTS: None

OTHER PROPOSED NATURAL TREATMENTS: Astragalus, Ayurvedic herbs, *Cordyceps*, lecithin, licorice, liver extracts, milk thistle, phosphatidylcholine, *Phyllanthus amarus*, reishi, SAMe, schisandra, taurine, thymus extract, traditional Chinese herbal medicine, vitamin C, whey protein

HERBS AND SUPPLEMENTS TO USE ONLY WITH CAUTION: Barberry, beta-carotene, blue-green algae, borage, chaparral, coltsfoot, comfrey, germander, germanium, greater celandine, kava, kombucha, mistletoe, pennyroyal, picrorhiza, pokeroot, sassafras, skullcap, spirulina, traditional Chinese herbal medicine, vitamin A, vitamin B$_3$

INTRODUCTION

Hepatitis is an infection of the liver caused by one of several viruses, the most common of which are named hepatitis A, B, and C. Hepatitis A is spread mainly through contaminated food and water, whereas hepatitis B is transmitted by sexual contact and by the use of contaminated needles. The route of transmission of hepatitis C is not completely clear but is believed to be similar to that of hepatitis B.

The first sign of hepatitis is called acute hepatitis. Hepatitis can also become a long-term disease known as chronic hepatitis. All forms of hepatitis cause jaundice, liver tenderness, and severe fatigue. Hepatitis A is the mildest form and seldom causes symptoms continuing longer than a couple of months. Hepatitis B and C produce more severe symptoms, which last two or three times longer and can become chronic.

Chronic hepatitis consists of persistent liver infection and inflammation that lingers long after the primary symptoms of the disease have disappeared. It can produce subtle symptoms of liver tenderness and continued fatigue and over time can gradually destroy the liver. Chronic hepatitis also appears to increase the risk of liver cancer.

The best treatment for hepatitis is prevention. One can avoid hepatitis A by practicing good hygiene and using the conventional preventive treatment, known as immunoglobulins, while traveling in areas where the disease is common. Hepatitis B can be prevented by immunization and by the same precautions used for preventing human immunodeficiency virus (HIV) infection. HIV precautions almost certainly decrease the transmission of hepatitis C too.

Conventional medicine has little in the way of treatment for the initial hepatitis infection once it has started. Treatment for chronic hepatitis is developing but is still quite imperfect. The most effective methods involve varieties of interferon.

PROPOSED NATURAL TREATMENTS

Traditional Chinese herbal medicine. Viral hepatitis has long been a serious problem in China and other parts of Asia, and for this reason many herbal formulas to treat it have been devised. The traditional Chinese herbal combination Shosaiko-to (minor *Bupleurum*) has been approved as a treatment for chronic hepatitis by the Japanese Health Ministry. However, a search of the literature uncovered only one large-scale, double-blind, placebo-controlled study supporting its effectiveness. In this twenty-four-week trial, the efficacy of Shosaiko-to was tested in 222 people with chronic active hepatitis using a double-blind, placebo-controlled, crossover design. Results showed that the use of Shosaiko-to significantly improved liver function measurements compared with placebo. Although these results are promising, an absence of long-term evaluation limits their meaningfulness. (The researchers followed participants for only three months.)

Other combination Chinese herbal therapies have also shown some promise for the treatment of chronic hepatitis, including those therapies named Bing Gan Tang, Yi Zhu decoction, Fuzheng Jiedu Tang, and Jianpi Wenshen recipe. However, the quality of most of these studies was again quite poor.

A well-designed, double-blind, placebo-controlled study evaluated a mixture of traditional Chinese herbs for people with hepatitis C and symptoms of fatigue. The tested mixture contained *Radix astragali* (6 percent), *R. acanthopanax* (8 percent), *R. bupleuir* (8 percent), *R. et tuber curcumae* (10 percent), *R. glycyrrhiza* (4 percent), *R. isatis* (14 percent), *R. paeoniae rubra* (14 percent), *R. salviae* (14 percent), *Rhizoma polygonum* (10 percent), and *Herba taraxaci* (12 percent). However, the mixture failed to prove more effective than placebo regarding symptoms or objective signs. Another complex Chinese herbal combination has also failed to prove effective. One Chinese herb widely advocated for chronic hepatitis B, *Sophorae flavescentis*, has not been shown effective, according to a comprehensive review of studies.

There are many incidents in which the use of Chinese herbs for treatment of hepatitis appears to have caused serious liver injury. Therefore, using Chinese herbs for hepatitis, except under the supervision of a physician, is not recommended.

Ayurvedic medicine. Ayurvedic medicine, the ancient medical system of India, has many traditional treatments for hepatitis. Some of these have undergone scientific evaluation. One such is a combination treatment called Kamalahar, which contains *Tecoma undulata*, *Phyllanthus urinaria*, *Embelia ribes*, *Taraxacum officinale*, *Nyctanthes arbortristis*, and *Terminalia arjuna*. In a double-blind, placebo-controlled study, fifty-two people with acute hepatitis were randomly assigned to receive placebo or this combination of herbal therapy at a dose of 500 milligrams (mg) three times daily for fifteen days. The results indicate that the herbal combination improved liver function to a significantly greater extent than did placebo.

Another combination therapy contains *Capparis spinosa*, *Cichorium intybus*, *Solanum nigrum*, *T. arjuna*, *Cassia occidentalis*, *Achillea millefolium*, and *Tamarix gallica*. In a poorly reported, five-week, double-blind, placebo-controlled study of thirty children with hepatitis A, the use of this combination formula apparently improved the rate of recovery compared with placebo. Benefits were also seen in a six-week study of thirty-four people with acute hepatitis. A third double-blind, placebo-controlled study evaluated the effectiveness of this combination in the treatment of a variety of liver conditions, including chronic and acute hepatitis, and found some evidence of benefit.

Single herbs also have been tried. In a double-blind trial of thirty-three people with acute viral hepatitis, the use of the herb *Picrorhiza kurroa* at a dose of 375 mg three times daily significantly speeded recovery time compared with placebo. The herb *P. amarus* has also been extensively studied as a treatment for chronic viral hepatitis, but it does not appear to be ef-

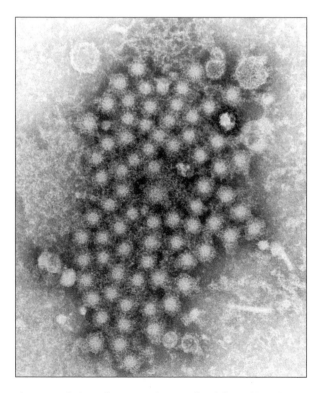

A transmission electron micrograph of hepatitis virions. (Centers for Disease Control and Prevention)

fective. Its close relative *P. urinaris* has also failed to prove effective. The quality of the reported studies remains poor, and Ayurvedic herbs cannot be regarded as a proven treatment for viral hepatitis.

Other herbs and supplements. The herb milk thistle has been proposed as a supportive treatment for viral hepatitis. However, study results are mixed, regarding both chronic and acute viral hepatitis. A 2007 review of all published and unpublished studies on milk thistle as a treatment for liver disease concluded that benefits were seen only in low-quality trials and, even in those, milk thistle did not show more than a slight benefit. A subsequent 2008 review of nineteen randomized trials failed to find evidence of a favorable effect on viral hepatitis.

Chronic hepatitis can cause cholestasis (backup of bile in the liver). In a two-week double-blind study of 220 persons with cholestasis, the use of the supplement S-adenosylmethionine at a dose of 1,600 mg daily significantly improved liver-related symptoms compared with placebo. Most participants in this study had chronic viral hepatitis.

The supplement phosphatidylcholine has shown some promise for hepatitis. In one double-blind study, it enhanced the effect of interferon in people with chronic hepatitis C, but not in those with chronic hepatitis B. However, in an open study, phosphatidylcholine failed to produce improvements in persons with acute hepatitis.

One small double-blind study found the herb picrorhiza more effective than placebo for reducing signs of liver damage in people with acute viral hepatitis. However, this study was preliminary and had numerous flaws. Another study failed to find N-acetylcysteine at a dose of 600 mg daily helpful for acute viral hepatitis.

In Japan, an injectable combination of the herb licorice and certain amino acids is used for chronic hepatitis. However, it is not clear whether the treatment actually works. Even if this were established, the results would not imply that oral licorice would have a similar effect; furthermore, the high dosages used for treatment of chronic hepatitis may cause an elevation of blood pressure and other serious medical problems. Licorice designed for oral use should not be injected.

Thymus extract has been tried as a treatment for hepatitis B and C. However, the results of small double-blind trials have not been positive. One study of antioxidant supplements also failed to find benefit.

Other common natural medicine recommendations for hepatitis include astragalus, *Cordyceps*, reishi, schisandra, taurine, vitamin C, and whey protein. However, there is no meaningful scientific evidence that these approaches work.

HERBS AND SUPPLEMENTS TO USE WITH CAUTION

Many natural products have the capacity to harm the liver. Furthermore, because of the generally inadequate regulation of dietary supplements, there are real risks that herbal products may contain liver-toxic contaminants even if the actual herbs listed on the label are safe. People with liver disease should not use any medicinal herbs except under the supervision of a physician.

All forms of vitamin B_3, including niacin, niacinamide (nicotinamide), and inositol hexaniacinate, may damage the liver when taken in high doses. (Nutritional supplementation at the standard daily requirement level should not cause a problem.)

Many herbs and supplements have known or suspected liver-toxic properties. These include barberry, borage, chaparral, coltsfoot, comfrey, germander, germanium (a mineral), greater celandine, kava, kombucha, mistletoe, pennyroyal, pokeroot, sassafras, and various herbs and minerals used in traditional Chinese herbal medicine.

In addition, herbs that are not liver-toxic in themselves are sometimes adulterated with other herbs of similar appearance that are accidentally harvested in a misapprehension of their identity (for example, germander found in skullcap products). Furthermore, blue-green algae species such as spirulina may at times be contaminated with liver-toxic substances called microcystins, for which no highest safe level is known.

Some scientific articles claim that the herb echinacea is potentially liver-toxic, but this concern appears to have been based on a misunderstanding of the herb's constituents. Echinacea contains substances in the pyrrolizidine alkaloid family. While many pyrrolizidine alkaloids are liver-toxic, those found in echinacea are not believed to have that property.

Whole valerian contains liver-toxic substances called valepotriates. Valepotriates, however, are thought to be absent from most commercial valerian products, and case reports suggest that even very high doses of valerian do not harm the liver.

EBSCO CAM Review Board

FURTHER READING

Chan, H. L., et al. "Double-Blinded Placebo-Controlled Study of *Phyllanthus urinaris* for the Treatment of Chronic Hepatitis B." *Alimentary Pharmacology and Therapeutics* 18 (2003): 339-345.

Gordon, A., et al. "Effects of *Silybum marianum* on Serum Hepatitis C Virus RNA, Alanine Aminotransferase Levels, and Well-Being in Patients with Chronic Hepatitis C." *Journal of Gastroenterology and Hepatology* 21 (2006): 275-280.

Groenbaek, K., et al. "The Effect of Antioxidant Supplementation on Hepatitis C Viral Load, Transaminases, and Oxidative Status." *European Journal of Gastroenterology and Hepatology* 18 (2006): 985-989.

Jakkula, M., et al. "A Randomized Trial of Chinese Herbal Medicines for the Treatment of Symptomatic Hepatitis C." *Archives of Internal Medicine* 164 (2004): 1341-6.

Mollison, L., et al. "Randomized Double Blind Placebo-Controlled Trial of a Chinese Herbal Therapy (CH100) in Chronic Hepatitis C." *Journal of Gastroenterology and Hepatology* 21 (2006): 1184-1188.

Rambaldi, A., B. Jacobs, and C. Gluud. "Milk Thistle for Alcoholic and/or Hepatitis B or C Virus Liver Diseases." *Cochrane Database of Systematic Reviews* (2007): CD003620. Available through *EBSCO DynaMed Systematic Literature Surveillance* at http://www.ebscohost.com/dynamed.

Yuen, M. F., et al. "Traditional Chinese Medicine Causing Hepatotoxicity in Patients with Chronic Hepatitis B Infection." *Alimentary Pharmacology and Therapeutics* 24 (2006): 1179-1186.

See also: Ayurveda; Cirrhosis; Hepatitis, alcoholic; Herbal medicine; Liver disease; Traditional Chinese herbal medicine.

Herbal medicine

CATEGORY: Therapies and techniques
RELATED TERMS: Herbology, traditional Chinese herbal medicine, Western herbal medicine
DEFINITION: Preventive medicine and therapy through the use of herbs.

OVERVIEW

Along with massage therapy, herbal treatment is one of the most ancient forms of medicine. By the time written history began, herbal medicine was already in full swing and being used all over the world.

There are several major surviving schools of herbal medicine. Two of the most complex systems are Ayurveda (the traditional herbal medicine of India) and traditional Chinese herbal medicine (TCHM). Both Ayurveda and TCHM make use of combinations of herbs. However, the herbal tradition in the West focuses more on individual herbs, sometimes known as simples. This is the form of herbology discussed here.

History of herbal medicine. Originally, herbal medicine in Europe was primarily a women's art. The classic image of witches boiling herbs in a cauldron stems to a large extent from this period. Beginning in about the thirteenth century, however, graduates of male-only medical schools and members of barber-surgeon guilds began to displace the traditional female village herbalists. Ultimately, much of the original lore was lost. (So-called traditional herbal compendiums, such as *Culpeper's Complete Herbal*, are actually of fairly recent vintage.)

Another major change took place in the nineteenth century, when chemistry had advanced far enough to allow extraction of active ingredients from herbs. The old French word for herb, *drogue*, became the name for chemical "drugs." Subsequently, these chemical extracts displaced herbs as the standard of care. Several forces led to the predominance of chemicals over herbs, but one of the most important of these forces remains a major issue today: the problem of reproducibility.

HERBAL MEDICINE'S GREATEST PROBLEM: REPRODUCIBILITY

In purchasing drugs, consumers generally know exactly what they are getting. Drugs are single chemicals that can be measured and quantified down to their molecular structure. Thus, a tablet of extra-strength Tylenol, for example, contains 500 milligrams of acetaminophen, regardless of where or when one buys it. Although it contains a vitamin, not a drug, the same is true of a vitamin C tablet, provided that it is correctly labeled.

Herbs, however, are living organisms comprising thousands of ingredients, and the proportions of all these ingredients may differ dramatically between two plants. Numerous influences can affect the nature of a given crop. Whether it was grown at the top or the

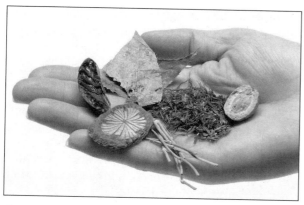

A variety of herbs can be used to prevent and treat illnesses. (PhotoDisc)

bottom of a hill, what the weather was like, what time of year it was picked, what other plants lived nearby, and what kind of soil predominated are only a few of the factors that can affect an herb's chemical makeup.

This presents a real problem for people who wish to use herbs medicinally (as opposed to, say, for taste or fragrance). Because so much variation is possible, it is difficult to know whether one batch of an herb is equivalent in effectiveness to another.

The desire to overcome this problem provided the main initial motivation for finding the active principles of herbs and purifying them into single-chemical drugs. However, by now, most of the common herbs that possess an identifiable active ingredient have long since been turned into drugs. Today's popular herbs do not contain any known, single, active ingredients. For this reason, there is no simple way to determine the effectiveness of a given herbal batch.

This difficulty can be partially overcome by a method called herbal standardization. In this process, manufacturers make an extract of the whole herb and boil off the liquid until the concentration of some ingredient reaches a certain percentage. Contrary to popular belief, this ingredient is not usually the active ingredient; it is merely a "tag" or "handle" used for standardization purposes.

The extract is then made into tablets or capsules or bottled as a liquid, with the concentration of the tag ingredient listed on the label. This method is far from perfect, because two products with the same concentration of tag ingredients may still differ widely in other unlisted or even unidentified active constituents. Nonetheless, this form of partial standardization is better than nothing, and it allows a certain amount of reproducibility. For this reason, it is recommended that whenever possible, one should use standardized herbal extracts. Even better, one should use the very same products that were tested in double-blind studies.

EFFECTIVENESS OF HERBS

There is no doubt that herbs can be effective treatments in principle, if for no other reason than that up through perhaps the 1970s, most drugs used in medicine came from herbs. Many of today's medicinal herbs have been studied in meaningful double-blind, placebo-controlled trials that provide a rational basis for believing them effective. Some of the best substantiated include *Ginkgo biloba* for Alzheimer's disease, St. John's wort for mild to moderate depression, and saw palmetto for benign prostatic hypertrophy.

However, even the best-documented herbs have less supporting evidence than the majority of drugs for one simple reason: An herb cannot be patented; therefore, no single company has the financial incentive to invest millions of dollars in research when another company can "steal" the product after it is proved to work. In addition, the problem of reproducibility always makes it difficult or impossible to know whether the batch of herbs a person is buying is as effective as the one tested in published studies.

The traditional uses of herbs are discussed here, but one should note that such uses are not reliable indicators of an herb's effectiveness. For many reasons, it simply is not possible to accurately evaluate the effectiveness of a medical treatment without performing double-blind, placebo-controlled studies, and many herbs lack these.

SAFETY ISSUES

There is a common belief that herbs are by nature safer and gentler than drugs. However, there is no rational justification for this belief. An herb is simply a plant that contains one or more drugs, and it is just as prone to side effects as any medicine, especially when taken in doses high enough to cause significant benefits.

Nonetheless, the majority of the most popular medicinal herbs are at least fairly safe. The biggest concern in practice tends to involve interactions with medications. Many herbs are known to interact with drugs, and as research into this area expands, more such interactions will be discovered.

EBSCO CAM Review Board

FURTHER READING

Bratman, S., and A. Girman, eds. *Mosby's Handbook of Herbs and Supplements and Their Therapeutic Uses.* St. Louis, Mo.: Mosby, 2003.

Dhanani, N. M., T. J. Caruso, and A. J. Carinci. "Complementary and Alternative Medicine for Pain." *Current Pain and Headache Reports* (November 10, 2010).

Pan, S. Y., et al. "New Perspectives on Innovative Drug Discovery." *Journal of Pharmacy and Pharmaceutical Sciences* 13 (2010): 450-471.

Schulz, V., R. Hansel, and V. Tyler. *Rational Phytotherapy: A Physician's Guide to Herbal Medicine.* 4th ed. New York: Springer, 2001.

Zhang, X., et al. "Chinese Medicinal Herbs for the Common Cold." *Cochrane Database of Systematic Reviews* (2007): CD004782. Available through *EBSCO DynaMed Systematic Literature Surveillance* at http://www.ebscohost.com/dynamed.

See also: Ayurveda; Chinese medicine; Folk medicine; Self-care; Traditional Chinese herbal medicine; Traditional healing.

Herpes

CATEGORY: Condition

RELATED TERMS: Cold sores, genital herpes, herpes simplex

DEFINITION: Treatment of blister-like lesions around the mouth and genitalia caused by the herpes virus.

PRINCIPAL PROPOSED NATURAL TREATMENTS:
- *Prevention:* L-lysine, *Melissa officinalis*
- *Treatment:* Aloe vera, *Melissa officinalis*, topical zinc

OTHER PROPOSED NATURAL TREATMENTS: Adenosine monophosphate, astragalus, bee propolis, cat's claw, echinacea, elderberry, *Eleutherococcus*, kelp, sage-rhubarb cream, sandalwood, tea tree oil, vitamin C, witch hazel

INTRODUCTION

The common virus herpes simplex, known as simply herpes, can cause painful blister-like lesions around the mouth and genitalia. Slightly different strains of herpes predominate in each of these two areas of the body, but the infections are essentially identical. In both areas, the herpes virus remains deep in the de-oxyribonucleic acid (DNA) of nerve ganglia, where it stays inactive for months or years. From time to time the virus reactivates, travels down the nerve, and starts an eruption. Common triggers include stress, dental procedures, infections, and trauma. Flare-ups usually become less severe over time.

Conventional medical treatment consists of antiviral drugs, such as Zovirax. Such medications can shorten the length and intensity of a herpes outbreak or, when taken consistently at lower dosages, reduce the frequency of flare-ups. In addition, they can reduce transmission of the disease.

PRINCIPAL PROPOSED NATURAL TREATMENTS

Several natural treatments have shown promise for treating herpes. However, while conventional treatments can reduce infectivity and thereby help prevent the spread of the disease, no natural treatment has been shown to do this. Commonsense methods used to prevent herpes transmission are not entirely effective: Many people are infectious even when they do not have obvious symptoms, and the use of a condom during sexual intercourse does not entirely prevent the spread of the virus. Therefore, if a person is sexually active with a noninfected partner who wishes to remain that way, the use of suppressive drug therapy is strongly recommended.

Melissa officinalis (lemon balm). More commonly known in the United States as lemon balm, *Melissa officinalis* is widely sold in Europe as a topical cream for the treatment of genital and oral herpes. One double-blind, placebo-controlled study followed sixty-six people who were just starting to develop a cold sore (oral herpes). Treatment with melissa cream produced significant benefits on day two, reducing intensity of discomfort, number of blisters, and the size of the lesion. (The researchers specifically looked at day two because, according to them, that is when symptoms are most pronounced.)

Another double-blind study followed 116 persons with oral or genital herpes. Participants used either melissa cream or placebo cream for up to ten days. The results showed that the use of the herb resulted in a significantly better rate of recovery than the use of placebo.

Aloe vera. The succulent aloe plant is well known as a treatment for burns and minor wounds. However, while there is little evidence it is effective for those purposes, two studies suggest that aloe has potential value in the treatment of herpes infections. A two-week, double-blind, placebo-controlled trial enrolled sixty men with active genital herpes. Participants applied aloe cream (0.5 percent aloe) or placebo cream three times daily for five days. The use of aloe cream reduced the time necessary for lesions to heal and also increased the percentage of persons who were fully healed by the end of two weeks.

An earlier double-blind, placebo-controlled study by the same author, enrolling 120 men with genital herpes, found that aloe cream was more effective than pure aloe gel or placebo. The author theorized that the oily constituents in the cream improved aloe absorption.

L-lysine. Another well-known treatment for herpes involves the amino acid L-lysine. Taken regularly in sufficient doses, lysine supplements appear to reduce the number and intensity of herpes flare-ups. However, a study evaluating lysine taken only at the onset of a herpes attack found no benefit. (One should consider using melissa for this latter purpose.)

One double-blind, placebo-controlled study followed fifty-two persons with a history of herpes flare-ups. While receiving 3 grams of L-lysine every day for six months, the treatment group experienced an average of 2.4 fewer herpes flare-ups than the placebo group; this was a significant difference. The lysine group's flare-ups were also significantly less severe, and they healed faster.

Another double-blind, placebo-controlled cross-over study of forty-one persons also found improvements in the frequency of attacks. This study found that 1,250 milligrams (mg) of lysine daily worked, but 624 mg did not. Other studies, including one that followed sixty-five persons, found no benefit, but these studies used lower dosages of lysine.

Zinc. Zinc lozenges or nasal sprays are thought to be effective for fighting the viruses that cause colds. A late study suggests that topical zinc also may be helpful for herpes infections of the mouth and face. In this trial, forty-six persons with cold sores were treated with a zinc oxide cream or placebo every two hours until cold sores resolved. The results showed that those using the cream experienced a reduction in severity of symptoms and a shorter time to full recovery.

OTHER PROPOSED NATURAL TREATMENTS

Eleutherococcus, also (incorrectly) called Russian or Siberian ginseng, has shown promise for the treat-ment of herpes. A six-month double-blind trial of ninety-three men and women with recurrent genital herpes infections found that treatment with *Eleutherococcus* (2 grams daily) reduced the frequency of infections by almost 50 percent.

A double-blind trial of 149 persons with recurrent oral herpes compared the effectiveness of cream containing Zovirax with cream containing the herbs sage and rhubarb and with cream containing sage alone. The combination of sage and rhubarb proved to be just as effective as Zovirax cream; sage by itself was less effective.

One study suggests that topical treatment with a vitamin C solution may speed healing of oral herpes outbreaks. Oral vitamin C combined with bioflavonoids has also shown some promise for genital herpes.

The results of a small, single-blind, controlled study suggests that the honeybee product propolis cream might cause attacks of genital herpes to heal faster. Other herbs and supplements that are sometimes recommended for herpes infections, but that lack meaningful supporting evidence, include adenosine monophosphate, astragalus, cat's claw, elderberry, kelp, sandalwood, tea tree oil, and witch hazel.

A product containing vitamins and minerals and the herbs paprika, rosemary, peppermint, milfoil, hawthorn, and pumpkin seed has been used in Scandinavia for many years as a treatment for various mouth-related conditions. However, a double-blind study of fifty people with recurrent oral herpes failed to find four months' treatment with this product more effective than placebo. Similarly, a one-year, double-blind, placebo-controlled study of fifty persons with

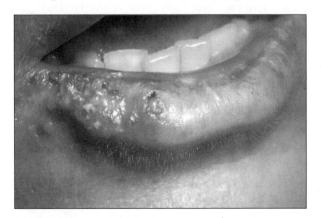

Herpes simplex virus on the lip. (©OJ Staats, MD/Custom Medical Stock Photo)

recurrent genital herpes failed to find the herb echinacea helpful for reducing the rate of flare-ups.

EBSCO CAM Review Board

FURTHER READING

Carson, C. F., et al. "*Melaleuca alternifolia* (Tea Tree) Oil Gel (6 Percent) for the Treatment of Recurrent Herpes Labialis." *Journal of Antimicrobial Chemotherapy* 48 (2001): 450-451.

Godfrey, H. R., et al. "A Randomized Clinical Trial on the Treatment of Oral Herpes with Topical Zinc Oxide/Glycine." *Alternative Therapies in Health and Medicine* 7 (2001): 49-54, 56.

Kane, Melissa, and Tatyana Gotovkina. "Common Threads in Persistent Viral Infections." *Journal of Virology* 84 (2010): 4116-4123.

Langlais, Robert P., and Craig S. Miller. *Color Atlas of Common Oral Diseases.* 4th ed. Philadelphia: Lippincott Williams & Wilkins, 2009.

Vonau, B., et al. "Does the Extract of the Plant *Echinacea purpurea* Influence the Clinical Course of Recurrent Genital Herpes?" *International Journal of STD and AIDS* 12 (2001): 154-158.

See also: Aloe; Canker sores; Herpes; Lemon balm; Lysine.

He shou wu

CATEGORY: Herbs and supplements
RELATED TERMS: Fo ti, *Polygonum multiflorum*
DEFINITION: Natural plant product used to treat specific health conditions.
PRINCIPAL PROPOSED USES: None
OTHER PROPOSED USES: Aging, constipation, enhancing mental function, graying hair, heart disease prevention, high cholesterol, immune support, insomnia

OVERVIEW

The name of this herb, He shou wu, means "Black-haired Mr. He," which is in reference to an ancient story of a Mr. He who restored his vitality, sexual potency, and youthful appearance by taking the herb now named for him. He shou wu is widely used in China for the traditional purpose of restoring black hair and other signs of youth.

Traditional Chinese herbal medicine ordinarily recommends the use of herbs in complex formulas, but He shou wu is also often taken as a single herb. He shou wu is often called fo ti; pure unprocessed root is named white fo ti, while herb boiled in black-bean liquid according to a traditional process is called red fo ti. The two forms are said to have somewhat different properties.

THERAPEUTIC DOSAGES

A typical dose of He shou wu is 3 grams of the raw herb three times daily, or according to the label for processed extracts. For most purposes, the processed or "red" fo ti is said to be superior. However, the raw herb is said to be more effective for constipation.

THERAPEUTIC USES

He shou wu is widely marketed today as a general antiaging herb, said to reduce cholesterol, prevent heart disease, prevent age-related loss of mental function, improve sleep, and extend life span. However, the evidence supporting these proposed uses is far too preliminary to meaningfully indicate effectiveness for any of them.

He shou wu is reputed to strengthen immunity. However, one constituent of the herb, emodin, has shown some promise as an immune system suppressant.

Finally, He shou wu has a traditional reputation as a mild laxative. In support of this, it has been pointed out that emodin belongs to a family of chemicals called anthraquinones; other members of this family act as laxatives. However, animal research has failed to find any evidence that emodin itself has a laxative effect.

SAFETY ISSUES

Detailed modern safety studies have not been performed on this herb. Immediate side effects are infrequent, primarily limited to mild diarrhea and the rare allergic reaction. Safety for young children, pregnant or nursing women, or those with severe kidney or liver disease has not been established.

Case reports relate use of a popular He shou wu product to liver inflammation. However, it is not clear whether the He shou wu herb itself was responsible; Asian herbal preparations of this type have frequently been found to contain unlisted toxic ingredients, either due to poor quality control or deliberate adulteration.

EBSCO CAM Review Board

FURTHER READING

Ernst, E. "Toxic Heavy Metals and Undeclared Drugs in Asian Herbal Medicines." *Trends in Pharmacological Sciences* 23 (2002): 136-139.

Koh, H. L., and S. O. Woo. "Chinese Proprietary Medicine in Singapore: Regulatory Control of Toxic Heavy Metals and Undeclared Drugs." *Drug Safety* 23 (2000): 351-362.

McRae, C. A., et al. "Hepatitis Associated with Chinese Herbs." *European Journal of Gastroenterology and Hepatology* 14 (2002): 559-562.

Park, G. J., et al. "Acute Hepatitis Induced by Shou-wu-pian, an Herbal Product Derived from *Polygonum multiflorum*." *European Journal of Gastroenterology and Hepatology* 16 (2001): 115-117.

See also: Aging; Cholesterol, high; Constipation; Herbal medicine; Immune support; Insomnia; Traditional Chinese herbal medicine.

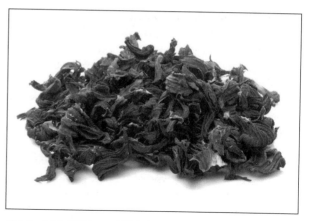

Petals of dried hibiscus. (©Mohamed Osama/Dreamstime.com)

Hibiscus

CATEGORY: Herbs and supplements
RELATED TERMS: *Hibiscus sabdariffa*, roselle
DEFINITION: Natural plant product used to treat specific health conditions.
PRINCIPAL PROPOSED USE: High blood pressure
OTHER PROPOSED USES: Antisepsis, cancer prevention, digestive upset, high cholesterol, liver protection

OVERVIEW

The red-flowered hibiscus shrub is a widely cultivated ornamental plant, and because of its pleasant, tangy taste, it is a common constituent of herbal beverage teas. Medicinally, hibiscus has been taken internally for the treatment of various forms of digestive upset, along with scurvy, anxiety, and fevers. It is said to have an antiseptic and astringent effect when used topically.

THERAPEUTIC DOSAGES

A typical adult dosage of hibiscus is 10 grams (g) of dried calyx (part of the flower), or an extract that provides 250 milligrams (mg) of anthocyanins daily.

THERAPEUTIC USES

Animal studies have suggested that hibiscus might help to lower blood pressure. Based on this, preliminary human studies have been conducted; however, all of these suffered from marked scientific flaws.

In one study, fifty-four people with hypertension were given either hibiscus tea or no extra treatment for two weeks. By the end of the study, people in the hibiscus group had significantly improved blood pressure, compared with those in the group receiving no extra treatment. These results mean little; for a variety of reasons, people who are enrolled in a study and given a treatment tend to improve, regardless of whether the treatment itself actually works. In order to actually show that a treatment works, it must be compared against a placebo.

Another flawed study enrolled ninety people with hypertension and compared the effectiveness of hibiscus (10 g dried hibiscus calyx in water daily) against the standard drug captopril (25 mg twice daily). The results showed equal benefit. However, once more the study is less meaningful than it sounds. This study also failed to use a placebo group. In addition, it was not conducted in a double-blind manner.

In one double-blind study of hibiscus for hypertension, 171 people were given either hibiscus extract (250 mg anthocyanins daily) or the standard drug lisinopril (10 mg daily). The results showed that hibiscus was less effective than the standard drug. Properly speaking, this is the only conclusion that can be drawn from the study. The researchers take pains to emphasize that people taking hibiscus showed blood pressure improvements. However, in the absence of a placebo against which to compare these improvements, they cannot be taken as indicating any specific effect of hibiscus itself. Thus, at present, there is no reliable evidence that hibiscus exerts any antihypertensive effect.

In another double-blind trial, hibiscus was compared to black tea among sixty persons with diabetes and mild hypertension. While subjects taking hibiscus significantly lowered their systolic (higher number) blood pressure over one month, those taking black tea significantly raised their systolic blood pressure over the same period. Again, without directly comparing hibiscus with a placebo, it is difficult to determine whether or not hibiscus effectively lowers blood pressure.

Finally, in a 2010 review of four trials involving 390 adults, investigators summarized the available research on *Hibiscus sabdariffa* for hypertension by concluding that there is insufficient evidence to support its effectiveness.

Hibiscus contains substances called anthocyanins, antioxidants similar to those found in bilberry, cranberry, and red wine. Weak evidence, too weak to be relied upon, hints that hibiscus or its anthocyanin constituents may have anticancer and liver-protective effects and might also improve one's cholesterol profile.

SAFETY ISSUES

As a widely used beverage tea, hibiscus is presumed to have a high degree of safety. However, comprehensive safety testing has not been performed. Maximum safe doses in pregnant or nursing women, young children, or individuals with severe liver or kidney disease have not been established. Some evidence suggests that hibiscus might slightly alter the metabolism of the drug acetaminophen, though the effect is probably not large enough to be very important.

EBSCO CAM Review Board

FURTHER READING

Chang, Y. C., et al. "Hibiscus Anthocyanins Rich Extract-Induced Apoptotic Cell Death in Human Promyelocytic Leukemia Cells." *Toxicology and Applied Pharmacology* 205 (2005): 201-212.

Herrera-Arellano, A., et al. "Clinical Effects Produced by a Standardized Herbal Medicinal Product of *Hibiscus sabdariffa* on Patients with Hypertension." *Planta Medica* 73 (2007): 6-12.

Kolawole, J. A., and A. Maduenyi. "Effect of Zobo Drink (*Hibiscus sabdariffa* Water Extract) on the Pharmacokinetics of Acetaminophen in Human Volunteers." *European Journal of Drug Metabolism and Pharmacokinetics* 29 (2004): 25-29.

Mozaffari-Khosravi, H, et al. "The Effects of Sour Tea (*Hibiscus sabdariffa*) on Hypertension in Patients with Type II Diabetes." *Journal of Human Hypertension* 23, no. 1 (2009): 48-54.

Wahabi, H. A., et al. "The Effectiveness of *Hibiscus sabdariffa* in the Treatment of Hypertension." *Phytomedicine* 17, no. 2 (2010): 83.

See also: Cancer risk reduction; Cholesterol, high; Herbal medicine; Hypertension; Liver disease.

Histidine

CATEGORY: Herbs and supplements
RELATED TERM: L-Histidine
DEFINITION: Natural substance of the human body used as a supplement to treat specific health conditions.
PRINCIPAL PROPOSED USES: None
OTHER PROPOSED USE: Rheumatoid arthritis

OVERVIEW

Histidine is a semi-essential amino acid, which means the body normally makes as much as it needs. Like most other amino acids, histidine is used to make proteins and enzymes. The body also uses histidine to make histamine, which causes the swelling and itching of an allergic reaction.

It appears that people with rheumatoid arthritis may have low levels of histidine in their blood. This has led to some speculation that histidine supplements might be a good treatment for this kind of arthritis, but so far no studies have confirmed this.

REQUIREMENTS AND SOURCES

Although histidine is not required in the diet, histidine deficiencies can occur during periods of very rapid growth. Dairy products, meat, poultry, fish, and other protein-rich foods are good sources of histidine.

THERAPEUTIC DOSAGES

A typical therapeutic dosage of histidine is 4 to 5 grams daily.

THERAPEUTIC USES

Although individuals with rheumatoid arthritis appear to have reduced levels of histidine in the blood, this by itself does not prove that taking histidine will help. One study designed to evaluate this question directly found no significant benefit.

SAFETY ISSUES

As a necessary nutrient, histidine is believed to be safe. However, maximum safe dosages of histidine have not been determined for young children, pregnant or nursing women, or those with severe liver or kidney disease. As with other supplements taken in large doses, it is important to purchase a quality product, as contaminants present even in very small percentages could conceivably add up and become toxic.

EBSCO CAM Review Board

FURTHER READING

Gerber, D. A., et al. "Free Serum Histidine Levels in Patients with Rheumatoid Arthritis and Control Subjects Following an Oral Load of Free L-Histidine." *Metabolism* 25 (1976): 655-657.

Pinals, R. S., et al. "Treatment of Rheumatoid Arthritis with L-Histidine." *Journal of Rheumatology* 4 (1977): 414-419.

See also: Allergies; Rheumatoid arthritis.

History of alternative medicine

CATEGORY: Issues and overviews

DEFINITION: An examination of a broad range of nontraditional healing therapies that rely on a balance of systems within the body and that avoid the use of drugs for treatment.

OVERVIEW

Alternative medicine (AM), often coupled with the term "complementary," is the practice of various healing techniques in place of traditional medicine. AM is not commonly taught in medical schools, and most AM practices are not covered by health insurance in the United States. AM practices are derived from ancient methods and beliefs and from social behaviors, spirituality, and newer approaches. AM bases good health on a balance of body systems (mental, spiritual, and physical), whereas conventional medicine views good health as the absence of disease.

Much of AM, with the exception of herbal supplements, is based on all aspects of the person being intertwined. This principle is called holism. It is believed that disharmony that undermines balance among these aspects can stress the body and lead to illness. Therefore, in an effort to alleviate sickness, therapies focus on bolstering the body's own defenses while restoring balance. Similar to Western medicine, however, AM emphasizes proper nutrition and preventive practices.

Before the 1990s, AM was dismissed by most American medical professionals, mostly because there was no supporting scientific evidence of its therapeutic effects. With an increasing number of AM practitioners, and with health consumer acceptance, it has become more common to integrate alternative therapies into mainstream health care. AM journals, organizations, courses of study, Web sites, and government-supported clinical trials are now common in the United States.

MECHANISMS OF ACTION

Only theories exist on the mechanisms of action for alternative remedies, so many advocates believe that the scientific method does not apply to this type of practice. Instead, AM advocates rely on anecdotes and theories, which include the theory that AM defies biologic mechanisms and should, therefore, be understood as less harmful than conventional methods. In many cases, simply publishing anecdotes in popular books and magazines is enough evidence for the general support of therapeutic claims.

Oftentimes, alternative remedies are discovered through trial and error. A specific alternative method may work for one person but not for another. Practitioners sometimes have to try several different approaches for the same issue in different persons. Also, one type of approach could be useful for several different health issues.

Language is another obstacle to understanding the way alternative therapies work. For instance, there are no direct translations for the types of energy in Ayurvedic medicine known as *vata*, *pitta*, and *kapha*, making it impossible to integrate these types of components into controlled scientific trials for the purpose of determining a mechanism of action.

USES

Alternative medicine is commonly used for relatively minor health problems (such as fatigue, insomnia, or back pain). For the most part, AM is utilized for health enhancement in a relatively healthy patient.

An increasingly popular application of alternative therapies is in integrative medicine, which is the combination of alternative and conventional remedies. Integrative medicine is emerging into mainstream medical practice because of supporting clinical evidence of its benefits. One example of integrated medicine is the use aromatherapy to minimize nausea after a course of chemotherapy.

EARLY HISTORY

The term "alternative medicine" has been in use since the late eighteenth century. The Greek physician Hippocrates, known as the founder of medicine, introduced this concept during a time when humans were questioning whether or not the practice of medicine is an art. Furthermore, Hippocrates believed the mind and body both play a role in the healing process. Ironically enough, the mind/body healing process is essentially the basis of many alternative therapies.

Several healing systems existed in the nineteenth century. Treatment procedures ranged from bleeding and purging to folk medicine and quackery. Many of these approaches were dangerous and often fatal, leading people to revolt against these extreme measures of medical practice. By midcentury, the general public showed its disappointment with standard therapies and began to turn to alternative methods. As a result, the first alternative medicine system in the West was implemented by Samuel Thomson, who used botanicals for healing. The plant drugs, he believed, either evacuated or heated the body. After his death in 1840, the Thomsonianism system fell from use.

Homeopathy was promoted by Samuel Hahnemann, a German physician who treated many disease symptoms with a series of drug dilutions. The term "allopathy" was coined by Hahnemann while he was in the United States. Mainstream medicine adopted allopathy as a standard medical term, and it has remained a part of health-care terminology.

Also at midcentury, Americans were introduced to hydropathy. This Austrian treatment called for a variety of baths (usually cold) to eliminate toxins and for strict lifestyle changes (such as in diet, exercise, and sleep). Several other popular remedies during this time were magnetism and hypnosis healing, which was introduced by Franz Mesmer.

Because of so many AM options, New York-based Wooster Beach decided to combine the various treatment approaches that were based on clinical expertise, calling his new approach eclectic medicine. Eclectic medicine advocated for care that incorporates more than one type of therapy or method. A modern form of eclectic medicine is acupuncture with chiropractic or osteopathic care. Eclectic medicine was well received from 1820 through the 1930s.

The second generation of alternative medical systems began in the second half of the nineteenth century. In the 1870s, Andrew Taylor Still pioneered the technique of musculoskeletal manipulation, better known as osteopathy. Following closely was Daniel David Palmer, who introduced chiropractic medicine. By the late nineteenth century, osteopathic and chiropractic schools were offering formal training. Naturopathy, using the body's natural healing powers, also became increasingly popular near the end of this century.

THE TWENTIETH CENTURY

By 1900, about 20 percent of all practitioners were AM physicians. Upon the discovery of novel drugs, such as antibiotics, in the 1930s and 1940s, the once highly acclaimed alternative therapies became nearly obsolete. Even doctors of osteopathic and chiropractic medicine were forced not to treat patients, and schools that once offered training in these disciples had to close their doors.

With immigration on the rise, especially in the 1970s, American physicians began to discover acupuncture, Chinese herbal medicine, and Ayurvedic medicine.

The philosophy of healing now faced much questioning by American physicians. Controversy erupted between medical doctors and AM practitioners. AM was denounced as unscientific, and AM practice was considered unethical. The American Medical Association's code of ethics even prohibited medical doctors from consulting with persons who used alternative remedies.

By the late twentieth century, physicians were again allowed to consult with AM practitioners, and osteopathy and chiropractic were more and more accepted by the medical mainstream. The general public had become dissatisfied with traditional medicine. Americans felt that health care was impersonal, that pharmaceuticals caused harm, and that medical care was costly.

In 1992, the National Institutes of Health established the Office of Alternative Medicine (now called the National Center for Complementary and Alternative Medicine) in an effort to examine and report on the efficacy of alternative methods. By 1995, the first journal dedicated to alternative therapies and health was in circulation. The notion of mind/body healing was regaining respect in mainstream medical practice.

A 1998 government report documented that four out of every ten American adults had used some type of alternative therapy in 1997. In addition, more than $20 billion was spent by Americans on alternative health care. By 2002, three out of four American adults had used some type of alternative remedy. With alternative medicine on the rise in the United States, the need for evidence-based alternative methods became clear.

Scientific Evidence

Testing alternative therapies for scientific relevance presents several challenges. First, many therapies existed long before the development of Western scientific, analytical methods. For instance, chiropractic procedures were discovered before scientific understandings of the nervous system. Second, mechanisms of action and proposed outcomes of alternative therapies are not clearly understood. Third, interventions may be a combination of treatments. For example, an Ayurvedic practitioner may prescribe herbal supplements, yoga, and dietary restrictions. The problem here is determining what intervention cured a certain problem. Finally, designing standardized placebo-controlled clinical trials is difficult. An example of this is the challenge of trying to create artificial yoga, chiropractic, or Tai Chi procedures.

New methods and study designs are needed to investigate alternative therapies for scientific support. It is encouraging to know, however, that thousands of trials are under way.

Conclusions

The combination of limited knowledge of the effects of AM and its increased use by health consumers produces a dangerous situation. Many products and procedures are not regulated, leading to the potential for risks. Herb-drug interactions may occur because of contamination or because of the poor quality of ingredients. Finally, not all AM practitioners are licensed or formally trained.

Jigna Bhalla, Pharm.D.

Further Reading

Alternative Medicine Center. http://www.altmed.net. A user-friendly guide to alternative medicine.

Goldberg, Burton. *Alternative Medicine: The Definitive Guide.* Tiburon, Calif.: Future Medicine, 1998. This book provides an overview of many different alternative medicine approaches.

Journal of Alternative and Complementary Medicine. http://www.liebertpub.com. A Web-based journal for practitioners seeking to integrate alternative medicine into their practice.

Marti, James E. *The Alternative Health and Medicine Encyclopedia.* 2d ed. Detroit: Visible Ink Press, 1997. This edition offers more than three hundred therapies for more than seventy disease states. It is easy to read and offers basic facts on a variety of alternative therapies.

Micozzi, Marc. *Fundamentals of Complementary and Alternative Medicine.* 3d ed. St. Louis, Mo.: Saunders/Elsevier, 2006. This book offers good background on the foundation and context of alternative therapies. Each entry also includes a list of further readings and related organizations.

Nash, Barbara. *From Acupressure to Zen: An Encyclopedia of Natural Therapies.* Upland, Pa.: Diane, 1998. This book provides an overview of basic information on many different alternative medicine approaches and natural therapies.

National Center for Complementary and Alternative Medicine. http://nccam.nih.gov. A U.S. government site that offers research-based information on complementary and alternative therapies.

See also: Alternative versus traditional medicine; History of complementary medicine; National Center for Complementary and Alternative Medicine; Traditional healing.

History of complementary medicine

CATEGORY: Issues and overviews

DEFINITION: An examination of the history of non-traditional or alternative medical practices that are complementary to traditional medicine.

OVERVIEW

The history of complementary medicine (CM) includes two distinct but overlapping narratives: the histories of the various complementary treatments and practices, themselves a collection of more than one hundred different approaches, and the history of their definition as complementary. One immediate problem is the lack of an agreed-upon definition of CM. The National Center for Complementary and Alternative Medicine (NCCAM) defines CM as "the use of a group of diverse medical and health care systems, practices, and products that are not generally considered part of conventional medicine . . . together with conventional medicine." The National Cancer Institute (NCI) defines CM as "any medical system, practice, or product that is not thought of as standard care" and that is used "with standard medicine."

The Institute of Medicine (IOM), however, notes that the identification of any treatment as complementary is in part a historical judgment; IOM defines CM as that which contrasts "the dominant health system of a particular society or culture in a given historical period." This essay will focus on the evolution of complementary medicine in the United States, which has been a unique historical laboratory for unconventional approaches to health care.

THE NINETEENTH CENTURY: INNOVATION AND COMPETITION

The term "complementary medicine" is a recent coinage, the result of two major changes in the landscape of health care in the United States. The first change was the transition in the nineteenth and early twentieth centuries from a range of patterns of medical education and competing philosophies of health care to the standardization of educational requirements for physicians and the establishment of Western scientific medicine as the yardstick against which all other approaches were measured. The second major change was the opposition to this standardization that began in the 1960s.

What is now considered the center of a physician's education, the university-related medical school, was the exception rather than the rule for the first century of the existence of the United States. Only two such schools had been founded before the American Revolution, one at the University of Pennsylvania (1765) and the other at Columbia University (1767). Because of the vast size of the continent and the difficulties of practicing medicine on the frontier, other ways of training physicians were adopted. Training now included apprenticeships with practicing physicians, at the end of which the fledgling practitioner was admitted to the local medical society on the basis of a letter of recommendation from the student's mentor. There were no state or national board examinations at this time.

Another development was the establishment of proprietary schools of medicine, so called because they were owned privately (usually by a group of local physicians) and operated for profit. Although some of the older East Coast institutions had founded schools of medicine separate from their undergraduate colleges (such as Harvard in 1782 and Yale in 1810), the proprietary schools met the needs of underserved rural areas in the Midwest and deep South. The proprietary schools also allowed for the emergence of alternatives to what had not yet been defined as mainstream scientific medicine.

Several competing approaches to health care flourished in the nineteenth century, ranging from such American innovations as Thomsonianism (1820s), osteopathy (1892), and chiropractic (1897) to such European imports as hydrotherapy (1844) and homeopathy (1848). Perhaps the most typically American development was eclectic medicine, which emerged in the 1830s and combined Thomsonianism with conventional medicine, physical therapy, and Native American herbalism. Its mix-and-match utilization of different therapies was a forerunner of CM as defined today.

THE TWENTIETH CENTURY: STANDARDIZATION AND NEW DIVERSIFICATION

In 1908, educator Abraham Flexner was asked by the Carnegie Foundation to evaluate the condition of medical education in the United States. Flexner's report, published in 1910, marked the end of the proprietary schools; their approach to medicine went underground for half a century, to reemerge in the wake of the counterculture of the 1960s. Flexner recommended the closure of half the 155 medical schools then operating in the United States; the establishment of the university-related school of medicine as the ideal pattern; the requirement of college-level preparation before admission to medical school; and strict adherence to mainstream science in teaching and research. Schools of homeopathy, naturopathy, and similar approaches were forced to abandon courses in these alternatives or to close down. The exception was osteopathy, which survived because the American Osteopathic Association was able to bring most schools of osteopathic medicine into line with Flexner's stipulations.

From the period following World War I until the 1960s, Western allopathic (conventional) medicine

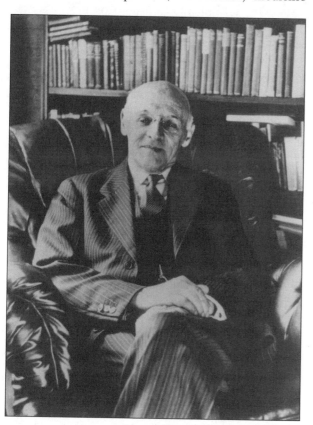

The Carnegie Foundation asked educator Abraham Flexner to evaluate the condition of medical education in the United States. (Getty Images)

was considered normative in the United States, with all other therapies classified as mere historical curiosities. The situation began to change in the 1960s for several reasons. First, mainstream medicine was discredited because of such emotionally painful episodes as the thalidomide disaster of 1961 and the withdrawal of diethylstilbestrol (DES) after 1971. The discovery that drugs developed to treat anxiety and the risk of miscarriage, respectively, had teratogenic or carcinogenic side effects led to skepticism regarding the benefits of so-called scientific medicine. Second, the bureaucratization of medicine spurred by the passage of the Health Maintenance Organization Act of 1973 and the rise of managed care caused widespread discontent among health consumers, who resented the denial of treatments they considered necessary; many also complained that medicine was becoming too impersonal.

The third factor that helped to revive interest in other approaches to health care was the emergence of new religious movements (NRMs) in the 1960s and 1970s. Some of these groups had affinities with Eastern religions and explored such ancient Asian medical systems as Ayurveda and traditional Chinese medicine. Others, influenced by the back-to-nature enthusiasm of the environmental movement, began to study Western herbalism and folk remedies in preference to the "artificial" prescription drugs produced in laboratories. Fourth, the emphasis of traditional Judaism and Christianity and NRMs on the importance of spiritual and physical well-being resonated with many who were dissatisfied with the assembly-line treatment they received in conventional health maintenance organizations. Part of the appeal of such therapies as chiropractic and naturopathy was that their practitioners spent time with their patients rather than rushing them through appointments as quickly as possible.

COMPLEMENTARY MEDICINE IN THE TWENTY-FIRST CENTURY

In the early twenty-first century, unconventional therapies were used much more often as complementary treatments than as strict alternatives to mainstream medicine. As a result, CAM's relationship to mainstream medicine is constantly changing. Three basic patterns define in the relationship of various complementary approaches to conventional medicine.

Defining ancient practices as complementary therapies. According to NCCAM, as of 2007, meditation and yoga were not only two of the most commonly used complementary approaches in the United States among adults but also among those that have shown the greatest increase in use since 2002. When prayer is included in NCCAM statistics, it appears to be the single complementary approach used most often in North America. Prayer for healing has been practiced by Jews and Christians since at least the first millennium B.C.E. Yoga as a spiritual discipline among Hindus goes back to about 600 B.C.E., although yoga was not widely practiced in North America until the 1970s and was added to college curricula in physical education departments rather than as a form of spirituality. What is significant about NCCAM's classification of these practices is its definition of them as therapies, given that they are far older than conventional medicine.

Mainstreaming of formerly unconventional treatments. Some approaches once considered unconventional are now regarded as mainstream practice. The most notable example is osteopathy, which began in the United States in the 1890s. Osteopathic schools chose to accept the recommendations of the 1910 Flexner report, reorganizing their curricula to increase the similarity of osteopathy to conventional medicine. By 1969, doctors of osteopathy (D.O.s) were accepted as members by the American Medical Association, and by 2000, they were accepted into almost all hospital postgraduate programs on an equal basis with medical doctors (M.D.s). The use of osteopathic manipulative medicine, the remaining distinctive feature of osteopathic training, is in decline; fewer osteopaths perform it today, and more recommend surgery as first-line treatment.

An example of an Asian therapy that is increasingly regarded as mainstream rather than complementary in the United States is acupuncture. Considered an exotic Chinese treatment until the early 1970s, acupuncture has been used by about 1 percent of the American population for pain relief as of 2007. The U.S. Food and Drug Administration (FDA) approved the use of properly manufactured acupuncture needles by licensed practitioners as early as 1996.

Complementary therapies in the United States considered mainstream elsewhere. Herbal medicine is an example of a therapy classified as complementary in the United States but regarded as mainstream practice

Complementary, Alternative, and Integrative Medicine Defined

- *Complementary medicine* is a type of therapy that is used with conventional medicine (for example, using massage therapy, a complementary therapy, and drug therapy, a conventional therapy, to reduce the discomfort of fibromyalgia).
- *Alternative medicine* replaces conventional medicine (for example, using a special diet to treat cancer instead of conventional cancer treatments such as chemotherapy, radiation, and surgery).
- *Integrative medicine* combines mainstream medical therapies with complementary and alternative therapies for which there is some high-quality scientific evidence of safety and effectiveness.

elsewhere, in this case in Europe and Japan. Herbal preparations are defined as dietary supplements in the United States and can be purchased over the counter. The Dietary Supplement Health and Education Act (DSHEA), passed by Congress in 1994, gave the FDA authority to monitor the safety of herbal products once on the market and to recall or impound those found to be contaminated or otherwise unsafe. Manufacturers of these products, however, are not required to demonstrate their safety or effectiveness before marketing them.

In Germany and Japan, by contrast, herbal preparations are prescribed by licensed physicians. In 1978, Commission E, a regulatory agency of the German government composed of pharmacists, physicians, and botanists, was formed to evaluate the safety and efficacy of more than three hundred herbs. The sale of prescription herbal medicines has been rising rapidly in Germany since the 1990s, driven by consumer demands for natural alternatives to synthetic drugs. The Japanese equivalent is Kampo, a group of 148 traditional herbal formulae originally derived from Chinese medicine and approved by the Japanese ministry of health beginning in 1967. The manufacture of Kampo formulae is rigorously supervised by the government, and the medicines must be obtained by prescription from licensed physicians.

Given the increasing fluidity of the boundaries between complementary and conventional therapies, many observers (particularly Edzard Ernst, the world's first professor of CM) are calling for an end to the classification of medicine as either mainstream or unconventional. Ernst stated in a 2008 interview, "There is no such thing as alternative medicine. There is either medicine that is effective or not, medicine that is safe or not."

Rebecca J. Frey, Ph.D.

FURTHER READING

Bodeker, G., et al. *WHO Global Atlas of Traditional, Complementary, and Alternative Medicine.* Kobe, Japan: WHO Kobe Centre, 2005. This two-volume publication consists of a map volume and a text volume. The map volume provides information not only on CAM therapies worldwide but also on legislation and professional regulation of CAM practitioners. The text volume offers detailed descriptions and analyses of the use of traditional and CAM therapies in twenty-three countries.

Ernst, Edzard, Max H. Pittler, and Barbara Wider, eds. *Complementary Therapies for Pain Management: An Evidence-Based Approach.* New York: Mosby/Elsevier, 2007. Coedited by a European expert on CM, this book offers concise summaries of complementary approaches to pain relief and analyses of clinical trial data for their effectiveness.

Institute of Medicine of the National Academies. *Alternative Medicine in the United States.* Washington, D.C.: National Academies Press, 2005. This report, originally commissioned by the National Academies of Science in 2002, discusses questions of public policy, identifies scientific issues regarding CM, and analyzes the populations that use complementary therapies most often.

National Center for Complementary and Alternative Medicine. http://nccam.nih.gov. A comprehensive site for basic information about CAM therapies and for demographic statistics about the use of CAM in the United States.

Office of Cancer Complementary and Alternative Medicine. http://www.cancer.gov/cam. Provides an introduction to the various complementary therapies for persons with cancer and information about clinical trials of CAM therapies.

Whorton, James C. *Nature Cures: The History of Alternative Medicine in America.* New York: Oxford University Press, 2002. This book is one of the few historical overviews of CAM therapies in the United States, as distinct from descriptions of the therapies themselves.

See also: Alternative versus traditional medicine; History of alternative medicine; Integrative medicine; National Center for Complementary and Alternative Medicine; Office of Cancer Complementary and Alternative Medicine; Traditional healing.

HIV/AIDS support

CATEGORY: Condition

RELATED TERMS: Acquired immunodeficiency syndrome, human immunodeficiency virus

DEFINITION: Treatment of symptoms of human immunodeficiency virus infection and acquired immunodeficiency syndrome.

PRINCIPAL PROPOSED NATURAL TREATMENTS: None

OTHER PROPOSED NATURAL TREATMENTS:

- *For inhibiting viral replication:* Aloe, astragalus, bacailin, boxwood extract, curcumin, elderberry, propolis, reishi, schisandra, spirulina
- *For enhancing the immune system:* Carnitine, coenzyme Q_{10}, dehydroepiandrosterone, echinacea, fish oil, ginseng, licorice, lipoic acid, maitake, massage therapy, methionine, *Momordica charantia*, N-acetylcysteine, omega-6 fatty acids, proteolytic enzymes, relaxation therapies, trichosanthin, whey protein
- *For fighting weight loss:* Glutamine, medium-chain triglycerides, whey protein
- *For treating other symptoms and opportunistic infections:* Bovine colostrum, Chinese herb combinations, cinnamon, dehydroepiandrosterone, tea tree oil
- *For treating medication side effects:* Carnitine, CoQ_{10}, glutamine, vitamin B_{12}, zinc
- *For general nutrition support:* Beta-carotene, iron, multivitamins, niacin, selenium, vitamin A, vitamin B_1, vitamin B_3, vitamin B_6, vitamin B_{12}, vitamin C, vitamin E, zinc

NATURAL TREATEMENTS TO AVOID: Garlic, St. John's wort

INTRODUCTION

The human immunodeficiency virus (HIV) is the virus that can lead to acquired immunodeficiency syndrome (AIDS). HIV progressively destroys or damages cells in the immune system, making its host vulnerable to certain cancers and infections. Opportunistic infections (those infections caused by microorganisms that do not ordinarily cause illness in healthy people) can have serious, and fatal, effects in people with AIDS.

HIV is spread most commonly through certain sexual practices and by intravenous drug use. Also, women can infect their fetuses before or during birth or later through breast-feeding.

Within a month or two of exposure, infection with HIV may cause short-term flulike symptoms, followed by a symptom-free period lasting months to years, during which the virus continues to multiply. After this stage, people with HIV may develop swollen lymph nodes, recurrent herpes sores, diarrhea, weight loss, and chronic yeast infections (oral or vaginal)–a state previously called AIDS-related complex (or ARC). Children may experience delayed development or fail to thrive. The infection is called AIDS when the number of immune cells known as CD4+, or helper T cells, drops below a certain level, or when opportunistic diseases such as pneumocystis pneumonia develop.

Today, both ARC and AIDS are collectively called symptomatic HIV infection. This condition is increasingly rare in the developed world because of the success of pharmaceutical treatments. For many people, HIV infection is a manageable, if challenging, chronic illness.

The most effective treatment for HIV is called HAART, or highly active antiretroviral therapy. This approach generally involves the combined use of three or more drugs, taken from various families of antiretroviral drugs, including non-nucleoside reverse transcriptase inhibitors, nucleoside reverse transcriptase inhibitors, fusion inhibitors, and protease inhibitors. Taken together, these medications can prevent the development of AIDS indefinitely.

HAART, however, causes numerous side effects. Surveys have shown that people with HIV often take natural remedies in addition to conventional medications, in hopes of reducing side effects and enhancing efficacy. Persons with HIV should consult their doctors about any natural substances being taken. Also, one should be alert to possible interactions. People with HIV should not use St. John's wort or garlic. Even vitamin C may pose risks.

PROPOSED NATURAL TREATMENTS

Among the many proposed natural treatments for HIV, none has more than preliminary supporting evidence.

Inhibiting viral replication. No natural remedies rival the effectiveness of antiretroviral drugs for inhibiting HIV replication in the body. However, preliminary research suggests that an extract of the leaves and stems of the boxwood shrub may have at least some efficacy. Many other herbs and supplements have been proposed, but there is little evidence that they work.

Boxwood. In a double-blind, placebo-controlled study of 145 people with HIV, French researchers studied the effects of two doses of a preparation made from the evergreen boxwood (*Buxus sempervirens*). The preparation was given in doses of 990 milligrams (mg) and 1,980 mg per day for periods ranging from four to sixty-four weeks.

When participants started the study, they had no symptoms of HIV and had never taken antiretroviral drugs. They were kept off anti-HIV drugs during the study. (This was before the use of anti-HIV drugs became widespread.) At the end, researchers found that among those taking the lower dose, fewer people developed AIDS, symptomatic HIV, or CD4+ counts below 200 compared with those taking the higher dose or placebo. Additionally, by the end of their treatment period, fewer people in the low-dose group had a large increase in the amount of HIV they carried compared with the other two groups.

The researchers had originally planned the study to continue for eighteen months (seventy-eight weeks). However, as the study progressed, a review committee decided to halt the study early when the average participant had taken boxwood or placebo for only thirty-seven weeks. The review committee felt it was unethical to continue to have some people take placebo, given the positive results among those taking the extract. Nonetheless, further research is necessary to confirm the effectiveness of boxwood extract for HIV, particularly with proven antiviral drugs, which have now become the standard of care for HIV infection.

No severe side effects were reported in this study, and the people taking boxwood had the same overall rate of side effects as those taking placebo. However, there are some safety concerns with this herb. A substance called cycloprotobuxine is believed to be one of the active ingredients in boxwood. High doses of this substance can cause vomiting, diarrhea, muscular spasms, and paralysis. The herb should only be taken under medical supervision. Safety in pregnant or nursing women, young children, and people with liver or kidney disease has not been established. In

The Connection Between HIV and Diet

HIV and many of its treatments can change the body's metabolism, or the way the body processes nutrients and other substances (like body fat). Some of these metabolic changes can lead to lipodystrophy, insulin resistance, and wasting syndrome, and can affect the way a person looks and feels. These three metabolic changes are defined here.

- *Lipodystrophy.* Also known as fat maldistribution or fat redistribution, lipodystrophy is a problem with the way the body produces, uses, and distributes fat. Lipodystrophy is associated with certain anti-HIV drugs. HIV-related lipodystrophy includes the body changes known as buffalo hump and protease paunch.
- *Insulin resistance.* Insulin resistance is an abnormal body response to insulin, a hormone that regulates glucose (sugar) levels. People with insulin resistance have abnormally high blood levels of insulin, which may lead to heart and cholesterol problems and obesity. Insulin resistance may occur in HIV-infected persons taking certain protease inhibitors.
- *Wasting syndrome.* Wasting syndrome is defined as the involuntary loss of more than 10 percent of one's body weight and experiencing more than thirty days of either diarrhea or weakness and fever. Wasting refers to the loss of muscle mass, although part of the weight loss may also be caused by loss of fat. HIV-associated wasting syndrome is considered an AIDS-defining condition.

addition, touching fresh boxwood leaves can occasionally cause skin irritation.

Only a special boxwood extract has been studied as a treatment for HIV infection. One should not try to use raw boxwood leaf because it might not be safe.

Other proposed natural treatments. One of the constituents of the herb aloe, acemannan, has shown some promise in test-tube and animal studies for stimulating immunity and inhibiting the growth of viruses. These findings have led to trials of acemannan (or whole aloe) for the treatment of HIV infection. However, a double-blind, placebo-controlled trial of acemannan failed to find any benefits for people with severe HIV infection. (There is some question whether the effects seen in these studies were actually caused by acemannan or by a contaminant called aloeride.)

Other substances that have been investigated for possible HIV suppression include bacailin (Chinese skullcap), curcumin, elderberry, schisandra, spirulina, and reishi. However, as with aloe, the evidence that they work is primarily limited to test-tube and animal studies; whether these results translate into real improvement among people with HIV has not been determined.

The herb St. John's wort contains a substance called hypericin, which has been investigated for possible anti-HIV effects. However, contrary to popular belief, neither hypericin nor St. John's wort is useful for treating HIV infection. In addition, St. John's wort seriously impairs the activity of standard HIV medications and might lead to treatment failure.

Enhancing the immune system. In test-tube studies, a number of substances have been found to improve measures of immunity in HIV infection, for example, by elevating CD4+ counts, changing the ratio between CD4+ cells and other immune cells, increasing amounts of other immune chemicals, or enhancing the body's ability to attack invading substances. However, there is relatively little information on whether they can actually help people with HIV infection.

N-acetylcysteine. One of the natural substances most widely used by people with HIV in hopes of enhancing immune system function is the antioxidant N-acetylcysteine (NAC), but evidence that it helps is somewhat conflicting. NAC is a specially modified form of the dietary amino acid cysteine. NAC supplements help the body make the important antioxidant enzyme glutathione. Early human trials, including a double-blind study of forty-five people, suggest that NAC may increase levels of CD4+ cells in healthy people and slow CD4+ cell decline in people with HIV infection. Another study of NAC combined with selenium had mixed results, affecting T-cell counts in some people but not in others. However, preliminary results of another study found that NAC had no effect on CD4+ counts or the amount of HIV in the blood. Whey protein also contains cysteine and may increase glutathione levels, but there is no evidence of any meaningful benefit.

Other proposed natural treatments. One study found evidence that the amino acid methionine taken at a dose of 2.4 g daily may mildly improve immune function in people with HIV infection. Other natural treatments that are sometimes recommended to boost immunity in HIV include andrographis, trichosanthin (compound Q), lipoic acid, coenzyme Q_{10}, maitake, a component of licorice known as glycyrrhizin, *Momordica charantia* (an herb also called bitter melon), echinacea, ginseng, omega-6 fatty acids, carnitine, and proteolytic enzymes. However, there is no real evidence that these treatments actually work. Garlic is sometimes recommended too, but for safety reasons it should be avoided by persons with HIV infection.

Fish oil is also sometimes recommended for enhancing immunity in HIV infection. However, one six-month, double-blind study found that a combination of the omega-3 fatty acids in fish oil plus the amino acid arginine was no more effective than placebo in improving immune function in people with HIV infection. Another study found that the hormone dehydroepiandrosterone (DHEA) does not improve immunity in people with HIV infection.

Study results are mixed on whether massage therapy can improve measures of immune function. A careful review of thirty-five randomized trials found that relaxation therapies may be generally helpful at improving the quality of life of HIV-positive persons and in reducing their anxiety, depression, stress, and fatigue. These interventions, though, had no significant effect on the growth of the virus, nor did they influence immunologic or hormonal activity. Subsequently, however, a small study involving forty-eight persons with HIV found that mindfulness meditation, a popular method for inducing the relaxation response, slowed the loss of the specific immune cells destroyed by the virus, though more research needs to be done to confirm this result.

Treating other symptoms and opportunistic infections. In addition to the foregoing treatments, a number of natural remedies have been proposed for symptoms of HIV or common opportunistic infections. Bovine colostrum has been suggested as a treatment for the chronic diarrhea that commonly occurs in people with HIV or AIDS, but the evidence that it works is weak at best.

Tea tree oil and cinnamon have been suggested as treatments for thrush (oral candida infection). There is some evidence that capsaicin cream applied topically is beneficial for limb pain caused by peripheral neuropathy associated with HIV infection.

DHEA is a hormone that seems to decrease in people with AIDS, possibly because of malnutrition and stress. One small double-blind trial suggests that DHEA (50 mg per day) may improve mood and fatigue scores in people with HIV; another small trial found

inconclusive results. A more substantial (145-participant) double-blind study found that DHEA at a dose of 100 to 400 mg daily improved symptoms of dysthymia (minor depression) in people with HIV, without significant adverse effects. DHEA does not appear to provide general benefits for people with HIV, such as improving immunity, suppressing virus levels, or aiding weight maintenance.

Chinese herbal combinations have been investigated for the treatment of HIV, but the results have not been very promising. In a twelve-week, double-blind, placebo-controlled trial, thirty HIV-infected adults with CD4+ counts of 200 to 500 were given a Chinese herbal formula containing thirty-one herbs. The results hint that the use of the herbal combination might have improved various symptoms compared with placebo, but none of the differences were statistically significant. People who believed they were taking the real treatment showed significant benefit regardless of whether they were in the placebo group or the real treatment group.

In another double-blind, placebo-controlled trial, sixty-eight HIV-positive adults were given either placebo or a preparation of thirty-five Chinese herbs for six months. The results indicate that the use of Chinese herbs did not improve symptoms or objective measurements of HIV severity. In fact, people using the herbs reported more digestive problems than those given placebo.

Fighting weight loss. Undesired weight loss is a frequent symptom of HIV and AIDS. Weight loss can be so extreme that the person seems to "waste away," hence the name "AIDS wasting syndrome," which is technically defined as the loss of more than 10 percent of body weight combined with either chronic diarrhea or weakness and fever. Many factors can contribute to this weight loss, including loss of appetite, nausea, malabsorption of nutrients, and mouth sores. Supplemental medium-chain triglycerides (MCTs), a particular type of fat, and glutamine may be helpful for this symptom, although there is no definitive evidence that they work.

MCTs. Fat malabsorption is particularly common in HIV infection and can lead to both diarrhea and weight loss. MCTs, which are more easily absorbed than ordinary fats (long-chain triglycerides), may help decrease diarrhea and wasting. Two small, double-blind studies have found that MCTs are more easily absorbed than long-chain triglycerides in people with

HIV or AIDS. However, there is no direct evidence that MCTs actually help people gain weight. In both of these studies, participants consumed nothing but a special nutritional formula containing MCTs. Taking MCTs in this way requires medical supervision to determine the dose. People with HIV or diabetes should not use MCTs (or any other supplement) without a doctor's supervision.

Glutamine. Another promising treatment for wasting is the amino acid glutamine, a substance that plays a role in maintaining the health of the immune system, digestive tract, and muscle cells. Although research is still preliminary, one double-blind, placebo-controlled study found that a combination of glutamine and antioxidants (vitamins C and E, beta-carotene, selenium, and N-acetylcysteine) led to significant weight gain in people with HIV who had lost weight. Another small, double-blind trial found that combination treatment with glutamine, arginine, and beta-hydroxy beta-methylbutyrate could increase muscle mass and possibly improve immune status.

Other natural treatments. Whey protein is sometimes recommended for weight gain in HIV, but evidence that it works is preliminary at best. One study found that while exercise improved weight gain, whey protein alone or with exercise offered no benefit. Fish oil might be helpful for weight gain, however.

Treating the side effects of medication. Several natural treatments have been proposed to treat side effects from various medications used in the treatment of HIV infection. Reverse transcriptase inhibitors, such as lamivudine and zidovudine, may damage mitochondria, the energy-producing subunits of cells. The supplement CoQ_{10} has been tried for minimizing side effects attributed to mitochondrial damage. In one study, the use of CoQ_{10} improved sense of well-being in asymptomatic people with HIV infection; however, it actually worsened pain symptoms in people with peripheral neuropathy.

Taking AZT (zidovudine, formerly called azidothymidine) can lead to zinc deficiency, which may interfere with immune function. One partially blinded study found that zinc supplements may benefit people on AZT. In the zinc-treated group, body weight increased or stabilized, CD4+ count rose, and participants had significantly fewer opportunistic infections.

Carnitine has also been proposed as a treatment for AZT side effects, based on early evidence that it may keep AZT from damaging muscle cells. Other weak evidence hints that the acetyl form of carnitine might reduce nerve-related side effects caused by HIV drugs in general.

Based on preliminary evidence, vitamin B_{12} has been suggested as a preventive for blood abnormalities caused by AZT. In one well-designed, double-blind study, the use of the amino acid glutamine at a dose of 30 grams (g) daily significantly reduced the diarrhea caused by the protease inhibitor nelfinavir. Presumably, glutamine would be helpful for other protease inhibitors.

It has been suggested that the supplement NAC might help prevent side effects from the antibiotic TMP-SMX (trimethoprim-sulfamethoxazole). However, two controlled studies found that NAC did not significantly decrease adverse reactions to TMP-SMX. Note, however, that TMP-SMX is known to decrease folate levels in the body, and folate supplements might therefore be useful.

The herb milk thistle is sometimes recommended for preventing liver problems related to the use of HIV medications. While there is no direct evidence that it is helpful for this purpose, there is fairly good evidence that the use of milk thistle does not adversely affect blood levels of indinavir.

General nutrition support. People infected with HIV may be particularly vulnerable to malnutrition because of decreased appetite, poor absorption, or possibly increased requirements for specific nutrients. Studies have found deficiencies of vitamins A, B_1, B_6, B_{12}, and E, beta-carotene, choline, folate, selenium, and zinc to be common among people with HIV infection. Many deficiencies become more common as the disease worsens. This suggests, but does not prove, that taking supplements of these nutrients may be helpful. One study evaluated whether the use of a multivitamin tablet might reduce infectivity of African women with HIV infection. Researchers unexpectedly found the opposite: Multivitamin tablets increase the levels of HIV in the genital area. The reason for this surprising finding is unknown. It is not clear whether the same response would occur among people living in developed countries who, presumably, have better underlying nutrition.

Vitamin A, beta-carotene, and mixed carotenoids. Vitamin A and beta-carotene are described together here because the body uses beta-carotene to produce vitamin A. Substances called carotenoids are closely related to vitamin A; this family includes lutein and lycopene.

Vitamin A deficiency may be linked to lower CD4+ counts and to higher death rates among HIV-positive people. A few preliminary studies have raised hopes that beta-carotene supplements might increase or preserve immune function or decrease symptoms among HIV-positive persons. One small, double-blind study suggested that taking beta-carotene might raise white blood cell count in people with HIV infection. However, two subsequent larger controlled trials found no significant differences between those taking beta-carotene or placebo in white blood cell count, CD4+ count, or other measures of immune function.

Two observational studies lasting six to eight years suggest that higher intakes of vitamin A or beta-carotene may be helpful, but they also found that caution is in order with regard to dosage. This group of researchers generally linked higher intake of vitamin A or beta-carotene to lower risk of AIDS and lower death rates, with an important exception: People with the highest intake of either nutrient (more than 11,179 international units [IU] per day of beta-carotene, more than 20,268 IU per day of vitamin A) did worse than those who took somewhat less. Excessive dosages of vitamin A can be toxic to the liver. One should consult with a physician about the right dose.

At one point it was thought that vitamin A supplements might decrease the rate of transmission of HIV from a pregnant woman to her newborn. However, it now appears that the reverse may be true: Vitamin A may increase the chance of such transmission.

One double-blind study found statistically weak evidence that the use of mixed carotenoids by persons with AIDS might prolong life.

B vitamins. An observational study found that HIV-positive men with the highest intakes of vitamins B_1, B_2, and B_6 and niacin had significantly longer survival rates, while a similar study found that those taking the most B_1 or niacin had a significantly lower rate of developing AIDS.

Vitamin B_{12} deficiencies in people infected with HIV have been linked to neurologic symptoms, including slower processing of information in studies of cognitive functioning; early research suggests that restoring B_{12} levels to normal may decrease these symptoms. Vitamin B_{12} deficiency has also been linked to lower CD4+ counts and more rapid development of AIDS.

Vitamin B_6 deficiency has been linked to impaired immune function in one study of people with HIV in-fection. Excessive intake of vitamin B_6 can cause neurologic problems.

Vitamins C and E. Massive doses of vitamin C have at times been popular among people with HIV based on preliminary evidence. An observational study linked high doses of vitamin C with slower progression to AIDS. High intake of vitamin E was also linked to decreased risk of progression to AIDS in a different observational study.

However, a double-blind study of forty-nine people with HIV who took combined vitamins C and E or placebo for three months did not show any significant effects on the amount of HIV detected or the number of opportunistic infections. It has been suggested that vitamin E may enhance the antiviral effects of AZT, but evidence for this is minimal.

Choline. The substance choline has been newly added to the list of essential nutrients. Evidence suggests that people with HIV who are low in choline may experience more rapid disease progression.

Iron. A study of seventy-one HIV-positive children noted a high rate of iron deficiency. One observational study of 296 men with HIV infection linked high intake of iron to a decreased risk of AIDS six years later. One should not take iron supplements, however, unless one is iron deficient.

Selenium. Selenium is required for a well-functioning immune system. Observational studies have linked higher levels of selenium in the blood with higher CD4+ counts and reduced risk of mortality from HIV disease. Selenium deficiency may also increase the infectiousness of women who are HIV positive.

In a double-blind, placebo-controlled study of 450 people with HIV, the use of selenium supplementation at a dose of 200 micrograms (mcg) per day appeared to reduce measures of viral load. However, the statistical method used in this study is somewhat questionable. Previous smaller studies using more standard statistical methods failed to find such effects.

In one double-blind, placebo-controlled study, the use of selenium at a dose of 200 mcg decreased anxiety in patients undergoing HAART. Selenium has also been proposed as a preventive or treatment for cardiomyopathy, a disorder of the heart muscle that can affect people with AIDS. Evidence of its benefits is weak.

Zinc. Some studies have found that HIV-positive people tend to be deficient in zinc, with levels dropping lower in more severe disease. It remains unclear whether taking zinc will help.

Higher zinc levels have been linked to better immune function and higher CD4+ cell counts, whereas zinc deficiency has been linked to increased risk of dying from HIV infection. One preliminary study among people taking AZT found that thirty days of zinc supplementation led to decreased rates of opportunistic infection over the following two years.

Other research has linked higher zinc intake to more rapid development of AIDS. In another study of HIV-positive people, those with higher zinc intake or those taking zinc supplements in any dosage had a greater risk of death within the following eight years. However, one study found that the use of zinc supplements could reduce diarrhea symptoms in people with HIV infection.

Multivitamins. Because so many nutrients are affected by HIV infection and treatments, multivitamin supplements are a logical choice. A double-blind study of forty people on HAART found that the use of a multinutrient supplement improved CD4 counts and possibly improved neuropathy symptoms. As indicated by a foregoing study that evaluated whether the use of a multivitamin tablet might reduce infectivity of African women with HIV, multivitamin tablets actually increased the levels of HIV in the genital area.

NATURAL TREATMENTS TO AVOID

People using HIV medications should not take St. John's wort. In a study of healthy volunteers, St. John's wort was found to decrease the blood concentration of indinavir, one of the most widely used protease inhibitors, by 49 to 99 percent. This could lead to treatment failure as well as the emergence of resistant HIV strains. St. John's wort also appears to interact with non-nucleoside reverse transcriptase inhibitors such as nevirapine.

Garlic may also combine poorly with certain HIV medications. Two people with HIV experienced severe gastrointestinal toxicity from the protease inhibitor ritonavir after taking garlic supplements, and another study found that garlic might interfere with the action of the protease inhibitor saquinavir, reducing blood levels of the medication. Another study found that vitamin C at a dose of 1 g daily substantially reduced blood levels of indinavir.

Other possible harmful effects discussed elsewhere in this article include the worsening of peripheral neuropathy symptoms by CoQ_{10} and an increase of infectivity attributable to the use of multivitamins. Persons with HIV should consult a doctor before using any herb or supplement. Given the large numbers of drugs, herbs, and supplements taken by many people with HIV, the possibility of interactions is high.

EBSCO CAM Review Board

FURTHER READING

Abrams, D. I., et al. "Dehydroepiandrosterone (DHEA) Effects on HIV Replication and Host Immunity." *AIDS Research and Human Retroviruses* 23 (2007): 77-85.

Agin, D., et al. "Effects of Whey Protein and Resistance Exercise on Body Cell Mass, Muscle Strength, and Quality of Life in Women with HIV." *AIDS* 15 (2001): 2431-2440.

Austin, J., et al. "A Community Randomized Controlled Clinical Trial of Mixed Carotenoids and Micronutrient Supplementation of Patients with Acquired Immunodeficiency Syndrome." *European Journal of Clinical Nutrition* 60 (2006): 1266-1276.

Baeten, J. M., et al. "Selenium Deficiency Is Associated with Shedding of HIV-1-infected Cells in the Female Genital Tract." *Journal of Acquired Immune Deficiency Syndromes* 26 (2001): 360-364.

Birk, T. J., et al. "The Effects of Massage Therapy Alone and in Combination with Other Complementary Therapies on Immune System Measures and Quality of Life in Human Immunodeficiency Virus." *Journal of Alternative and Complementary Medicine* 6 (2000): 405-414.

Cárcamo, C., et al. "Randomized Controlled Trial of Zinc Supplementation for Persistent Diarrhea in Adults with HIV-1 Infection." *Journal of Acquired Immune Deficiency Syndromes* 43 (2006): 197-201.

Creswell, J. D., et al. "Mindfulness Meditation Training Effects on CD4+ T Lymphocytes in HIV-1 Infected Adults." *Brain, Behavior, and Immunity* 23 (2009): 184-188.

Diego, M. A., et al. "HIV Adolescents Show Improved Immune Function Following Massage Therapy." *International Journal of Neuroscience* 106 (2001): 35-45.

Hurwitz, B. E., et al. "Suppression of Human Immunodeficiency Virus Type 1 Viral Load with Selenium Supplementation." *Archives of Internal Medicine* 167 (2007): 148-154.

Kaiser, J. D., et al. "Micronutrient Supplementation Increases CD4 Count in HIV-Infected Individuals on Highly Active Antiretroviral Therapy." *Journal of Acquired Immune Deficiency Syndromes* 42 (2006): 523-528.

McClelland, R. S., et al. "Micronutrient Supplementation Increases Genital Tract Shedding of HIV-1 in Women." *Journal of Acquired Immune Deficiency Syndromes* 37 (2004): 1657-1663.

Mehta, S., and W. Fawzi. "Effects of Vitamins, Including Vitamin A, on HIV/AIDS Patients." *Vitamins and Hormones* 75 (2007): 355-383.

Piscitelli, S. C., A. H. Burstein, and D. Chaitt, et al. "Indinavir Concentrations and St. John's Wort." *The Lancet* 355 (2000): 547-548.

Piscitelli, S. C., A. H. Burstein, and N. Welden, et al. "The Effect of Garlic Supplements on the Pharmacokinetics of Saquinavir." *Clinical Infectious Diseases* 34 (2002): 234-238.

Rabkin, J. G., et al. "Placebo-Controlled Trial of Dehydroepiandrosterone (DHEA) for Treatment of Nonmajor Depression in Patients with HIV/AIDS." *American Journal of Psychiatry* 163 (2006): 59-66.

Scott-Sheldon, L. A., et al. "Stress Management Interventions for HIV+ Adults." *Health Psychology* 27 (2008): 129-139.

Shor-Posner, G., et al. "Psychological Burden in the Era of HAART: Impact of Selenium Therapy." *International Journal of Psychiatry in Medicine* 33 (2003): 55-69.

Simpson, D. M., S. Brown, and J. Tobias. "Controlled Trial of High-Concentration Capsaicin Patch for Treatment of Painful HIV Neuropathy." *Neurology* 70 (2008): 2305-2313.

Weber, R., et al. "Randomized, Placebo-Controlled Trial of Chinese Herb Therapy for HIV-1-Infected Individuals." *Journal of Acquired Immune Deficiency Syndromes and Human Retrovirology* 22 (1999): 56-64.

Youle, M., and M. Osio. "A Double-Blind, Parallel-Group, Placebo-Controlled, Multicentre Study of Acetyl L-Carnitine in the Symptomatic Treatment of Antiretroviral Toxic Neuropathy in Patients with HIV-1 Infection." *HIV Medicine* 8 (2007): 241-250.

See also: ACE inhibitors; Diet-based therapies; Herbal medicine; Immune support; Medium-chain triglycerides; Protease inhibitors; Reverse transcriptase inhibitors; Vitamins and minerals; Weight loss, undesired; Wellness, general.

HIV support: Homeopathic remedies

RELATED TERMS: Acquired immunodeficiency syndrome, human immunodeficiency virus

CATEGORY: Homeopathy

DEFINITION: Homeopathic treatment of infection caused by the human immunodeficiency virus.

STUDIED HOMEOPATHIC REMEDY: Classical homeopathic remedy

INTRODUCTION

HIV, or human immunodeficiency virus, is the virus that causes acquired immunodeficiency syndrome (AIDS). First identified in 1983, this virus progressively destroys or damages cells in the immune system, making its host vulnerable to certain cancers and infections. These opportunistic infections, caused by microorganisms that do not ordinarily cause illness in healthy people, can have serious, even fatal, effects on those with human immunodeficiency virus infection.

Within one or two months of exposure, a person with HIV may have short-term flulike symptoms, followed by a symptom-free period lasting months to years, during which the virus continues to multiply. After this stage, people with HIV may develop swollen lymph nodes, recurrent herpes sores, diarrhea, weight loss, and chronic yeast infections (oral or vaginal)–a state previously called AIDS-related complex or ARC. Children may experience delayed development or failure to thrive. The infection is called AIDS when the number of immune cells known as CD4+ or helper T-cells drops below a certain level, or when opportunistic diseases such as pneumocystis pneumonia develop. Today, both ARC and AIDS are sometimes collectively called symptomatic HIV infection.

HIV is spread most commonly through sexual activity or by intravenous drug abuse. Also, pregnant women can infect their fetuses before or during birth, and after birth through breast-feeding.

Effective medications have helped to turn HIV infection from an always-fatal illness into a manageable illness. None of the homeopathic treatments described here can substitute for standard care, however.

SCIENTIFIC EVALUATIONS OF HOMEOPATHIC REMEDIES

The outcome of one study suggests that individualized homeopathic treatment might be helpful in HIV infection. However, these results were too preliminary to be relied upon. A six-month, double-blind, placebo-controlled study of eighty people evaluated the effects of treatment with an individualized homeopathic remedy on the progression of HIV infection. The remedy was assigned based on the classic homeopathic symptom picture. Participants took the remedy or placebo for six months. Researchers then performed blood tests to measure CD4+ and CD8+ counts (standard indicators of HIV progression).

The group of participants with more advanced symptoms (persistent generalized lymphadenopathy, which is stage III of symptoms as classified by the Centers for Disease Control and Prevention, or CDC) showed a significant increase in CD4+ counts with homeopathic treatment. However, homeopathic treatment did not benefit a group without symptoms (CDC stage II). The investigators suggest that the study time was too short to evaluate effectiveness in asymptomatic HIV because the CD4+ counts can change very slowly over time.

In any case, because of the division into small subgroups with more and less severe illness, the results of this study are difficult to rely upon. Larger trials are necessary to reliably identify a benefit with homeopathic treatment.

TRADITIONAL HOMEOPATHIC TREATMENTS

HIV is a complex illness with many possible symptoms. For this reason, there is no group of homeopathic remedies representative of common classical approaches.

EBSCO CAM Review Board

FURTHER READING

Fritts, M., et al. "Traditional Indian Medicine and Homeopathy for HIV/AIDS." *AIDS Research and Therapy* 5 (2008): 25.

Mills, E., P. Wu, and E. Ernst. "Complementary Therapies for the Treatment of HIV: In Search of the Evidence." *International Journal of STD and AIDS* 16 (2005): 395-403.

Rastogi, D. P., et al. "Homeopathy in HIV Infection." *British Homeopathic Journal* 88 (1999): 49-57.

Ullman, D. "Controlled Clinical Trials Evaluating the Homeopathic Treatment of People with Human Immunodeficiency Virus or Acquired Immune Deficiency Syndrome." *Journal of Alternative and Complementary Medicine* 9 (2003): 133-141.

See also: Herbal medicine; HIV support; Homeopathy; Immune support; Traditional healing.

Hives

CATEGORY: Condition

RELATED TERMS: Angioedema, cholinergic urticaria, dermographism, prickly heat, urticaria

DEFINITION: Treatment of inflammation of the surface layers of the skin.

PRINCIPAL PROPOSED NATURAL TREATMENTS: None

OTHER PROPOSED NATURAL TREATMENTS: Acupuncture, food allergen elimination diet, quercetin, sublingual immunotherapy, vitamin B_{12}, vitamin C

INTRODUCTION

Hives, the common name for a condition called urticaria, is an inflammation of the surface layers of the skin and is characterized by small, itchy red or white welts (wheals). Urticaria is usually caused by an allergic reaction; however, the allergenic trigger is often unknown. When a cause can be identified, it is frequently something taken by mouth, such as shellfish or other fish, dairy products, peanuts or other legumes, chocolate, fresh fruit, or medications. Sometimes other allergens, such as pollens, molds, or animal dander, can produce hives. Hives can also be caused by heat (cholinergic urticaria, or prickly heat), cold (cold urticaria), pressure (dermographism and pressure urticaria), light (solar urticaria), exercise, and certain infections such as hepatitis B.

In most acute cases, urticaria disappears within hours or days without any treatment. Sometimes, however, it may continue for a prolonged period or recur frequently. Such chronic cases are often difficult to treat.

Urticaria is closely related to another condition called angioedema, which involves swelling in the deeper layers of the skin. When swelling occurs in the throat or tongue, angioedema can be life-threatening. Urticaria and angioedema are also closely related to anaphylaxis, an extremely dangerous condition that can lead to death within minutes or hours.

Anaphylaxis is an overwhelming allergic reaction that may lead to swelling of internal organs, collapse of blood circulation, shock, or suffocation. It may be caused by all the same factors that trigger hives; one of the best-known causes is bee sting allergy.

Conventional treatments for urticaria and angioedema include avoidance of triggering factors, the use of antihistamines, and, occasionally, corticosteroids. When breathing is threatened, epinephrine shots and hospitalization may be needed.

PROPOSED NATURAL TREATMENTS

Sublingual immunotherapy (SLIT) has shown (in one small, double-blind, placebo-controlled trial) some promise for treating urticaria caused by latex allergies. Based on the theory that urticaria may be caused by delayed-type food allergies, food allergen elimination diets have been tried as a treatment for chronic symptoms. However, the evidence that it works remains preliminary.

There are many forms of the elimination diet. One of the most common involves starting with a highly restricted diet consisting only of foods that are seldom allergenic, such as rice, yams, and turkey. Other proponents of the elimination diet allow a greater range of foods at the outset. If dietary restriction leads to resolution or improvement of symptoms, foods are then reintroduced one by one to see which, if any, will trigger urticaria.

In China, urticaria is often treated with acupuncture; however, the evidence that acupuncture works for this condition is far too weak. Vitamins C and B_{12}, and the flavonoid quercetin, have also been suggested for treatment, but there is no evidence that they work for treating urticaria.

EBSCO CAM Review Board

FURTHER READING

Chen, C. J., and H. S. Yu. "Acupuncture Treatment of Urticaria." *Archives of Dermatology* 134 (1998): 1397-1399.

Nettis, E., et al. "Double-Blind, Placebo-Controlled Study of Sublingual Immunotherapy in Patients with Latex-Induced Urticaria." *British Journal of Dermatology* 156 (2007): 674-681.

Supramaniam, G., and J. O. Warner. "Artificial Food Additive Intolerance in Patients with Angio-oedema and Urticaria." *The Lancet* 2 (1986): 907-909.

Zuberbier, T., et al. "Pseudoallergen-Free Diet in the Treatment of Chronic Urticaria." *Acta Dermato-venereologica* 75 (1995): 484-487.

See also: Acne; Allergies; Eczema; Food allergies and sensitivities; Seborrheic dermatitis.

Home health

CATEGORY: Issues and overviews
RELATED TERMS: Home cleanliness, home hygiene, housecleaning, housekeeping, indoor air pollution
DEFINITION: The recognition and removal of allergens, pathogens, and other pollutants found in the home or other living environment.

NATURAL POLLUTANTS

Every home contains natural pollutants that require regular removal to reduce health risks, prevent offensive odors, and eliminate stains and structural damage that devalue the structure. Most of these pollutants become airborne and are inhaled, creating subsequent health problems that range in severity from sneezing to difficulty breathing. Other pollutants may be unintentionally ingested, causing illness.

Airborne pollutants are collectively called dust. The most common component of dust in a home is dead skin particles shed by the home's residents. Dust also contains hair, ash, pollen, fibers, and minerals from outdoor soil. Overexposure to dust can lead to allergies, respiratory diseases, and asthma. Dust mites feed on the organic matter in dust. They most commonly live on mattresses, sheets, and pillows. Their excrement contains substances that can cause severe allergic reactions. Companies are now making tightly woven anti-allergy encasings for mattresses and pillows. The use of air filters in the furnace, air conditioner, and vacuum cleaner reduces airborne contaminants.

The inhabitants of a house, such as humans, pets, and occasionally rodents, naturally shed hair, dander, saliva, urine, and feces. Such substances may trigger an allergic reaction in people or may carry bacteria, viruses, or parasites that infect humans. Hair and dander may be removed by frequent vacuuming and dusting; excretions should be cleaned up with soap and water. Toilets should be disinfected regularly;

closing the lid before flushing prevents the contents from being dispersed into the room as an aerosol.

Also living in homes may be insects such as flies, termites, ants, spiders, fleas, lice, cockroaches, and bedbugs. Many of these insects feed on garbage, food spills and crumbs that are not cleaned up, and food supplies that are not adequately packaged. Insects can transmit diseases to humans either directly by biting or indirectly by contaminating food with eggs or droppings. Insects may be eliminated from the home by natural or chemical pesticides or by swatting or vacuuming, or with flypaper. Adequate containment of garbage, keeping kitchen floors swept and counters wiped clean, and storing food in airtight containers will discourage their return.

Pollen from houseplants and cut flower arrangements may diminish indoor air quality. Pollen may also drift inside through open windows and doors and be brought in on shoes and clothing, especially from plants next to the house. Indoor pollen may be reduced by keeping houseplants and floral arrangements well hydrated. Outdoor plants near windows and doors should be trimmed away from openings. Although silk floral arrangements do not contain pollen, their complex surfaces trap dust, so they should be cleaned regularly by spraying with compressed air.

Mold, which is a fungus, grows in warm, damp areas such as inadequately ventilated bathrooms, kitchens, and basements. Mold releases spores into the air, which, when inhaled, may cause symptoms such as a dry cough, nasal congestion, eye irritation, and wheezing. Mold may be visible, but it is usually detected initially by its musty odor. It may be destroyed by scrubbing first with a detergent without ammonia in hot water and then with a 10 percent bleach solution. Porous materials such as carpeting and insulation that remain damp should be discarded.

Bacteria and viruses may make a person ill when ingested or inhaled. They may be found on unwashed, uncooked fruits and vegetables and on uncooked meats. Raw foods should be thoroughly washed before they are eaten. Handling raw meat and neglecting to wash one's hands and the food preparation surface afterward may result in the contamination of other foods and subsequent pathogen ingestion. Surfaces that come in contact with raw meat juices should be thoroughly disinfected.

Bacteria and viruses may also be transmitted on surfaces that are commonly used by many people, surfaces such as doorknobs and telephones. Such surfaces should be wiped with a disposable disinfectant cloth regularly and more frequently during cold and flu season.

CHEMICAL POLLUTANTS

Among other causes, the degassing of synthetic materials in newer homes, and poor ventilation that keeps the house airtight, may lead to sick building syndrome. Symptoms of sick building syndrome include eye irritation, scratchy or sore throat, nasal congestion, skin rash, and difficulty concentrating. The symptoms typically begin within one hour of entering a polluted structure and disappear within one hour of leaving the structure.

Another chemical pollutant is tobacco smoke. The ash becomes a component of dust; the odor lingers in soft surfaces such as curtains, upholstery, and clothing; and the secondhand smoke is inhaled by the other residents of the home, causing increased respiratory problems.

Carbon monoxide is an odorless, colorless gas that may be given off by faulty furnaces or space heaters. Exposure may cause flulike symptoms, severe headache, dizziness, trouble breathing, and even death. Carbon monoxide detectors in the home are recommended and may be found in combination with smoke detectors.

Radon is another invisible, odorless gas that is also radioactive. It results from the decay of uranium in the soil and seeps into a home through the foundation, where it can build up to dangerous levels. Radon increases the risk of lung cancer for those who breathe it. The U.S. Environmental Protection Agency recommends that all homes be tested for radon below the third floor. Commercial radon reduction systems are available too.

Asbestos, used as pipe insulation, may be a pollutant in homes that were built between 1920 and 1978. Breathing high levels of exposed asbestos may result in an increased risk of cancer and lung disease. Homes built before 1978 may also contain lead paint. Flakes of this paint have a sweet taste, making the paint tempting to children. If they ingest the paint flakes, they can become ill with lead poisoning.

Bethany Thivierge, M.P.H.

FURTHER READING

U.S. Department of Homeland Security, Federal Emergency Management Agency. "Dealing with Mold and

Mildew in Your Flood Damaged Home." Available at http://www.fema.gov/pdf/rebuild/recover/fema_mold_brochure_english.pdf. A clear, authoritative explanation of how to improve home health by finding and removing mold and mildew.

U.S. Environmental Protection Agency. "A Citizen's Guide to Radon." Available at http://www.epa.gov/radon/pubs/citguide.html. Information on what homeowners can do to protect themselves from radon.

_____, Office of Air and Radiation. "The Inside Story: A Guide to Indoor Air Quality." Available at http://www.epa.gov/iaq/pubs/insidest.html#iaqhome1. A complete discussion of home air quality, common pollutants, and improvement measures.

See also: Allergies; Allergies: Homeopathic remedies; Feng shui; Folk medicine; Herbal medicine; Homeopathy; Whole medicine.

Homeopathy: Overview

CATEGORY: Homeopathy

DEFINITION: An alternative therapy based on the belief that a substance that provokes symptoms in a healthy person can also treat a sick person who has those same symptoms.

INTRODUCTION

In the opinion of most medical professionals in the United States, homeopathy is nothing but quackery. Even though the use of herbs and supplements has remained largely outside mainstream medicine, physicians tend to accept in principle that herbs and supplements could have effects in the body. In contrast, homeopathy is an approach to healing that sounds quasi-magical. Indeed, homeopathic remedies are so phenomenally diluted that they contain no material substance in them except pure sugar. Proponents of homeopathy believe that these "high potency" remedies possess some sort of healing energy field, an unbelievable concept for medical professionals accustomed to seeing the world from a scientific perspective.

Nonetheless, homeopathy is still used widely, especially in the United Kingdom but also in the United States and other countries. Some studies seem to provide evidence that homeopathic remedies can be effective.

The term "homeopathy" is formed from the combination of two Greek words: *omio*, meaning "same," and *pathos*, meaning "suffering." This etymology reflects the homeopathic belief that a substance that causes certain symptoms in a healthy person can cure an ailing person who has similar symptoms. Although this theory sounds superficially similar to the principle behind vaccines, homeopathy actually functions in a distinctly different manner. The homeopathic theory has some relationship to ancient healing traditions, but in many ways it stands uniquely on its own, unrelated to other approaches.

THE ORIGIN OF HOMEOPATHY

Homeopathy was developed by Samuel Christian Hahnemann, born in 1755 in Dresden, Germany, and

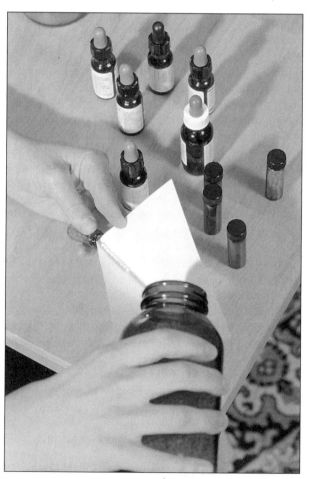

A homeopathist prepares remedies for a patient. (PhotoDisc)

educated as a physician. The medical practices of the eighteenth century were remarkably unhelpful and invasive. A good example is bloodletting. Doctors commonly bled their patients of a pint of blood or more per treatment, in the belief that doing so would accelerate healing. More likely, however, bloodletting impaired the patients' ability to recover, rather than strengthened it, and the practice is undoubtedly responsible for many deaths.

Physicians also used strong laxatives to "cleanse" the body. These purgatives included toxic drugs containing mercury or arsenic, and they too contributed to the great danger of being visited by a doctor.

Hahnemann quickly became disillusioned by the standard medical procedures of his time; he gave up his medical practice and supported his family in part by translating old scientific and medical texts into German. In 1790, while translating William Cullen's *Materia Medica*, he was struck by the lack of experimental basis for Cullen's suggested uses for drugs. Hahnemann wondered how doctors could justify prescribing toxic substances without even knowing their effects on healthy people. He came to believe there was a correlation between the resulting symptoms of toxic doses of a given substance and the symptoms that the substance was being used to cure.

To explore his new theory, Hahnemann began collecting reports of accidental poisonings. Later, he tested various substances on himself and documented his reactions to them. For example, he had read that *Cinchona officinalis*, or Peruvian bark, was used by South American Indians to treat malaria. Hahnemann took a high dose of *C. officinalis* and his body reacted by breaking out in fever. Because malaria is characterized by fever, he perceived his own fever as evidence that a substance used to treat an ailment produced similar symptoms in a healthy person.

Hahnemann then set out to experiment systematically with this hypothesis, ingesting other substances and carefully noting his reactions to them. He also gave substances to other healthy people. Hahnemann took detailed notes of the reactions. He recorded not only major physical symptoms, such as fever, but also any sensation experienced by the person, including such details as a desire to lie down on one's left side and restlessness that is worse in the early evening. These "provings," as he called them, were recorded in homeopathic medical texts (such as the *Homeopathic Materia Medica*) and became the basis for homeopathic treatment.

Provings are now done in a different manner, using homeopathic dilutions of substances rather than the substances themselves. Also, provings are more often done using high dilutions of substances; in other words, the homeopathic remedy is tested, not the underlying substance. This method is safer, even if not entirely consistent with the original theory.

The three laws. Based on his observations, Hahnemann postulated three major laws of homeopathy, the first two proposed early in his practice and the third after twenty years of practice. (Homeopathy also has a minimum of six other relatively minor laws.) The first law is known as the Law of Similars, or "like cures like." This law states that "a substance that produces a certain set of symptoms in a healthy person has the power to cure a sick person manifesting those same symptoms." The second law, or Law of Infinitesimals, states that diluting a remedy makes it more powerful.

These two laws in combination define the method of creating homeopathic remedies. The following is an example: The substance ipecac (today an over-the-counter household remedy for poisoning) causes vomiting. According to the first and second laws of homeopathy, diluted ipecac would potentially treat vomiting, and the more it is diluted, the more it is effective.

Hahnemann's third law, the Law of Chronic Disease, states that "when disease persists despite treatment, it is the result of one or more conditions that affect many people and have been driven deep inside the body by earlier allopathic therapy."

The word "allopathic," which is sometimes used to describe conventional medicine, was also a creation of Hahnemann and was used as the opposite of "homeopathic." Allopathic means "other than the disease," while homeopathic means "same as the disease." In other words, homeopathy uses remedies that, when taken in high doses by healthy people (according to the first law), cause symptoms similar to those of the disease they are intended to treat. The allopathic remedies used by conventional physicians, such as prednisone for asthma, do not have the same relationship. They simply relieve the symptoms, and for that reason (according to homeopathic theory) do not get to the heart of the problem.

Hahnemann believed that allopathic treatments were actually harmful. A skin rash provides an example. To Hahnemann, such a condition represents the body's attempt to release a deeper illness.

Two Main Principles, or Laws, of Homeopathy

Principle of Similars. The Principle of Similars (or "like cures like") states that a disease can be cured by a substance that produces similar symptoms in healthy people. This idea, which can be traced to Hippocrates, was further developed by physician Samuel Hahnemann after he repeatedly ingested cinchona bark, a popular treatment for malaria, and found that he developed the symptoms of the disease. Hahnemann theorized that if a substance could cause disease symptoms in a healthy person, small amounts could cure a sick person who had similar symptoms.

Principle of Dilutions. The Principle of Dilutions (also known as the Law of Minimum Dose or the Law of Infinitesimals) states that the lower the dose of the medication, the greater its effectiveness. In homeopathy, substances are diluted in a stepwise fashion and are shaken vigorously between each dilution. This process, referred to as potentization, is believed to transmit some form of information or energy from the original substance to the final diluted remedy. Most homeopathic remedies are so dilute that no molecules of the healing substance remain. However, in homeopathy, it is believed that the substance has left its imprint or essence, which stimulates the body to heal itself (this theory is called the memory of water).

Homeopathic treatment would seek to facilitate such a release. In contrast, allopathic remedies, like cortisone cream, suppress the rash and thereby drive the illness back into the body.

Herbal remedies are also allopathic, according to this principle. Taking St. John's wort for depression, according to homeopathy, is just as likely to worsen the underlying problem as using the antidepressant drug Prozac. Furthermore, herbs, like drugs, are said to interfere with the effectiveness of homeopathic remedies. Thus, contrary to popular opinion, homeopathy and herbal medicine are not compatible.

In further work developing the third law, Hahnemann elaborated on the various types of deeply buried diseases that could be the roots of many illnesses. He focused ultimately on psoriasis and syphilis as the primary underlying "miasms" beneath many health problems. However, this feature of his theory is less popular with today's practitioners of homeopathy.

HOMEOPATHIC DILUTIONS

The second law of homeopathy requires that a homeopathic treatment be diluted for maximum effect. Hahnemann developed techniques to control the concentration, or dilution, of substances to create homeopathic remedies. First, he took the substance and preserved it in a solvent, usually alcohol. The substances he used were plants and minerals. After letting the substance stand for one month, he poured off the liquid, which became the "mother tincture." Next, he took one drop of tincture and added it to ninety-nine drops of pure alcohol. He then mixed the liquid by banging the container on a hard surface, a process called succussion. Homeopathic practitioners believe that succussion is essential to creating an effective remedy.

This first step creates a remedy with a dilution of one part in 10^2, or 100. This dilution would be noted by adding the letter c, for centesimal (indicating a dilution of two factors of 10), or by adding 2x or D2 (x and D each indicate one factor of 10). The dilution is then continued, always adding one part of tincture to ninety-nine parts alcohol, and succussing at each step. Such a process carried out six times leads to a 6c remedy (or 12x or D12), and so forth.

Homeopathic remedies sometimes are made with substances that are insoluble. In this case, the substances are ground up, mixed with lactose, and then made into remedies. At times, people make homeopathic remedies by diluting one part of tincture to nine drops of alcohol at each step, to make a 1x or D1 dilution.

The complete process of creating homeopathic remedies is called "potentization," based on the theory that each successive dilution makes the remedy more potent. Today, a person can buy homeopathic remedies that consist of small, white milk-sugar pills into which the potentized solution has been absorbed. Other remedies are in the form of liquids to ingest or creams to use externally.

Special forms of homeopathic remedies. In addition to standard homeopathic remedies that use unrelated substances that happen to produce a similar symptom, there are two special forms of homeopathic remedies (isopathic and nosode) that use substances specifically related to the condition. Isopathic remedies are made from the actual substance that causes the condition. For example, homeopathically prepared cat dander (containing zero molecules of cat dander) might be used to treat cat allergy. Nosodes are made from infected animal tissues or bodily secretions. For example, tuberculosis-infected glands from a cow could be homeopathically diluted to create a remedy for human tuberculosis.

THE PRACTICE OF HOMEOPATHY: CONSTITUTIONAL AND DISEASE-ORIENTED HOMEOPATHY

Hahnemann's theory of homeopathy is now known as constitutional (or classical) homeopathy. This holistic art looks at the symptom picture of a person, including psychological, emotional, physical, and hereditary information, and tries to choose an appropriate remedy. A simplified form of homeopathy has developed too: disease-oriented (or symptomatic) homeopathy, in which remedies are given based solely on specific diseases. Both types of homeopathy have been studied scientifically, although disease-oriented homeopathy has received more attention for the simple reason that it is easier to study.

MODERN HOMEOPATHY

Homeopathy is highly respected in Great Britain, where it is part of the national health-care system. It is also widely used in India and, to a lesser extent, France, Germany, the Netherlands, Greece, South Africa, and South America. In the United States, homeopathy is again becoming more widespread after a period of decline.

In the United States, over-the-counter homeopathic remedies are available in pharmacies and health-food stores. Unlike herbs and supplements, manufacturers of homeopathic products are allowed to make strong healing claims on the labels, in part because one of the founders of the organization that became the U.S. Food and Drug Administration, Royal Copeland, was a homeopathic physician. He made sure that homeopathic medicines were given a specially protected status.

SCIENTIFIC EVALUATION OF HOMEOPATHY

Despite its widespread acceptance in some countries, most modern scientific experts do not take homeopathy seriously, putting it in the same category as perpetual motion machines, ghosts, and extra sensory perception. There are several reasons for this intense skepticism, but the most important focuses on a basic fact of chemistry. Simply put, there is absolutely nothing material in a high-potency homeopathic

remedy; some force of nature unknown to modern science would have to be involved if homeopathy were effective.

In the process of making a 30x homeopathic remedy, the original substance is diluted by a factor of one part in 10^{30}. This is such an enormous dilution that not even one single molecule is likely to remain. Such a remedy is merely pure sugar (if the form is a sugar pill) or pure water (if the form is a tincture). Even higher dilutions are in use, some so vast that one could use, for example, the entire earth as the starting material and still not end up with a single molecule of the original material in the resulting remedy.

Because of this chemical reality, the comparison of homeopathy to vaccinations, as advanced by many homeopathic practitioners, falls short. Vaccinations contain a great deal of substance, an amount that can be measured and weighed and which stimulates the immune system. High-potency homeopathic remedies, by contrast, contain nothing. (Low-potency remedies do contain a measurable amount of substance, but they are supposedly less effective than the high-potency forms, which are physically content-free.)

Some researchers have speculated that homeopathic remedies produce subtle alterations in the structure of the water in which they are dissolved. However, studies with highly sensitive equipment have failed to find any evidence of such structural changes, and chemistry, as it has been understood both before and after the development of quantum mechanics, makes it highly implausible that liquid water could retain any changes of the type hypothesized.

There are other problems with homeopathy. For one, it is difficult to understand why a substance that produces certain symptoms when taken in overdose should cure a disease that just coincidentally happens to possess the same symptoms. This hypothesis appears too tidy and perfect to reflect the messy world of human illness.

Furthermore, the detailed symptom pictures upon which constitutional homeopathy are based seem to be far too specific and personal to offer any likelihood of universal truth. For example, the homeopathic remedy sulphur is said to be useful for people who have red lips, stooped posture, and a tendency toward untidiness in personal affairs. A small selection of other supposed characteristics of this remedy include midmorning hunger and a tendency for increased discomfort of whatever physical symptoms they may be experiencing between 10 and 11 A.M. and after exposure to cold air or motion.

As noted, these symptoms were assembled through multiple experiences of overdose (homeopathic provings). However, from a scientific perspective, it is difficult to believe that the majority of people who overdose on sulphur experience symptoms largely similar to these (and to the several pages of other symptoms commonly associated with the remedy). In any case, modern knowledge of the difficulties involved in evaluating the effects of medical treatments indicates that provings must be conducted in a double-blind and placebo-controlled manner to be valid. Otherwise, participants are likely to experience symptoms simply because they expect to, and observers will tend to observe the expected symptom picture too. Few of the provings used to define the treatments chosen by homeopaths were performed in a scientifically reliable way. Large, rigorous studies have failed to find any difference in symptoms or biochemical measures between healthy people given homeopathic treatments and people given a placebo.

Thus, homeopathy seems to be a method that should not have a chance of being true. However, some studies have found evidence that homeopathic remedies do relieve symptoms of illness. Many of these were double-blind, placebo-controlled studies, the most meaningful kind of study. This presents a conundrum to impartial scientists. How can this contradiction be resolved?

One possibility is to agree that homeopathy operates through some mysterious force that science has yet failed to discover. Another, less optimistic interpretation is that the positive trials may be too flawed to mean anything, even though they were double-blind.

In 1997, scientists Klaus Linde, Nicola Clausius, and others published a groundbreaking review of all placebo-controlled trials of homeopathic remedies. This article appeared in a prestigious British journal, *The Lancet*. The authors wanted to determine whether there was enough evidence in total to say that homeopathy has benefits beyond the placebo effect. The results of this meta-analysis were positive and have been widely quoted by advocates of homeopathy to conclude that the method has been proven effective.

However, not all double-blind, placebo-controlled trials are created equal. Fairly subtle design flaws can invalidate the results of a study that, on first glance, seems rigorous. In 1999 the authors reanalyzed the data and noticed a direct relationship between the quality of the study and the amount of benefit seen: The higher the quality, the less the benefit. Based on this, Linde and colleagues concluded that their original meta-analysis overestimated the extent to which homeopathy had been proven more effective than placebo. A 2005 evaluation of all the evidence regarding homeopathy also failed to find convincing evidence that homeopathy is more effective than placebo.

Since then, however, further positive studies have been reported, some of which appear to be quite well designed. So does homeopathy actually work? Maybe, but when a method seems scientifically impossible, it properly requires a high level of evidence before it can be accepted as true. Homeopathy has not yet achieved this level of evidence and, therefore, should be regarded as unproven therapy.

WHAT TO EXPECT DURING TREATMENT

To understand how a visit to a homeopathic physician works, one should consider the following imaginary scenario: Sam has felt tense and nervous for months. His workload has increased dramatically since he started a new job last year. He has not been sleeping well and he has lost weight. His conventional physician recommends a stress-reduction program consisting of gentle exercise and regular relaxation, but Sam decides to try classical homeopathy instead.

Sam's initial homeopathic consultation consists of a lengthy interview. The homeopath makes note of small nuances that would not be considered important by a conventional physician. Aside from his nervousness, Sam has been suffering from frequent nosebleeds, easy bruising, dry cough, hoarseness of voice at times, and occasional diarrhea and stomach aches.

The doctor asks whether cold drinks relieve his stomach pain, and Sam nods. Next, the homeopath asks him several questions about his family history, personality, and psychological tendencies. Sam says that he is outgoing and friendly and likes company. "You wouldn't happen to be afraid of thunderstorms," the doctor asks, and Sam answers that he is. The interview continues for one hour.

Based on her analysis of Sam's "constitution" as revealed by close questioning, the homeopath carefully selects a homeopathic remedy that matches it, based on the classic description in the *Homeopathic Materia Medica*. This encyclopedic reference reports the symptoms to be expected when taking an overdose of various substances. These descriptions are complex and elaborate, covering physical and psychological symptoms that developed in the people who undertook the experiment; taken together, they represent the "symptom picture" of the remedy.

Sam's homeopath chooses the remedy phosphorus because its symptom picture matches him closely. He is told to take the remedy for three months. During the period of treatment, he is advised to avoid the use of any pharmaceutical drugs, medicinal herbs (such as St. John's wort), or foods with druglike properties (such as coffee) because they have properties that might antidote (counteract) the effect of treatment. At the end of three months, Sam is advised to call for a follow-up visit, at which point he may be given a new remedy to treat "deeper" problems that may emerge.

This description applies to practitioners using classical or constitutional homeopathy. Many alternative practitioners use homeopathic remedies to treat particular diseases and use herbs and supplements in conjunction with them.

SAFETY ISSUES

Although serious objections remain regarding the possible efficacy of homeopathy, there is little doubt that in one respect, Hahnemann achieved his aim when he invented the treatment: Even if it does not work, it cannot possibly cause direct harm.

Homeopathy came into being during a period in history when conventional medicine was often more harmful than helpful. It was the age of "heroic medicine," during which treatments were chosen more for the drama of their effects than for any evidence of efficacy. The most dramatic effects, however, were frequently the most dangerous. Bleeding sick patients or inducing vomiting or diarrhea were more likely to kill people than to help them.

Modern conventional medicine is far safer (not to mention more effective). Nonetheless, most pharmaceutical medications present some risk. Not so with homeopathic treatments. On a chemical basis, there is nothing in them (or, for low-potency formulations, next to nothing); for this reason, it is as difficult to conceive of any manner in which homeopathic remedies could cause harm as it is to believe that they can cure. Homeopathic tablets are, by nature, completely nontoxic.

However, according to the principles of classical (or constitutional) homeopathy versus disease-ori-

ented (or symptomatic) homeopathy, these remedies can cause problems. On the way toward a cure, temporary exacerbation of symptoms is said to occur frequently. Such "homeopathic aggravations" are supposed to indicate a release of underlying problems, and they are therefore seen as ultimately helpful, if temporarily unpleasant. However, there is no meaningful scientific evidence that such aggravations take place at any higher rate than could be accounted for by chance (and patient expectation).

CONCLUSION

Because the theories of homeopathy seem to contradict basic laws of physics, it appears reasonable to insist that homeopathy meet a higher standard of proof than other forms of alternative medicine, and it has not done so. Some apparently rigorous studies do appear to have found homeopathic methods effective. However, many more studies have failed to find it effective, and overall, the body of supporting evidence is too weak to overcome the reasonable presumption that homeopathy does not work. Proponents of homeopathy have considerable work to do before their method can be given scientific credence.

EBSCO CAM Review Board

FURTHER READING

Altunc, U., M. H. Pittler, and E. Ernst. "Homeopathy for Childhood and Adolescence Ailments." *Mayo Clinic Proceedings* 82 (2007): 69-75.

Anick, D. J. "High Sensitivity 1H-NMR Spectroscopy of Homeopathic Remedies Made in Water." *BMC Complementary and Alternative Medicine* 4 (2004): 15.

Brien, S., G. Lewith, and T. Bryant. "Ultramolecular Homeopathy Has No Observable Clinical Effects: A Randomized, Double-Blind, Placebo-Controlled Proving Trial of Belladonna 30C." *British Journal of Clinical Pharmacology* 56 (2003): 562-568.

Dantas, F., and P. Fisher. "A Systematic Review of Homeopathic Pathogenetic Trials ('Provings') Published in the United Kingdom from 1945 to 1995." In *Homeopathy: A Critical Appraisal*, edited by E. Ernst and E. G. Hahn. Boston: Butterworth Heinemann, 1998.

Ernst, E. "Homeopathy: What Does the 'Best' Evidence Tell Us?" *Medical Journal of Australia* 192 (2010): 458-460.

_____. "Is Homeopathy a Clinically Valuable Approach?" *Trends in Pharmacological Sciences* 26 (2005): 547-548.

Grabia, S., and E. Ernst. "Homeopathic Aggravations." *Homeopathy* 92 (2003): 92-98.

Gray, B. *Homeopathy: Science or Myth?* Berkeley, Calif.:
North Atlantic Books, 2000.

Haller, John S. *The History of American Homeopathy: The
Academic Years, 1820-1935.* New York: Pharmaceutical Products Press, 2005.

_____. *The History of American Homeopathy: From Ra-
tional Medicine to Holistic Healthcare.* New Brunswick,
N.J.: Rutgers University Press, 2009.

Kraft, K. "Complementary/Alternative Medicine in the
Context of Prevention of Disease and Maintenance
of Health." *Preventive Medicine* 49 (2009): 88-92.

Lewith, G., et al. "The Context and Meaning of Placebos for Complementary Medicine." *Forschende
Komplementärmedizin* 16 (2009): 404-412.

Linde, K., N. Clausius, et al. "Are the Clinical Effects
of Homeopathy Placebo Effects?" *The Lancet* 350
(1997): 834-843.

Linde, K., M. Scholz, et al. "Impact of Study Quality
on Outcome in Placebo-Controlled Trials of Homeopathy." *Journal of Clinical Epidemiology* 52
(1999): 631-636.

Walach, H., et al. "Research on Homeopathy: State of
the Art." *Journal of Alternative and Complementary
Medicine* 11 (2005): 813-829.

See also: Hahnemann, Samuel; Herbal medicine;
History of alternative medicine; Naturopathy; Pseudoscience; Traditional Chinese herbal medicine.

Homocysteine, high

CATEGORY: Condition

RELATED TERM: Hyperhomocysteinemia

DEFINITION: Treatment of abnormally high levels of
homocysteine, a substance produced when the body
breaks down the amino acid methionine.

PRINCIPAL PROPOSED NATURAL TREATMENTS: Folate, vitamin B_6, vitamin B_{12}

OTHER PROPOSED NATURAL TREATMENTS: Phosphatidylcholine, trimethylglycine

INTRODUCTION

Beginning in the late 1990s, medical researchers
began to suspect that high levels of homocysteine (a
substance produced when the body breaks down the
amino acid methionine) may accelerate atherosclerosis, the primary cause of heart attacks, strokes, and
intermittent claudication. During a brief period, it
was widely proclaimed that homocysteine was an even
more important risk factor for heart disease than cholesterol. However, it now appears that reducing homocysteine provides minimal benefits.

Most of the supporting evidence for a homocys-
teine-atherosclerosis connection comes from observational studies that found an association between high
levels of homocysteine and increased atherosclerosis.
Observational studies, however, do not show cause
and effect. It is quite possible that unknown underlying factors increase homocysteine levels and also accelerate atherosclerosis, rather than that high homocysteine causes accelerated atherosclerosis. Only
intervention trials (studies in which people are actually given a treatment) can show whether a treatment
is effective.

Several massive studies of this type were initiated in
response to the observational data. The results of five
such trials have been reported, involving a total of
more than eighteen thousand men and women. In
these studies, high doses of supplementary vitamin
B_6, vitamin B_{12}, and folate were used to lower homocysteine levels. None of these studies found significant benefit for preventing stroke, heart attack, or
heart-related death.

A smaller study failed to find that these same homocysteine-lowering vitamins preserved mental function in people with the loss of mental function caused
by atherosclerosis in the brain. Another study failed to
find that lowering homocysteine with B vitamins can
improve mental function in the elderly. On one of the
few positive notes, one substantial trial found that the
use of these homocysteine-lowering nutrients helped
prevent restenosis (recurrent vessel clogging) after
angioplasty.

In addition to atherosclerosis, correlations have
also been found between high homocysteine levels
and numerous other diseases, including Alzheimer's
disease, osteoporosis, complications of pregnancy,
deep venous thrombosis, and pulmonary embolism.
Again, however, most of the supporting evidence for
a connection comes from observational studies; the
results of double-blind studies are less encouraging.
One very substantial double-blind, placebo-controlled
study failed to find that reducing homocysteine levels
can help prevent recurrent deep venous thrombosis

or pulmonary embolism. Data gathered in another study also failed to show benefit for preventing these two conditions. Four double-blind studies failed to find benefit for Alzheimer's disease or other forms of dementia. In addition, double-blind studies of B vitamins for reducing osteoporosis risk have not produced convincing evidence of benefit.

On a positive note, a double-blind, placebo-controlled study in Denmark of 728 elders with high homocysteine and relatively low folate intake found that the use of folate supplements slowed the progression of age-related hearing loss. Folate may also improve mental function in elders with high homocysteine.

Another study found that in people who had already had a stroke and were partially paralyzed, supplementation with vitamin B_{12} and folate reduced the risk of falls leading to hip fractures. Participants were elderly Japanese with high levels of homocysteine and low levels of folate and vitamin B_{12}. It is not clear how the treatment produced this benefit: It might have reduced the tendency for recurrent strokes or might have strengthened bones, improved balance, or produced benefit by some other means. Another study used blood tests to look at effects on bone but failed to find that reducing homocysteine levels had any effect.

People with diabetes or inflammatory bowel disease (Crohn's disease or ulcerative colitis) and those undergoing kidney dialysis may be at higher than normal risk for elevated homocysteine levels. A simple blood test can determine homocysteine levels. Both conventional and alternative practitioners use the natural substances described here to treat elevated homocysteine.

PRINCIPAL PROPOSED NATURAL TREATMENTS

Three nutrients act together to help the body reduce homocysteine levels: vitamin B_6, vitamin B_{12}, and folate. Many Americans are at least marginally deficient in vitamin B_6. Vitamin B_{12} deficiency occurs primarily in the elderly and in people who take drugs that suppress stomach acid. Folate deficiency is thought to have become fairly uncommon in the United States because of the enrichment of grains that began in the late 1990s. However, it appears that the dose of folate required to achieve maximum homocysteine reduction is 800 micrograms daily, higher than the usual nutritional recommendations. Nonetheless, studies utilizing high doses of these vitamins for lowering homocysteine and therefore preventing

cardiovascular disease have generally failed to find benefit.

OTHER PROPOSED NATURAL TREATMENTS

Some people develop extraordinarily high levels of homocysteine because of a genetic defect. The supplement trimethylglycine (TMG) is a treatment for this condition approved by the U.S. Food and Drug Administration. TMG also seems to be effective for milder forms of high homocysteine. However, the nutrients mentioned in the foregoing section are less expensive and probably equally, if not more, effective at lowering homocysteine. Furthermore, TMG might raise cholesterol levels, thereby potentially undoing whatever benefit that might result from lowering homocysteine.

Phosphatidylcholine might also reduce homocysteine. Another study failed to find soy isoflavones helpful for reducing homocysteine levels.

EBSCO CAM Review Board

FURTHER READING

Aisen, P. S., et al. "High-Dose B Vitamin Supplementation and Cognitive Decline in Alzheimer Disease." *Journal of the American Medical Association* 300 (2008): 1774-1783.

Albert, C. M., et al. "Effect of Folic Acid and B Vitamins on Risk of Cardiovascular Events and Total Mortality Among Women at High Risk for Cardiovascular Disease." *Journal of the American Medical Association* 299 (2008): 2027-2036.

Ebbing, M., et al. "Mortality and Cardiovascular Events in Patients Treated with Homocysteine-Lowering B Vitamins After Coronary Angiography." *Journal of the American Medical Association* 300 (2008): 795-804.

Lin, P. T., et al. "Low-Dose Folic Acid Supplementation Reduces Homocysteine Concentration in Hyperhomocysteinemic Coronary Artery Disease Patients." *Nutrition Research* 26 (2006): 460-466.

McMahon, J. A., et al. "A Controlled Trial of Homocysteine Lowering and Cognitive Performance." *New England Journal of Medicine* 354 (2006): 2764-2772.

Sato, Y., et al. "Effect of Folate and Mecobalamin on Hip Fractures in Patients with Stroke." *Journal of the American Medical Association* 293 (2005): 1082-1088.

Van Uffelen, J. G., et al. "The Effect of Walking and Vitamin B Supplementation on Quality of Life in Community-Dwelling Adults with Mild Cognitive Impairment." *Quality of Life Research* 16 (2007): 1137-1146.

See also: Folate; Vitamin B_6; Vitamin B_{12}.

Honey

CATEGORY: Functional foods

DEFINITION: Natural food promoted as a dietary supplement for specific health benefits.

PRINCIPAL PROPOSED USES: Burns, wounds

OTHER PROPOSED USES: Alcohol intoxication, constipation, gingivitis, hay fever, high cholesterol

OVERVIEW

Honey has been appreciated as a food since the dawn of human history. Its medicinal use also is ancient. The Greek physician Hippocrates recommended topical application of honey for infected wounds and for ulcers of the lips. Roman physicians used honey as an oral medication for constipation, diarrhea, upset stomach, sore throat, and coughs.

USES AND APPLICATIONS

Honey consists largely of fructose and glucose, two related forms of sugar. Its sugar concentration is high enough to kill microorganisms in the same manner as the sugar in jams and jellies. This would appear to be

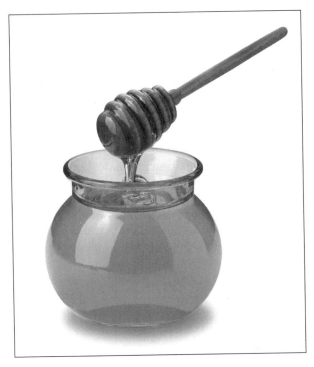

Honey has been used orally and topically since ancient times.
(©Danny Smythe/Dreamstime.com)

the primary basis for honey's most-studied use: as a topical application to treat or prevent infection.

In some controlled trials, honey has shown some promise for treating abscesses, diabetic foot ulcers, venous leg ulcers, minor abrasions, and postoperative wound infections, and for preventing infections following surgery and catheter infections in people undergoing hemodialysis. In most of these studies, honey was used not alone but combined with standard treatments, such as oral or topical antibiotics or surgical debridement (removal of dead tissue). Not all studies show clear benefit, however. One trial found that antibacterial honey (Medihoney) did not significantly improve wound healing in 105 persons with mostly leg ulcers. The best evidence is probably for the acute treatment of minor burns, though the studies supporting this use remain inconclusive.

Sugar paste too has shown promise as a wound treatment. However, some evidence hints that honey may be more effective than concentrated sugar. If true, this suggests that additional, nonsugar constituents of honey provide benefit. It is often stated in honey-related literature that honey produces hydrogen peroxide and that this explains additional benefit. However, there is no evidence that honey produces sufficient hydrogen peroxide to have any meaningful effect. Another theory is that honey might stimulate healing.

Other uses of honey have also shown some promise. In one study, when participants with gum inflammation (gingivitis) regularly chewed "honey leather," their inflammation decreased.

The oral consumption of honey might have a slight laxative effect. Honey taken by mouth might also increase the body's ability to metabolize alcohol, thereby limiting intoxication and more rapidly reducing alcohol blood levels. Finally, one study hints that honey might improve cholesterol profile and blood sugar levels.

It has been suggested that the consumption of honey can reduce symptoms of hay fever. However, the one published study designed to test this suggestion failed to find benefit. A small study of forty people suggests topical honey may help prevent development of oral mucositis (painful inflammation of mucus membranes in the mouth) in persons having radiochemotherapy for head and neck cancer.

DOSAGE

When used topically to treat burns, honey is generally applied either directly to the wound in a thin coat or in the form of a honey-soaked dressing. Oral dosages of honey for medicinal purposes range from 1 to 5 tablespoons several times daily.

Safety Issues

As a widely consumed food, honey is believed to be quite safe. However, infants younger than twelve months of age should not consume honey because of the risk of infant botulism. Honey may contain slight amounts of pollen. However, it appears that allergy to honey is uncommon among persons allergic to pollen.

EBSCO CAM Review Board

Further Reading

Gethin, G., and S. Cowman. "Manuka Honey vs. Hydrogel: A Prospective, Open Label, Multicentre, Randomised Controlled Trial to Compare Desloughing Efficacy and Healing Outcomes in Venous Ulcers." *Journal of Clinical Nursing* 18 (2009): 466-474.

Jull, A. B., A. Rodgers, and N. Walker. "Honey as a Topical Treatment for Wounds." *Cochrane Database of Systematic Reviews* (2008): CD005083. Available through *EBSCO DynaMed Systematic Literature Surveillance* at http://www.ebscohost.com/dynamed.

Okeniyi, J. A., et al. "Comparison of Healing of Incised Abscess Wounds with Honey and EUSOL Dressing." *Journal of Alternative and Complementary Medicine* 11 (2005): 511-513.

Robson, V., S. Dodd, and S. Thomas. "Standardized Antibacterial Honey (Medihoney) with Standard Therapy in Wound Care." *Journal of Advanced Nursing* 65 (2009): 565-575.

See also: Burns, minor; Functional foods: Introduction; Wounds, minor.

Hoodia

Category: Herbs and supplements
Related term: *Hoodia gordonii*
Definition: Natural plant product used to treat specific health conditions.
Principal proposed use: Weight loss

Overview

Hoodia is a cactus-like plant that grows in the Kalahari Desert of South Africa and Namibia. Advertising

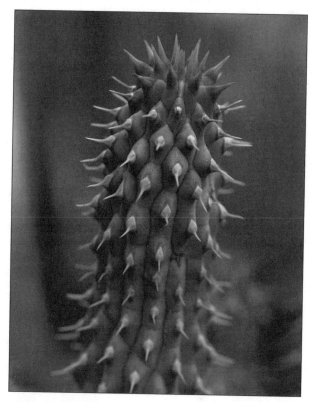

Around 2002, hoodia began to be heavily marketed as a supplement for weight loss. However, there is no reliable evidence that it offers any benefit. (Getty Images)

literature associated with hoodia claims that the herb has been used for thousands of years by the San people (commonly, though inappropriately, known as Bushmen) to stave off hunger and thirst during long desert treks. However, this claim has not been independently verified. Other sources state that the plant was used by the San rarely, and only as a food (as a disfavored food consumed only when better-tasting food sources were not available).

Therapeutic Dosages

A typical dose of hoodia is 400 milligrams twice daily.

Therapeutic Uses

Around 2002, hoodia began to be heavily marketed as a supplement for weight loss. However, there is no reliable evidence that it offers any benefit.

The manufacturer Phytopharm cites a double-blind, placebo-controlled study of 18 overweight people in the United Kingdom who were given either hoodia or placebo for fifteen days. Reportedly, people in the hoodia group consumed one thousand fewer calories daily than those in the placebo group, despite remaining sedentary. If true, this would be an enormous effect. However, this study was small, it was performed by the manufacturer without outside supervision, and it has never been published. Only if a larger, independent study verifies these results will it be possible to say that there is meaningful evidence supporting the use of hoodia for weight loss.

The only published evidence on hoodia is far too preliminary to be relied upon. One animal study found that when the presumed active ingredient of hoodia is injected into the brains of rats their appetite decreases. The authors conclude from their research that hoodia may work by affecting metabolism in the brain. However, injections in the brain are quite a different matter from oral consumption and could suppress appetite simply by being traumatic. Potentially more meaningful animal studies compared hoodia against placebo when fed to rats. Supposedly, benefits were again seen. However, these studies were published only in abstract form, and therefore the results cannot be independently evaluated. In any case, numerous products cause weight loss in animals but do not prove to be useful treatments when tested in people.

The purported active ingredient of hoodia is a substance christened P57. For a time, the drug company Pfizer investigated P57 as a possible weight-loss drug, but the company ceased research in 2003.

SAFETY ISSUES

There are no known safety issues regarding hoodia. However, no meaningful independent studies of hoodia's safety have been reported. Safety in pregnant or nursing women, young children, or people with liver or kidney disease has not been established.

EBSCO CAM Review Board

FURTHER READING

MacLean, D. B., and L. G. Luo. "Increased ATP Content/Production in the Hypothalamus May Be a Signal for Energy-Sensing of Satiety: Studies of the Anorectic Mechanism of a Plant Steroidal Glycoside." *Brain Research* 1020 (2004): 1-11.

See also: Herbal medicine; Obesity and excess weight.

Hopkins, Frederick

CATEGORY: Biography
IDENTIFICATION: English biochemist who postulated the idea of "accessory factors," or vitamins, contained in foods
BORN: June 20, 1861; Eastbourne, Sussex, England
DIED: May 16, 1947; Cambridge, England

OVERVIEW

Frederick Hopkins, an English biochemist, believed that some foods contained "accessory factors," or vitamins, that were necessary for the functions of the human body. With Christiaan Eijkman, another researcher in biochemistry, Hopkins was awarded the Nobel Prize in Physiology or Medicine in 1929 for their discovery of several vitamins. In particular, Hopkins was credited with discovering growth-stimulating vitamins.

Hopkins was said to have childhood interests in both literary and scientific topics, and he excelled in many school subjects, especially chemistry. As a teenager, he scored well on an examination at the College of Preceptors, which yielded him a prize in the field of science. At the age of seventeen, he completed his secondary education and went on to publish his first scientific article (on the beetle) in *The Entomologist*.

After his early successes in academia, Hopkins worked as an insurance clerk for a short time. During his work in the field, he was assigned to work with a chemist, which ultimately led Hopkins back to a life in scientific research after a few years of taking part in a number of important legal cases. He eventually obtained a bachelor's degree in science in his early twenties, and he finally earned a medical degree from Guy's Hospital in London when he was around thirty-two years old. After completing his medical training, Hopkins taught physiology and toxicology at his medical alma mater for a few years and thereafter transferred to Cambridge to study in the field that eventually came to be known as biochemistry (or the chemical aspects of physiology).

Hopkins had a number of successes in research. Of note, he is known for discovering the amino acid tryptophan and elucidating its structure in 1901. His pioneering efforts lay the groundwork for many other notable scientists, including Nobel laureates. Hopkins was knighted in 1925 and received many other prestigious awards during his career, including a Royal Medal in 1918, a Copley Medal in 1926, and admission into the Order of Merit in 1935.

Brandy Weidow, M.S.

FURTHER READING

Ellis, H. "Sir Frederick Gowland Hopkins." *British Journal of Hospital Medicine*, n.s. 72, no. 7 (2011): 414.

Gilman, Sander L. "Hopkins, Frederick Gowland." In *Diets and Dieting: A Cultural Encyclopedia*. New York: Routledge, 2008.

Hopkins, Frederick. "Feeding Experiments Illustrating the Importance of Accessory Food Factors in Normal Dietaries." *Journal of Physiology* 44 (1912): 425-460.

Thomas, Nigel J. T. "The Life and Scientific Work of Sir Frederick Gowland Hopkins." In *The Biographical Encyclopedia of Scientists*, edited by Richard Olson and Roger Smith. New York: Marshall Cavendish, 1998.

See also: Diet-based therapies; Vitamins and minerals.

Hops

CATEGORY: Herbs and supplements
RELATED TERM: *Humulus lupulus*
DEFINITION: Natural plant product used to treat specific health conditions.
PRINCIPAL PROPOSED USES: None
OTHER PROPOSED USES: Allergic rhinitis, anxiety, breast enhancement, cavities, digestive problems, insomnia, menopausal symptoms, periodontal disease

OVERVIEW

Hops, the fruiting bodies of the hop plant, is most famous as the source of beer's bitter flavor, but it also has a long history of use in herbal medicine. In Greece and Rome, hops was used as a remedy for poor digestion and intestinal disturbances. The Chinese used the herb for these purposes and to treat leprosy and tuberculosis.

As the cultivation of hops for beer spread through Europe, it gradually became obvious that workers in hop fields tended to fall asleep on the job, more so than could be explained by the tedious work. This observation led to enthusiasm for using hops as a seda-

tive. However, subsequent investigation suggests that much of the sedative effect seen in hop fields is caused by an oil that evaporates quickly in storage.

Despite the absence of this oil, dried hop preparations do appear to be somewhat calming. While the exact reason is not clear, it seems that a sedating substance known as methylbutenol develops in the dried herb over a period of time. It may also be manufactured in the body from other constituents of dried hops.

THERAPEUTIC DOSAGES

The standard dosage of hops is 0.5 grams taken one to three times daily.

THERAPEUTIC USES

Germany's Commission E authorizes the use of hops for "discomfort due to restlessness or anxiety and sleep disturbances." However, scientists have had difficulty proving that hops causes sedation. Because its sedative effect is mild at most, the herb is often combined with other natural treatments, such as valerian, for anxiety and insomnia. One small, double-blind study found evidence that a proprietary combination of hops and valerian extract is more effective as a sleep aid than placebo; the results of this trial also hint that hops plus valerian is more effective than valerian alone, but this possible finding did not reach statistical significance.

In addition, hops has fairly strong estrogen-like properties, making it a phytoestrogen. The basis for this activity is a constituent called 8-prenyl naringenin. Like soy, another phytoestrogen, hops has been proposed as a treatment for menopausal symptoms. It is also marketed as a breast enhancement product. However, there is no direct evidence that it works for either of these purposes.

For reasons that are not clear, a water extract of hops, called hop water, has shown promise for reducing allergic reactions. In a small, double-blind, placebo-controlled study, use of hop water at a dose of 100 milligrams daily significantly reduced symptoms of allergy to the Japanese cedar. (The Japanese cedar is a strong allergen, similar in its sensitizing power to ragweed.)

A special extract of the hop plant called hop bract polyphenols has shown promise for preventing cavities and treating or preventing periodontal disease. Like other bitter plants, hops is also used to improve appetite.

Hop Water and Allergies

Hops (the fruiting bodies of the hop plant) are most famous as the source of the bitter flavor in beer. However, hops also have a long history of use in herbal medicine. Hops as herbs are most commonly used today as a mild sedative, possibly helpful for anxiety and insomnia. In addition, hops have a constituent with strong estrogen-like properties, and for that reason hops have been proposed as a treatment for menopausal symptoms. However, neither of these proposed uses is supported by reliable scientific evidence.

In recent years, an entirely novel and rather surprising potential use of hops has come to light: treating hay fever. For reasons that are not clear, a water extract of hops (hop water) may reduce allergic reactions. The first evidence came from an animal study performed in Japan in 2005. Based on these results, and on subsequent animal studies, Japanese researchers conducted a double-blind, placebo-controlled human trial.

In this study, thirty-nine people were given a daily drink containing either 100 milligrams of hop water or placebo. All of these study participants were known to have allergies to the plant Japanese cedar. This plant is a strong allergen—as famous in Japan for causing hay fever symptoms as ragweed is in the United States. The results of this small trial were promising. Over the weeks of the study, the use of the hop water extract significantly reduced nasal symptoms, compared with placebo.

Steven Bratman, M.D.

SAFETY ISSUES

Hops is believed to be nontoxic. However, as with all herbs, some people are allergic to it. Interestingly, some species of dogs, greyhounds in particular, appear to be sensitive to hops with reports of deaths occurring. The mechanism of this toxicity is not known. Those taken with the popular hobby of brewing beer at home are advised to keep pets away from the relatively large quantity of hops used in this process.

As noted, hops has estrogen-like effects. Like estrogen itself, hops might stimulate the growth of breast cancer cells. On this basis, women who have had breast cancer, or who are at high risk for it, should probably avoid hops until more is known. (Beer does not appear to contain enough of the active phytoes-

trogen in hops, 8-prenyl naringenin, to matter). Children should also probably abstain from hops to avoid its unwanted estrogen-like effects. Safety in pregnant or nursing women, and in people with severe liver or kidney disease, has not been established.

IMPORTANT INTERACTIONS

One animal study suggests that hops might increase the effect of sedative drugs, so individuals should not take hops with other medications for insomnia or anxiety, except under a physician's supervision. Individuals who are taking sedative drugs should also not take hops except under a physician's supervision.

EBSCO CAM Review Board

FURTHER READING

Koetter, U., et al. "A Randomized, Double-Blind, Placebo-Controlled, Prospective Clinical Study to Demonstrate Clinical Efficacy of a Fixed Valerian Hops Extract Combination (ZE 91019) in Patients Suffering from Non-organic Sleep Disorder." *Phytotherapy Research* 21, no. 9 (2007): 847-851.

Segawa, S., et al. "Clinical Effects of a Hop Water Extract on Japanese Cedar Pollinosis During the Pollen Season." *Bioscience, Biotechnology, Biochemistry* 71, no. 8 (2007): 1955-1962.

Shinada, K., et al. "Hop Bract Polyphenols Reduced Three-Day Dental Plaque Regrowth." *Journal of Dental Research* 86 (2007): 848-851.

See also: Allergies; Anxiety and panic attacks; Cavity prevention; Dyspepsia; Herbal medicine; Insomnia; Menopause; Periodontal disease.

Horehound

CATEGORY: Herbs and supplements
RELATED TERM: *Marrubium vulgare*
DEFINITION: Natural plant product used to treat specific health conditions.
PRINCIPAL PROPOSED USE: Cough
OTHER PROPOSED USES: Asthma, loss of appetite, sore throat

OVERVIEW

The herb horehound has been used since Roman times as a treatment for coughs and other respiratory

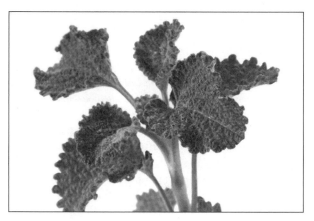

Horehound is taken as a dry herb or as pressed juice. (©Czuber/ Dreamstime.com)

problems, as well as for rabies. It was also popular among native North Americans. Teas and syrups of horehound continued to be used through the nineteenth century for coughs and lung complaints, as well as for menstrual problems. Although the herb itself has a strong bitter taste, horehound candy is considered pleasant by some, and it is still available in traditional candy stores.

THERAPEUTIC DOSAGES

A typical dose of horehound is 1.5 grams three times daily of the dry herb or 2 to 6 tablespoons daily of the pressed juice.

THERAPEUTIC USES

Horehound is recommended by some current herbalists as a treatment for cough, asthma, and sore throat. In addition, like other bitter herbs, horehound is thought to enhance appetite, and Germany's Commission E has approved it for this use. However, there is no reliable scientific evidence to support these uses. Only double-blind, placebo-controlled studies can prove a treatment effective, and none have been performed on horehound.

It is commonly stated that horehound loosens bronchial mucus, but there is no meaningful or substantial evidence to support this claim. Weak evidence (far too weak to be relied upon), hints that horehound or its constituents marrubenol and marrubiin might have smooth-muscle relaxant, antidiabetic, blood-pressure-lowering, and non-narcotic pain-reducing effects.

SAFETY ISSUES

Horehound is thought to be relatively nontoxic, but it has not undergone any meaningful safety study. Horehound is traditionally not recommended for use by pregnant women. Safety in young children, nursing women, and people with severe liver or kidney disease has not been evaluated.

EBSCO CAM Review Board

FURTHER READING

Novaes, A. P., et al. "Preliminary Evaluation of the Hypoglycemic Effect of Some Brazilian Medicinal Plants." *Therapie* 56 (2001): 427-430.

See also: Asthma; Colds and flu; Cough; Herbal medicine.

Horny goat weed

CATEGORY: Herbs and supplements
RELATED TERMS: *Epimedium grandiflorum, E. sagittatum*
DEFINITION: Natural plant product used to treat specific health conditions.
PRINCIPAL PROPOSED USES: Female sexual dysfunction, male sexual dysfunction
OTHER PROPOSED USE: Menopausal symptoms

OVERVIEW

Horny goat weed is an ornamental plant that also has a long history of traditional use in Asian herbal medicine. Its whimsical name is said to derive from folk observations that goats who grazed on the herb became unusually sexually active. Horny goat weed is said to "tonify the kidney yang"; this is an expression whose meaning cannot be fully explained without entering into the theoretical framework of traditional Chinese medicine, but in a loose sense it signifies warming and invigorating the core energy of the body. Traditional uses of the herb (generally in formulas involving several other herbs as well) include treatment of male sexual dysfunction, prostate and urinary problems, low back pain, knee pain, poor memory, emotional timidity, and general symptoms of aging. The aboveground portion of the plant is used medicinally.

THERAPEUTIC DOSAGES

A typical dose of horny goat weed is 250-1,000 milligrams daily.

THERAPEUTIC USES

Horny goat weed is currently marketed as a sexual stimulant for both men and women and also as a treatment for menopausal symptoms. However, there is no meaningful scientific evidence to support these proposed uses. Statements on multiple Web sites claim that it increases testosterone levels, inhibits acetylcholinesterase (a chemical important in the function of the nervous system), and has been shown to act as an aphrodisiac in mice. However, the references cited on these sites do not support these statements. What limited scientific evidence is available is at best far too preliminary to prove anything.

According to test-tube studies and preliminary human trials, a different species in the same family, *Epimedium brevicornum*, may have estrogenic activity. However, even if this were to also apply to horny goat weed, it would not indicate effectiveness for menopausal symptoms. Many herbs with estrogenic effects in the test tube do not appear to help menopausal symptoms. (The one herb that most reliably appears to affect menopausal symptoms, black cohosh, does not have estrogenic effects in the test tube.)

A study of yet another distinct species, *E. koreanum*, seems to be the source of the widespread claim that horny goat weed affects acetylcholinesterase.

In fact, only double-blind, placebo-controlled studies can begin to prove a treatment effective, and none have been performed on horny goat weed taken by itself. The only study of this type tested a combination of horny goat weed, maca, *Lepidium meyenii*, *Mucuna pruriens*, and *Polypodium vulgare*. It supposedly found benefit, but its design and reporting were markedly inadequate, and the results are unreliable.

SAFETY ISSUES

The safety of horny goat weed is unknown. There is one case report in which use of a horny goat weed product caused rapid heart rate and maniclike mood changes in a sixty-six-year-old man. It is not clear whether the herb itself caused the symptoms, as it is possible the product used by this individual might have been adulterated or contaminated with an unlisted active substance. Safety in young children, pregnant or nursing women, and people with severe liver or kidney disease has definitely not been established.

EBSCO CAM Review Board

FURTHER READING

Lin, C. C., et al. "Cytotoxic Effects of Coptis Chinensis and Epimedium Sagittatum Extracts and Their Major Constituents (Berberine, Coptisine, and Icariin) on Hepatoma and Leukaemia Cell Growth." *Clinical and Experimental Pharmacology and Physiology* 31 (2004): 65-69.

Meng, F. H., et al. "Osteoblastic Proliferative Activity of Epimedium Brevicornum Maxim." *Phytomedicine* 12 (2005): 189-193.

Oh, M. H., et al. "Screening of Korean Herbal Medicines Used to Improve Cognitive Function for Anti-cholinesterase Activity." *Phytomedicine* 11 (2004): 544-548.

Partin, J. F., and Y. P. Pushkin. "Tachyarrhythmia and Hypomania with Horny Goat Weed." *Psychosomatics* 45 (2004): 536-537.

Wang, S., et al. "Angiogenesis and Anti-angiogenesis Activity of Chinese Medicinal Herbal Extracts." *Life Sciences* 74 (2004): 2467-2478.

Wu, H., et al. "Chemical and Pharmacological Investigations of Epimedium Species." *Progress in Drug Research* 60 (2003): 1-57.

Yap, S. P., et al. "New Estrogenic Prenylflavone from *Epimedium brevicornum* Inhibits the Growth of Breast Cancer Cells." *Planta Medica* 71 (2005): 114-119.

Zhang, C. Z., et al. "In Vitro Estrogenic Activities of Chinese Medicinal Plants Traditionally Used for the Management of Menopausal Symptoms." *Journal of Ethnopharmacology* 98 (2005): 295-300.

See also: Herbal medicine; Menopause; Men's health; Sexual dysfunction in men; Sexual dysfunction in women; Women's health.

Horse chestnut

CATEGORY: Herbs and supplements
RELATED TERM: *Aesculus hippocastanum*
DEFINITION: Natural plant product used as a dietary supplement for specific health benefits.
PRINCIPAL PROPOSED USE: Venous insufficiency
OTHER PROPOSED USES: Hemorrhoids, minor injuries, phlebitis

OVERVIEW

The horse chestnut tree is widely cultivated for its bright white, yellow, or red flower clusters. Closely related to the Ohio buckeye, this tree produces large seeds known as horse chestnuts. A superstition in many parts of Europe suggests that carrying these seeds in one's pocket will ward off rheumatism. More serious medical use dates back to nineteenth-century France, where extracts were used to treat hemorrhoids.

THERAPEUTIC DOSAGES

The most common dosage of horse chestnut is 300 mg twice daily, standardized to contain 50 mg aescin per dose, for a total daily dose of 100 mg aescin. Horse chestnut preparations should certify that a toxic constituent called esculin has been removed. Also, a delayed-release formulation should be used to prevent gastrointestinal upset.

THERAPEUTIC USES

German research of this herb began in the 1960s and ultimately led to the approval of a horse chestnut extract for vein diseases of the legs. Horse chestnut is the third most common single-herb product sold in Germany, after ginkgo and St. John's wort. In Japan, an injectable form of horse chestnut is widely used to reduce inflammation after surgery or injury; however, it is not available in the United States, and it may present safety risks.

The active ingredients in horse chestnut appear to be a group of chemicals called saponins, of which aescin is considered the most important. Aescin appears to reduce swelling and inflammation. It is not clear how aescin might work, but theories include "sealing" leaking capillaries, improving the elastic strength of veins, preventing the release of enzymes (known as glycosaminoglycan hydrolases) that break down collagen and open holes in capillary walls, decreasing inflammation, and blocking other various physiological events that lead to vein damage.

Horse chestnut is most often used as a treatment for venous insufficiency. This is a condition associated with varicose veins, when the blood pools in the veins of the leg and causes aching, swelling, and a sense of heaviness. While horse chestnut appears to reduce these symptoms, no studies have evaluated whether it can make visible varicose veins disappear or prevent new ones from developing.

Because hemorrhoids are actually a form of varicose veins, horse chestnut is used for them as well, and one double-blind, placebo-controlled study suggests that it may be effective. Another double-blind study found that a topically applied gel made from horse chestnut may be helpful for bruises. Oral horse chestnut also has been proposed for minor injuries and surgery, but published studies on this potential use were not double-blind.

Finally, horse chestnut is sometimes used with conventional treatment in cases where the veins of the lower legs become seriously inflamed (called phlebitis). Note, however, that phlebitis is potentially dangerous and requires a doctor's supervision.

SCIENTIFIC EVIDENCE

Venous insufficiency. More than 800 persons have been involved in double-blind, placebo-controlled studies of horse chestnut for treating venous insufficiency.

One of the largest of these trials followed 212 people for 40 days. In this crossover study, participants

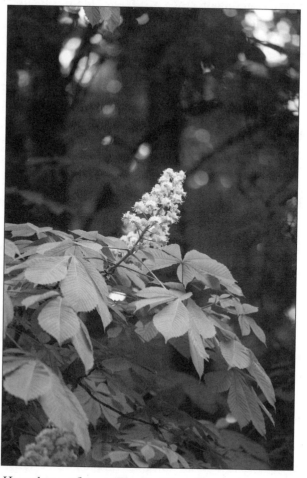

Horse chestnut flowers. (Phanie/Photo Researchers, Inc.)

initially received horse chestnut or placebo and then were crossed over to the other treatment (without their knowledge) after twenty days. The results showed that horse chestnut produced significant improvement in leg edema, pain, and sensation of heaviness. However, the design of this study was not quite up to modern standards.

A better-designed double-blind study of 74 persons also found benefit. Good results also were seen in a partially double-blind, placebo-controlled study, which compared the effectiveness of horse chestnut to that of compression stockings, a standard treatment. This study followed 240 people for twelve weeks. Compression stockings worked faster at reducing swelling, but by the end of the study the results were equivalent, and both treatments were better than placebo. However, a small double-blind trial suggests that oligomeric proanthocyanidins (OPCs) from pine bark are more effective than horse chestnut for the treatment of venous insufficiency.

Hemorrhoids. A double-blind, placebo-controlled study of eighty people with symptomatic hemorrhoids evaluated the use of a horse chestnut product providing 40 milligrams (mg) of aescin three times daily. The results indicated that the use of horse chestnut produced noticeable subjective improvements in pain, bleeding, and swelling within one week; within two weeks, the benefits were visible by objective examination.

Bruises. A double-blind study of seventy people found that about 10 grams of 2 percent aescin gel, applied externally to bruises in a single dose five minutes after they were induced, reduced bruise tenderness.

SAFETY ISSUES

Whole horse chestnut is classified as an unsafe herb by the U.S. Food and Drug Administration. Eating the nuts or drinking a tea made from the leaves can cause horse chestnut poisoning, the symptoms of which include nausea, vomiting, diarrhea, salivation, headache, breakdown of red blood cells, convulsions, and circulatory and respiratory failure, possibly leading to death. However, manufacturers of the typical European standardized extract formulations remove the most toxic constituent (esculin) and standardize the quantity of aescin. To prevent stomach irritation caused by another ingredient of horse chestnut, the extract is supplied in a controlled-release product, which reduces the incidence of irritation to below 1 percent, even at higher doses.

Properly prepared horse chestnut products appear to be quite safe. After decades of wide usage in Germany, there have been no reports of serious harmful effects, and even mild reported reactions have been few in number.

In animal studies, horse chestnut and its principal ingredient aescin have shown a low degree of toxicity, producing no measurable effects when taken at dosages seven times higher than normal. Dogs and rats have been treated for thirty-four weeks with this herb without harmful effects.

Persons with severe kidney problems should avoid horse chestnut. In addition, injectable forms of horse chestnut can be toxic to the liver. The safety of horse chestnut in children and pregnant or nursing women has not been established. However, thirteen pregnant women were given horse chestnut in a controlled study without noticeable harm. Furthermore, studies in pregnant rats and rabbits found no injury to embryos at doses up to ten times the human dose and changes of questionable significance at thirty times the dose.

Finally, horse chestnut should not be combined with anticoagulant, or blood-thinning, drugs, as it may amplify their effect.

IMPORTANT INTERACTIONS

One should not use horse chestnut without medical supervision if also taking aspirin, clopidogrel (Plavix), ticlopidine (Ticlid), pentoxifylline (Trental), or anticoagulant drugs such as warfarin (Coumadin) or heparin.

EBSCO CAM Review Board

FURTHER READING

Diehm, C., et al. "Comparison of Leg Compression Stocking and Oral Horse-Chestnut Seed Extract Therapy in Patients with Chronic Venous Insufficiency." *The Lancet* 347 (1996): 292-294.

Koch, R. "Comparative Study of Venostasin and Pycnogenol in Chronic Venous Insufficiency." *Phytotherapy Research* 16, suppl. 1 (2002): S1-S5.

Pittler, M. H., and E. Ernst. "Horse-Chestnut Seed Extract for Chronic Venous Insufficiency." *Archives of Dermatology* 134 (1998): 1356-1360.

Sirtori, C. R. "Aescin: Pharmacology, Pharmacokinetics, and Therapeutic Profile." *Pharmacology Research* 44 (2001): 183-193.

See also: Hemorrhoids; Phlebitis and deep vein thrombosis; Varicose veins.

Horseradish

CATEGORY: Herbs and supplements
RELATED TERMS: *Armoracia lapathifolia, A. rusticana, Cochlearia armoracia*
DEFINITION: Natural plant product used as a dietary supplement for specific health benefits.
PRINCIPAL PROPOSED USES: Acute bronchitis, common cold, sinusitis, urinary tract infection

OVERVIEW

The spicy root of the horseradish plant is a widely used condiment. Native to southeast Europe, it is widely cultivated in Germany. In Japan, it is called wasabi, and it forms a ubiquitous part of sushi cuisine.

Horseradish root also has a long history of medicinal use. Taken internally, it was thought to be effective for bladder infections and other bladder and kidney problems. (Horseradish oil once formed a part of a drug licensed in the United States for treatment of bladder infection; however, contrary to statements made on some Web sites, this drug is no longer in use.) Horseradish also was taken internally as a treatment for respiratory infections and for joint pain. It was also applied externally in the form of a poultice to wounds, painful joints, and strained muscles.

THERAPEUTIC DOSAGES

A typical recommended dose of horseradish is 3 to 5 grams (g) of the freshly grated root taken three times daily, or 2 to 3 milliliters (ml) daily of horseradish tincture. For external use, freshly grated root is wrapped in thin gauze and applied to the skin until a sensation of warmth develops. The combined nasturtium-horseradish product should be taken according to label instructions.

THERAPEUTIC USES

There are no scientific studies of horseradish that have attained even the minimum level of scientific reliability. Only double-blind, placebo-controlled studies can show a treatment effective, and no such studies of horseradish taken by itself have been reported.

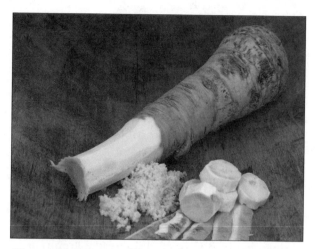

The root of the horseradish plant has a long medicinal history. (©Joerg Mikus/Dreamstime.com)

Germany's Commission E has approved horseradish for supportive treatment of urinary tract infections and for treatment of respiratory infections such as acute bronchitis, colds, sore throat, and sinusitis; however, this approval is based more on tradition than on science.

Test-tube studies performed in the 1950s indicated that horseradish essential oil has antimicrobial properties. However, it is a long way from test-tube studies to actual efficacy in humans; virtually all essential oils have antimicrobial properties in the test tube, but none have gone on to show value as antibiotics.

Constituents of horseradish essential oil include the substance families glucosinolate, gluconasturtiin, and sinigrin. These and similar substances are also found in the plant nasturtium. A preliminary, double-blind, placebo-controlled study published in 2007 found some evidence that a standardized combination of nasturtium and horseradish might prevent new bladder infections among people with a history of recurrent bladder infections. This study, however, had numerous problems in design and statistical analysis. An even less reliable human trial found weak evidence that this combination could be helpful for children with sinusitis, bronchitis, or urinary tract infections.

SAFETY ISSUES

As a commonly consumed condiment, horseradish is believed to be relatively safe. However, because of its spicy nature, it can cause burning mouth pain, sweating, and gastrointestinal distress. Left too long in contact in the skin, marked irritation may develop. Maximum safe doses of horseradish have not been established for pregnant or nursing women, for young children, or for people with serious liver or kidney disease.

EBSCO CAM Review Board

FURTHER READING

Albrecht, U., K. H. Goos, and B. Schneider. "A Randomised, Double-blind, Placebo-Controlled Trial of a Herbal Medicinal Product Containing *Tropaeoli majoris herba* (Nasturtium) and *Armoraciae rusticanae radix* (Horseradish) for the Prophylactic Treatment of Patients with Chronically Recurrent Lower Urinary Tract Infections." *Current Medical Research and Opinion* 23 (2007): 2415-2422.

Goos, K. H., U. Albrecht, and B. Schneider. "On-going Investigations on Efficacy and Safety Profile of a Herbal Drug Containing Nasturtium Herb and Horseradish Root in Acute Sinusitis, Acute Bronchitis, and Acute Urinary Tract Infection in Children in Comparison with Other Antibiotic Treatments." *Arzneimittel-Forschung* 57 (2007): 238-246.

Williams, G., and J. C. Craig. "Prevention of Recurrent Urinary Tract Infection in Children." *Current Opinion in Infectious Diseases* 22 (2009): 72-76.

See also: Bladder infection; Bronchitis; Colds and flu; Sinusitis.

Horsetail

CATEGORY: Herbs and supplements
RELATED TERM: *Equisetum arvense*
DEFINITION: Natural plant product used to treat specific health conditions.
PRINCIPAL PROPOSED USES: Brittle nails, osteoporosis, rheumatoid arthritis

OVERVIEW

Horsetail is a living fossil, the sole descendent of primitive plants eaten by dinosaurs one hundred million years ago. Horsetail contains unusually high levels of the element silicon, making the herb so abrasive that it can be used for polishing. In addition, the plant can incorporate dissolved gold and other minerals into its structure. Medicinally, horsetail has been used for treating urinary disorders, wounds, gonorrhea, nosebleeds, digestive disorders, gout, and many other conditions.

THERAPEUTIC DOSAGES

The standard dosage of horsetail is 1 gram in capsule or tea form up to three times daily, as needed. Medicinal horsetail should not be confused with its highly toxic relative, the marsh horsetail (*Equisetum palustre*).

THERAPEUTIC USES

Silicon plays a role in bone health, and for this reason, horsetail has been recommended to prevent or treat osteoporosis and to strengthen brittle nails. The famous German herbalist Rudolf Weiss also suggests that horsetail can relieve symptoms of rheumatoid arthritis. However, there is no real scientific evidence for these proposed uses.

SAFETY ISSUES

Noticeable side effects from standard dosages of horsetail tea are rare. However, horsetail contains an enzyme that damages vitamin B_1 (thiamin) and has caused severe illness and even death in livestock that consumed too much of it. In Canada, horsetail products are required to undergo heating or other forms of processing to inactivate this harmful constituent.

In addition, perhaps because horsetail contains low levels of nicotine, children have been known to become seriously ill from using horsetail branches as blow guns. This plant can also concentrate toxic metals present in its environment. For all of these reasons, horsetail is not recommended for young children, pregnant or nursing women, or those with severe kidney or liver disease.

Persons taking the medication lithium should use herbal diuretics, such as horsetail, only under the supervision of a physician, as becoming dehydrated while taking this medication can be dangerous. Horsetail may also cause loss of potassium, which may be dangerous for people taking drugs in the digitalis family.

Individuals taking drugs in the digitalis family or taking lithium should use horsetail only under medical supervision.

EBSCO CAM Review Board

FURTHER READING

Brinker, F. *Herb Contraindications and Drug Interactions.* 2d ed. Sandy, Oreg.: Eclectic Medical, 1998.

Pyevich, D., and M. P. Bogenschutz. "Herbal Diuretics and Lithium Toxicity." *American Journal of Psychiatry* 158 (2001): 1329.

See also: Herbal medicine; Nails, brittle; Osteoporosis; Rheumatoid arthritis.

Hufeland, Cristoph Wilhelm

CATEGORY: Biography

IDENTIFICATION: German physician who introduced the term "macrobiotic" and promoted a natural health approach, including dietetics, physical therapy, and other natural practices

BORN: August 12, 1762; Langensalza, Thuringia (now in Germany)

DIED: August 25, 1836; Berlin, Prussia (now in Germany)

OVERVIEW

Cristoph Wilhelm Hufeland, a German physician and notable researcher and writer, introduced the term "macrobiotic" in his book *Makrobiotik: Oder, Die Kunst, das menschliche Leben zu verlängern* (1797; *The Art of Prolonging Life*, 1797) in the context of preventive medicine. The concept of macrobiotics plays a prominent role in many forms of complementary and alternative medicine. Hufeland also is noted for his pioneering contributions to many then-emerging fields, including public health, therapeutics, pediatrics, child-rearing, and medical education. He also is credited for his groundbreaking discussion of the body's natural cycle consisting of twenty-four-hour increments, making him an early contributor to the field of chronobiology.

Hufeland was from a family of physicians (both his father and his grandfather were personal physicians to members of the royal court of Weimer), and he too went on to attend medical school in 1783. Like the generations before him, Hufeland practiced medicine in Weimar for some time, after taking over his ailing father's practice.

Hufeland also acted as an honorary professor, lecturer, and writer for many years. In 1801, he moved to Berlin to treat the Prussian royal family and eventually

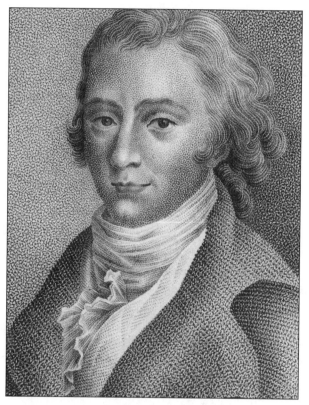

Christoph Wilhelm Hufeland. (Hulton Archive/Getty Images)

to direct a university department of medicine and the ministry of health. He was reportedly acquainted with Samuel Hahnemann, the founder of homeopathy, although the two openly disagreed on the utility of some clinical approaches. Hufeland was known to support a natural healing power approach, in contrast to harsh and invasive strategies. In particular, he promoted dietetics, physical therapy, and other forms of natural medicine.

Hufeland's first book promoted the use of smallpox vaccines; this stance was quite controversial at the time. The development of this vaccine was in its infancy; about 2 percent of vaccine recipients died as a result. Hufeland also had an interest in improving public health and was concerned about the discrepancies in treatment between the wealthy and impoverished populations.

In an effort to improve the sanitary conditions of public water, Hufeland encouraged bathing in the sea. He also investigated the conditions of German spas, which he feared housed unsanitary and potentially dangerous conditions. He made efforts to enforce educational reform, and he wrote several books to promote public understanding of pediatric and maternal health. He also published books covering some aspects of pharmacology.

Brandy Weidow, M.S.

FURTHER READING

Kushi, Michio, and Stephen Blauer. *The Macrobiotic Way.* 3d ed. New York: Avery, 2004.

"Macrobiotics." In *Complementary and Alternative Medicine Sourcebook*, edited by Amy L. Sutton. Detroit: Omnigraphics, 2010.

See also: Diet-based therapies; Ishizuka, Sagen; Macrobiotic diet; Ohsawa, George.

Humor and healing

CATEGORY: Therapies and techniques

RELATED TERMS: Humor therapy, laughter medicine, laughter therapy

DEFINITION: Therapy that uses humor to relieve physical and emotional problems.

PRINCIPAL PROPOSED USES: Circulatory system, immune system, oxygen intake, pain relief, relaxation, well-being

OTHER PROPOSED USES: Blood pressure, digestion, improvement of mental functions

OVERVIEW

The Old Testament references the healing properties of humor: "A merry heart doeth good like a medicine." Throughout the centuries, court jesters have been hired by monarchs to relieve the stress of governmental duties. As early as the thirteenth century, surgeons used humor to distract patients from pain.

In modern times, a systematic approach appears to be developing, consisting of exposure to true mirthful laughter in a supportive environment, under the guidance of a qualified leader or therapist, and combined with attitudinal healing and conventional medicine.

MECHANISM OF ACTION

Laughter is thought to trigger the release of endorphins, the body's natural painkillers. Laughter relaxes muscles, which may then also reduce four neuroendocrine hormones associated with the stress response: epinephrine, cortisol, dopac, and growth hormone.

Laughter moves lymph fluid around the body because of the convulsions that come from the process of laughing. This process helps clear waste products from organs and tissues and boosts the immune system. Laughter is also thought to boost the immune system by increasing both salivary immunoglobulin (IgA) and blood levels of IgA, along with IgM and IgG, a substance called complement 3, which helps antibodies destroy infected cells. Laughter boosts the immune system also by helping the body increase the number and activity of natural killer cells, the number and level of activation of helper T cells, and the ratio of helper to suppressor T cells. Laughter also is thought to increase levels of gamma interferon, a complex substance that plays an important role in the maturation of B cells, the growth of cytotoxic T cells, and the activation of natural killer cells.

Finally, laughter appears to cause the tissue that forms the inner lining of blood vessels, the endothelium, to dilate or expand to increase blood flow.

USES AND APPLICATIONS

Researchers have described different types of humor. Passive humor is created through entertainment, such as watching a film or reading a book. Humor production involves finding humor in stressful situations.

Hospitals and ambulatory care centers have incorporated spaces where humorous materials can be accessed, and they often have clowns and comedians perform or interact with patients to help make them laugh. Other hospitals create what are called laughter clubs or use volunteer groups to visit hospitalized persons to provide laughter. Another type of laughter therapy is laughter yoga.

SCIENTIFIC EVIDENCE

No double-blind studies have been conducted on laughter therapy, but many observational studies exist. The most well-known record of the benefits of laughter and humor healing is the book *Anatomy of an Illness as Perceived by the Patient* by Norman Cousins. In 1964, Cousins was diagnosed with a debilitating inflammatory condition. He experimented with laughter (among other complementary therapies) by systematically watching the television show *Candid Camera*, by watching Marx Brothers films, and by reading humorous books. He wrote "I made the joyous discovery that ten minutes of genuine belly laughter had an anesthetic effect and would give me at least two hours of pain-free sleep."

The first study to prove that laughter helps heart health was performed by researchers at the University of Maryland and published in 2000. In this study, persons with heart disease were 40 percent less likely to laugh in a variety of situations, compared with people of the same age without heart disease. In the study, researchers compared the humor responses of three hundred people, one-half of whom either had suffered a heart attack or had undergone coronary artery bypass surgery. The other one-half were healthy, age-matched participants who did not have heart disease.

In another study at the University of Maryland (2005), some patients were shown disturbing films and others were shown humorous films. The funny films enhanced blood vessel health.

In a five-year study of persons with leg ulcers, researchers at the University of Leeds' School of Healthcare showed that laughing gets the diaphragm moving, playing a vital part in moving blood around the body. In a separate study by Loma Linda University in Southern California, researchers studied men and women taking medication for diabetes, high blood pressure, and high cholesterol and proved that those prescribed mirthful laughter in the form of thirty minutes of comedy every day showed considerable reduction in stress hormone levels.

CHOOSING A PRACTITIONER

Usually a person does not choose a single practitioner but is placed in a group when already being treated at an institution. It also is plausible that a person could self-treat.

SAFETY ISSUES

Laughter therapy is cost-effective and noninvasive.
Stephanie Eckenrode, L.L.B., B.A.

FURTHER READING

Cancer Treatment Centers of America. http://www.cancercenter.com/complementary-alternative-medicine/laughter-therapy.cfm.

Cousins, Norman. *Head First: The Biology of Hope and the Healing Power of the Human Spirit.* New York: Penguin Books, 1989.

Laughter Heals Foundation. http://www.laughterheals.org.

Stewart, Susan M. "Laughter: Nature's Healing Refrain." In *Healing with Art and Soul: Engaging One's Self Through Art Modalities,* edited by Kathy Luethje. Newcastle upon Tyne, England: Cambridge Scholars, 2009.

See also: Art therapy; Color therapy; Depression, mild to moderate; Guided imagery; Mind/body medicine; Music therapy; Pet ownership; Seasonal affective disorder; Self-care.

Huperzine A

CATEGORY: Herbs and supplements
DEFINITION: Natural plant product used to treat specific health conditions.
PRINCIPAL PROPOSED USES: Age-related memory loss, Alzheimer's disease and other forms of dementia

OVERVIEW

Huperzine A is a potent chemical derived from a particular type of club moss (*Huperzia serrata* [Thumb] *Trev.*). Like caffeine and cocaine, huperzine A is a medicinally active, plant-derived chemical that belongs to the class known as alkaloids. It was first isolated in 1948 by Chinese scientists. This substance is really more a drug than an herb, but it is sold over the counter as a dietary supplement for memory loss and mental impairment.

Studies in animals suggested that huperzine A could improve memory skills. These findings led to human trials and the subsequent marketing of the huperzine A as a treatment for Alzheimer's disease and related conditions. It is also sold as a "brain booster" for enhancing memory and mental function in people without Alzheimer's disease.

Huperzine A inhibits the enzyme acetylcholinesterase. This enzyme breaks down acetylcholine, a substance that plays an important role in mental function. When the enzyme that breaks it down is inhibited, acetylcholine levels in the brain tend to rise. Drugs that inhibit acetylcholinesterase (such as tacrine and donepezil) improve memory and mental functioning in people with Alzheimer's and other severe conditions.

The research on huperzine A indicates that it works in much the same way. The chemical action of huperzine A is very precise and specific. It "fits" into a niche on the enzyme where acetylcholine is supposed to attach. Because huperzine A is in the way, the enzyme cannot grab and destroy acetylcholine. This mechanism has been demonstrated by considerable scientific work, including sophisticated computer modeling of the shape of the molecule. Huperzine A may also help protect nerve cells from damage.

While huperzine A is sold as a dietary supplement, in all essential ways it is simply a typical drug. Huperzine A is highly purified in a laboratory and is just a single chemical. It is simply not much like an herb. Herbs contain hundreds or thousands of chemicals. Huperzine A resembles drugs such as digoxin, codeine, Sudafed, and vincristine (a chemotherapy drug), which are also highly purified chemicals taken from plants. If huperzine A is called a "natural" treatment, it would also be necessary to also call these drugs, and dozens of other standard drugs, "natural."

THERAPEUTIC DOSAGES

Huperzine A is a highly potent compound with a recommended dose of only 100 to 200 micrograms twice a day for age-related memory loss. Individuals should use it only under a doctor's supervision.

SCIENTIFIC EVIDENCE

All clinical trials of huperzine to date were performed in China and reported in Chinese. A double-blind, placebo-controlled study evaluated 103 people with Alzheimer's disease who received either huperzine A or placebo twice daily for eight weeks. About 60 percent of the treated participants showed improvements in memory, thinking, and behavioral functions compared to 36 percent of the placebo-treated group, and the difference was significant. Benefits were also seen in an earlier double-blind trial using injected huperzine in 160 individuals with dementia or other memory disorders.

However, not all studies have been positive. Another double-blind trial of sixty individuals with Alzheimer's disease found no significant difference in symptoms between the treated group and the placebo group. Such contradictory results are common when a treatment is only modestly effective, as may be the case here. In a 2008 detailed review of six randomized controlled trials, researchers concluded that, on balance, huperzine A appears to have some beneficial effects. However, the variable quality of these studies suggests that the evidence to date is not strong. Huperzine is also promoted for improving memory in healthy individuals, but the supporting evidence for this claim appears to be limited to one small, poorly designed trial.

SAFETY ISSUES

Perhaps because it works so specifically, huperzine A appears to have few side effects. However, children, pregnant or nursing women, or those with high blood pressure or severe liver or kidney disease should not take huperzine A except on a doctor's recommendation. Experts do not know for sure whether huperzine A interacts adversely with any drugs; however, it seems likely that huperzine might interact with drugs that function in a similar fashion, such as standard drugs for Alzheimer's disease.

EBSCO CAM Review Board

FURTHER READING

Cheng, D. H., and X. C. Tang. "Comparative Studies of Huperzine A, E2020, and Tacrine on Behavior and Cholinesterase Activities." *Pharmacology, Biochemistry, and Behavior* 60 (1998): 377-386.

Sun, Q. Q., et al. "Huperzine-A Capsules Enhance Memory and Learning Performance in Thirty-Four Pairs of Matched Adolescent Students." *Zhongguo Yao Li Xue Bao* 20 (1999): 601-603.

See also: Aging; Alzheimer's disease and non-Alzheimer's dementia; Herbal medicine; Memory and mental function impairment.

Hydralazine

CATEGORY: Drug interactions
DEFINITION: Medication that causes dilation of the walls of blood vessels and is sometimes used to treat hypertension.
INTERACTIONS: Coenzyme Q_{10}, *Coleus forskohlii*, vitamin B_6
Trade name: Apresoline

VITAMIN B_6

Effect: Supplementation Likely Helpful

Hydralazine is known to deplete the blood of vitamin B_6. Taking vitamin B_6 supplements may prevent or reverse side effects of the medication.

COENZYME Q_{10} (CoQ_{10})

Effect: Supplementation Possibly Helpful

There is some evidence that hydralazine might impair the body's ability to manufacture the substance CoQ_{10}. This suggests (but does not prove) that taking CoQ_{10} supplements may produce a beneficial effect.

Coleus forskohlii

Effect: Theoretical Interaction

The herb *Coleus forskohlii* relaxes blood vessels and might have unpredictable effects if combined with hydralazine.

EBSCO CAM Review Board

FURTHER READING

Brunton, Laurence L., et al., eds. *Goodman and Gilman's The Pharmacological Basis of Therapeutics.* 11th ed. New York: McGraw-Hill Medical, 2011.

Kishi, H., et al. "Bioenergetics in Clinical Medicine: Inhibition of Coenzyme Q10 Enzymes by Clinically Used Anti-hypertensive Drugs." *Research Communications in Chemical Pathology and Pharmacology* 12, no. 3 (1975): 533-540.

Shils, M., et al., eds. *Modern Nutrition in Health and Disease.* 9th ed. Baltimore: Williams and Wilkins, 1999.

See also: Coenzyme Q_{10}; *Coleus forskohlii*; Food and Drug Administration; Heart attack; Hypertension; Supplements: Overview; Vitamin B_6; Vitamins and minerals.

Hydrotherapy

CATEGORY: Therapies and techniques

RELATED TERMS: Aquatic therapy, balneotherapy, hydrothermal therapy

DEFINITION: Treatment and therapy involving the use of water.

PRINCIPAL PROPOSED USES: Circulation, inflammation, muscle strengthening and relaxation, pain, swelling

OTHER PROPOSED USES: Digestion, fibromyalgia, gallbladder disease, headaches, immune system, liver disease, lung disease, nervous disorders, paralysis

OVERVIEW

Hydrotherapy has been used throughout history by many different cultures. The Old Testament mentions the healing powers of mineral waters, and the use of water as a healing agent was well established in ancient Greece. The early Roman and Turkish baths remain popular tourist attractions today.

The modern use of hydrotherapy is associated with Vincent Preissnitz, who established the Graefenberg cure in the nineteenth century for treating a variety of ailments. This treatment involved the use of hot and cold water in every conceivable way.

Traditional Native American healing uses sweat lodges as a type of remedy. Sweating is thought to be a form of cleansing that purges poisons from the body. This belief is similar to that of the Scandinavians, who commonly use saunas as therapy.

MECHANISM OF ACTION

A physiological basis exists for hydrotherapy. Cold is stimulating, and it causes superficial blood vessels to constrict, shunting the blood to internal organs. Hot water is relaxing, causes blood vessels to dilate, and removes wastes from body tissues. Alternating hot and cold water also improves elimination, decreases inflammation, and stimulates circulation.

The recuperative and healing properties of hydrotherapy are based on its mechanical and thermal effects. It exploits the body's reaction to hot and cold stimuli, to the protracted application of heat, and to pressure exerted by water. The nerves carry impulses felt at the skin deeper into the body, where they are instrumental in stimulating the immune system, influencing the production of stress hormones, invigorating circulation and digestion, encouraging blood flow, and decreasing pain sensitivity. Generally, heat quiets and soothes the body, slowing the activity of internal organs. Cold, in contrast, stimulates and invigorates, increasing internal activity.

Hydrotherapy can soothe sore or inflamed muscles and joints, rehabilitate injured limbs, lower fevers, soothe headaches, promote relaxation, treat burns and frostbite, and ease labor pains. The temperature of the water used affects the therapeutic properties of the treatment. Hot water is chosen for its relaxing properties. It is also thought to stimulate the immune system. Tepid water can also be used for stress reduction and may be particularly relaxing in hot weather. Cold water is used to reduce inflammation.

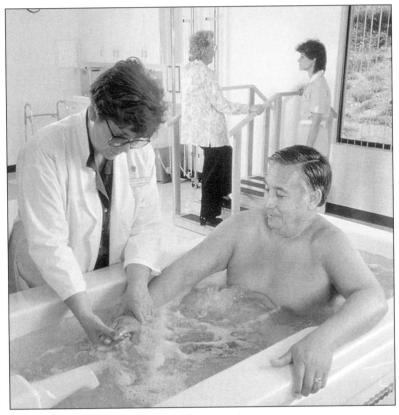

A patient receives a therapeutic bath. (Digital Stock)

SCIENTIFIC EVIDENCE

Case reports, observational studies, and a number of controlled studies provide evidence of success in the use of hydrotherapy. Hydrotherapy is an accepted way to treat symptoms for many conditions, although many forms of the therapy have not been studied carefully. Some types of hydrotherapy, such as ice packs for slight sprains and hot compresses for sore muscles, are well-proven conventional therapies. Warm compresses or warm water soaks are also sometimes used in mainstream medicine to help treat local skin conditions, such as infection. Cold is known to reduce blood flow to the part of the body where it is applied, while heat does the opposite.

Certain types of hydrotherapy can be useful for persons with severe burns, rheumatoid arthritis, spinal cord injuries, and bone injuries. An analysis of studies done on hydrotherapy for lower back pain suggested that it might be helpful, although further studies are needed. Physical therapy is a mainstream

treatment that is sometimes given in a pool, where the water can help to support the person's body weight and reduce impact on joints.

One study was designed to evaluate the effectiveness of hydrotherapy in persons with osteoarthritis (OA) of the knee. Persons with OA using hydrotherapy were compared with subjects with OA of the knee who performed land-based exercises instead of hydrotherapy. Hydrotherapy was superior to land-based exercise in relieving pain before and after walking during the last follow-up. The study concluded that water-based exercises are suitable and effective alternatives for managing OA of the knee.

SAFETY ISSUES

Most forms of hydrotherapy are considered safe. However, people who are frail, elderly, or very young may become dehydrated or develop serious blood chemistry imbalances in very warm water or saunas. Persons with diabetes or poor sensation may be at higher risk of scalding or burning from hot soaks or compresses. Pregnant women and persons with heart or lung problems may have trouble with very hot or very cold water. Those with poor circulation or problems such as Raynaud's phenomenon or frostbite may find that these conditions worsen with the application of cold water, ice, or cold wraps. Excessive heat or cold applied directly to the skin for long periods of time may cause pain, skin drying, and even tissue damage.

Gerald W. Keister, M.S.

FURTHER READING

Burns, S. B., and J. L. Burns. "Hydrotherapy." *Journal of Alternative and Complementary Medicine* 3 (1997): 105-107.

Cassileth, B. *The Alternative Medicine Handbook: The Complete Reference Guide to Alternative and Complementary Therapies.* New York: W. W. Norton, 1998.

Harmer, A. R., et al. "Land-Based Versus Water-Based Rehabilitation Following Total Knee Replacement." *Arthritis and Rheumatism* 61, no. 2 (2009): 184-191.

McVeigh, J. G., et al. "The Effectiveness of Hydrotherapy in the Management of Fibromyalgia Syndrome." *Rheumatology International* 29 (2008): 119-130.

Silva, L. E., et al. "Hydrotherapy Versus Conventional Land-Based Exercise for the Management of Patients with Osteoarthritis of the Knee." *Physical Therapy* 88, no. 1 (2008): 12-21.

See also: Balneotherapy; Cryotherapy; Magnet therapy; Osteoarthritis; Pain management; Rheumatoid arthritis; Soft tissue pain.

Hydroxycitric acid

CATEGORY: Herbs and supplements
RELATED TERMS: *Garcinia cambogia*, gorikapuli, hydroxycitrate, Malabar tamarind
DEFINITION: Natural plant product used to treat specific health conditions.
PRINCIPAL PROPOSED USES: None
OTHER PROPOSED USE: Weight loss

OVERVIEW

Hydroxycitric acid (HCA), a derivative of citric acid, is found primarily in a small, sweet, purple fruit called the Malabar tamarind, or, as it is most commonly called, *Garcinia cambogia*. Test-tube and animal research suggests that HCA may be helpful in weight loss because of its effects on metabolism. However, studies in humans have found mixed results.

REQUIREMENTS AND SOURCES

HCA is not an essential nutrient for the body. The Malabar tamarind is the only practical source of this supplement.

THERAPEUTIC DOSAGES

A typical dosage of HCA is 250 to 1,000 milligrams (mg) three times daily. Supplements are available in many forms, including tablets, capsules, powders, and even snack bars. Products are often labeled *G. cambogia* and standardized to contain a fixed percentage of HCA. Various proprietary forms of HCA are also available and are often claimed by their promoters to be more effective.

THERAPEUTIC USES

Although animal and test-tube studies, as well as two human trials, suggest that HCA might encourage weight loss, other studies have found no benefit.

SCIENTIFIC EVIDENCE

It remains unclear whether HCA offers any weight-loss benefits. In an eight-week double-blind, placebo-controlled trial of sixty overweight individuals, use of HCA at a dose of 440 mg three times daily produced significant weight loss, compared with placebo. In contrast, a twelve-week, double-blind, placebo-controlled trial of 135 overweight persons, who were given either placebo or 500 mg of HCA (as *G. cambogia* extract standardized to contain 50 percent HCA) three times daily, found no effect on body weight or fat mass. However, this study has been criticized for using a high-fiber diet, which is thought to impair HCA absorption.

A twelve-week double-blind trial of eighty-nine individuals found that HCA had no effect on appetite. Another study tested HCA to see if it could cause weight loss by altering metabolism, but no effects on metabolism were found.

SAFETY ISSUES

The Malabar tamarind, from which HCA is extracted, is a traditional food and flavoring in Southeast Asia. No serious side effects have been reported from animal or human studies involving either fruit extracts or the concentrated chemical. A proprietary calcium-potassium salt of HCA appears to have undergone considerable formal safety study, without evidence of toxicity appearing. However, maximum safe doses have not been established, especially for pregnant or nursing women, young children, or people with severe liver or kidney disease.

EBSCO CAM Review Board

FURTHER READING

Badmaev, V., et al. "*Garcinia cambogia* for Weight Loss." *Journal of the American Medical Association* 282 (1999): 233-234.

Mattes, R. D., and L. Bormann. "Effects of (–)-Hydroxycitric Acid on Appetitive Variables." *Physiology and Behavior* 71 (2000): 87-94.

Preuss, H. G., et al. "An Overview of the Safety and Efficacy of a Novel, Natural (–)-Hydroxycitric Acid

Extract (HCA-SX) for Weight Management." *Journal of Medicine* 35 (2004): 33-48.

Vasques, C. A., et al. "Evaluation of the Pharmacotherapeutic Efficacy of *Garcinia cambogia* Plus *Amorphophallus konjac* for the Treatment of Obesity." *Phytotherapy Research* 22 (2008): 1135-1140.

See also: Diet-based therapies; Obesity and excess weight.

Hydroxymethyl butyrate

CATEGORY: Herbs and supplements

RELATED TERMS: Beta-hydroxy beta-methylbutyric acid, HMB

DEFINITION: Natural substance of the human body used as a supplement to treat specific health conditions.

PRINCIPAL PROPOSED USE: Muscle building for strength in athletes and bodybuilders

OTHER PROPOSED USE: Enhancing recovery from heavy exercise

OVERVIEW

Technically called beta-hydroxy beta-methylbutyric acid, the chemical hydroxymethyl butyrate (HMB) is found naturally in the human body when the amino acid leucine breaks down. Leucine is found in particularly high concentrations in muscles, especially. During athletic training, damage to the muscles leads to the breakdown of leucine and to increased HMB levels.

Evidence suggests that taking HMB supplements might signal the body to slow down the destruction of muscle tissue. However, while promising, the research record is contradictory and marked by an absence of large studies.

REQUIREMENTS AND SOURCES

HMB is not an essential nutrient, so there is no established requirement. HMB is found in small amounts in citrus fruit and catfish. In order to get a therapeutic dosage, however, individuals need to take a supplement in powder or pill form.

THERAPEUTIC DOSAGES

A typical therapeutic dosage of HMB is 3 grams (g) daily. One should not confuse HMB with gamma hydroxybutyrate (GHB), a similar supplement. GHB can cause severe sedation, especially when combined with other sedating substances, such as alcohol or antianxiety drugs.

THERAPEUTIC USES

According to some but not all of the small double-blind trials performed thus far, HMB may improve response to weight training. One small double-blind, placebo-controlled trial found hints that HMB might help prevent muscle damage during prolonged exercise, thereby potentially enhancing recovery during athletic training; however, a follow-up study failed to find this benefit. A small study found evidence that HMB might improve aerobic exercise capacity. Weak evidence suggests that HMB might improve blood pressure and cholesterol levels.

SCIENTIFIC EVIDENCE

In a controlled study, forty-one male volunteers, nineteen to twenty-nine years old, were given either 0 g, 1.5 g, or 3 g of HMB daily for three weeks. The participants also lifted weights three days a week for ninety minutes. The results suggest that HMB can enhance strength and muscle mass in direct proportion to intake.

In another controlled study reported in the same article, thirty-two male volunteers took either 3 g of HMB daily or placebo and then lifted weights for two or three hours daily, six days a week for seven weeks. The HMB group saw a significantly greater increase in its bench-press strength than the placebo group. However, there was no significant difference in body weight or fat mass by the end of the study. Similarly, a double-blind, placebo-controlled trial of thirty-nine men and thirty-six women found that within four weeks, HMB supplementation improved response to weight training.

Two placebo-controlled studies in women found that 3 g of HMB had no effect on lean body mass and strength in sedentary women, but it did provide an additional benefit when combined with weight training. In addition, a double-blind study of thirty-one men and women, seventy years old, undergoing resistance training, found significant improvements in fat-free mass attributable to the use of HMB (3 g daily). However, other small studies have found marginal or no benefits with HMB for enhancing body composition or strength.

When the results of small studies contradict one another, it often means that the studied treatment produces minimal benefits at most, and this may be the case with HMB. Larger trials will be necessary to truly determine the extent of its effect.

SAFETY ISSUES

HMB seems to be safe when taken at standard doses. Clinical trials have not found any significant adverse effects with short-term HMB use. Short- and long-term toxicological studies in animals have also found no evidence of harm. However, full safety studies have not been performed, so HMB should not be used by young children, pregnant or nursing women, or those with severe liver or kidney disease, except on the advice of a physician.

As with all supplements taken in very large doses, it is important to purchase a quality product, as an impurity present even in very small percentages could add up to a real problem.

EBSCO CAM Review Board

FURTHER READING

Hoffman, J. R., et al. "Effects of Beta-Hydroxy Beta-Methylbutyrate on Power Performance and Indices of Muscle Damage and Stress During High-Intensity Training." *Journal of Strength and Conditioning Research* 18 (2004): 747-752.

Jowko, E., et al. "Creatine and Beta-Hydroxy Beta-Methylbutyrate (HMB) Additively Increase Lean Body Mass and Muscle Strength During a Weight-Training Program." *Nutrition* 17 (2001): 558-566.

Lamboley, C. R., et al. "Effects of Beta-Hydroxy Beta-Methylbutyrate on Aerobic-Performance Components and Body Composition in College Students." *International Journal of Sport Nutrition and Exercise Metabolism* 17 (2007): 56-69.

Ransone, J., Neighbors, K, et al. "The Effect of Beta-Hydroxy Beta-Methylbutyrate on Muscular Strength and Body Composition in Collegiate Football Players." *Journal of Strength and Conditioning Research* 17 (2003): 34-39.

Slater, G., et al. "Beta-Hydroxy Beta-Methylbutyrate (HMB) Supplementation Does Not Affect Changes in Strength or Body Composition During Resistance Training in Trained Men." *International Journal of Sport Nutrition and Exercise Metabolism* 11 (2001): 384-396.

Thomson, J. S. "Beta-Hydroxy Beta-Methylbutyrate (HMB) Supplementation of Resistance Trained Men." *Asia Pacific Journal of Clinical Nutrition* 13 (2004): S59.

See also: Exercise; Sports and fitness support: Enhancing performance; Sports and fitness support: Enhancing recovery.

Hypertension

CATEGORY: Condition
RELATED TERMS: High blood pressure
DEFINITION: Treatment of the conditions that cause blood pressure to rise to abnormal, dangerous levels.
PRINCIPAL PROPOSED NATURAL TREATMENTS: Coenzyme Q_{10}, relaxation therapies, *Stevia rebaudiana*
OTHER PROPOSED NATURAL TREATMENTS: Acupuncture, Ayurvedic herbal combinations, bacailin, barberry, biofeedback, black tea, calcium, chocolate, *Cordyceps*, fiber, fish oil, *Eclipta alba*, gamma-aminobutyric acid, garlic, glucomannan, green coffee bean extract, grape juice, hibiscus, *Achillea wilhelmsii*, maca, magnesium, melatonin, milk fermented by probiotics, olive leaf, potassium, qigong, quercetin, soy, Tai Chi, vitamin C
HERBS AND SUPPLEMENTS TO USE ONLY WITH CAUTION: *Citrus aurantium*, soy isoflavones, vitamin C plus oligomeric proanthocyanidins, vitamin E

INTRODUCTION

Most people cannot tell when their blood pressure is high, which is why hypertension is called the "silent killer." Elevated blood pressure can lead to a greatly increased risk of heart attack, stroke, and many other serious illnesses. Along with high cholesterol and smoking, hypertension is a major cause of atherosclerosis. In turn, atherosclerosis causes heart attacks, strokes, and other diseases of impaired circulation.

The mechanism by which high blood pressure produces atherosclerosis is somewhat similar to what happens in a hose fitted with a high-pressure nozzle. All such nozzles come with a warning label that states that pressure in the hose should be discharged after use. Many people, however, leave the hose with full pressure after using it. This rather common practice does not produce any immediate consequences. The

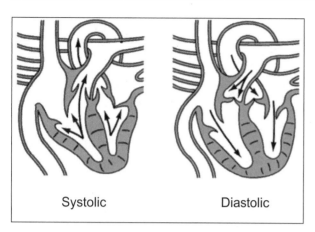

Systolic   Diastolic

Blood pressure is measured in two numbers: systolic pressure over diastolic pressure. Readings greater than 140 systolic over 90 diastolic indicate the presence of hypertension.

hose does not develop leaks at the seams or burst outright on the first occasion it is left untended. However, a garden hose that is frequently left under pressure will begin to age more rapidly than it would otherwise. Its lining will begin to crack, its flexibility will diminish, and within a season or two the hose will develop and show leaks.

When human blood vessels are exposed to constant high pressure, a similar process is set in motion. Blood pressure that elevates to, for example, a reading of 220/170 (systolic pressure/diastolic pressure), which is quite common during certain physical activities such as weight lifting, do no harm. Only when excessive pressure is sustained do blood vessel linings begin to be injured and undergo the unhealthy changes known as atherosclerosis.

Although it is important to lower blood pressure, only rarely does it need to be lowered instantly. In most situations, a person has plenty of time to work on bringing down blood pressure. However, this does not mean that one should ignore it. Over time, high blood pressure can damage nearly every organ in the body.

The best way to determine one's blood pressure is to take several readings at different times during the day and on different days of the week. Blood pressure readings will vary from moment to moment; what matters most is the average blood pressure. Thus, if many low readings balance out a few high readings, the net result may be satisfactory. However, it is essential not to ignore a high value that may have been caused by stress, for example. To record an accurate

number, all measurements must be included in the calculations.

In most cases, the cause of hypertension is unknown. The kidneys play an important role in controlling blood pressure, and the level of squeezing tension in the blood vessels also makes a large contribution.

Lifestyle changes, such as quitting cigarettes, losing weight, and increasing exercise, can dramatically reduce blood pressure. One study found that engaging in aerobic exercise sixty to ninety minutes weekly may be sufficient for producing maximum benefits. Another study found that taking ten-minute brisk walks four times per day significantly improves blood pressure.

For many years doctors advised persons with hypertension to cut down on salt in the diet. Today, however, the value of this dietary change has undergone significant questioning. Considering how rapidly knowledge is evolving, it is suggested that one consult a physician to learn the latest recommendations.

If lifestyle changes fail to reduce blood pressure, or if one cannot make these alterations, many effective drugs are available. Sometimes experimentation with a few drugs helps in finding the most effective one.

PRINCIPAL PROPOSED NATURAL TREATMENTS

There are no herbs or supplements for hypertension with solid scientific support. However, the supplement coenzyme Q_{10} and extracts from the herb *Stevia rebaudiana* have shown some promise in preliminary trials.

Coenzyme Q_{10}. The supplement coenzyme Q_{10} (CoQ_{10}) has shown promise as a treatment for high blood pressure, but the evidence that it works is not strong. An eight-week, double-blind, placebo-controlled study of fifty-nine men already taking medication for high blood pressure found that 120 milligrams (mg) daily of CoQ_{10} reduced blood pressure by about 9 percent compared with placebo. In addition, a twelve-week, double-blind, placebo-controlled study of eighty-three people with isolated systolic hypertension (a type of high blood pressure in which only the "top" number is high) found that the use of CoQ_{10} at a dose of 60 mg daily improved blood pressure measurements to a similar extent.

Also, in a twelve-week, double-blind, placebo-controlled trial of seventy-four people with diabetes, the use of CoQ_{10} at a dose of 100 mg twice daily significantly reduced blood pressure compared with

Lifestyle Changes for Hypertension

Considerable scientific evidence exists showing that adopting the following lifestyle modifications can help a person avoid, reduce, or even eliminate the need for medicines to treat high blood pressure:

Achieve and maintain a healthy weight. If a person is to make just one lifestyle modification, it should be to lose weight if one is overweight. Not only is obesity a major contributor to hypertension, it is also associated with other cardiovascular risks, including high cholesterol and diabetes. The best way to lose weight is to combine a moderate exercise program with a healthy diet. A personal trainer and a registered dietician can help one get started.

Limit salt intake. Not everyone responds to salt in the same way, but blood pressure is affected in some persons by the amount of salt they eat. Because there is no easy way to determine who is salt-sensitive and who is not, the best advice is to reduce one's salt intake. Some nutritionists advise keeping sodium intakes below 1,500 milligrams per day. This can be difficult in an era of processed foods, which tend to be high in salt. One should check the Nutrition Facts label on foods to see how much sodium they contain. The best way to limit sodium is to eat a diet rich in fruits, vegetables, and freshly prepared foods, which are naturally low in sodium.

Eat plenty of fruits, vegetables, and nonfat dairy. One may want to talk to a dietician about the DASH diet, which is rich in fruits, vegetables, and low-fat dairy foods and is low in saturated fat, total fat, and cholesterol. This diet was designed to help people lower their blood pressure.

Exercise regularly. Even independent of its favorable effects on weight, regular aerobic exercise can lower blood pressure. A person can get the most benefit from participating in an activity like walking briskly for thirty minutes every day.

Moderate alcohol consumption. While moderate alcohol consumption may, on balance, be beneficial to your health, excessive alcohol is clearly associated with increased blood pressure. Men should restrict their alcohol consumption to two drinks per day and women to one drink.

Quit smoking. Smoking is bad for one's health in many ways. It increases the risk of having heart disease, among other health problems. Quitting smoking does not directly lower blood pressure, but it is very important for persons with high blood pressure to reduce their overall risk of death.

Richard Glickman-Simon, M.D.;
reviewed by Brian Randall, M.D.

placebo. Antihypertensive effects were also seen in earlier smaller trials, but most of them were not double-blind, so they mean little.

Stevia rebaudiana. The herb *Stevia rebaudiana* is best known as a sweetener. Its active ingredients are known as steviosides. In a one-year, double-blind, placebo-controlled study of 106 people in China with moderate hypertension (approximate blood pressure of 165/103), steviosides at a dose of 250 mg three times daily reduced blood pressure by approximately 10 percent. Full benefits took months to develop. However, this study is notable for finding no benefits in the placebo group. This is unusual and tends to cast doubt on the results.

Benefits also were reported in a two-year, double-blind, placebo-controlled study, also in China, of 174 people with milder hypertension (average initial blood pressure of approximately 150/95). This study used twice the dose of the previous study: 500 mg three times daily. A reduction in blood pressure of approximately 6 to 7 percent was seen in the treatment group compared with the placebo group, beginning within one week and enduring throughout the two years of the study. At the end of the study, 34 percent of those in the placebo group showed heart damage from high blood pressure (left ventricular hypertrophy), while only 11.5 percent of the stevioside group did, a difference that was statistically significant. No significant adverse effects were seen. However, once again, no benefits were seen in the placebo group. This is a red flag for problems in study design. Furthermore, a study by an independent set of researchers failed to replicate these findings.

Another study involving people with diabetes and healthy persons found that stevia, at a dose of 250 mg three times daily, had no significant effect on blood pressure after three months of treatment. A study by an independent set of researchers failed to replicate these findings.

Relaxation therapies. Although it seems intuitive that relaxation should lower blood pressure, the evidence for the benefits of relaxation therapies for treating hypertension is far from convincing. In a review of twenty-five studies investigating various relaxation therapies (totaling 1,198 participants), researchers found that those studies employing a control group reported no significant effect on lowering blood pressure compared to sham (placebo) therapies.

More specifically, biofeedback is widely advocated for treating hypertension. However, in an analysis of twenty-two studies, real biofeedback when used alone was found to be no more effective than sham (fake) biofeedback. A subsequent review of thirty-six trials with 1,660 participants found inconsistent evidence for the effectiveness of biofeedback for treatment of hypertension in comparison to drug therapy, sham biofeedback, no intervention, or other relaxation techniques.

However, some studies have been supportive. A review of nine randomized trials concluded that the regular use of Transcendental Meditation significantly reduced both systolic and diastolic blood pressure compared to a control. Similarly, an analysis of seventeen randomized controlled trials of various relaxation therapies found that only Transcendental Meditation resulted in significant reductions in blood pressure. Biofeedback, progressive muscle relaxation, and stress management training produced no such benefit. In addition, a trial of eighty-six persons with hypertension suggested that daily, music-guided, slow breathing reduced systolic blood pressure measured in a twenty-four-hour period.

OTHER PROPOSED NATURAL TREATMENTS

The Iranian herb *Achillea wilhelmsii* was tested in a double-blind trial of sixty men and women with mild hypertension. The results showed that treatment with an *A. wilhelmsii* extract significantly reduced blood pressure readings. Also, in a double-blind study of forty-three men and women with hypertension, the use of a proprietary Ayurvedic herbal combination containing *Terminali arjuna* and about forty other herbs proved almost as effective for controlling blood pressure as the drug methyldopa.

Although the research record is mixed, it appears that fish oil may reduce blood pressure, at least slightly. Fish oil contains two major active ingredients, DHA (docosahexaenoic acid) and EPA (eicosapentaenoic acid). Some evidence suggests that it is the DHA in fish oil, not the EPA, that is responsible for this benefit.

Several studies have found that glucomannan, a dietary fiber derived from the tubers of *Amorphophallus konjac*, may improve high blood pressure. Other forms of fiber also may be helpful.

Milk fermented by certain probiotics (friendly bacteria) may provide a small blood-pressure-lowering effect. Also, growing evidence supports the use of a green coffee bean extract for high blood pressure. Three preliminary double-blind studies found that chocolate (high in polyphenols) might help mild hypertension. A review including several additional studies drew a similar conclusion.

Numerous studies have found weak evidence that garlic lowers blood pressure slightly, perhaps 5 to 10 percent more than placebo. It remains unclear whether garlic supplements can help persons with high blood pressure safely eliminate or avoid antihypertensive medications.

People who are deficient in calcium may be at great risk of developing high blood pressure. Among people who already have hypertension, increased intake of calcium might slightly decrease blood pressure, according to some studies. In an extremely large, randomized, placebo-controlled trial involving 36,282 postmenopausal women, 1,000 mg of calcium plus 400 international units of vitamin D given daily did not significantly reduce blood pressure in seven years in women with or without hypertension. Weak evidence hints that the use of calcium by pregnant women might reduce the risk of hypertension in their children. Also, study results are mixed on whether magnesium or potassium supplements can improve blood pressure. At most, the benefit is likely quite small.

In a thirty-day, double-blind, placebo-controlled study of thirty-nine people taking medications for hypertension, treatment with 500 mg of vitamin C daily reduced blood pressure by about 10 percent. Smaller benefits were seen in studies of people with normal blood pressure or borderline hypertension. One double-blind study compared 500, 1,000, and 2,000 mg of vitamin C and found an equivalent level of benefit in all three groups. (Because of the lack of a placebo group, this study cannot be used as proof of effectiveness, only as a demonstration of the equivalence of the doses.) However, other studies have failed to find evidence of benefit with vitamin C. This mixed evidence suggests, on balance, that if vitamin C does have any blood-pressure-lowering effect, it is at most quite modest.

Unexpectedly, one study found that a combination of vitamin C (500 mg daily) and grape seed oligomeric proanthocyanidins (1,000 mg daily) slightly increased blood pressure. Whether this was a fluke of statistics or a real combined effect remains unclear.

Other studies suggest possible benefit with the Ayurvedic herb *Eclipta alba* (also known as Bhringraja or Keshraja), beta-hydroxy-beta-methylbutyrate, theanine from black tea, blue-green algae products, chitosan, concord grape juice, garlic, gamma-aminobutyric acid, various forms of the herb hawthorn, kelp, lipoic acid combined with carnitine, quercetin, *Salvia hispanica* (a grain), and sweetie fruit (a hybrid between grapefruit and pummelo, high in citrus bioflavonoids). However, the supporting evidence cannot be considered reliable for any of these treatments.

There is mixed evidence on whether soy protein and its associated isoflavones are helpful for blood pressure. A comprehensive review of studies investigating the influence of phytoestrogens (including soy) on blood pressure found no meaningful effect. However, another review found that soy protein alone could significantly reduce blood pressure.

Three small, double-blind, placebo-controlled studies found evidence that melatonin may slightly reduce nighttime blood pressure. Getting adequate vitamin D may help prevent the development of hypertension. The vitamin folate may help decrease blood pressure (and might provide other heart-healthy effects) in smokers.

The herbs astragalus, barberry, *Coleus forskohliibacailin*, hibiscus, maitake, maca, and olive leaf, and the supplements beta-carotene, *Cordyceps*, flaxseed oil, royal jelly, and taurine, are sometimes recommended for high blood pressure, but there is no meaningful evidence that they work. Also, reducing homocysteine with B vitamins does not appear to reduce blood pressure in healthy people with high homocysteine.

One study was quoted as having showed that a traditional Chinese herbal formula can reduce blood pressure, but the study actually failed to find any effect on blood pressure. In a review of twenty-six published studies examining the effectiveness of Tai Chi for high blood pressure, 85 percent demonstrated a reduction in blood pressure. However, only five of these twenty-six studies were of acceptable quality.

A substantial study (192 participants) failed to find acupuncture helpful for high blood pressure. However, another study, this one enrolling 160 people, did report benefit, but the study was small and had problems in its use of statistics. In a review of eleven randomized-controlled trials on the subject, researchers determined that acupuncture's ability to lower blood pressure remains inconclusive.

The alternative therapies hatha yoga, qigong, and Tai Chi have shown some potential benefit for high blood pressure, the mechanism of action probably being similar for each. A later review of multiple studies investigating the effectiveness of self-practiced qigong, for example, concluded that this therapy was more effective at lowering blood pressure than no-treatment controls. However, it was no more effective than standard treatments for hypertension: antihypertensive medications or conventional exercise.

In a twelve-week study of 140 men and women with stage I hypertension, chiropractic spinal manipulation plus dietary change did not produce any greater benefit than dietary change alone. For many years, the American Heart Association and other major foundations have recommended reducing saturated fat and increasing carbohydrates in one's diet. However, growing evidence suggests that it is preferable to keep carbohydrate levels relatively low while replacing saturated fat with monounsaturated fats such as olive oil.

HERBS AND SUPPLEMENTS TO USE ONLY WITH CAUTION

There is one highly credible case report of severe, dangerous hypertension caused by consumption of isoflavones made from soy during the course of a clinical trial on this supplement. This is most likely a rare, highly individual response, but if it could occur with one person, it also could occur with another.

As noted, in one study, a combination of vitamin C and grape seed oligomeric proanthocyanidins mildly increased blood pressure. In another study, the use of vitamin E raised blood pressure in people with type 2 diabetes.

The herb *Citrus aurantium* (bitter orange) may increase blood pressure. In addition, various herbs and supplements may interact adversely with drugs used to treat hypertension.

EBSCO CAM Review Board

FURTHER READING

Anderson, J. W., C. Liu, and R. J. Kryscio. "Blood Pressure Response to Transcendental Meditation." *American Journal of Hypertension* 21 (2008): 310-316.

Erkkila, A. T., et al. "Effects of Fatty and Lean Fish Intake on Blood Pressure in Subjects with Coronary Heart Disease Using Multiple Medications." *European Journal of Nutrition* 47 (2008): 319-328.

Greenhalgh, J., R. Dickson, and Y. Dundar. "Biofeedback for Hypertension." *Journal of Hypertension* 28 (2010): 644-652.

Heather, O. D., et al. "Relaxation Therapies for the Management of Primary Hypertension in Adults." *Cochrane Database of Systematic Reviews* (2008): CD004935. Available through *EBSCO DynaMed Systematic Literature Surveillance* at http://www.ebscohost.com/dynamed.

Hooper, L., et al. "Flavonoids, Flavonoid-Rich Foods, and Cardiovascular Risk." *American Journal of Clinical Nutrition* 88 (2008): 38-50.

Lee, H., et al. "Acupuncture for Lowering Blood Pressure." *American Journal of Hypertension* 22 (2009): 122-128.

Margolis, K. L., et al. "Effect of Calcium and Vitamin D Supplementation on Blood Pressure." *Hypertension* 52 (2008): 847-855.

Modesti, P. A., et al. "Psychological Predictors of the Antihypertensive Effects of Music-Guided Slow Breathing." *Journal of Hypertension* 28 (2010): 1097-1103.

Ried, K., et al. "Effect of Garlic on Blood Pressure." *BMC Cardiovascular Disorders* 9 (2008): 13.

Rogers, P. J., et al. "Time for Tea: Mood, Blood Pressure, and Cognitive Performance Effects of Caffeine and Theanine Administered Alone and Together." *Psychopharmacology* 195 (2008): 569-577.

Wahabi, H. A., et al. "The Effectiveness of *Hibiscus sabdariffa* in the Treatment of Hypertension." *Phytomedicine* 17 (2010): 83-86.

See also: Atherosclerosis; Calcium channel blockers; Coenzyme Q$_{10}$; Heart attack; Low-carbohydrate diet; Stevia.

Hypertension: Homeopathic remedies

Category: Homeopathy

Definition: The use of highly diluted remedies to treat high blood pressure.

Studied homeopathic remedies: *Aurum, Baryta carbonica, Lachesis*

Scientific Evaluations of Homeopathic Remedies

Researchers have completed two studies of homeopathic remedies for treating hypertension. However, neither study yielded encouraging results. A four-week, double-blind, placebo-controlled study enrolling thirty-two participants evaluated the possible efficacy of *Baryta carbonica* 15c (centesimals) in the treatment of hypertension. This study found no statistically significant difference between the treatment and control groups.

A small, double-blind, crossover study enrolled ten people with essential hypertension and compared individualized homeopathic treatment to standard drug therapy. These participants were examined on a weekly basis for sixteen weeks. Homeopathic treatment proved ineffective.

Traditional Homeopathic Treatments

Classical homeopathy offers possible homeopathic treatments for hypertension. These therapies are chosen based on various specific details of the person seeking the treatment. *Baryta carbonica* is traditionally used for people with hypertension who are extremely shy, lack concentration, and often display immature behavior. The symptom picture of this remedy includes high blood pressure that is made worse by exertion or by lying on the left side, along with a tendency toward gripping pains in the stomach that improve when one lies on one's stomach.

Aurum is often recommended for people whose high blood pressure is caused by slow-burning, long-term stress, which is often associated with one's career or ambition. *Lachesis* may be used for a person with high blood pressure who has a flushed look to the face, whose behavior is overactive, and who has a tendency to engage in compulsive talking, as if an inner boiler were always about to explode.

EBSCO CAM Review Board

Further Reading

Bignamini, M., et al. "Controlled Double Blind Trial with *Baryta carbonica* 15CH Versus Placebo in a Group of Hypertensive Subjects Confined to Bed in Old People's Home." *British Homeopathic Journal* 76 (1987): 114-119.

Loizzo, M. R., et al. "Hypotensive Natural Products: Current Status." *Mini Reviews in Medicinal Chemistry* 8 (2008): 828-855.

Teut, M., et al. "Homeopathic Treatment of Elderly Patients." *BMC Geriatrics* 10 (2010): 10.

Tirapelli, C. R., et al. "Hypotensive Action of Naturally Occurring Diterpenes: A Therapeutic Promise for the Treatment of Hypertension." *Fitoterapia* 81 (2010): 690-702.

See also: Hypertension; Preeclampsia and pregnancy-induced hypertension.

Hyperthyroidism

CATEGORY: Condition
RELATED TERMS: Graves' disease, subacute thyroiditis, thyroid hormone, excess, thyrotoxicosis
DEFINITION: Treatment for excessive amounts of thyroid hormone released by the thyroid gland.
PRINCIPAL PROPOSED NATURAL TREATMENTS: None
OTHER PROPOSED NATURAL TREATMENTS: Bugleweed, L-carnitine, glucomannan, motherwort, royal jelly
HERBS AND SUPPLEMENTS TO AVOID: Ashwaghanda, bladderwrack, kelp

INTRODUCTION

Hyperthyroidism is a condition in which the thyroid gland releases excessive amounts of thyroid hormone. Symptoms include weight loss, fatigue, fast heart rate, heart palpitations, intolerance to heat, insomnia, anxiety, frequent bowel movements, scant menstruation, bone thinning, hair loss, changes in the appearance of the eye (bulging or staring), and goiter (a visible enlargement of the neck caused by a swollen thyroid gland).

The most common form of hyperthyroidism is Graves' disease. In this condition, the body manufactures antibodies that have the unintended effect of stimulating the thyroid gland. (In another condition, Hashimoto's thyroiditis, the body produces antibodies that decrease thyroid output.) In addition, benign tumors of the thyroid can secrete excessive thyroid hormone on their own (cancerous tumors seldom do). Viral infection of the thyroid (subacute thyroiditis) causes short-lived hyperthyroidism followed by a more prolonged period of hypothyroidism.

Medical treatment of hyperthyroidism is highly effective. In most cases of ongoing hyperthyroidism, radioactive iodine is used to destroy thyroid tissue. This approach is both safe and effective, because almost all the iodine in the body ends up in the thyroid; the ra-

dioactive treatment, therefore, does not damage any other tissues. Other approaches to hyperthyroidism include drugs to block the effects of high thyroid hormone or to slow thyroid hormone production, and, in relatively rare cases, surgery.

PROPOSED NATURAL TREATMENTS

Physician supervision is necessary to determine why the thyroid is overactive to design a specific treatment plan. None of the treatments discussed in this section actually get to the root of the problem, nor have they been proven effective. Self-treatment of hyperthyroidism is not recommended.

Test-tube and animal studies suggest that the herb bugleweed may reduce thyroid hormone by decreasing levels of TSH (the hormone that stimulates the thyroid gland) and by impairing thyroid hormone synthesis. In addition, bugleweed may block the action of thyroid-stimulating antibodies found in Graves' disease.

The supplement L-carnitine has shown promise for treating a special form of hyperthyroidism that may occur during the treatment of benign goiter. People with benign goiter often take thyroid hormone pills as treatment. Sometimes, successful treatment of this condition requires taking slightly more thyroid hormone than the body needs, resulting in symptoms of mild hyperthyroidism. A double-blind, placebo-controlled trial found evidence that the use of the supplement L-carnitine could alleviate many of these symptoms. This six-month study evaluated the effects of L-carnitine in fifty women who were taking thyroid hormone for benign goiter. The results showed that a dose of 2 grams (g) or 4 g of carnitine daily protected participants' bones and reduced other symptoms of hyperthyroidism. Carnitine is thought to affect thyroid hormone by blocking its action in cells. A preliminary trial found some evidence that when the supplement glucomannan is added to standard treatment, normal thyroid hormone levels are restored more rapidly.

For many people, the most problematic symptom of hyperthyroidism is rapid or irregular heartbeat. In cases of temporary high thyroid hormone levels (as in the form of a viral infection), conventional treatment may involve simply protecting the heart. Germany's Commission E (the herbal regulating body in that country) has authorized the use of the herb motherwort as part of an overall treatment plan for an overactive thyroid (hyperthyroidism). Motherwort is said to calm the heart; however, there is no meaningful evidence to indicate that it is effective for the heart-related symptoms of hyperthyroidism (or any other heart-related symptoms). Royal jelly has been proposed for use in Graves' disease, but there is no meaningful evidence that it is effective.

HERBS AND SUPPLEMENTS TO AVOID

According to one study in animals, the herb ashwaghanda may raise thyroid hormone levels. For this reason, it should not be used by people with hyperthyroidism. Taking excessive kelp, bladderwrack, or other forms of seaweed can cause hyperthyroidism by overloading the body with iodine.

EBSCO CAM Review Board

FURTHER READING

Azezli, A. D., T. Bayraktaroglu, and Y. Orhan. "The Use of Konjac Glucomannan to Lower Serum Thyroid Hormones in Hyperthyroidism." *Journal of the American College of Nutrition* 26 (2007): 663-668.

Benvenga, S., M. Lakshmanan, and F. Trimarchi. "Carnitine Is a Naturally Occurring Inhibitor of Thyroid Hormone Nuclear Uptake." *Thyroid* 10 (2000): 1043-1050.

Benvenga, S., et al. "Usefulness of L-carnitine, a Naturally Occurring Peripheral Antagonist of Thyroid Hormone Action, in Iatrogenic Hyperthyroidism." *Journal of Clinical Endocrinology and Metabolism* 86 (2001): 3579-3594.

Erem, C., et al. "The Effects of Royal Jelly on Autoimmunity in Graves' Disease." *Endocrine* 30 (2006): 175-183.

See also: Fatigue; Hypothyroidism; Thyroid hormone; Weight loss, undesired.

Hypnotherapy

CATEGORY: Therapies and techniques
RELATED TERMS: Ericksonian hypnosis, hypnosis, neurolinguistic programming, self-hypnosis
DEFINITION: Technique involving hypnosis to produce a therapeutic benefit.
PRINCIPAL PROPOSED USES: Cancer treatment (reducing side effects), surgery support, warts

OTHER PROPOSED USES: Asthma, burn injury (reducing pain), fibromyalgia, hay fever, irritable bowel syndrome, labor and delivery, nocturnal enuresis, psoriasis, smoking cessation, tension and other forms of headache, weight loss

OVERVIEW

Hypnotherapy is a poorly understood technique that has multiple definitions, descriptions, and forms. It is generally agreed that the hypnotic state is different from both sleep and ordinary wakefulness, but just exactly what it consists of remains unclear. Hypnosis is sometimes described as a form of heightened attention combined with deep relaxation, uncritical openness, and voluntarily lowered resistance to suggestion. Thus, one might say that when a person watches an engrossing film and allows himself or herself to surrender to it as if it were reality, then that person is undergoing something indistinguishable from hypnosis.

In therapeutic hypnosis, the hypnotherapist uses one of several techniques to induce a hypnotic state. The best-known (but dated) technique is the swinging watch accompanied by the suggestion to fall asleep. Such "fixed gaze" hypnosis is no longer the mainstay.

More often, hypnotists use progressive relaxation methods. Other methods include mental misdirection (as when a person is fooled during a suspenseful film) and deliberate mental confusion. The net effect is the same; the person being hypnotized is in a state of heightened willingness to accept outside suggestions.

Once the person is in this state, the hypnotherapist can make a suggestion aimed at producing therapeutic benefit. At its most straightforward, this involves direct affirmation of the desired health benefit, such as, "You are now relaxing the muscles of your neck, and you will keep them relaxed." Indirect or paradoxical suggestions may be used too, especially in schools of hypnotherapy such as Ericksonian hypnosis and neurolinguistic programming. It is also possible to learn to give oneself suggestions by inducing a state of hypnosis; this is called self-hypnosis.

USES AND APPLICATIONS

Hypnotherapy is commonly used for the treatment of addictions and for reducing fear and anxiety surrounding stressful situations, such as surgery or severe illness. Other relatively common uses for

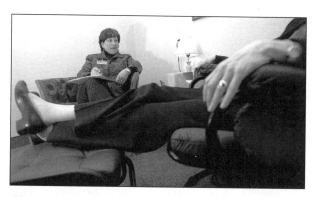

Ohio therapist Jane Ehrman uses hypnosis and imagery to help her patient relax and manage pain in 2006. (AP Photo)

hypnotherapy include insomnia, childbirth, pain control in general, and nocturnal enuresis (bedwetting). However, the evidence that hypnotherapy is effective for these uses remains incomplete at best.

SCIENTIFIC EVIDENCE

It is more difficult to ascertain the effectiveness of a therapy like hypnosis than a drug or a pill for one simple reason: It is difficult to design a proper double-blind, placebo-controlled study of this therapy. Researchers studying the herb St. John's wort, for example, can use placebo pills that are indistinguishable from the real thing. However, it is difficult to conceive of a form of placebo hypnosis that cannot be detected as such by both practitioners and participants. For this reason, all studies of hypnosis have made various compromises to the double-blind design. Some studies randomly assigned participants to receive either hypnosis or no treatment. In the best of these studies, results were rated by examiners who did not know which participants were in which group (in other words, the examiners were blinded observers). However, it is not clear whether benefits reported in such studies come from the hypnosis or less specific factors, such as mere attention.

Other studies have compared hypnosis with various psychological techniques, including relaxation therapy and cognitive psychotherapy. However, the same issues arise when trying to study these latter therapies as with hypnosis, and the results of a study that compares an unproven treatment to an unproven treatment are not meaningful.

In some studies, participants were allowed to choose whether they received hypnosis or some other therapy. Such nonrandomized studies are highly unreliable; the people who chose hypnosis, for example, might have been different in another way.

Even less meaningful studies of hypnotism simply involved giving people hypnosis and monitoring them to see whether they improved. Studies of this type have been used to support the use of hypnotherapy for hundreds of medical conditions. However, for many reasons, such open-label trials prove nothing.

In studies of most medical therapies, researchers must be sure to eliminate the possibility of a placebo effect. This concern, however, loses its relevance when hypnotism is in question. It is not a criticism of a study on hypnosis if an observed benefit turns out to be caused by the power of suggestion. After all, hypnosis consists precisely of the power of suggestion. (The placebo effect is only one of many problems with open-label studies, however.) Given these caveats, this article discusses what science knows about the medical benefits of hypnotherapy.

Possible benefits of hypnotherapy. A minimum of twenty controlled studies, enrolling more than fifteen hundred people in total, evaluated the potential benefit of hypnosis for people undergoing surgery. The combined results of the studies suggest that hypnosis may provide benefits both during and after surgery, benefits including reducing anxiety, pain, and nausea; normalizing blood pressure and heart rate; minimizing blood loss; speeding recovery; and shortening hospitalization. Many of these studies, however, were of poor quality.

Hypnosis has also shown some promise for reducing nausea, pain, and anxiety in adults and children undergoing treatment for cancer. It also may be useful in persons with breast cancer who also have hot flashes.

Numerous anecdotal reports suggest that warts can sometimes disappear in response to suggestion. In three controlled studies enrolling a total of 180 people with warts, the use of hypnosis showed superior results compared to no treatment. In one of these studies, hypnosis also was superior to salicylic acid (a standard treatment for warts). In that trial, hypnosis also was better than fake salicylic acid, hinting that the power of suggestion is greater with hypnosis than with an ordinary placebo.

Many smokers have tried hypnotherapy to break their addiction. While hypnotherapy benefits some smokers, it does not appear to be superior to other methods. In a review of nine studies, researchers found no consistent evidence that hypnotherapy was better than fourteen other interventions for nicotine addiction. Also, a later trial found that, when combined with a nicotine patch, hypnotherapy was no better than cognitive behavioral therapy.

Other conditions for which hypnosis has shown promise in controlled trials include the following: asthma, burn injury (reducing pain), fibromyalgia, hay fever, irritable bowel syndrome, labor and delivery and other gynecologic procedures, nocturnal enuresis, chest pain of unknown cause (unrelated to the heart), peptic ulcers, psoriasis, pain associated with diagnostic procedures, tension headache and other forms of headache, and vertigo and headache caused by head injury. However, the quality of many of the supporting studies was poor, and their results were frequently inconsistent.

Hypnosis is particularly popular as an aid to weight loss. However, a careful analysis of published studies shows that hypnosis is not effective for this condition; at best, the evidence points toward only a marginal benefit.

WHAT TO EXPECT DURING TREATMENT

Hypnotherapy sessions usually last thirty to sixty minutes. They typically involve some questions and answers, followed by the hypnosis itself. Some hypnotists teach their clients self-hypnosis so they can reinforce the formal session.

CHOOSING A PRACTITIONER

As with all medical therapies, it is best to choose a licensed practitioner in states where a hypnotherapy license is available. Where licensure is not available, one should seek a referral from a qualified and knowledgeable medical provider.

SAFETY ISSUES

In the hands of a competent practitioner, hypnotherapy should present no more risks than any other form of psychotherapy. These risks might include worsening of the original problem and temporary fluctuations in mood.

Contrary to various works of fiction, hypnosis does not give the hypnotist absolute power over his or her subject. However, as with all forms of psychotherapy, the hypnotherapist does gain some power over the client through the client's trust; an unethical therapist can abuse this power.

EBSCO CAM Review Board

FURTHER READING

Abbot, N. C., L. F. Stead, and A. R. White. "Hypnotherapy for Smoking Cessation." *Cochrane Database of Systematic Reviews* (2000): CD001008. Available through *EBSCO DynaMed Systematic Literature Surveillance* at http://www.ebscohost.com/dynamed.

Carmody, T. P., et al. "Hypnosis for Smoking Cessation." *Nicotine and Tobacco Research* 10 (2008): 811-818.

Elkins, G., et al. "Randomized Trial of a Hypnosis Intervention for Treatment of Hot Flashes Among Breast Cancer Survivors." *Journal of Clinical Oncology* 26 (2008): 5022-5026.

Jones, H., et al. "Treatment of Non-cardiac Chest Pain." *Gut* 55 (2006): 1403-1408.

Langewitz, W., et al. "Effect of Self-Hypnosis on Hay Fever Symptoms." *Psychotherapy and Psychosomatics* 74 (2005): 165-172.

Marc, I., et al. "Hypnotic Analgesia Intervention During First-Trimester Pregnancy Termination." *American Journal of Obstetrics and Gynecology* 199 (2008): 469.

Richardson, J., et al. "Hypnosis for Nausea and Vomiting in Cancer Chemotherapy." *European Journal of Cancer Care* 16 (2007): 402-412.

Slack, D., et al. "The Feasibility of Hypnotic Analgesia in Ameliorating Pain and Anxiety Among Adults Undergoing Needle Electromyography." *American Journal of Physical Medicine and Rehabilitation* 88 (2009): 21-29.

See also: Cancer treatment support; Guided imagery; Meditation; Surgery support; Transcendental Meditation; Warts.

Hypothyroidism

CATEGORY: Condition

RELATED TERMS: Hashimoto's thyroiditis, thyroid hormone, low, thyroiditis, Hashimoto's

DEFINITION: Treatment of the thyroid gland's failure to produce adequate levels of thyroid hormone.

Principal proposed natural treatments: Armour Thyroid

Other proposed natural treatments: *Bacopa monniera* (brahmi), selenium, traditional Chinese herbal medicine, vitamin B$_3$, zinc

Herbs and supplements to use only with caution: Bladderwrack, genistein, iodine, iron, isoflavones, kelp, soy

Introduction

In hypothyroidism, the thyroid gland fails to produce adequate levels of thyroid hormone. Symptoms include sluggishness, sensitivity to cold, weight gain, depression, dry skin, loss of hair, excessive menstruation, hoarseness, and goiter (a visible enlargement of the neck caused by a swollen thyroid gland).

Hashimoto's thyroiditis is the most common natural cause of low thyroid hormone levels. In this autoimmune condition, the body develops antibodies that attack and gradually destroy the thyroid. A viral infection of the thyroid can also decrease thyroid hormone production, but the effect is generally mild and temporary. Finally, iodine deficiency can cause hypothyroidism, but this seldom occurs in the developed world, where iodine is routinely added to salt.

In addition to these natural causes, there is still one more common cause of hypothyroidism: medical treatment for hyperthyroidism (excessive production of thyroid hormone). People with certain forms of hyperthyroidism receive treatment with radioactive iodine to inactivate the thyroid gland. This treatment causes hypothyroidism, which requires lifelong treatment with thyroid replacement therapy.

Until the 1990s, doctors commonly diagnosed hypothyroidism by conducting laboratory tests to measure thyroid hormone levels in the blood (the T4 level). Normal thyroid levels vary widely among people, so this method could not always correctly identify the disease. A much better lab test, which became available in the 1990s, involves measurement of a hormone called TSH, or thyroid stimulating hormone.

TSH is released by the pituitary gland to control the thyroid gland. The pituitary gland constantly measures the level of thyroid hormone in the blood and adjusts TSH levels as necessary to get it right. When thyroid hormone levels are high, it turns TSH levels down. When thyroid hormone levels are too low, the pituitary raises TSH levels to stimulate the thyroid. If the thyroid gland does not respond by raising thyroid hormone levels, the pituitary turns up the TSH levels even higher. When TSH levels are higher than normal limits, this means that the thyroid gland is having trouble producing enough thyroid hormone for the body's needs. In other words, the person has entered a hypothyroid state or is about to enter such a state. This method of determining thyroid status has proved reliable.

Medical treatment for low-thyroid conditions is safe and very effective. Treatment involves the use of a hormone called levothyroxine, or T4. The body actually uses two forms of thyroid, T4 and T3, but in most cases the body easily and automatically converts T4 to T3 in the right proportions. The drug dosage is adjusted by monitoring TSH levels. When the pituitary gland is satisfied, the dose is most likely correct.

Other Proposed Treatments

So-called natural thyroid hormone is popular in alternative medicine. Sold by prescription only under the name Armour Thyroid, this extract of pig thyroid contains both T4 and T3. There is no doubt that Armour Thyroid is as effective as standard synthetic thyroid hormone, and it is a satisfactory choice for those who prefer to use natural treatments. However, there is no evidence that Armour Thyroid is any more effective than standard medications, and there are some concerns that variations in stomach absorption may produce slightly erratic results.

One double-blind study failed to find a combination of synthetic T3 and T4 more effective than synthetic T4 as a treatment for hypothyroidism in regard to well-being, quality of life, or mental function. Another double-blind study failed to find any difference between T4 alone or T3 plus T4 in people whose thyroid had been removed because of thyroid cancer. Another study also failed to find discernible differences between the two treatments regarding mood, fatigue, well-being, or mental function; however, for reasons that are unclear, persons given T3 plus T4 were significantly more likely to prefer the new treatment to their previous care than those who were continued on T4. Unless this was merely a statistical accident, people who received the combined treatment were apparently able to detect some subtle benefit that they could not quite understand.

Other than Armour Thyroid, there are no natural therapies with documented efficacy for the treatment of hypothyroidism. Treatments that are sometimes

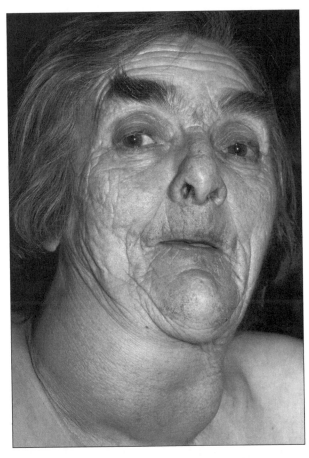

Woman suffering from hypothyroidism. (Dr. P. Marazzi/ Photo Researchers, Inc.)

recommended but lack any meaningful scientific support include *Bacopa monniera* (brahmi), selenium, traditional Chinese herbal medicine, vitamin B_3, and zinc.

Far too frequently, people with low thyroid levels consume seaweed or iodine supplements in hopes that these supplements will help. However, while iodine deficiency does cause low thyroid levels, taking iodine will not help if one is not deficient in it. (The vast majority of people living in the developed world have plenty of iodine.) Excessive iodine intake can occasionally cause hypothyroidism.

Theory of widespread marginal hypothyroidism. There is little doubt that many cases of marginal hypothyroidism go unidentified, and that occasional tests for thyroid adequacy should be part of routine medical care. However, some proponents of alternative medicine go further and suggest that undiagnosed hypothyroidism is a serious epidemic, causing a high percentage of all the illnesses afflicting modern humans. (One of the best-known books on this theory is *Solved: The Riddle of Illness* by Stephen E. Langer and James F. Scheer, which was published in 1984.) Supposedly, laboratory tests for thyroid hormone levels are not reliable, and many people have marginally low thyroid levels despite normal lab readings.

These thyroid enthusiasts recommend that people use measurements of basal body temperature and not blood tests to determine whether thyroid levels are adequate. Basal body temperature is measured by placing a thermometer under the armpit before arising in the morning. According to proponents of the marginal hypothyroidism theory, a measurement of lower than about 97.5° Fahrenheit indicates a problem. People with basal body temperature readings below this level and symptoms consistent with hypothyroidism are advised to use Armour Thyroid (or various other animal-source thyroid gland supplements that can be obtained with a bit of work). The net result is supposed to be a great improvement in overall health and the resolution of many illnesses.

However, there are a number of problems with this theory. One is that the majority of women have basal body temperature readings below 97.5° Fahrenheit in the time before ovulation, a fact used in the symptothermal method of natural family planning. Many healthy men have normal basal body temperatures below 97.5° Fahrenheit too. Because symptoms consistent with hypothyroidism (such as fatigue, depression, and weight gain) occur in many people, this approach is guaranteed to recommend that enormous numbers of people take thyroid supplements.

Furthermore, the basal body temperature method was developed in the days before TSH levels could be measured, a time in which doctors could measure T4 levels only; there is too great a variation in the normal level of T4 for such tests to have been reliable. However, now that the TSH test has become available, the situation has changed. TSH measurements indicate the body's own determination of its thyroid hormone level. It is difficult to justify ignoring the body's own "opinion" in favor of an arbitrary reading on a thermometer. Indeed, when people with normal TSH levels are given thyroid medication, the body responds by lowering its own production of thyroid hormone, essentially fighting this supposedly natural therapy.

Nonetheless, the enthusiasm for thyroid medication continues unabated, and some alternative medicine physicians continue to maintain that thyroid hormone supplementation is useful even in the presence of a normal TSH test. In 2001, a double-blind, placebo-controlled, crossover trial attempted to evaluate the validity of this theory. Researchers enrolled twenty-two people with symptoms consistent with hypothyroidism but with normal TSH measurements, and nineteen healthy people. About one-half of each group was given standard synthetic thyroid hormone (thyroxine 100 micrograms [this is T4]) for twelve weeks and placebo for another twelve weeks; the other half received placebo for the first period and thyroid hormone for the second. Improvement was measured through questionnaires evaluating general health, emotional well-being, and mental function.

The results showed that participants with symptoms of low thyroid hormone improved significantly. However, those taking placebo improved just as much. In other words, thyroid hormone proved no more effective than placebo. (The healthy participants showed little response to either placebo or thyroid hormone.)

This study indicates that synthetic human thyroid hormone supplementation (T4) is not helpful for people who have normal TSH but have symptoms that are reminiscent of low thyroid hormone. It did not evaluate the effectiveness of the animal-source thyroid recommended by proponents of the hypothyroid theory and, therefore, does not entirely settle the controversy.

HERBS AND SUPPLEMENTS TO USE WITH CAUTION

Supplementation with iodine will not help the thyroid gland except in people who are iodine-deficient. In Japan, the excessive use of seaweed (such as kelp or bladderwrack) is a fairly common cause of hypothyroidism. For this reason, people with low thyroid hormone levels should not consume excessive amounts of these iodine-rich foods.

Soy and its isoflavones (such as genistein) appear to have numerous potential effects involving the thyroid gland. When given to people with impaired thyroid function, soy products have been observed to reduce absorption of thyroid medication. In addition, some evidence hints that soy isoflavones may directly inhibit the function of the thyroid gland, although this inhibition may be significant only in people who are deficient in iodine. However, to make matters more confusing, studies of healthy humans and animals given soy isoflavones or other soy products have generally found that soy either had no effect on thyroid hormone levels or actually increased levels. In view of soy's complex effects regarding the thyroid, people with impaired thyroid function should not take large amounts of soy products except under the supervision of a physician. Iron supplements may also interfere with thyroid hormone absorption.

EBSCO CAM Review Board

FURTHER READING

Bell, D. S., and F. Ovalle. "Use of Soy Protein Supplement and Resultant Need for Increased Dose of Levothyroxine." *Endocrine Practice* 7 (2001): 193-194.

Persky, V. W., et al. "Effect of Soy Protein on Endogenous Hormones in Postmenopausal Women." *American Journal of Clinical Nutrition* 75 (2002): 145-153.

Pollock, M. A., et al. "Thyroxine Treatment in Patients with Symptoms of Hypothyroidism but Thyroid Function Tests Within the Reference Range." *British Medical Journal* 323 (2001): 891-895.

Regalbuto, C., et al. "Effects of Either LT4 Monotherapy or LT4/LT3 Combined Therapy in Patients Totally Thyroidectomized for Thyroid Cancer." *Thyroid* 17 (2007): 323-331.

Walsh, J. P., et al. "Combined Thyroxine/Liothyronine Treatment Does Not Improve Well-Being, Quality of Life, or Cognitive Function Compared to Thyroxine Alone." *Journal of Clinical Endocrinology and Metabolism* 88 (2003): 4543-4550.

See also: Depression, mild to moderate; Fatigue; Hyperthyroidism; Obesity and excess weight; Thyroid hormone.

Hyssop

CATEGORY: Herbs and supplements
RELATED TERM: *Hyssop officinalis*
DEFINITION: Natural plant product used to treat specific health conditions.
PRINCIPAL PROPOSED USES: None
OTHER PROPOSED USES: Asthma, common cold, cough, sore throat

OVERVIEW

The herb hyssop (*Hyssop officinalis*) has a long history of use in both religion and medicine. The biblical phrase "purge me with Hyssop, and I shall be clean" echoes the ancient Greek use of this herb for cleansing sacred sites. Various preparations of hyssop have been used medicinally for respiratory problems, including cough, chest congestion, sore throat, and bronchitis. Hyssop has also been used to treat a variety of digestive problems, including stomach pain and intestinal gas. The fragrant essential oil of hyssop is an ingredient in the liqueur Chartreuse.

THERAPEUTIC DOSAGES

A typical dose of hyssop essential oil is 1 to 2 drops daily. Hyssop tea is made by steeping 2 to 3 teaspoons of herb in a cup of hot water and may be taken two to three times daily for sore throat.

THERAPEUTIC USES

The essential oil of hyssop is still recommended by herbalists today for treatment of respiratory and digestive problems, such as the common cold, asthma, acute bronchitis and cough, stomach upset, and intestinal gas. Hyssop tea is recommended as a gargle for sore throat. However, there is no meaningful evidence that it is effective for any of these purposes.

Preliminary evidence, too weak to rely upon, hints that extracts of hyssop might have anti-HIV (human immunodeficiency virus) activity. Other preliminary evidence weakly suggests that constituents in hyssop might reduce absorption of carbohydrates from the digestive tract. This has led to statements that hyssop is helpful for treating diabetes and aiding weight loss, but in reality the evidence is far too weak to draw any such conclusion.

SAFETY ISSUES

Hyssop has undergone no more than minimal evaluation for safety. Hyssop tea is thought to be relatively benign, but hyssop essential oil, like most essential oils, is toxic in excessive doses. Some of its constituents might increase risk of seizures. For this reason, hyssop essential oil should not be used by people with epilepsy. It should also not be used by young children, pregnant or nursing women, or people with severe liver or kidney disease.

EBSCO CAM Review Board

FURTHER READING

Hold, K. M., et al. "Metabolism and Mode of Action of Cis- and Trans-3-Pinanones (The Active Ingredients of Hyssop Oil)." *Xenobiotica* 32 (2002): 251-265.

Matsuura, H., et al. "Isolation of Alpha-Glusosidase Inhibitors from Hyssop (*Hyssopus officinalis*)." *Phytochemistry* 65 (2003): 91-97.

Miyazaki, H., et al. "Inhibitory Effects of Hyssop (*Hyssopus officinalis*) Extracts on Intestinal Alpha-Glucosidase Activity and Postprandial Hyperglycemia." *Journal of Nutritional Science and Vitaminology* 49 (2004): 346-349.

See also: Asthma; Common cold: Homeopathic remedies; Colds and flu; Cough; Herbal medicine.

I

Immune support

CATEGORY: Therapies and techniques

RELATED TERMS: Frequent infections, immunity boosting, immunomodulation, weak immunity

DEFINITION: Therapies to increase the effectiveness of the immune system in fighting infection.

OVERVIEW

The body must contend with constant attacks by microscopic organisms. To defend itself, it has a wide range of defenses that together are called the immune system.

Persons with diseases that cause immune deficiency, such as acquired immunodeficiency syndrome (AIDS), are harmed by infectious microorganisms that a healthy person could ward off easily. However, even healthy people get sick from time to time, as infectious agents manage to sneak by the defenses. Also, some apparently healthy people nonetheless get sick quite often. Any explanation of why it is so difficult to improve resistance to illness should include a discussion of the nature of immunity.

The immune system. The immune system consists primarily of various types of white blood cells and the chemicals that they manufacture (such as antibodies). In certain conditions, such as AIDS, many of these white blood cells are damaged or dead. In such cases, the term "immune deficiency" is clearly appropriate. The circumstance is analogous to an army that lacks, say, weaponry.

However, careful examination of most people who frequently get colds (or bladder infections or herpes attacks, for example) fails to turn up any visible deficits in the immune system. They have all the immune cells and antibodies they need in roughly the right amounts, and all the various parts appear to work just fine. It is not known why some people get sick so often.

One can hypothesize that in some people the immune system fails to function properly for a relatively subtle, invisible reason, much as a well-equipped army might lose its fighting form because of apathy or disunity. However, even people who develop frequent colds manage to fight off thousands of other infections every day.

For this reason, an alternative hypothesis comes to mind: that over-susceptibility to a particular type of infection may be caused by something more specific than general immune weakness. As an example, chronically inflamed mucous membranes might lead to frequent colds, because an inflamed mucous membrane may be more porous to cold viruses. Similarly, a woman's bladder wall might allow particularly easy attachment of bacteria, leading to frequent bladder infections. In reality, though, these are all speculations. It is not known why some people frequently develop minor infections. For this reason, it is very difficult to find a way to fix the problem.

Immunomodulation. Many natural products are said to boost general immunity. However, while science can study the effect of a single treatment on a single illness, it is not known how a treatment strengthens the immune system in general. Scientists can measure the effects of an herb on individual white blood cell types and note changes in activity, but they do not know how to interpret the results of those measurements as a whole. After all, the immune system is a system, and systems are notoriously complicated to analyze. Current knowledge does not allow science to predict the ultimate effect of fine changes in the system's parts.

To acknowledge this limitation, scientists tend to use the term "immunomodulatory" rather than "immune-stimulating" when they refer to a substance that causes measurable alterations in immune function. This terminology notes a change (modulation) but does not assume the change is good, bad, or indifferent.

Hundreds or thousands of herbs have immunomodulatory effects. In many cases, these may represent nothing more than the body's reaction to the herb as a foreign presence–an immune reaction to the herb itself, in other words, with no special benefits.

Zinc and Immune Function

Severe zinc deficiency depresses immune function, and even mild to moderate degrees of zinc deficiency can impair macrophage and neutrophil functions, natural-killer-cell activity, and complement activity. The body requires zinc to develop and activate T-lymphocytes. Persons with low zinc levels have shown reduced lymphocyte proliferation response to mitogens and other adverse alterations in immunity that can be corrected by zinc supplementation.

Zinc toxicity can occur in both acute and chronic forms. Acute adverse effects of high zinc intake include nausea, vomiting, loss of appetite, abdominal cramps, diarrhea, and headaches. One case report cited severe nausea and vomiting within thirty minutes of ingesting 4 grams of zinc gluconate (570 milligrams [mg] elemental zinc). Intakes of 150 to 450 mg of zinc per day have been associated with such chronic effects as low copper status, altered iron function, reduced immune function, and reduced levels of high-density lipoproteins.

In some cases, observed immunomodulatory effects could indicate an alteration in immune function with potential benefits under certain conditions, but it is impossible to know.

Theoretically, it is possible that some natural substance could boost all aspects of immunity. However, if it did, it would be a highly dangerous substance. The immune system is finely balanced. An immune system that is too relaxed fails to defend against infections; an immune system that is too active attacks healthy tissues, causing autoimmune diseases (such as AIDS). A universal immune booster might cause lupus, Crohn's disease, asthma, Graves' disease, Hashimoto's thyroiditis, multiple sclerosis, or rheumatoid arthritis, among other problems.

Rather than preferring an immune booster, one might rather prefer a treatment that somehow fine-tunes the immune system. It is not known, however, if such a treatment exists.

NATURAL MEDICINE

Herbs and supplements. There is no doubt that good general nutrition is necessary for strong immunity. However, excessive intake of some nutrients (zinc, for example) may weaken immunity. Still, there is some specific scientific evidence that multivitamin/multimineral supplements may help certain people stay well. A number of herbs and supplements have shown promise for preventing or treating certain specific infections, including bladder infection, colds and flus, diarrhea, fungal infection, herpes infection, middle ear infection, and vaginal yeast infection.

Immunizations are widely used to strengthen the immune response to specific illnesses, such as influenza. However, some people (especially the elderly) may not respond adequately to immunizations. Certain natural products, such as ginseng, vitamin E, and multivitamin/multimineral supplements, may enhance the immune response.

Echinacea is widely claimed to be an immune-strengthening herb, but evidence suggests that its regular use does not help prevent colds or other infections. Echinacea may, however, help colds that have already begun.

The fungi products *Coriolus versicolor*, active hexose correlated compound, maitake, reishi, and shiitake are widely believed by the Japanese to help support the immune system during cancer treatment. However, there is no reliable evidence to indicate that they are effective for this purpose.

Substances that enhance the growth of friendly bacteria in the large intestine have been studied for their favorable effects on the immune system, with mixed results. Probiotics (such as acidophilus) consist of various bacterial species capable of rebalancing the healthy population of bacteria in the gut. Certain types of starches, called prebiotics, are not fully digested and, therefore, remain in the intestine and feed healthy bacteria. There is some evidence that probiotics and, to a lesser extent, prebiotics may lead to a reduction in allergic symptoms and possibly minor infections, especially in children.

Lifestyle issues. There is little doubt that if one lives a healthy lifestyle with good nutrition and plenty of exercise, one will approach more closely a state of optimum health. However, the key to this health is moderation. Too much exercise (as in marathon running) can weaken the immune system, leading to infections. (Heavy endurance exercise can benefit from the use of vitamin C, beta-sitosterol, and glutamine to prevent the "post-marathon sniffle.")

Although it is commonly said that high levels of sugar intake weaken immunity, there is no meaningful evidence to support this view. Similarly, while severe alcohol abuse clearly damages immune function, there is no evidence that moderate alcohol consumption increases the risk of infection.

Some persons believe that getting cold causes colds, but this claim has not been proven. There is also no reliable evidence that reducing intake of dairy products will prevent respiratory infections. Finally, contrary to popular belief, early antibiotic treatment of children with ear infections does not seem to damage the child's immunity and thereby cause a greater rate of ear infections.

Alternative therapies. Various alternative therapies are said to be able to enhance overall health and thereby prevent illness in general. These include methods such as acupuncture, Ayurveda, chiropractic spinal manipulation, naturopathy, Reiki, Tai Chi, therapeutic touch, traditional Chinese herbal medicine, and yoga. However, there is little to no meaningful scientific evidence to indicate that these methods have any specific positive effect on immunity.

EBSCO CAM Review Board

FURTHER READING

Grimm, W., and H. Muller. "A Randomized Controlled Trial of the Effect of Fluid Extract of *Echinacea purpurea* on the Incidence and Severity of Colds and Respiratory Infections." *American Journal of Medicine* 106 (1999): 138-143.

Jiang, M. H., L. Zhu, and J. G. Jiang. "Immunoregulatory Actions of Polysaccharides from Chinese Herbal Medicine." *Expert Opinion on Therapeutic Targets* 14 (2010): 1367-1402.

Majdalawieh, A. F., and R. I. Carr. "In Vitro Investigation of the Potential Immunomodulatory and Anti-Cancer Activities of Black Pepper (*Piper nigrum*) and Cardamom (*Elettaria cardamomum*)." *Journal of Medicinal Food* 13 (2010): 371-381.

Senchina, D. S., et al. "Herbal Supplements and Athlete Immune Function–What's Proven, Disproven, and Unproven?" *Exercise Immunology Review* 15 (2009): 66-106.

Turner, R. B., D. K. Riker, and J. D. Gangemi. "Ineffectiveness of Echinacea for Prevention of Experimental Rhinovirus Colds." *Antimicrobial Agents and Chemotherapy* 44 (2000): 1708-1709.

Vonau, B., et al. "Does the Extract of the Plant *Echinacea purpurea* Influence the Clinical Course of Recurrent Genital Herpes?" *International Journal of STD and AIDS* 12 (2001): 154-158.

See also: Allergies; Fructo-oligosaccharides; Herbal medicine; HIV support: Homeopathic remedies; Probiotics; Sublingual immunotherapy.

Indigo

RELATED TERMS: *Indigofera oblongifolia, I. tinctoria*
CATEGORY: Herbs and supplements
DEFINITION: Natural plant product used to treat specific health conditions.
PRINCIPAL PROPOSED USES: None
OTHER PROPOSED USES: Antiseptic, liver protection

OVERVIEW

The leaflets and branches of the indigo plant yield an exquisite blue dye; people around the globe have used it to color textiles and clothing for centuries. Before the development of synthetic blue dyes, indigo was cultivated for this pigment rather than for medicinal use.

In the traditional medicine of India and China, indigo was used in the treatment of conditions now known as epilepsy, bronchitis, liver disease, and psychiatric illness. However, there is no real scientific evidence for any of these uses.

THERAPEUTIC DOSAGES

No standard dosage of indigo has been established.

THERAPEUTIC USES

Based on its traditional use for liver problems, researchers have investigated whether indigo might protect the liver against chemically induced injury. Animal studies do suggest that extracts of the indigo species *Indigofera tinctoria* protect the liver from damage by toxic chemicals. No human trials, however, have been performed to examine indigo's effects on the liver.

The species *I. oblongifolia* has been tested for its antibacterial and antifungal activity. In a test-tube trial, this plant showed significant activity against certain types of bacteria and fungi. This research is still in its preliminary stages, so it is too early to tell whether *I. oblongifolia* will prove useful for the treatment of any infectious diseases.

A different plant called wild indigo (*Baptisia tinctoria*), in combination with echinacea and white cedar, has been studied as a possible immune stimulant. However, wild indigo is not part of the *Indigofera* family of plants and is not discussed here.

SAFETY ISSUES

The indigo species *I. tinctoria* has a history of use in traditional medical systems, and it is regarded by herbalists as safe; occasional allergic reactions have been reported. However, comprehensive safety tests have not been performed. For this reason, indigo should not be used by pregnant or nursing women, young children, or persons with severe liver or kidney disease. Safety in other persons is unknown.

The species *I. spicata* (formerly *I. endecaphylla*), however, is poisonous: It has killed cattle and other animals and has caused birth defects in rats. Other indigo species have also been found to be lethal. For this reason, it is important to avoid ingesting indigo internally unless one is certain that it has been harvested and processed expertly and reliably.

Reviewed by EBSCO CAM Review Board

FURTHER READING

Dahot, M. U. "Antibacterial and Antifungal Activity of Small Protein of *Indigofera oblongifolia* Leaves." *Journal of Ethnopharmacology* 64 (1999): 277-282.

Wustenberg, P., et al. "Efficacy and Mode of Action of an Immunomodulator Herbal Preparation Containing Echinacea, Wild Indigo, and White Cedar." *Advances in Therapy* 16 (1999): 51-70.

See also: Herbal medicine; Liver disease; Traditional healing.

Indole-3-carbinol

CATEGORY: Herbs and supplements
RELATED TERM: I3C
DEFINITION: Natural substance promoted as a dietary supplement for specific health benefits.
PRINCIPAL PROPOSED USE: Cancer prevention
OTHER PROPOSED USES: Liver protection, respiratory papillomatosis

OVERVIEW

Indole-3-carbinol (I3C), a chemical found in vegetables of the broccoli family, is thought to possess properties against cancer and appears to work in several ways, including the following: facilitating the conversion of estrogen to a less cancer-promoting form; partially blocking the effects of estrogen on cells; directly killing or inhibiting cancer cells; and reducing levels of free radicals, which can promote cancer by damaging deoxyribonucleic acid (DNA).

SOURCES

I3C is found in cruciferous vegetables (*Brassica* plants), such as cabbage, broccoli, Brussels sprouts, cauliflower, kale, kohlrabi, and turnips. A typical Japanese diet provides the equivalent of about 112 milligrams (mg) of I3C daily; intake in Western diets is lower.

THERAPEUTIC DOSAGES

A four-week, double-blind, placebo-controlled trial of fifty-seven women found that a minimum dose of 300 mg of I3C daily may be necessary to reduce the risk of estrogen-promoted cancers. Another study found benefits with 400 mg of I3C per day. However, until the overall effects of I3C are better understood, it is recommend that one obtain this substance through the consumption of broccoli family vegetables rather than by taking it as a supplement.

THERAPEUTIC USES

I3C is being studied as a chemopreventive agent, that is, a substance that helps prevent cancer. Numerous animal studies suggest that I3C might help reduce the risk of estrogen-sensitive cancers and other types of cancer. One double-blind, placebo-controlled study in humans suggests that it can help reverse cervical dysplasia, a precancerous condition. Weaker evidence hints at benefits for vulvar intraepithelial neoplasia, a precancerous condition of the vulva. (Note that one should not attempt to treat cervical dysplasia, or any other precancerous or cancerous condition, without physician supervision.)

Some evidence indicates that I3C might also help prevent recurrences of a rare condition called respiratory papillomatosis. This disease involves benign tumors in the lungs, mouth, and vocal chords. I3C has additionally been investigated as a liver protectant.

Further evidence suggests that I3C must be exposed to stomach acid to exert its full effects. For this reason, persons with low stomach acid, such as those taking H_2 blockers (such as ranitidine, or Zantac) or proton pump inhibitors (such as omeprazole, or Prilosec), may not benefit as much from I3C.

SCIENTIFIC EVIDENCE

A twelve-week, placebo-controlled trial of thirty women with stage 2 or 3 cervical dysplasia found that treatment with I3C at a daily dose of 200 or 400 mg significantly improved the rate at which the cervix spontaneously returned to normal.

SAFETY ISSUES

Studies in rats, chickens, guinea pigs, mice, and dogs suggest that I3C is safe at recommended doses. Human trials have found no significant side effects with I3C. However, one study in rats found increased abnormalities in male offspring, specifically related to their fertility. For this reason, I3C supplements should not be used by pregnant women.

There are other concerns with I3C too. For example, despite its overall anticancer effects, there is some evidence that I3C has tumor-promoting properties under certain circumstances. For this reason, the long-term use of concentrated I3C supplements may not be safe. In addition, persons who have already had cancer should not use I3C (or any other supplement) except under physician supervision.

In addition, because it facilitates the inactivation of estrogen, it is possible that I3C might tend to promote osteoporosis in postmenopausal women and could interfere with estrogen therapies (such as birth control pills and hormone replacement therapy). However, this concern is purely theoretical.

IMPORTANT INTERACTIONS

Persons who are taking any medication that contains estrogen (including birth control pills) should be aware that I3C might interfere with the action of this type of medication.

EBSCO CAM Review Board

FURTHER READING

Auborn, K. J. "Therapy for Recurrent Respiratory Papillomatosis." *Antiviral Therapy* 7 (2002): 1-9.

Broadbent, T. A., and H. S. Broadbent. "The Chemistry and Pharmacology of Indole-3-Carbinol (Indole-3-Methanol) and 3-(Methoxymethyl)Indole." *Current Medicinal Chemistry* 5 (1998): 469-491.

Hong, C., G. L. Firestone, and L. F. Bjeldanes. "Bcl-2 Family-Mediated Apoptotic Effects of 3,3'-Diindolyl-

methane (DIM) in Human Breast Cancer Cells." *Biochemical Pharmacology* 63 (2002): 1085-1097.

Naik, R., et al. "A Randomized Phase II Trial of Indole-3-Carbinol in the Treatment of Vulvar Intraepithelial Neoplasia." *International Journal of Gynecological Cancer* 16 (2006): 786-790.

See also: Cancer risk reduction; Cervical dysplasia; Diindolylmethane; Estrogen; Women's health.

Infertility, female

CATEGORY: Condition

DEFINITION: Treatment of the inability of a woman (or a girl) to become pregnant.

PRINCIPAL PROPOSED NATURAL TREATMENTS: None

OTHER PROPOSED NATURAL TREATMENTS: Acupuncture, ashwagandha, bee propolis, beta-carotene, black cohosh, calcium, chasteberry, false unicorn, maca, multivitamins, N-acetylcysteine, reducing stress, traditional Chinese herbal medicine, vitamin C, vitamin D

INTRODUCTION

There are many possible causes of female infertility. Tubal disease and endometriosis (a condition in which uterine tissue begins to grow where it should not) account for 50 percent of female infertility; failure of ovulation is the cause of about 30 percent; and cervical factors cause another 10 percent.

An immense industry has sprung up around correcting female infertility, using techniques that range from hormone therapy to in vitro (test-tube) babies. Although these methods have their occasional stunning successes, there is considerable controversy about the high cost and low rate of effectiveness of fertility treatments in general. The good news is that apparently infertile women often become pregnant eventually with no medical intervention.

PROPOSED NATURAL TREATMENTS

Women with a condition known as polycystic ovary syndrome (PCOS) may be infertile. A double-blind, placebo-controlled study evaluated the effectiveness of N-acetylcysteine (NAC) in 150 women with PCOS who had previously failed to respond to the fertility drug clomiphene, a commonly used medication to induce ovulation. Participants were given clomiphene

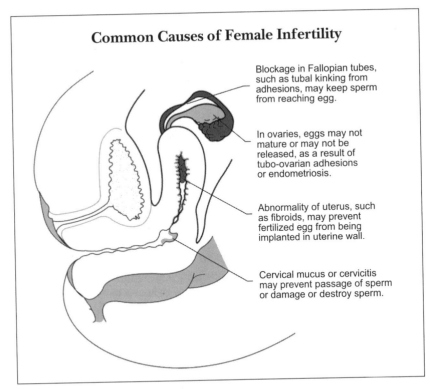

Common Causes of Female Infertility

Blockage in Fallopian tubes, such as tubal kinking from adhesions, may keep sperm from reaching egg.

In ovaries, eggs may not mature or may not be released, as a result of tubo-ovarian adhesions or endometriosis.

Abnormality of uterus, such as fibroids, may prevent fertilized egg from being implanted in uterine wall.

Cervical mucus or cervicitis may prevent passage of sperm or damage or destroy sperm.

plus placebo or clomiphene plus 1.2 grams daily of NAC. The results indicated that combined treatment with NAC plus clomiphene was markedly more effective than clomiphene taken with placebo. Almost 50 percent of the women in the combined treatment group ovulated compared to about 1 percent in the clomiphene-alone group. The pregnancy rate in the combined treatment group was 21 percent, compared to 0 percent in the clomiphene-alone group.

Black cohosh (*Cimicifuga racemosa*), an herb with estrogen-like effects, drew the attention of researchers who were interested in whether it might be helpful for women with unexplained infertility who were also being treated with clomiphene but had yet to conceive. Roughly 120 women were randomly divided into two groups. Both groups continued to receive clomiphene, but the women in one of the groups also received 120 milligrams (mg) of black cohosh. Pregnancy rates were significantly higher in the black cohosh plus clomiphene group compared to the clomiphene-only group.

In a small, double-blind, placebo-controlled trial, the use of bee propolis at a dose of 500 mg twice daily resulted in a pregnancy rate of 60 percent, compared to 20 percent in the placebo group. This difference was statistically significant.

Because of its effects on the hormone prolactin, the herb chasteberry has been tried as a fertility treatment. However, the only properly designed study of this potential use was too small to return conclusive results. A larger study evaluated a combination containing chasteberry, green tea, arginine, and multiple vitamins and minerals. In this double-blind study, ninety-three women experiencing infertility were given either the combination treatment or the placebo for three months. After three months, 26 percent of the women given the real treatment were pregnant compared to 10 percent of those in the placebo group, a difference that was statistically significant.

Weak evidence hints that vitamin D and calcium may also be helpful for infertility. Another small study found some evidence that supplements containing isoflavones may increase the effectiveness of in vitro fertilization (IVF). Another study reported that vitamin C supplements slightly improved pregnancy rates in women with a condition called luteal phase defect, but because researchers failed to give the control group a placebo and instead merely left them untreated, the results are not meaningful. Another study that had severe defects in design reported that multivitamin supplements may slightly increase fertility. Stress may lead to infertility, and treatments for reducing stress might help increase fertility. The herb maca (*Lepidium meyenii*) is widely advocated as a fertility-enhancing herb. However, the only basis for this claim are a few animal studies.

Caffeine avoidance has also been recommended for improving fertility, but there is no evidence that it helps. Acupuncture has a long history of traditional use for infertility, but the supporting evidence for its use is weak. A few open trials appeared to show that acupuncture can enhance the success rate of IVF. Two better-designed studies, however, failed to find acupuncture more effective than placebo. A 2008 analysis of seven randomized trials, involving a total of 1,366 women, found that, on balance, acupuncture may significantly improve the odds of pregnancy in

Chasteberry for Female Infertility

Chasteberry is the fruit of the chaste tree (*Vitex agnus-castus*), a small shrub-like tree native to Central Asia and the Mediterranean region. The name is thought to come from a belief that the plant promoted chastity. Common names for chasteberry include chaste-tree berry, vitex, and monk's pepper.

Chasteberry has been used for thousands of years, mostly by women to ease menstrual problems and to stimulate the production of breast milk. Chasteberry is still used for menstrual problems, such as premenstrual syndrome, and for symptoms of menopause, for some types of infertility, and for acne.

Certain hormone levels may be affected by chasteberry. Women who are pregnant, who are taking birth control pills, or who have a hormone-sensitive condition (such as breast cancer) should not use chasteberry.

women undergoing IVF. However, because not all seven studies used sham (fake) acupuncture as a control, the reliability of this conclusion is questionable. Moreover, a second analysis in the same year of thirteen randomized-control trials investigating the effectiveness of acupuncture in 2,500 women undergoing a specialized IVF procedure, in which sperm is injected directly into the egg, found no evidence of any benefit. In a subsequent review of thirteen trials, a different group of researchers concluded that acupuncture may improve the success rate of IVF, but only if it is used on the day of embryo transfer (when the fertilized egg is placed into the womb). According to this study, acupuncture is not effective when used up to three days after embryo transfer or when eggs are being retrieved from the ovaries.

Traditional Chinese herbal medicine also has a long history of use for infertility, but there is no meaningful evidence to indicate that it is effective. One case report has linked the use of a Chinese herbal product with reversible ovarian failure. Other treatments sometimes recommended for female infertility include ashwagandha, false unicorn, and beta-carotene, but there is no evidence that these treatments work.

EBSCO CAM Review Board

FURTHER READING

Ali, A. F. M., and A. Awadallah. "Bee Propolis Versus Placebo in the Treatment of Infertitily Associated with Minimal or Mild Endometriosis." *Fertility and Sterility* 80, suppl. 3 (2003): S32.

Domar, A. D., et al. "The Impact of Acupuncture on In Vitro Fertilization Outcome." *Fertility and Sterility* 91 (2009): 723-726.

El-Toukhy, T., et al. "A Systematic Review and Meta-analysis of Acupuncture in In Vitro Fertilisation." *BJOG: An International Journal of Obstetrics and Gynaecology* 115 (2008): 1203-1213.

Manheimer, E., et al. "Effects of Acupuncture on Rates of Pregnancy and Live Birth Among Women Undergoing In Vitro Fertilisation." *British Medical Journal* 336 (2008): 545-549.

Shahin, A. Y., et al. "Adding Phytoestrogens to Clomiphene Induction in Unexplained Infertility Patients." *Reproductive Biomedicine Online* 16 (2008): 580-588.

Unfer, V., et al. "Phytoestrogens May Improve the Pregnancy Rate in In Vitro Fertilization-Embryo Transfer Cycles." *Fertility and Sterility* 82 (2004): 1509-1513.

Westergaard, L. G., et al. "Acupuncture on the Day of Embryo Transfer Significantly Improves the Reproductive Outcome in Infertile Women." *Fertility and Sterility* 85 (2006): 1341-1346.

Westphal, L. M., M. L. Polan, and A. S. Trant. "Double-Blind, Placebo-Controlled Study of Fertilityblend: A Nutritional Supplement for Improving Fertility in Women." *Clinical and Experimental Obstetrics and Gynecology* 33 (2006): 205-208.

See also: Cervical dysplasia; Endometriosis; Estrogen; Infertility, male; Menopause; Pregnancy support; Sexual dysfunction in women; Women's health.

Infertility, male

CATEGORY: Condition

RELATED TERM: Sperm motility

DEFINITION: Treatment of a man's inability to impregnate a woman.

PRINCIPAL PROPOSED NATURAL TREATMENTS: None

OTHER PROPOSED NATURAL TREATMENTS: Antioxidants, astaxanthin, carnitine, coenzyme Q_{10}, lycopene, maca (*Lepidium meyenii*), *Panax ginseng*, selenium, vitamin B_{12}, vitamin C, vitamin E, zinc plus folate

HERBS AND SUPPLEMENTS TO USE ONLY WITH CAUTION: Andrographis, licorice, melatonin, soy, stevia

INTRODUCTION

Male infertility, the inability of a man to produce a pregnancy in a woman, is often caused by measurable deficits in sperm function or sperm count. In about one-half of all cases, however, the source of the problem is never discovered.

Without any treatment, about 25 percent of reportedly infertile men help bring about a pregnancy within one year of the time they first visit a physician for treatment. In other words, infertility is often only low fertility.

PROPOSED NATURAL TREATMENTS

Carnitine. Growing, if not entirely consistent, evidence suggests that various forms of the supplement L-carnitine may improve sperm function and thereby provide benefit in male infertility. In one double-blind study, sixty men with abnormal sperm function were given either carnitine (as L-carnitine at 2 grams [g] per day and as acetyl-L-carnitine at 1 g per day) or placebo for six months. The results showed significant improvement in sperm function in the treated group compared with the placebo group.

A six-month, double-blind, placebo-controlled study of similar size, which involved men with low sperm counts, found benefits with carnitine taken alone or as carnitine combined with the anti-inflammatory drug cinnoxicam. In addition, a two-month, double-blind, placebo-controlled, crossover study of one hundred men with various forms of infertility found probable benefits with 2 g daily of L-carnitine.

Zinc plus folate. A twenty-six-week, double-blind, placebo-controlled trial compared the effects of treatment with zinc (66 milligrams (mg) of zinc sulfate, supplying 15 mg of zinc), folate (5 mg), and zinc plus folate with placebo. A total of 108 fertile men and 103 men with impaired fertility (subfertile men) participated in the study. The two supplements combined significantly improved the sperm count and the percentage of healthy sperm in the subfertile men; neither supplement alone produced this effect, and there was little effect of the combined therapy on fertile men. Another study also found potential benefit with zinc plus folate.

Vitamin B_{12}. Mild vitamin B_{12} deficiencies are relatively common in people over the age of sixty years. Such deficiencies lead to reduced sperm counts and

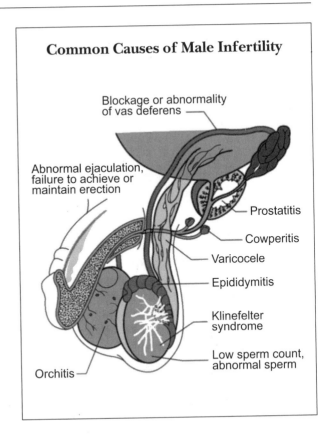

Common Causes of Male Infertility

Blockage or abnormality of vas deferens

Abnormal ejaculation, failure to achieve or maintain erection

Prostatitis

Cowperitis

Varicocele

Epididymitis

Klinefelter syndrome

Low sperm count, abnormal sperm

Orchitis

lowered sperm mobility. Thus, vitamin B_{12} supplementation has been tried for improving fertility in men with abnormal sperm production.

In one double-blind study of 375 infertile men, supplementation with vitamin B_{12} produced no benefits on average in the group as a whole. However, in a particular subgroup of men with sufficiently low sperm count and sperm motility, vitamin B_{12} appeared to be helpful. Such "dredging" of the data is suspect from a scientific point of view, however, and this study cannot be taken as proof of effectiveness.

Antioxidants. Free radicals, dangerous chemicals found naturally in the body, may damage sperm. For this reason, a number of studies have evaluated the benefits of antioxidants for male infertility.

In a double-blind, placebo-controlled study of 110 men whose sperm showed subnormal activity, daily treatment with 100 international units of vitamin E resulted in improved sperm activity and increased rate of pregnancy in their partners. Preliminary studies suggest that vitamin C may improve sperm count and function. However, a late double-blind study of thirty-one persons that tested both vitamin C and vitamin E found no benefit. The dosages studied ranged from 200 to 1,000 mg daily.

According to one small double-blind study, the antioxidant carotenoid astaxanthin might enhance male fertility. Other antioxidants that have shown some promise include lycopene, coenzyme Q_{10}, and selenium.

A major pharmaceutical company tested a miscellaneous mixture of antioxidants and reported success for male infertility. However, there is no reason to believe that either the components of this product or their exact proportions were chosen with any particular insight; any such insight regarding the optimum formulation does not exist.

Other herbs and supplements. Preliminary evidence suggests improvements in sperm function or pregnancy rates with the use of the herb *Panax ginseng.* Also, the herb *Lepidium meyenii* (maca) is claimed to enhance fertility, but the supporting evidence is limited to animal studies and one small uncontrolled study in humans conducted by a single research group. Contrary to what is stated on numerous Web sites, maca does not appear to raise testosterone levels.

In a double-blind trial of twenty-eight men with impaired sperm activity, the use of docosahexaenoic acid, a component of fish oil, failed to improve sperm health. Another double-blind study failed to find L-arginine effective for improving pregnancy rates. One very small study failed to find magnesium helpful for infertility.

Many other substances have been suggested as treatments for poor sperm function and infertility, including the herbs ashwagandha, *Eleutherococcus*, pygeum, saw palmetto, and suma, and the supplements S-adenosylmethionine and calcium, but there is no meaningful supporting evidence for these treatments.

HERBS AND SUPPLEMENTS TO USE ONLY WITH CAUTION

Soy or soy isoflavones, and the herb licorice, may reduce testosterone levels in men. For this reason, men with impotence, infertility, or decreased libido may want to avoid these natural products.

One report claims that both tea tree oil and lavender oil have estrogenic (estrogen-like) and antiandrogenic (testosterone-blocking) effects. If this is true, men with infertility should avoid the use of these herbs. However, a literature search failed to find any other published reports that corroborate this claim.

According to a preliminary double-blind study, the supplement melatonin affects testosterone and estrogen metabolism in men, and when taken at a dose of 3 mg daily for six months, it may impair sperm function.

Preliminary evidence from animal studies hints that the use of some forms of peppermint at high doses might impair fertility. There is contradictory evidence from animal studies on whether the herb andrographis may impair fertility. The same is true of the herb stevia.

EBSCO CAM Review Board

FURTHER READING

Balercia, G., et al. "Placebo-Controlled Double-Blind Randomized Trial on the Use of L-carnitine, L-acetylcarnitine, or Combined L-carnitine and L-acetylcarnitine in Men with Idiopathic Asthenozoospermia." *Fertility and Sterility* 84 (2005): 662-671.

Ebisch, I. M., et al. "Does Folic Acid and Zinc Sulphate Intervention Affect Endocrine Parameters and Sperm Characteristics in Men?" *International Journal of Andrology* 29 (2006): 339-345.

Henley, D. V., et al. "Prepubertal Gynecomastia Linked to Lavender and Tea Tree Oils." *New England Journal of Medicine* 356 (2007): 479-485.

See also: Carnitine; Folate; Sexual dysfunction in men; Vitamin B_{12}; Zinc.

Influenza: Homeopathic remedies

CATEGORY: Homeopathy
RELATED TERM: Flu
DEFINITION: Homeopathic treatment of the illness caused by a viral infection.
STUDIED HOMEOPATHIC REMEDIES: Oscillococcinum, L52 (a combination of *Eupatorium* perf., aconite, *Bryonia, Arnica, Gelsemium*, China, belladonna, *Drosera, Polygala*, and eucalyptus)

INTRODUCTION

Influenza, more commonly called the flu, is caused by three main types of viruses: type A, type B, and type C. Of the three, type A is the most common and the most potentially severe, type B is the second most common, and type C is relatively uncommon.

The symptoms of influenza are similar to those of the common cold but almost always more severe. The onset is usually sudden, with a fever up to 103° Fahrenheit (39° Celsius), severe exhaustion, and muscle and joint aches (especially in the back and legs). Symptoms also include a prominent headache, runny nose, sore throat, and cough. As the illness progresses, the muscle aches tend to get worse and the cough becomes more prominent. Influenza also can lead to sensitivity to light, watery eyes, nausea, and vomiting. While the majority of these symptoms should abate in a few days to one week, the fatigue and weakness could linger; the body can also continue to sweat easily for weeks.

Although it is annoying to everyone who gets it, influenza can be dangerous for the very young and very old, for women in the third trimester of pregnancy, and for those with lung disease, heart disease, kidney disease, diabetes, blood diseases (such as sickle cell anemia), or immunosuppression (as with acquired immunodeficiency syndrome or leukemia). Flu can also worsen chronic respiratory illnesses such as asthma and bronchitis, possibly leading to hospitalization. Other possible complications include inflammation of the brain, heart, or nervous system. Homeopathic treatment should not be relied upon to prevent dangerous complications of influenza.

SCIENTIFIC EVALUATIONS OF HOMEOPATHIC REMEDIES

Two widely used homeopathic flu remedies have been studied in scientific trials; evidence is quite promising for the first remedy, oscillococcinum.

Oscillococcinum. Oscillococcinum is a widely available homeopathic treatment for flu. It is made from the tissue of ducks. Thus, this remedy is much like a homeopathic nosode. Oscillococcinum is of 200c (centesimal) potency, meaning that it is diluted to one part in 10^{400} (a dilution so high that even if one started with a chunk of duck the size of the sun, not one molecule would remain).

A double-blind, placebo-controlled study involving nearly five hundred people found that participants who took oscillococcinum recovered faster from the flu than those persons taking only placebo. This study was performed during an influenza epidemic in 1989 in France.

Participants who received oscillococcinum rather than placebo demonstrated a significantly greater percentage of early recovery (within forty-eight hours of the onset of symptoms). Overall, about 61.2 percent of participants in the oscillococcinum treatment group gave it a favorable judgment, whereas only 49.3 percent in the placebo group rated their "treatment" favorably. This difference in positive perception by the treatment group was statistically significant. Furthermore, the treatment group used significantly fewer optional symptomatic medications (such as acetaminophen) than the control group. This suggests that their symptoms were less severe.

In a similar double-blind study performed in Germany, investigators gave 334 people who had flulike symptoms (within twenty-four hours of administering the treatment) either oscillococcinum or placebo three times daily for three days. Again, significant benefits were seen. However, while these results are apparently positive, the published reports are scant on detail, making the quality of these studies difficult to fully assess.

L52. Another widely used flu treatment, L52, is a liquid homeopathic formula of ten ingredients: *Eupatorium* perf., aconite, *Bryonia*, *Arnica*, *Gelsemium*, China, belladonna, *Drosera*, *Polygala*, and eucalyptus. A large, double-blind, placebo-controlled study of about twelve hundred participants evaluated the effectiveness of L52 for preventing the flu rather than for treating it. No benefits were seen, but L52 has shown some promise for treatment of the flu.

TRADITIONAL HOMEOPATHIC TREATMENTS

Classical homeopathy offers many possible homeopathic treatments for the flu. These therapies are chosen based on various specific details of the person seeking treatment.

For example, a person who experiences chills up and down the spine and who feels tired and weak but not thirsty might be given homeopathic *Gelsemium*. Further details of this remedy's symptom picture include headache, runny nose, sore throat, and a desire to be left alone.

However, different auxiliary symptoms might indicate a different choice of remedy. For example, suppose a person has the flu and is very thirsty, especially for cold drinks, and feels better in a cool room than in a warm room. The person also has pain with motion and is irritable. These symptoms fit with the homeopathic treatment *Bryonia*.

EBSCO CAM Review Board

FURTHER READING

Ferley, J. P., et al. "A Controlled Evaluation of a Homeopathic Preparation in the Treatment of Influenza-Like Symptoms." *British Journal of Clinical Pharmacology* 27 (1989): 329-335.

Guo, R., M. H. Pittler, and E. Ernst. "Complementary Medicine for Treating or Preventing Influenza or Influenza-Like Illness." *American Journal of Medicine* 120 (2007): 923-929.

Kirkby, R., and P. Herscu. "Homeopathic Trial Design in Influenza Treatment." *Homeopathy* 99 (2010): 69-75.

Kirkby, R., et al. "Methodological Considerations for Future Controlled Influenza Treatment Trials in Complementary and Alternative Medicine." *Journal of Alternative and Complementary Medicine* 16 (2010): 275-283.

Papp, R., et al. "Oscillococcinum in Patients with Influenza-Like Syndromes." *British Homeopathic Journal* 87 (1989): 69-76.

See also: Bronchitis; Colds and flu; Common colds: Homeopathic remedies; Cough; Influenza vaccine; Sinusitis.

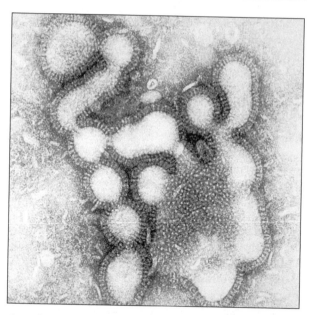

An enlarged view of the influenza virus. (Digital Stock)

Influenza vaccine

CATEGORY: Drug interactions
DEFINITION: A vaccine that decreases the risk of infection with the virus that causes influenza.
INTERACTION: Ginseng
TRADE NAMES: FluShield, Fluvirin, Fluzone

GINSENG

Effect: May Increase Effectiveness of Vaccine

A double-blind study of 227 persons found that ginseng might help the influenza vaccine work more effectively, increasing antibody production and decreasing the frequency of colds and flu. The dose used in the study was 100 milligrams of Asian ginseng (*Panax ginseng*) taken twice daily for one month before and two months after the vaccine was administered.

EBSCO CAM Review Board

FURTHER READING

Olivares, M., et al. "Oral Intake of *Lactobacillus fermentum* CECT5716 Enhances the Effects of Influenza Vaccination." *Nutrition* 23 (2007): 254-260.

Scaglione, F., et al. "Efficacy and Safety of the Standardised Ginseng Extract G115 for Potentiating Vaccination Against the Influenza Syndrome and Protection Against the Common Cold." *Drugs Under Experimental and Clinical Research* 22, no. 2 (1996): 65-72.

See also: Colds and flu; Elderberry; Food and Drug Administration; Ginseng; Immune support; Influenza: Homeopathic remedies.

Injuries, minor

CATEGORY: Condition
RELATED TERMS: Bruises, contusions, joint injuries, ligament injuries, minor sports injuries, muscle injuries, sports injuries, sprains, strains
DEFINITION: Treatment of minor injuries, specifically bruises, minor fractures, and sprains.
PRINCIPAL PROPOSED NATURAL TREATMENT: Proteolytic enzymes
OTHER PROPOSED NATURAL TREATMENTS: Bioflavonoids (citrus bioflavonoids and oxerutins), calcium

and vitamin D, comfrey (topical only), creatine, glucosamine, homeopathic *Arnica*, horse chestnut, oligomeric proanthocyanidins, vitamin C

INTRODUCTION

All people are likely to injure themselves sometime during their lives. Although minor injuries such as bruises and sprains will heal without treatment, they can be quite unpleasant. Discussed here are injuries such as bruises, minor fractures, and sprains. There are other forms of minor injury, however, including minor burns, minor wounds, back pain, and more chronic soft tissue injuries.

Conventional treatment for minor sprains and strains involves anti-inflammatory drugs, icing, and, in some cases, physical therapy. Bruises are sometimes treated with ultrasound, although there is no meaningful evidence that it really helps.

PRINCIPAL PROPOSED NATURAL TREATMENTS

Proteolytic enzymes. Proteolytic enzymes help digest the proteins in food. The pancreas produces the proteolytic enzymes trypsin and chymotrypsin, and others, such as papain and bromelain, are found in foods. Proteolytic enzymes are primarily used as digestive aids for people who have trouble digesting proteins. When taken by mouth, proteolytic enzymes appear to be absorbed internally to a certain extent, and they might reduce inflammation and swelling. Several small studies have found proteolytic enzyme combinations helpful for the treatment of minor injuries. However, the best and largest trial failed to find benefit. Most studies have involved proteolytic enzymes combined with citrus bioflavonoids, which are also thought to decrease swelling.

A double-blind, placebo-controlled study of forty-four persons with sports-related ankle injuries found that treatment with a proteolytic enzyme and bioflavonoid combination resulted in faster healing and reduced the time away from training by about 50 percent. Based on these and other results, a large (721-participant) double-blind, placebo-controlled trial of people with ankle sprains was undertaken to compare placebo with bromelain, trypsin, or rutin (a bioflavonoid), separately or in combination. None of the treatments, alone or together, proved more effective than placebo.

Three other small double-blind studies, involving about eighty athletes, found that treatment with pro-teolytic enzymes significantly speeded healing of bruises and other mild athletic injuries compared with placebo. In another double-blind trial, one hundred people were given an injection of their own blood under the skin to simulate bruising following an injury. Researchers found that treatment with a proteolytic enzyme combination significantly speeded recovery. However, most of these older studies fall beneath modern standards in design and reporting.

OTHER PROPOSED NATURAL TREATMENTS

Oligomeric proanthocyanidins (OPCs), substances found in grape seed and pine bark, have shown promise for the treatment of minor injuries. A ten-day, double-blind, placebo-controlled study of fifty people found that OPCs improved the rate at which edema disappeared following sports injuries. Also, a double-blind, placebo-controlled study of sixty-three women with breast cancer found that 600 milligrams of OPCs daily for six months reduced postoperative edema and pain. Similarly, in a double-blind, placebo-controlled study of thirty-two people who had cosmetic surgery of the face, swelling disappeared much faster in the treated group.

Preliminary evidence from a somewhat poorly reported double-blind trial of forty college football players suggests that a combination of vitamin C and citrus bioflavonoids taken before practice can reduce the severity of athletic injuries. Another small placebo-controlled study suggests that an oral combination product containing vitamin C, calcium, potassium, proteolytic enzymes, rutin, and OPCs can slightly accelerate healing of skin wounds. A double-blind study of people recovering from minor injuries, including minor surgery, found that the bioflavonoid-like substances called oxerutins have similar effects.

The herb horse chestnut is thought to have properties similar to those of citrus bioflavonoids. The active ingredient in horse chestnut is a substance called aescin. One double-blind study of seventy people found that about 10 g of 2 percent aescin gel, applied externally to bruises in a single dose five minutes after the bruises were induced, reduced the tenderness of those bruises.

The herb comfrey is unsafe for internal use because of the presence of liver-toxic pyrrolizidine alkaloids. However, topical use is believed to be safe. In a double-blind, placebo-controlled study of 142 people with an ankle sprain, the use of comfrey gel resulted

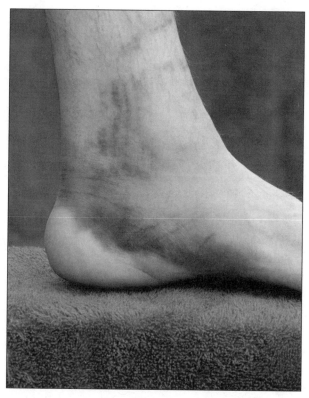

A severe ankle sprain caused bruising. (Stephen J. Krasemann/Photo Researchers, Inc.)

in more rapid recovery than placebo gel, according to measurements of pain, swelling, and mobility.

The supplement creatine has shown some promise for preventing the muscle weakness that commonly occurs when a limb is immobilized following injury or surgery. However, one study failed to find creatine helpful for restoring strength following arthroscopic knee surgery.

The supplement glucosamine might be helpful for people who experience knee pain from cartilage injury. In addition, one study found somewhat inconsistent evidence hinting that glucosamine might aid recovery from acute knee injuries experienced by competitive athletes. A small, double-blind, placebo-controlled study suggests that the use of calcium (1 g daily) plus vitamin D (800 international units daily) may speed bone healing after fracture in people with osteoporosis. Another study found that the use of relaxation therapies to manage stress reduced the number of injury and illness days among competitive athletes.

One study failed to find that onion extract can help reduce scarring in the skin. Also, homeopathic forms of the herb *Arnica* are popular as a treatment for injuries, but studies suggest they are no more effective than placebo.

EBSCO CAM Review Board

FURTHER READING

Braham, R., B. Dawson, and C. Goodman. "The Effect of Glucosamine Supplementation on People Experiencing Regular Knee Pain." *British Journal of Sports Medicine* 37 (2003): 45-49.

Brown, S. A., et al. "Oral Nutritional Supplementation Accelerates Skin Wound Healing." *Plastic and Reconstructive Surgery* 114 (2004): 237-244.

Hespel, P., et al. "Oral Creatine Supplementation Facilitates the Rehabilitation of Disuse Atrophy and Alters the Expression of Muscle Myogenic Factors in Humans." *Journal of Physiology* 536 (2001): 625-633.

Kerkhoffs, G. M., et al. "A Double Blind, Randomised, Parallel Group Study on the Efficacy and Safety of Treating Acute Lateral Ankle Sprain with Oral Hydrolytic Enzymes." *British Journal of Sports Medicine* 38 (2004): 431-435.

Ostojic, S. M., et al. "Glucosamine Administration in Athletes: Effects on Recovery of Acute Knee Injury." *Research in Sports Medicine* 15 (2007): 113-124.

Perna, F. M., et al. "Cognitive Behavioral Stress Management Effects on Injury and Illness Among Competitive Athletes." *Annals of Behavioral Medicine* 25 (2003): 66-73.

Stevinson, C., et al. "Homeopathic *Arnica* for Prevention of Pain and Bruising." *Journal of the Royal Society of Medicine* 96 (2003): 60-65.

Tyler, T. F., et al. "The Effect of Creatine Supplementation on Strength Recovery After Anterior Cruciate Ligament (ACL) Reconstruction." *American Journal of Sports Medicine* 32 (2004): 383-388.

See also: Bromelain; Proteolytic enzymes.

Innate intelligence

CATEGORY: Therapies and techniques
RELATED TERMS: Homeostasis, law of life, universal intelligence
DEFINITION: The premise that inherent knowledge

acquired at birth guides the human body and determines health.

PRINCIPAL PROPOSED USES: General health, well-being

OVERVIEW

The concept of innate intelligence was developed by the founder of chiropractic, D. D. Palmer (1845-1913) and elaborated by his son, B. J. Palmer (1882-1961). The Palmers drew upon nineteenth century medical theories, spiritualist philosophies, and psychoanalytic theory for the concept. By innate intelligence they meant a fundamental, inborn knowledge that tells an organism how to grow, how to adapt to its environment, and how to remain healthy. With innate energy and innate matter, innate intelligence forms the chiropractic triune of life.

MECHANISM OF ACTION

Innate intelligence is not physiological. Instead, it is a guiding principle. More specifically, innate energy links the guidance from innate intelligence to innate matter, the substance of the body. When there is no interruption or interference in this natural process, the body remains healthy. The process can be impaired, however, and according to the Palmers, this fact gives rise to all disease.

USES AND APPLICATIONS

Conservative chiropractic theory holds that stressors cause a subluxation, a dysfunctional segment of the spinal column. Through the nervous system, the subluxation disrupts the triune of life, resulting in disease. Treatment involves manipulating the spine so that the nervous system is unimpaired and innate energy can properly link innate intelligence to innate matter.

SCIENTIFIC EVIDENCE

No evidential-based study, either experimental or observational, supports the existence of innate intelligence. As chiropractic theory developed, some theorists retreated from the spiritualist overtones of the Palmers and equated innate intelligence either with homeostasis, the body's natural metabolic base state or equilibrium, or simply with any unknown force that acts on the body. It has also been argued that innate intelligence is the basis of epigenetics, mechanisms other than the genetic blueprint in deoxyribo-nucleic acid (DNA) that influence the expression of genes.

CHOOSING A PRACTITIONER

Innate intelligence belongs to the traditionalist or "straight" school of chiropractic and proposes to treat disease solely through spinal column manipulation. (Information on straight chiropractic care can be obtained from the Federation of Straight Chiropractors and Organizations at http://www.straightchiropractic.com.) The "mixing" school of chiropractic blends manipulation and other treatments and considers innate intelligence an outmoded concept.

SAFETY ISSUES

While spinal manipulation may relieve symptoms of some disorders, the medical community in general regards it as inappropriate for most disease and as potentially deleterious if employed to the exclusion of mainstream medical treatment.

Roger Smith, Ph.D.

FURTHER READING

Gatterman, Meridel I. *Chiropractic, Health Promotion, and Wellness.* Sudbury, Mass.: Jones and Bartlett, 2007.

Keating, Joseph C., Jr., Alana K. Callender, and Carl. S. Cleveland III. *A History of Chiropractic Education in North America.* Davenport, Iowa: Association for the History of Chiropractic, 1998.

Lenarz, Michael. *Chiropractic Way: How Chiropractic Care Can Stop Your Pain and Help You Regain Your Health Without Drugs or Surgery.* New York: Bantam Books, 2003.

Morgan, L. "Innate Intelligence: Its Origins and Problems." *Journal of the Canadian Chiropractic Association* 42 (1998): 35-41.

Senzon, Simon A. *The Spiritual Writings of B. J. Palmer.* Vol. 1. Ashville, N.C.: Author, 2004.

Rondberg, Terry A. "Innate Intelligence." World Chiropractic Alliance. Available at http://www.worldchiropracticalliance.org/resources/greens/green5.htm.

See also: Chiropractic; Faith healing; Integrative medicine; Meditation; Palmer, Daniel David; Qigong; Spirituality; Traditional healing.

Inosine

Category: Herbs and supplements
Definition: Natural substance of the human body used as a supplement to treat specific health conditions.
Principal proposed uses: None
Other proposed uses: Heart attack recovery, irregular heartbeat, sports performance enhancement, Tourette's syndrome

Overview

Inosine is an important chemical found throughout the body. It plays many roles, one of which is helping to make ATP (adenosine triphosphate), the body's main form of usable energy. Based primarily on this fact, inosine supplements have been proposed as an energy-booster for athletes, as well as a treatment for various heart conditions.

Requirements and Sources

Inosine is not an essential nutrient. However, brewer's yeast and organ meats, such as liver and kidney, contain considerable amounts. Inosine is also available in purified form.

Therapeutic Dosages

When used as a sports supplement, a typical dosage of inosine is 5 to 6 grams daily.

Therapeutic Uses

Inosine has been proposed as a treatment for various forms of heart disease, from irregular heartbeat to recovery from heart attacks. However, the evidence that it offers any benefit to the heart remains far too preliminary to rely upon.

Inosine is better known as a performance enhancer for athletes, although most of the available evidence suggests that it does not work for this purpose. Inosine has also been suggested as a possible treatment for Tourette's syndrome, a neurological disorder.

Safety Issues

Although no side effects have been reported with the use of inosine, long-term use should be avoided. A very preliminary double-blind crossover study that enrolled seven participants suggests that high doses of inosine (5,000 to 10,000 milligrams per day for five to ten days) may increase the risk of uric acid-related problems, such as gout or kidney stones.

The safety of inosine for young children, pregnant or nursing women, or those with serious liver or kidney disease has not been established. As with all supplements taken in multigram doses, it is important to purchase a reputable product, because a contaminant present even in small percentages could add up to a real problem.

EBSCO CAM Review Board

Further Reading

McNaughton, L., et al. "Inosine Supplementation Has No Effect on Aerobic or Anaerobic Cycling Performance." *International Journal of Sport Nutrition* 9 (1999): 333-344.

Starling, R. D., et al. "Effect of Inosine Supplementation on Aerobic and Anaerobic Cycling Performance." *Medicine and Science in Sports and Exercise* 28 (1996): 1193-1198.

See also: Heart attack; Sports and fitness support: Enhancing performance.

Inositol

Category: Herbs and supplements
Related terms: Inositol hexaphosphate, IP6, myo-inositol, phytic acid, vitamin B_8
Definition: Natural substance promoted as a dietary supplement for specific health benefits.
Principal proposed uses: Depression, panic disorder
Other proposed uses: Alzheimer's disease, attention deficit disorder, bipolar disorder, bulimia, cancer prevention, diabetic neuropathy, obsessive-compulsive disorder, premenstrual syndrome, polycystic ovarian syndrome, psoriasis caused by treatment with lithium

Overview

Inositol, unofficially referred to as vitamin B_8, is present in all animal tissues, with the highest levels in the heart and brain. It is part of the membranes (outer coverings) of all cells. It plays a role in helping the liver process fats and in contributing to the function of muscles and nerves.

Inositol may also be involved in depression. People who are depressed may have lower-than-normal levels of inositol in their spinal fluid. In addition, inositol participates in the action of serotonin, a neurotransmitter known to be a factor in depression. (Neurotransmitters are chemicals that transmit messages between nerve cells.) For these two reasons, inositol has been proposed as a treatment for depression, and preliminary evidence suggests that it may be helpful. Inositol also has been tried for other psychological and nerve-related conditions.

SOURCES

Inositol is not known to be an essential nutrient. However, nuts, seeds, beans, whole grains, cantaloupe, and citrus fruits supply a substance called phytic acid (inositol hexaphosphate, or IP6), which releases inositol when acted on by bacteria in the digestive tract. The typical American diet provides an estimated 1,000 milligrams daily.

THERAPEUTIC DOSAGES

Experimentally, inositol dosages of up to 18 grams (g) daily have been tried for various conditions.

THERAPEUTIC USES

Inositol has been studied for depression, bipolar disorder, panic disorder, bulimia, and obsessive-compulsive disorder, but the evidence remains far from conclusive. Other potential uses include Alzheimer's disease and attention deficit disorder. According to two double-blind studies enrolling almost four hundred people, inositol may help improve various symptoms of polycystic ovary syndrome, including infertility and weight gain. Another small double-blind study found that inositol supplements could help reduce symptoms of psoriasis triggered or made worse by the use of the drug lithium. A small double-blind study failed to find inositol helpful for premenstrual dysphoric disorder, a severe form of premenstrual syndrome.

Inositol is sometimes proposed as a treatment for diabetic neuropathy, but there have been no double-blind, placebo-controlled studies on this subject, and two uncontrolled studies had mixed results. Inositol has also been investigated for potential cancer-preventive properties.

SCIENTIFIC EVIDENCE

Depression. Small double-blind studies have found inositol helpful for depression. In one such trial, twenty-eight depressed persons were given a daily dose of 12 g of inositol for four weeks. By the fourth week, the group receiving inositol showed significant improvement compared with the placebo group. However, a double-blind study of forty-two people with severe depression that was not responding to standard antidepressant treatment found no improvement when inositol was added.

Panic disorder. People with panic disorder frequently develop panic attacks, often with no warning. The racing heartbeat, chest pressure, sweating, and other physical symptoms can be so intense that they are mistaken for a heart attack. A small double-blind study (twenty-one participants) found that people given 12 g of inositol daily had fewer and less severe panic attacks compared with the placebo group.

A double-blind, crossover study of twenty people compared inositol to the antidepressant drug fluvoxamine (Luvox), a medication related to Prozac. The results of four weeks of treatment showed that the supplement was, at minimum, just as effective as the drug.

Bipolar disorder. In a six-week, double-blind study, twenty-four people with bipolar disorder received either placebo or inositol (2 g three times daily for a week, then increased to 4 g three times daily) in addition to their regular medical treatment. The results of this small study failed to show statistically significant benefits; however, promising trends were seen that suggest a larger study is warranted.

Polycystic ovary syndrome. Polycystic ovary syndrome (PCOS) is a chronic endocrine disorder in women that leads to infertility, weight gain, and many other problems. In a double-blind, placebo-controlled trial, 136 women with PCOS were given inositol at a dose of 100 mg twice daily, while 147 were given placebo. During the study period of fourteen weeks, participants given inositol showed improvement in ovulation frequency compared with those given placebo. Benefits were also seen in terms of weight loss and levels of HDL (good) cholesterol. A subsequent study of ninety-four women found similar results. However, both of the studies were performed by the same research group. Independent confirmation is necessary before inositol can be considered an effective treatment for PCOS.

SAFETY ISSUES

No serious side effects have been reported for inositol, even with a therapeutic dosage that equals about eighteen times the average dietary intake. However, no long-term safety studies have been performed.

Although inositol has sometimes been recommended for bipolar disorder, there is evidence to suggest inositol may trigger manic episodes in people with this condition. Persons with bipolar disorder should not take inositol unless under a doctor's supervision.

Safety has not been established in young children, women who are pregnant or nursing, and those with severe liver and kidney disease. As with all supplements used in very large doses, it is important to purchase a reputable product, because a contaminant present even in small percentages could be harmful.

EBSCO CAM Review Board

FURTHER READING

Allan, S. J., et al. "The Effect of Inositol Supplements on the Psoriasis of Patients Taking Lithium." *British Journal of Dermatology* 150 (2004): 966-969.

Gerli, S., et al. "Randomized, Double-Blind, Placebo-Controlled Trial: Effects of Myo-Inositol on Ovarian Function and Metabolic Factors in Women with PCOS." *European Review for Medical and Pharmacological Sciences* 11 (2007): 347-354.

Nemets, B., et al. "Myo-Inositol Has No Beneficial Effect on Premenstrual Dysphoric Disorder." *World Journal of Biological Psychiatry* 3 (2002): 147-149.

Palatnik, A., et al. "Double-Blind, Controlled, Crossover Trial of Inositol Versus Fluvoxamine for the Treatment of Panic Disorder." *Journal of Clinical Psychopharmacology* 21 (2001): 335-339.

See also: Alzheimer's disease and non-Alzheimer's dementia; Attention deficit disorder; Anxiety and panic attacks; Bipolar disorder; Depression, mild to moderate; Mental health.

Insect bites and stings

CATEGORY: Condition
RELATED TERM: Insect repellants
DEFINITION: Treatment of the bites and stings of insects.
PRINCIPAL PROPOSED NATURAL TREATMENTS: None
OTHER PROPOSED NATURAL TREATMENTS: *Insect repellant (topical):* Proprietary products containing soybean oil and germanium oil, proprietary bath

lotions, garlic, essential oils (citronella grass, *Ocimum americanum, Citrus hystrix,* lemongrass, turmeric, and vanilla)

• *Insect repellant (local):* Citronella candles, incense
• *Insect repellant (oral):* Garlic
• *Insect bite treatment:* Topical creams containing such herbs as aloe, *Calendula,* chamomile, goldenseal, licorice, and marshmallow

OTHER PROPOSED NATURAL TREATMENTS: Sonic wrist strap repellants, vitamin B_1

INTRODUCTION

Insects are the most successful group of creatures on Earth, greatly outdoing mammals in number of species and sheer mass of life. Furthermore, despite great effort, human attempts to eliminate certain insects, such as mosquitoes, have failed.

In trying to avoid insect bites, however, humans are doing a bit better. The chemical DEET (N,N-diethyl-3-methylbenzamide), which is found in almost all insect repellants, is highly successful, especially against mosquitoes, flies, fleas, and ticks. Contrary to popular belief, DEET appears to be a safe substance when used in a normal fashion. After many decades of use

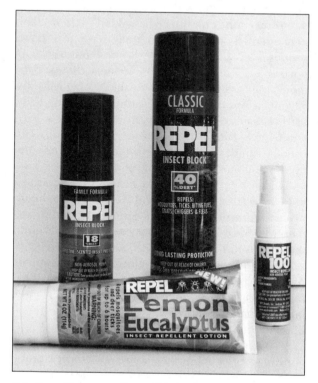

Selection of insect repellents. (PR Newswire)

by millions of people, DEET has been associated with only a small number of adverse reactions, and those side effects that have been reported seem to represent unusual personal responses rather than toxicity in the ordinary sense. Medical treatment for bites that have already occurred consists primarily of soothing topical treatments.

PROPOSED NATURAL TREATMENTS

Because of fears about the safety of DEET (probably unfounded), many natural products have been marketed as safer substitutes. However, while some of these may be effective to a certain extent, none matches the power of the chemical.

One of the best of these natural treatments appears to be a proprietary product containing soybean oil and geranium oil. In a small but well-designed study, this product, when applied to the skin, prevented insects from biting for an average of about ninety minutes. This benefit was equivalent to that of a low-strength DEET repellant (4.75 percent). However, researchers found that high-strength DEET repellants (24 percent) provided about three hundred minutes of protection.

Proprietary bath lotions marketed to repel insects do not appear to provide more than a slight level of bite protection (unless DEET is added to them). Various essential oils, applied topically, have also shown promise for preventing insect bites, but the supporting evidence remains preliminary. Some commonly used essential oils include the oil of eucalyptus, citronella grass (*Cymbopogon winterianus*), clove, hairy basil (*Ocimum americanum*), kaffir lime (*Citrus hystrix*), lemongrass, *Patchouli*, pine, turmeric, and vanilla. Citronella candles and incense appear to reduce the number of bites by less than 50 percent.

The herb garlic, when taken by mouth, may act as a mild insect repellant. A twenty-week, double-blind, placebo-controlled trial followed eighty Swedish soldiers and measured the number of tick bites received during the garlic and the placebo treatments. The results showed a modest but statistically significant reduction in tick bites when soldiers consumed 1,200 milligrams of garlic daily. However, another study failed to find one-time use of garlic helpful for repelling mosquitoes.

Wrist bands containing mosquito repellants do not appear to offer more than marginal efficacy. Sonic mosquito repellers do not appear to work. Oral vitamin B_1 also appears to be completely ineffective.

For people who have already been bitten, topical creams containing such herbs as aloe, *Calendula*, chamomile, goldenseal, licorice, and marshmallow are often recommended, but there is no evidence that they are effective.

EBSCO CAM Review Board

FURTHER READING

Coro, F., and S. Suarez. "Review and History of Electronic Mosquito Repellers." *Wing Beats* 11 (2000): 6-7, 30-32.

Fradin, M. S., and J. F. Day. "Comparative Efficacy of Insect Repellents Against Mosquito Bites." *New England Journal of Medicine* 347 (2002): 13-18.

Oyedele, A. O., et al. "Formulation of an Effective Mosquito-Repellent Topical Product from Lemongrass Oil." *Phytomedicine* 9 (2002): 259-262.

Rajan, T. V., et al. "A Double-Blinded, Placebo-Controlled Trial of Garlic as a Mosquito Repellant." *Medical and Veterinary Entomology* 19 (2005): 84-89.

Trongtokit, Y., et al. "Comparative Repellency of Thirty-Eight Essential Oils Against Mosquito Bites." *Phytotherapy Research* 19 (2005): 303-309.

See also: Aloe; Allergies; Calendula; Chamomile, Garlic; Goldenseal; Injuries, minor; Insect bites and stings: Homeopathic remedies; Licorice; Marshmallow; Turmeric; Wounds, minor.

Insect bites and stings: Homeopathic remedies

CATEGORY: Homeopathy
DEFINITION: The use of highly diluted remedies to treat symptoms caused by insect bites and stings.
STUDIED HOMEOPATHIC REMEDIES: Echinacea; isopathic remedies; *Ledum*; topical homeopathic remedy containing *Echinacea augustifolia*, *Ledum palustre*, *Urtica urens*, and citronella and eucalyptus oils; *Urtica*

SCIENTIFIC EVALUATIONS OF HOMEOPATHIC REMEDIES

In a randomized, single-blind, placebo-controlled study, researchers used a homeopathic gel manufactured and marketed in the Netherlands as a topical treatment for insect bites. The gel was made from a mixture of homeopathic medicines that included

Echinacea augustifolia, Ledum palustre, Urtica urens, and citronella and eucalyptus oils. The researchers found sixty-eight healthy people who were willing to let mosquitoes bite them on the forearm in three different places. The bites were then treated with both the homeopathic gel and placebo that was identical to the treatment except that it lacked the homeopathic medicines. The homeopathic remedy proved no more effective than placebo.

It is worthwhile to note that many homeopaths object to the formulation of this gel because it includes strongly aromatic oils (citronella and eucalyptus). According to the principles of classical homeopathy, these oils would be expected to "antidote" (block) the effects of the homeopathic ingredients.

TRADITIONAL HOMEOPATHIC TREATMENTS

Classical homeopathy often recommends homeopathic echinacea for insect bites and stings with venom. *Ledum* is commonly used for puncture wounds and insect bites, and *Urtica* is used as a remedy for itching. Other common homeopathic treatments for insect bites and stings include isopathic remedies made from the offending insect. These remedies include *Apis mellifica* from the honey bee and *Vespa crabro* from the wasp.

EBSCO CAM Review Board

FURTHER READING

Altunc, U., M. H. Pittler, and E. Ernst. "Homeopathy for Childhood and Adolescence Ailments." *Mayo Clinic Proceedings* 82 (2007): 69-75.

Hill, N., et al. "A Placebo Controlled Clinical Trial Investigating the Efficacy of a Homeopathic After-Bite Gel in Reducing Mosquito Bite Erythema." *European Journal of Clinical Pharmacology* 49 (1995): 103-108.

Trongtokit, Y., et al. "Comparative Repellency of Thirty-Eight Essential Oils Against Mosquito Bites." *Phytotherapy Research* 19 (2005): 303-309.

Ullman, D., and M. Frass. "A Review of Homeopathic Research in the Treatment of Respiratory Allergies." *Alternative Medicine Review* 15 (2010): 48-58.

See also: Allergies; Echinacea; Homeopathy; Wounds, minor.

Insomnia

CATEGORY: Condition
RELATED TERM: Sleeplessness
DEFINITION: Treatment of the inability to fall asleep or to get restful sleep.
PRINCIPAL PROPOSED NATURAL TREATMENTS: Melatonin, valerian (alone or with hops or melissa)
OTHER PROPOSED NATURAL TREATMENTS: Acupuncture or acupressure, ashwagandha, astragalus, biofeedback, chamomile, 5-hydroxytryptophan, gamma-aminobutyric acid, He shou wu, hops, kava, lady's slipper orchid, magnesium, passionflower, probiotics, relaxation therapies, St. John's wort, skullcap

INTRODUCTION

Many people have a serious problem getting a good night's sleep. Lives have become simply too busy for many to get the eight hours really needed. To make matters worse, many people have insomnia. When a person does get to bed, he or she may stay awake thinking for hours. Sleep itself may be restless instead of refreshing.

Most people who sleep substantially less than eight hours a night experience a variety of unpleasant symptoms. The most common are headaches, mental confusion, irritability, malaise, immune deficiencies, depression, and fatigue. Complete sleep deprivation can lead to hallucinations and mental collapse.

The best way to improve sleep involves making lifestyle changes: eliminating caffeine and sugar from one's diet, avoiding stimulating activities before bed, adopting a regular sleeping time, and gradually turning down the lights. More complex behavioral approaches to improving sleep habits can be adopted too.

Many drugs can also help with sleep. Such medications as Sonata, Lunesta, Ambien, Restoril, Ativan, and Xanax are widely used for sleep problems. Of these, only Lunesta has been tested for long-term use. All of these medications are in essence tranquilizers and, therefore, have a potential for dependence and abuse; the newer sleep-inducing drug Rozerem (ramelteon) acts like an enhanced version of the supplement melatonin and is not thought to have such potential.

Other Herbal Supplements for Insomnia

Catnip. The leaves of the catnip plant (*Nepeta cataria*) may produce sleepiness in humans. However, there are no clinical trials to prove its effectiveness or to determine the optimal dose. Catnip is safe to consume at reasonable doses. However, it can be dangerous if taken in very large quantities. Do not use catnip if you are pregnant.

Chamomile. The chamomile herb is the dried or fresh flowers of a small, daisy-like plant (*Matricaria recutita*). Chamomile has been used for thousands of years to treat insomnia. Apigenin is a chemical in chamomile that works in the brain to produce muscle relaxation and initiate sleep. It has been shown to produce a sedative and antianxiety effect in mice. However, there are no human clinical studies proving the sedative effects of chamomile. The exact dose of chamomile that produces sedation is not known.

Chamomile is safe to consume. However, women who are pregnant or who are breast-feeding should consult a doctor before consuming chamomile for therapeutic purposes. If you are allergic to ragweed, you may also be allergic to chamomile. Highly concentrated chamomile tea may induce vomiting.

Hops. The hops plant (*Humulus lupulus*) is typically used to flavor beer. Historically, the flowers have been used to treat mild insomnia. Sleeping on pillows filled with hops flowers is said to promote sleep. Hops, in combination with valerian, is mildly sedating. The most effective dose is not known. Hops are relatively safe, but there are reports of allergic skin rash after handling the plant. Do not use hops if you have depression.

Kava. Kava is extracted from the root of a deciduous shrub called *Piper methysticum*. South Pacific Island cultures have used kava for centuries. However, in some countries, kava has been abused and is a serious social and health problem. To help insomnia, take kava one hour before bedtime.

The dose depends on the amount of the active ingredients, called kavalactones, in the product. It is recommended that people use kava extract standardized to 30 percent kavalactones. Do not take kava if you are preg-nant, are breast-feeding, or have clinical depression. Kava may affect judgment or reflexes during the operation of machinery and may enhance the effects of alcohol and psychiatric drugs.

Kava may cause problems with the liver. If you are taking kava, you should be monitored by your doctor for liver problems.

Lavender. Lavender (*Lavandula angustifolia*) is a flowering plant with a pleasant odor. The flower oil is calming and may help insomnia. One study of elderly people with sleeping difficulties found that inhaling lavender oil was as effective as some sleeping pills. Internal use of the essential oil can cause severe nausea and should be avoided.

Lemon balm. Lemon balm is a plant (*Melissa officinalis*) with a pleasant lemon smell. It can be grown in most gardens. The leaves are used in traditional medicine to treat sleep disturbances. There is not enough evidence to recommend lemon balm as the sole treatment for insomnia. Therefore, there is no recommended dose. Lemon balm appears to be safe but may cause excessive sedation.

Passionflower. Passionflower (*Passiflora incarnata*) was used historically and is used currently as a mild sedative. In studies of mice, passionflower produced sedation. There is not enough evidence to recommend it for the treatment of insomnia. It seems to be safe, although it may increase the effect of other drugs, especially sedatives.

Skullcap. Skullcap is an herb (*Scutellaria lateriflora*) that was used historically as a sedative. It is currently found in insomnia products. There is no evidence to support its effectiveness or to recommend dosages. It has not been proven to be safe, and there is debate over whether it can cause liver toxicity.

Valerian. For centuries, Europeans have used valerian as a sedative and sleep aid. The valerian plant has thick roots with a foul smell. Valerian extract is made from the dried roots and is currently used for relaxation and for promoting sleep. Clinical research studies have shown inconsistent evidence for the effectiveness of valerian for insomnia. Valerian appears safe to use, but it may impair the ability to drive or operate machinery.

Antidepressants can also be used to correct sleep problems. Low doses of certain antidepressants immediately bring on sleep because their side effects include drowsiness. However, this effect tends to wear off with repeated use. For chronic sleeping problems, full doses of antidepressants can sometimes be helpful. Antidepressants are believed to work by actually altering brain chemistry, which produces a beneficial effect on sleep. Trazadone and amitriptyline are two of the most commonly prescribed antidepressants when improved sleep is desired, but most other antidepressants also can be helpful.

PRINCIPAL PROPOSED NATURAL TREATMENTS

Although the scientific evidence is not definitive, the herb valerian and the hormone melatonin are widely accepted as treatments for certain forms of insomnia.

Valerian. Valerian has a long traditional use for insomnia, and today it is an accepted over-the-counter treatment for insomnia in Germany, Belgium, France, Switzerland, and Italy. However, the evidence that it really works remains inconsistent and incomplete. A systematic review concluded that valerian is safe but probably not effective for treating insomnia. However, there have been some positive results, with both valerian alone and valerian combined with other herbs.

Valerian is most commonly recommended to be used as needed for occasional insomnia. However, the results of the largest and best-designed positive study found benefits only regarding long-term improvement of sleep. In this double-blind, placebo-controlled trial, one-half of the participants took 600 milligrams (mg) of an alcohol-based valerian extract one hour before bedtime, while the other one-half took placebo. Valerian did not work right away. For the first couple of weeks, valerian and placebo had similar affects. However, by day twenty-eight, valerian's effectiveness increased. Effectiveness was rated as good or very good by participant evaluation in 66 percent of the valerian group and in 61 percent by doctor evaluation, whereas in the placebo group, only 29 percent were so rated by participants and doctors.

Although positive, these results are a bit confusing, because in another large study, valerian was effective immediately. Other studies, most of relatively low quality, found immediate benefits too. To further confuse the matter, four later studies of valerian failed to find evidence of any benefit; one was a four-week study that included 135 people given valerian and 135 given placebo. The most recent trial, a two-week study of 405 people, reported "modest benefits at most."

A study of 184 people that tested a standardized combination of valerian and hops had mixed results. Researchers tested quite a few aspects of sleep (such as time to fall asleep, length of sleep, and number of awakenings) and found evidence of benefit in a few. This use of multiple outcome measures makes the results somewhat unreliable.

Other studies have compared valerian (either alone or with hops or melissa) with benzodiazepine drugs. Most of these studies found the herbal treatment approximately as effective as the drug, but because of the absence of a placebo group, these results are less than fully reliable. Mixed results like these suggest that valerian is at most modestly helpful for improving sleep.

Melatonin. The body uses melatonin as part of its normal control of the sleep-wake cycle. The pineal gland makes serotonin and then turns it into melatonin when exposure to light decreases. Strong light (such as sunlight) slows melatonin production more than does weak light, and a completely dark room increases the amount of melatonin made. Taking melatonin as a supplement seems to stimulate sleep when the natural cycle is disturbed. It may also have a direct sedative effect.

Although not all studies were positive, reasonably good evidence indicates that melatonin is helpful for insomnia related to jet lag. One of the best supporting studies was a double-blind, placebo-controlled study that enrolled 320 travelers crossing six to eight time zones. The participants were divided into four groups and given a daily dose of 5 mg of standard melatonin, 5 mg of slow-release melatonin, 0.5 mg of standard melatonin, or placebo. The group that received 5 mg of standard melatonin slept better, took less time to fall asleep, and felt more energetic and awake during the day than the other three groups. Mixed results have been seen in studies involving the use of melatonin for ordinary insomnia, insomnia in swing-shift workers, and insomnia in elderly people.

A four-week double-blind trial evaluated the benefits of melatonin for children with difficulty falling asleep. A total of forty children who had experienced this type of sleep problem for at least one year were given either placebo or melatonin at a dose of 5 mg. The results showed that the use of melatonin helped participants fall asleep significantly more easily. Benefits were also seen in a similar study of sixty-two children with this condition. The long-term safety of melatonin usage has not been established. One should not give a child melatonin except under physician supervision.

Many persons stay up late on Friday and Saturday nights and then find it difficult to go to sleep at a reasonable hour Sunday night. A small, double-blind, placebo-controlled study found evidence that the use of melatonin 5.5 hours before the desired Sunday bedtime improved the ability of participants to fall asleep.

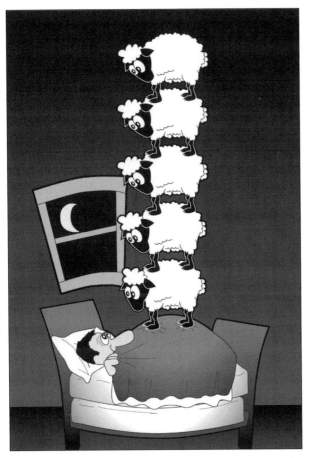

Complete sleep deprivation can lead to hallucinations and mental collapse. (©Robert Balazik/Dreamstime.com)

Benefits were seen in a small double-blind trial of persons in a pulmonary intensive care unit. It is difficult to sleep in an ICU, and the resulting sleep deprivation is not helpful for those recovering from disease or surgery. In this study of eight hospitalized persons, 3 mg of controlled-release melatonin significantly improved sleep quality and duration.

Blind people often have trouble sleeping on any particular schedule because there are no light cues available to help them get tired at night. A small, double-blind, placebo-controlled crossover trial found that the use of melatonin at a dose of 10 mg per day synchronized participants' sleep schedules.

Some people find it impossible to fall asleep until early morning, a condition called delayed sleep phase syndrome. Melatonin may be beneficial for this syndrome.

In addition, people trying to stop using sleeping pills in the benzodiazepine family may find melatonin helpful. A double-blind, placebo-controlled study of thirty-four persons who regularly used such medications found that melatonin at a dose of 2 mg nightly (controlled-release formulation) could help them discontinue the use of the drugs. There can be risks in discontinuing benzodiazepine drugs, however, so persons should consult a physician for advice.

OTHER PROPOSED NATURAL TREATMENTS

Acupressure or acupuncture may be helpful for insomnia, but the supporting evidence remains weak. A single-blind, placebo-controlled study involving 84 nursing home residents found that real acupressure was superior to sham acupressure for improving sleep quality. Treated participants fell asleep faster and slept more soundly. In a similar study, researchers found that performing acupressure on a single point on both wrists for five weeks improved sleep quality among residents of long-term-care facilities more than did lightly touching the same point. Another single-blind, controlled study reported benefits with acupuncture but failed to include a proper statistical analysis of the results. For this reason, no conclusions can be drawn from the report. In a third study, ninety-eight people with severe kidney disease were divided into three groups: no extra treatment, twelve sessions of fake acupressure (not using actual acupressure points), or twelve sessions of real acupressure. Participants receiving real acupressure experienced significantly improved sleep compared to those receiving no extra treatment. However, fake acupressure was just as effective as real acupressure. Also, a small placebo-controlled trial involving sixty adults with insomnia found that three weeks of electroacupuncture improved sleep efficiency and decreased wake time after sleep onset.

In a trial involving twenty-eight women, six weeks of auricular acupuncture, in which needles are placed in the outer ear, was more effective than sham acupuncture. However, in a carefully conducted review of ten randomized trials involving auricular acupuncture or acupressure (using magnetic pellets), researchers were unable to draw conclusions because of the poor quality of the studies.

Preliminary evidence suggests that Tai Chi, an ancient Chinese practice involving graceful movements combined with meditation, may benefit some people who have trouble sleeping. In one randomized study, a certain form of Tai Chi was more effective than health education after twenty-five weeks in persons with moderate insomnia.

Numerous controlled studies have evaluated relaxation therapies for the treatment of insomnia. These studies are difficult to summarize because many of the trials involved therapy combined with other methods, such as biofeedback, sleep restriction, and paradoxical intent (trying not to sleep). The type of relaxation therapy used in the majority of these trials was progressive muscle relaxation. Overall, the evidence indicates that relaxation therapies may be somewhat helpful for insomnia, although not dramatically so. For example, in a controlled study of seventy people with insomnia, participants using progressive relaxation showed no meaningful improvement in the time taken to fall asleep or in the duration of sleep, but they reported feeling more rested in the morning. In another study, twenty minutes of relaxation practice was required to increase sleeping time by thirty minutes.

One small double-blind study found a particular Ayurvedic herbal combination helpful for insomnia. Herbs used for anxiety are commonly recommended for insomnia too. As noted, hops and lemon balm have been studied in combination with valerian. One double-blind study found that the antianxiety herb kava taken alone may aid sleep for people whose insomnia is associated with anxiety and tension. However, a fairly large study failed to find kava helpful for ordinary insomnia. There are serious concerns that kava may occasionally cause severe liver disorders.

The substance GABA (gamma-aminobutyric acid) is a naturally occurring neurotransmitter that is used within the brain to reduce the activity of certain nerve systems, including those related to anxiety. For this reason, GABA supplements are sometimes recommended for treatment of anxiety-related conditions, such as insomnia. However, there are no studies whatsoever supporting the use of GABA supplements for this purpose. It appears that, when taken orally, GABA cannot pass the blood-brain barrier and, therefore, does not even enter the brain.

One small study hints that the fragrance of lavender essential oil might aid sleep. Slight evidence exists to support the use of magnesium or probiotics (healthy bacteria) for insomnia in the elderly.

The herb St. John's wort and the supplement 5-hydroxytryptophan have shown promise as treatments for depression. Because prescription antidepressants can aid sleep, these natural substances have been suggested for insomnia. However, there is no direct evidence that they are effective. A double-blind trial of twelve persons without insomnia found no sleep-promoting benefit with St. John's wort.

Other herbs reputed to offer both antianxiety and anti-insomnia benefits include ashwagandha, astragalus, chamomile, He shou wu, lady's slipper, passionflower, and skullcap. However, there is no supporting evidence to indicate that any of these really work. Finally, a number of supplements might offer benefits for improving mental function during periods of sleep deprivation.

EBSCO CAM Review Board

FURTHER READING

Bent, S., et al. "Valerian for Sleep." *American Journal of Medicine* 119 (2006): 1005-1012.

Buscemi, N., et al. "The Efficacy and Safety of Exogenous Melatonin for Primary Sleep Disorders." *Journal of General Internal Medicine* 20 (2006): 1151-1158.

Edwards, B. J., et al. "Use of Melatonin in Recovery from Jet-Lag Following an Eastward Flight Across Ten Time-Zones." *Ergonomics* 43 (2000): 1501-1513.

Irwin, M. R., R. Olmstead, and S. J. Motivala. "Improving Sleep Quality in Older Adults with Moderate Sleep Complaints: A Randomized Controlled Trial of Tai Chi Chih." *Sleep* 31 (2008): 1001-1008.

Lewith, G. T., et al. "A Single-Blinded, Randomized Pilot Study Evaluating the Aroma of *Lavandula augustifolia* as a Treatment for Mild Insomnia." *Journal of Alternative and Complementary Medicine* 11 (2005): 631-637.

Sadeghniiat-Haghighi, K., et al. "Efficacy and Hypnotic Effects of Melatonin in Shift-Work Nurses." *Journal of Circadian Rhythms* 6 (2008): 10.

Sjoling, M., M. Rolleri, and E. Englund. "Auricular Acupuncture Versus Sham Acupuncture in the Treatment of Women Who Have Insomnia." *Journal of Alternative and Complementary Medicine* 14 (2008): 39-46.

Sun, J. L., et al. "Effectiveness of Acupressure for Residents of Long-Term Care Facilities with Insomnia." *International Journal of Nursing Studies* 47 (2010): 798-805.

Yeung, W. F., et al. "Electroacupuncture for Primary Insomnia." *Sleep* 32 (2009): 1039-1047.

See also: Chronic fatigue syndrome; Fatigue; Fibro-myalgia: Homeopathic remedies; Melatonin; Memory and mental function impairment; Mental health; Valerian.

Insulin

CATEGORY: Drug interactions

DEFINITION: Injections used to regulate blood sugar in persons with type 1 diabetes and in persons with severe type 2 diabetes.

INTERACTIONS: Various herbs and supplements

TRADE NAMES: Humalog, Humulin, Iletin, Novolin, Velosulin

HERBS AND SUPPLEMENTS

Effect: Might Require Reduced Insulin Dosage

Meaningful preliminary evidence suggests that the use of certain herbs and supplements could potentially improve blood sugar control and require one to reduce his or her insulin dosage. These herbs and supplements are aloe, chromium, fenugreek, ginseng, gymnema, coenzyme Q_{10}, and vanadium.

Weaker evidence suggests that the following herbs and supplements could potentially have the same effect under certain circumstances: *Anemarrhena asphodeloides*, arginine, *Azadirachta indica* (neem), bilberry leaf, biotin, bitter melon, carnitine, *Catharanthus roseus*, *Coccinia indica*, coenzyme Q_{10}, conjugated linoleic acid, *Cucumis sativus*, *Cucurbita ficifolia*, *Cuminum cyminum* (cumin), *Euphorbia prostrata*, garlic, glucomannan, *Guaiacum coulteri*, *Guazuma ulmifolia*, guggul, holy basil, *Lepechinia caulescens*, lipoic acid, *Medicago sativa* (alfalfa), *Musa sapientum* L. (banana), niacinamide, nopal cactus, onion, *Phaseolus vulgaris*, *Psacalium peltatum*, pterocarpus, *Rhizophora mangle*, salt bush, *Spinacea oleracea*, *Tournefortia hirsutissima*, *Turnera diffusa*, and vitamin E.

EBSCO CAM Review Board

FURTHER READING

Pi-Sunyer, F. X. "How Effective Are Lifestyle Changes in the Prevention of Type 2 Diabetes Mellitus?" *Nutrition Reviews* 65 (2007): 101-110.

Wang, E., and J. Wylie-Rosett. "Review of Selected Chinese Herbal Medicines in the Treatment of Type 2 Diabetes." *Diabetes Educator* 34, no. 4 (2008): 645-654.

Xie W., Y. Zhao, and Y. Zhang. "Traditional Chinese Medicines in Treatment of Patients with Type 2 Diabetes Mellitus." *Evidence-Based Complementary and Alternative Medicine* (March 17, 2011).

See also: Aloe; Chromium; Coenzyme Q_{10}; Diabetes; Diabetes, complications of; Fenugreek; Food and Drug Administration; Ginseng; Gymnema; Herbal medicine; Low-glycemic index diet; Vanadium.

Insurance coverage

CATEGORY: Issues and overviews

DEFINITION: The approval by a health insurance carrier for payment of services by a complementary or alternative medicine provider.

CRITERIA FOR COVERAGE

There are many complementary and alternative medicine (CAM) therapies, but only a few have been accepted by traditional medicine and are covered by health insurance plans, even when ordered by a medical doctor or an osteopathic doctor. A covered CAM therapy is reimbursed directly to either the provider or the patient by the patient's health insurance company. If the payment goes directly to the CAM provider, then the patient is responsible for a copayment (the patient's up-front share of the cost of treatment). Other health insurance companies have negotiated a discount with selected CAM providers. The patient pays this discounted amount out-of-pocket. This discounted payment, however, is not considered insurance coverage.

Several factors are considered by health insurance companies when deciding whether to cover a CAM service. These factors include whether the treatment is experimental; whether it is ordered by a medical doctor or an osteopathic doctor; whether the CAM provider is licensed by his or her respective state; whether the treatment provided is generally known; and whether the treatment has been adequately researched and found to be effective. Treatments or therapies that are considered experimental are rarely covered by health insurance, and services ordered by a medical doctor or an osteopath are more likely to be covered.

CAM providers who are licensed by their states have had their education and training validated and meet the standards of their states of practice. Licensing standards vary from state to state. Therapies that have been adequately researched are those that have been proven effective by a body of research. The therapy does not have to be 100 percent effective, but it should demonstrate a reasonable amount of effectiveness in treating patient conditions. Medical doctors and osteopaths are more likely to accept therapies that have been adequately researched. Often medical doctors reject CAM therapies because they are not knowledgeable about them.

COVERAGE FOR SPECIFIC TYPES OF CAM

Some CAM services are accepted by traditional medicine and covered by health insurance. Biofeedback and nutritional therapy are covered if they are ordered by a medical doctor. Midwives and osteopathic physicians are covered in most states. The midwife, for example, must be a registered nurse midwife with a master's degree in midwifery and must be working in a hospital or office with a medical doctor. Midwives who are not registered nurses are not covered. Osteopaths, because they have been educated in ways similar to medical doctors, are considered to be physicians, and they function like medical doctors within their medical specialty. Another CAM service, pet therapy, is usually provided at no charge. The pets, usually dogs, visit patients in hospitals or extended care facilities.

The CAM therapies that are most often covered by health insurance are chiropractic, acupuncture, and massage. Chiropractic is almost universally covered by insurance, although there are often limits on the number of office visits that will be covered.

Acupuncture and massage therapy are covered less often, and they may be covered only for certain conditions. Acupuncture is often covered only for pain management for persons with cancer, and massage therapy may be covered only for persons with fibromyalgia.

IMPLICATIONS OF LIMITED COVERAGE

Despite the limited insurance coverage for CAM services, the services remain popular with consumers. Annually, the CAM industry earns about $34 billion in the United States. It seems, then, that a lack of insurance coverage for CAM has not interfered with the use of these providers. People who use CAM do tend to be wealthier and better educated. They also seem to feel that CAM treatment is helpful to them.

One effect of limited insurance coverage for CAM services is the relatively low cost for these services. This is good for consumers but not necessarily good for providers. CAM providers often earn much less than their counterparts in traditional medicine and are more likely to keep their business expenses low with, for example, a small staff and a small leased office.

Christine M. Carroll, R.N.

FURTHER READING

Cleary-Guida, Maria B., et al. "A Regional Survey of Health Insurance Coverage for Complementary and Alternative Medicine: Current Status and Future Ramifications." *Journal of Alternative and Complementary Medicine* 7, no. 3 (2001): 269-273.

Lafferty, William E., et al. "Insurance Coverage and Subsequent Utilization of Complementary and Alternative Medical (CAM) Providers." *American Journal of Managed Care* 12, no. 7 (2006): 397-404.

Nahin, Richard L., et al. "Costs of Complementary and Alternative Medicine (CAM) and Frequency of Visits to CAM Practitioners: United States, 2007." National Health Statistics Reports: Department of Health and Human Services, July 30, 2009. Available at http://www.cdc.gov/nchs/data/nhrs018.pdf.

National Center for Complementary and Alternative Medicine. "Paying for CAM Treatment." Available at http://nccam.nih.gov/health/financial.

White House Commission on Complementary and Alternative Medicine. "Coverage and Reimbursement." Available at http://www.whccamp.hhs.gov/fr7.html.

See also: Clinical trials; Double-blind, placebo-controlled studies; Health freedom movement; Licensing and certification for CAM practitioners; Pseudoscience; Regulation of CAM; Scientific method.

Integrative medicine

CATEGORY: Therapies and techniques

RELATED TERMS: Acupuncture, Ayurveda, complementary and alternative medicine, cross-cultural medicine, functional medicine, homeopathy, hypnosis, guided imagery, integrated health care, manual therapy, meditation, mind/body therapy, nutritional medicine, psychosomatic medicine, relaxation training, self-healing, spirituality, traditional Chinese medicine, yoga

DEFINITION: A relationship-centered care system that combines mainstream medical and alternative therapeutic methods to potentiate the body's innate capacity to heal.

PRINCIPAL PROPOSED USES: Allergies, anxiety, cardiovascular disorders, depression, endocrine dysfunction, infections, metabolic dysfunction, pain management, respiratory diseases, skin and joint diseases

OTHER PROPOSED USES: Cancer, diabetes, hypertension, osteoporosis, pregnancy-related conditions, menopause-related conditions, stroke, substance abuse

OVERVIEW

According to Andrew Weil, a prominent physician and a proponent of this system, integrative medicine (IM) works with the body's natural potential for healing. In the human body, many pathways and

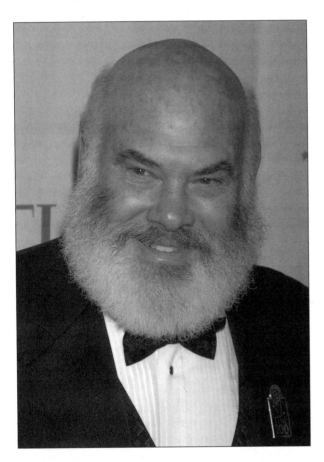

Andrew Weil, a proponent of integrative medicine. (AP Photo)

mechanisms serve to maintain health and promote healing. The IM perspective recognizes that treatment, often a combination of allopathic and alternative medicine, should unblock and enhance these mechanisms.

In practice, the therapeutic process addresses the whole person and relies on the main pillars of a person's well-being: mind, body, spirit, and community. This paradigm emphasizes the importance of a sound physician-patient relationship for a successful healing process. Developing rapport and empathy greatly facilitates the efficacy of lifestyle changes and the use of therapies such as pharmaceuticals, homeopathy, dietary supplements, traditional Chinese medicine, Ayurveda, manual methods, mind/body techniques, and movement therapy.

Until the 1970s, little was done to connect traditional, ancient healing modalities to biomedicine. At that time, the holistic health movement in the United States and in Western Europe started a "dynamic alliance" of therapists, including Native American healers, yoga teachers, and homeopaths. Modern medicine began taking steps to reduce the excessive use of technology and the inherent disconnect from the patient, while rediscovering more natural, less invasive avenues of healing.

The Consortium of Academic Health Centers for Integrative Medicine, founded in 2000, brings together many highly esteemed academic medical centers dedicated to promoting IM through educational opportunities, health policies, research, and collaborative initiatives. The term "integrative medicine" will most likely be used until the value of this balanced approach becomes widely recognized as simply good medicine.

MECHANISM OF ACTION

Integrative medicine combines conventional medical treatments with carefully selected alternative therapies that are proven to be safe and effective. The goal of the integrative movement is to bring back the art of healing and to address the root of the pathological process, not just the symptoms. In addition to acquiring the foundations of medical knowledge, physicians should be able to release, explore, and exploit the intrinsic healing responses of the body. Practitioners are therefore encouraged to become familiar with, and critically assess, the modalities of complementary and alternative medicine (CAM).

Core areas of education include the philosophy of science, cross-cultural medicine, principles of mind/body medicine, self-healing, and spirituality. The practitioner's ability to self-explore and maintain his or her own health balance are considered essential for the therapeutic act. The physician strives to become a partner and a mentor, who understands the important coordinates of his or her patient's life events, culture, beliefs, and relationships. By acknowledging a person's uniqueness, the processes of health maintenance and healing are tailored to best address a person's background and conditions. Matching the patient's belief system can, especially in chronic illness, lead to the activation of an internal healing response, often known as the placebo effect. Far from being a useless phenomenon based on deception, this response ultimately results in enhanced health.

USES AND APPLICATIONS

Overall, IM is a combination of art and science that seeks health maintenance and disease prevention and treatment using the most natural, least invasive interventions available. Virtually all categories of disorders, and especially chronic diseases, can benefit from an integrated approach.

Cardiovascular disorders. Cardiovascular disorders such as congestive heart failure, coronary artery disease, hypertension, and peripheral vascular disease can be treated with conventional methods and with lifestyle modifications, nutrition, dietary supplements (omega-3 fatty acids, coenzyme Q_{10}, carnitine, arginine, hawthorn, and garlic), relaxation, meditation, and hydrotherapy. Primary prevention is critical in coronary artery disease and hypertension.

Cancer. Cancer can be treated with the synergistic reduction of the sequellae and by limiting the toxicity or trauma of conventional therapies and by alleviating psychological distress. Nutritional changes, dietary supplements (vitamins, immunomodulators, ginger, marijuana, and St. John's wort), acupuncture, mind/body techniques, and group support are often recommended. Preventive approaches (for breast cancer, for example) involve lifestyle changes (exercise, nutrition, limiting toxins, and breast-feeding), botanicals (seaweed, rosemary, and green tea), and mind/body methods.

Endocrine and metabolic disorders. Endocrine and metabolic disorders are also amenable to integrated therapies. Insulin resistance is often treated with metformin

---

Integrative Medicine and Health Care Reform

Integrative medicine proponent Andrew Weil spoke before the U.S. Senate Committee on Health, Education, Labor, and Pensions in 2009 on the place of integrative medicine in health care reform in the United States. Part of his testimony is presented here.

Everyone agrees that functional, cost-effective health care must be built on a foundation of disease prevention and health promotion. The main reason for the impending collapse of the American health care system is its lopsided focus on intervention in established disease, much of which is lifestyle related and therefore preventable.

It is less obvious that meaningful health care reform also requires a transformation of medicine. The high-tech interventions that conventional medicine primarily uses, including pharmaceutical drugs, are simply too expensive. American health professionals are not trained to use low-tech, cost-effective treatments that work well for many common disease conditions.

Integrative Medicine (IM) can solve both of these problems. As developed and taught by the University of Arizona Center for Integrative Medicine, it [IM] addresses all aspects of lifestyle to promote health and alleviate illness. . . .

Our [the United States'] long-term goal must be to shift our health care efforts from disease intervention to health promotion and disease prevention. That does not mean withholding treatment from those who need it; those with existing conditions need to be treated effectively and compassionately. But my concept of prevention goes well beyond immunization, sanitation, and diagnostic screenings. I am suggesting that the time has come for a new paradigm of preventive medicine and a society-wide effort to educate our citizens about health and self-care.

---

hydrochloride, lifestyle changes, and a low-carbohydrate diet. Supplements such as chromium, vanadium, alpha-lipoic acid, American ginseng, and fenugreek can provide benefits too. In persons with diabetes mellitus, essential care includes diet, exercise, and pharmaceuticals. Dietary supplements, such as vitamins, bilberry, and *Ginkgo biloba*, and mind/body techniques (for example, relaxation and yoga) may mitigate vascular disease and even lower glucose levels. Alternative therapies to consider in persons with hypothyroidism include dietary supplements such as vitamins, zinc, selenium, and traditional Chinese botanicals, and practices such as yoga. Pharmaceuticals are available for the treatment of osteoporosis, and vitamin D, ipriflavone, and exercise constitute useful adjuvants.

Gastrointestinal disorders. Gastroesophageal reflux, peptic ulcer disease, and irritable bowel syndrome can be treated with lifestyle changes and with botanicals (licorice, chamomile, and marshmallow root), homeopathics, and mind/body therapies (including stress management and guided imagery).

Neurological disorders. Stroke, multiple sclerosis, Alzheimer's disease, Parkinson's disease, seizures, and migraine have been linked to oxidative stress, neurotoxic factors, and inflammatory processes. Thus, they can greatly benefit from integrative methods. The complementary therapies include, but are not limited to, dietary and nutritional supplementation (omega-3 fatty acids, glutathione, coenzyme Q_{10}, alpha-lipoic acid, N-acetylcysteine, niacin, vitamins, melatonin, and magnesium), herbal supplementation (*Ginkgo biloba*, milk thistle, turmeric, vinpocetine, and skullcap), meditation, yoga, and exercise.

Asthma and allergies. Asthma and allergies respond well to alternative methods that include nutritional and environmental changes, exercise, botanicals (ginkgo, coleus, licorice, kanpo, bioflavonoids, and stinging nettle), vitamins and minerals, homeopathics, massage, inhalation, breathing techniques, and mind/body therapy.

Upper respiratory infections and sinusitis. Upper respiratory infections and sinusitis can be treated with pharmaceuticals, dietary changes, hydration, steam inhalation, supplements (vitamins, antioxidants, zinc, magnesium, garlic, and echinacea), and homeopathic remedies.

Depression and anxiety. Depression and anxiety represent a spectrum of disorders ideally suited for IM. In addition to pharmaceuticals, persons can benefit from lifestyle changes, physical activity, nutritional remedies (omega-3 fatty acids, B vitamins, folic acid, and hydroxytryptophan), botanical remedies (St. John's wort, kava kava, and ginkgo), psychotherapy, relaxation training, yoga, acupuncture, and transcranial stimulation.

Pain. Pain management represents a challenge for both the physician and the person in pain. Truly integrating allopathic and alternative medicines can offer relief and reduce frustration. Reassurance and lifestyle changes are often the first step of the therapeutic plan. A vast array of useful approaches includes pharmacotherapy, exercise, supplements (arnica and omega-3 fatty acids), homeopathy, manual methods, acupuncture, transcutaneous nerve stimulation, and mind/body therapy. Surgery is considered after conservative therapies have failed.

Pregnancy and menopause. The integrative approach to pregnancy and menopause reaches beyond the use of combined mainstream and alternative therapies. These conditions require a careful initial encounter and subsequent consideration of the mind, body, spirit, and community context. The patient-practitioner interaction is oriented toward health rather than disease, and listening to the person seeking care is essential. In pregnancy especially, the need for noninvasive, natural approaches becomes crucial. Nausea and vomiting, for example, are treated with supplements (vitamin B_6, red raspberry leaf, ginger root, and chamomile), homeopathics, acupuncture, and mind/body therapies.

Alcoholism and substance abuse. Therapeutic options for alcoholism and substance abuse include botanicals (valerian, kudzu, kava kava), acupuncture, mind/body therapies, and spirituality. The options also include twelve-step programs.

SCIENTIFIC EVIDENCE

Integrative practice is committed to the scientific method and is rooted in evidence. At the same time, the integrative practitioner aims to transcend the confines of "scientific truth" and connect with the people he or she serves on multiple levels.

A number of CAM therapies have proved effective as complements to conventional medical treatments. These CAM therapies include dietary and herbal supplements, acupuncture, manual therapy, biofeedback, relaxation training, and movement therapy. When a strong evidence base is developed for a particular complementary method, it can become part of the integrative armamentarium. After it reviewed the evidence base, for example, the Society for Integrative Oncology supported the use of acupuncture in cases in which cancer-related pain is poorly controlled.

According to the American Academy of Pediatrics, a review conducted in 2002 found more than fourteen hundred randomized-control trials of pediatric CAM; the quality of these trials was determined to be as good as those focusing on conventional therapies. It is important to note that different levels of evidence are required to prove the safety and efficacy of complementary therapies, depending on the goals of the treatment. Lower levels of evidence (that is, nonrandomized and observational studies) are acceptable for preventive or supportive goals and for noninvasive approaches. Furthermore, integrating represents more than combining; it involves holistic treatment and the synergistic application of an array of treatments. Thus, the extent of the combination or integration varies. This leads to unique challenges for the scientific validation of integrative methods. Traditional research models often appear inadequate. More studies are needed that examine the appropriateness and manner of integration for specific diseases and conditions.

CHOOSING A PRACTITIONER

Approximately 70 percent of medical schools in the United States have courses in CAM. Integrative medicine centers and fellowship programs exist at many prominent universities and hospitals in the United States, including the University of Arizona, Duke University, Harvard University, the University of Michigan, and the Mayo Clinic. These centers tend to be directed by conventional physicians (doctors of medicine and doctors of osteopathy) and staffed by various practitioners.

The American Board of Integrative Holistic Medicine establishes standards for the application of IM principles and offers certification. The American Association of Integrative Medicine provides an accreditation program. Even so, qualified IM practitioners are still difficult to find, and the demand greatly exceeds the supply. Oftentimes, the collaboration between conventional physicians of various specialties and certified CAM practitioners provides the foundation and benefits of integrative care. The American Holistic Medical Association maintains a directory of integrative and holistic practitioners holding relevant degrees.

SAFETY ISSUES

When implemented by physicians and CAM practitioners who are well versed in the integrative method, IM is safe and beneficial.

Mihaela Avramut, M.D., Ph.D.

FURTHER READING

American Association of Integrative Medicine. http://www.aaimedicine.com. Promotes the development of IM.

American Board of Integrative Holistic Medicine. http://integrativeholisticdoctors.org. Establishes and maintains standards of care.

American Holistic Medical Association. http://www.holisticmedicine.org. Promotes holistic and integrative principles.

Consortium of Academic Health Centers for Integrative Medicine. http://www.imconsortium.org. Advances the principles and practice of integrative health care within academic institutions.

Baer, Hans. *Toward an Integrative Medicine: Merging Alternative Therapies with Biomedicine.* Walnut Creek, Calif.: Altamira Press, 2004. A comprehensive overview of the holistic movement and its journey into mainstream medicine.

Kurn, Sidney, and Sheryl Shook. *Integrated Medicine for Neurologic Disorders.* Albuquerque, N.Mex.: Health Press, 2008. Review of nutritional and herbal therapies for practitioners who treat persons with neurological disorders.

Leis, A. M., L. C. Weeks, and M. J. Verhoef. "Principles to Guide Integrative Oncology and the Development of an Evidence Base." *Current Oncology* 15, suppl. 2 (2008): S83-S87. Discusses the need for evidence to support the overall practice of integration and the challenges posed by the validation process.

Rakel, David, ed. *Integrative Medicine.* 2d ed. Philadelphia: Saunders/Elsevier, 2007. An authoritative textbook that discusses the philosophy and method of integrative medicine and details therapeutic modalities for numerous diseases and conditions.

Rees, L., and A. Weil. "Integrated Medicine [Editorial]." *British Medical Journal* 322 (2001): 119-120. Defines the basic tenets of IM.

See also: Alternative versus traditional medicine; Acupuncture; Ayurveda; Guided imagery; Homeopathy; Hypnotherapy; Meditation; Mind/body medicine; Naturopathy; Popular practitioners; Self-care; Spirituality; Traditional Chinese herbal medicine; Traditional healing.

Intermittent claudication

CATEGORY: Condition

RELATED TERM: Peripheral vascular disease

DEFINITION: Treatment of severe muscle pain caused by blocked arteries in the legs.

PRINCIPAL PROPOSED NATURAL TREATMENTS: *Ginkgo biloba*, inositol hexaniacinate, L-carnitine, mesoglycan

OTHER PROPOSED NATURAL TREATMENTS: Arginine, beta-carotene or vitamin E, or a combination of the two, policosanol

INTRODUCTION

The arteries supplying the legs with blood may become seriously blocked in advanced stages of atherosclerosis (commonly, if somewhat incorrectly, known as hardening of the arteries). This can lead to severe, cramping pain when walking more than a short distance, because the muscles are starved for oxygen. This condition is called intermittent claudication. The intensity of intermittent claudication is often measured in the distance a person can walk without pain.

Conventional treatment for intermittent claudication consists of measures to combat atherosclerosis and the use of the drug Trental (pentoxifylline) and other medications. In advanced cases, surgery to improve blood flow may be necessary.

PRINCIPAL PROPOSED NATURAL TREATMENTS

A number of natural treatments may be helpful for intermittent claudication, but it is not clear whether it is safe to combine them with the medications that may be prescribed at the same time. Medical supervision is definitely necessary for this serious disease.

Ginkgo. Many studies support the effectiveness of ginkgo for intermittent claudication. According to nine double-blind, placebo-controlled trials, ginkgo can significantly increase pain-free walking distance, presumably by increasing circulation.

One study enrolled 111 persons and followed them for twenty-four weeks. Participants were measured for pain-free walking distance by walking up a 12 percent slope on a treadmill at two miles per hour. At the beginning of treatment, both the placebo and ginkgo (120 milligrams [mg]) groups were able to walk about 350 feet without pain. At the end of the trial, although both groups had improved, the ginkgo group had improved significantly more, showing about a 40 percent increase in pain-free walking distance compared to only a 20 percent improvement in the placebo group. Similar improvements were seen in a double-blind, placebo-controlled trial of sixty persons who had achieved maximum benefit from physical therapy.

Taking a higher dose of ginkgo may provide enhanced benefits in intermittent claudication. A twenty-four-week, double-blind, placebo-controlled study of seventy-four persons found that ginkgo at a dose of 240 mg per day was more effective than 120 mg per day. A 2009 review of eleven trials with 477 persons suggested that those who took ginkgo could walk farther than control subjects, but these results are limited by differences among the trials.

However, not all studies have been positive. In another randomized trial involving sixty-two persons (averaging seventy years of age), 300 mg of ginkgo per day was no better than placebo at improving pain-free walking distance in four months of treatment.

L-carnitine. The vitamin-like substance L-carnitine also appears to be of some benefit in intermittent claudication. Although it does not increase blood flow, carnitine appears to increase walking distance by improving energy utilization in the muscles.

A twelve-month, double-blind, placebo-controlled trial of 485 persons with intermittent claudication evaluated the potential benefits of a special form of carnitine called propionyl-L-carnitine. Participants with relatively severe disease showed a 44 percent improvement in walking distance compared with placebo. However, no improvement was seen in those with mild disease. Benefits were seen in most other studies using L-carnitine or propionyl-L-carnitine.

Inositol hexaniacinate. The supplement inositol hexaniacinate, a special form of vitamin B_3, appears to be helpful for intermittent claudication. Double-blind studies involving about four hundred persons found that the supplement can improve walking distance for people with intermittent claudication. For example, in one study, one hundred persons were given either placebo or 4 grams of inositol hexaniacinate daily. In three months, participants improved significantly in the number of steps they could take on a special device before experiencing excessive pain.

Mesoglycan. Mesoglycan is a substance found in many tissues in the body, including the joints, intestines, and the lining of blood vessels. A twenty-week, double-blind, placebo-controlled trial that enrolled

242 people evaluated the effects of mesoglycan in intermittent claudication. Significantly more participants in the mesoglycan group responded to treatment (defined as a greater than 50 percent improvement in walking distance) than in the placebo group.

OTHER PROPOSED NATURAL TREATMENTS

The supplement arginine has been tried for treatment of intermittent claudication. Two poorly designed studies had suggested benefit. However, the most recent, largest, and best-designed trial not only failed to find arginine effective, but the results suggested that arginine can actually increase symptoms of intermittent claudication.

Various antioxidants have been suggested for the treatment of intermittent claudication. However, a double-blind, placebo-controlled trial of 1,484 persons with intermittent claudication found no benefit from vitamin E (50 mg daily), beta-carotene (20 mg daily), or a combination of the two.

According to a few studies performed in Cuba, the sugarcane-derived substance policosanol is helpful for intermittent claudication. Numerous other Cuban studies reported that sugarcane policosanol lowers cholesterol. However, all these studies were performed by a single set of researchers, and they are financially connected to the product. Several independent studies that attempted to replicate the cholesterol-related results failed to find benefit. For this reason, all claims associated with policosanol are in doubt. One small study found weak preliminary evidence that lipoic acid might improve symptoms in intermittent claudication.

HERBS AND SUPPLEMENTS TO USE WITH CAUTION

Various herbs and supplements may interact adversely with drugs used to treat intermittent claudication.

EBSCO CAM Review Board

FURTHER READING

Castano, G., et al. "Effects of Policosanol and Lovastatin in Patients with Intermittent Claudication." *Angiology* 54 (2003): 25-38.

Gardner, C. D., et al. "Effect of *Ginkgo biloba* (EGb 761) on Treadmill Walking Time Among Adults with Peripheral Artery Disease." *Journal of Cardiopulmonary Rehabilitation and Prevention* 28 (2008): 258-265.

Hiatt, W. R., et al. "Propionyl-L-Carnitine Improves Exercise Performance and Functional Status in Patients with Claudication." *American Journal of Medicine* 110 (2001): 616-622.

Nenci, G. G., et al. "Treatment of Intermittent Claudication with Mesoglycan." *Thrombosis and Haemostasis* 86 (2001): 1181-1187.

Nicolai, S., et al. "*Ginkgo biloba* for Intermittent Claudication." *Cochrane Database of Systematic Reviews* (2009): CD006888. Available through *EBSCO DynaMed Systematic Literature Surveillance* at http://www.ebscohost.com/dynamed.

Vincent, H. K., et al. "Effects of Alpha-Lipoic Acid Supplementation in Peripheral Arterial Disease." *Journal of Alternative and Complementary Medicine* 13 (2007): 577-584.

Wilson, A. M., et al. "L-Arginine Supplementation in Peripheral Arterial Disease: No Benefit and Possible Harm." *Circulation* 116 (2007): 188-195.

See also: Carnitine; Ginkgo; Mesoglycan; Pain management; Policosanol; Venous insufficiency: Homeopathic remedies; Vitamin B_3.

The Internet and CAM

CATEGORY: Issues and overviews
DEFINITION: Overview of online resources on complementary and alternative medicine.

OVERVIEW

The Internet, also called the Web, is an extremely popular source of information on countless topics, including complementary and alternative medicine (CAM). The Internet provides current, comprehensive, and searchable information on any CAM topic, which gives the Internet an advantage over traditional forms of media, such as print. However, because virtually anyone can publish information on the Internet through personal Web sites and blogs, Web-based information can be worthless, and relying on it can even be detrimental.

The most reliable information can be obtained from sources such as university medical centers; from PubMed, the public research database that includes millions of citations for biomedical literature, run by the National Center for Biotechnology Information of the National Institutes of Health (NIH); from the Centers for Disease Control and Prevention (CDC); and from the World Health Organization (WHO).

Although focused on conventional medicine, these entities and others like them are paying increasing attention to CAM, which is gaining popularity throughout

---

Researching CAM on the Web

Dietary supplements—vitamins, minerals, herbs or other botanicals, amino acids, and substances such as enzymes, organ tissues, and metabolites—compose a significant portion of the complementary and alternative medicine (CAM) industry. Information on these products abounds on CAM-related Web sites. Yet the effectiveness of many of these supplements remains unproven. The following guidelines can help one prepare in searching the Web for information on CAM.

- *What Is On the Web?* There is no shortage of data regarding dietary supplements on the Web. Many sites dedicated to oral health supplements are retail sites selling products or are sites that link directly to a vendor. Many of these sites claim to treat, prevent, diagnose, or even cure specific diseases. How credible are these claims? Other sites are personal sites without links to vendors; government, industry, or academic sites describing particular supplements; and sites containing referenced articles about the supplements.

- *False Claims.* Web-based health claims about supplements are not always true. Researchers have found that many Web sites contain incorrect or misleading statements, some of which can directly result in serious harm to health consumers.

- *Failure to Disclose Information.* However, it is not only the claims made on these Web sites that can be misleading. The information many sites choose *not* to disclose can be equally dangerous. Some retail CAM sites omit the standard federal disclaimer, which informs the user that the site's information is general in nature and that it cannot take the place of medical evaluation, diagnosis, and treatment by a health care provider.

  Many sites do not disclose potential adverse health effects such as heart attacks, strokes, arrhythmias, increased blood pressure, and heart palpitations; and others leave out the recommended dosage of supplements. Essentially, the information, or lack thereof, presented on CAM-related Web sites, which are intended to enhance one's health, may actually jeopardize it.

- *Lack of Federal Regulation.* The 1994 passage of the Dietary Supplement and Health and Education Act (DSHEA), which states that manufacturers do not

have to prove the safety or efficacy of a dietary supplement before it is placed on the market, limited the U.S. Food and Drug Administration's (FDA's) control over dietary supplements. The act also made it easier for less-than-reliable information regarding dietary supplements to reach consumers through the Web.

Although the DSHEA stripped some of the FDA control over dietary supplements and placed the burden of determining the safety and efficacy of these supplements more heavily on the consumer, it did not leave consumers completely without guidance.

- *Government Supports Research on Dietary Supplements.* When the DSHEA passed, the U.S. Congress established the Office of Dietary Supplements (ODS) at the National Institutes of Health (NIH) to promote a greater understanding of dietary supplements. To this end, the ODS evaluates scientific information on supplements, stimulates and supports research, and disseminates results to the public. The ODS Web site contains a database of federally funded research projects on dietary supplements. The site offers information about the ingredients found in dietary supplements and about related health outcomes and biological effects.

- *Tips for Navigating CAM Web Sites.* Paying close attention to the language CAM Web sites use to describe supplements can also alert the user to false or misleading information. One should be aware of the following:

  - Vague claims, such as "breakthrough," "miracle cure," and "magical," which present no legitimate research to support them

  - Use of pseudomedical jargon, such as "detoxify" or "purify," to describe a product's effects

  - Claims that a product is backed by scientific studies, without references to those studies

  - Failure to list side effects

  - Accusations that the government, the medical profession, or drug companies are suppressing information about a given supplement

Elizabeth Heubeck, M.A.;
reviewed by Brian P. Randall, M.D.

the United States and Europe. On PubMed, one can limit searches to citations related to CAM.

CAM's POPULARITY

The information available on the Internet would have little impact if interest in CAM were lacking; in fact, interest is surging. A 2011 study conducted by researchers at the University of Texas evaluated the reasons for CAM's increasing popularity. One of the study's researchers, Dejun Su, noted that "The rising cost of healthcare is outpacing inflation and salaries, and there's a good possibility that that is linked to increasing CAM use." Su added that CAM usage has been increasing in acceptance for a number of years. In 1990, one-third of all Americans had tried some form of CAM; by 2002, that number had nearly doubled, and the numbers are continuing to increase.

The study compared data from the 2002 and 2007 National Health Interview Surveys, which are conducted annually by the National Center for Health Statistics (a subsidiary of the CDC), which tracks the health-care status of Americans and tracks their access to the system. Overall, the United States saw a 14 percent increase in the use of CAM from 2002 to 2007. Among the most popular forms of CAM were massage and chiropractic care.

In June 2010, representatives of the Chinese ministry of health visited the University of California, Los Angeles (UCLA), to learn how traditional Chinese medicine and integrative medicine are practiced in the United States as a new health-care model. Also, UCLA's Center for East-West Medicine is collaborating with China to develop an online informational library on integrative medicine. The Center is also creating an Internet-based multimedia resource for clinicians, educators, and consumers.

PURCHASING CAM PRODUCTS ON THE WEB

Herbal products, for example, are widely available for sale through commercial Web sites. The herbal product digitalis, which is used for the treatment of heart conditions, is derived from the foxglove shrub (*Digitalis lanata*). Quinine, which has a number of medicinal uses (as, for example, an antimalarial and an analgesic) is derived from the bark of the cinchona tree (*Cinchona* species).

Because herbal products are natural products, they do not fall under the jurisdiction of government agencies such as the U.S. Food and Drug Administration (FDA). The FDA requires a rigorous testing process before a drug can be made available to the general public. No such oversight occurs with herbal products. Medical experts fear that some persons with serious medical conditions, such as malignant cancers, will purchase worthless products through the Web and fail to seek conventional medical care for life-threatening illnesses.

INTERNET RESOURCES

Much of the Internet is devoted to the marketing of products or services. One can purchase natural products and can locate CAM practitioners (such as acupuncturists and massage therapists) and instructors (such as in yoga and meditation). Also, Web sites exists for persons seeking general information about CAM. The simplest method for information gathering is via a search engine. For example, searching on the phrase "prostate and saw palmetto" reveals information on the use of saw palmetto for benign prostatic hypertrophy. Search results will include links to scientific papers, but also to anecdotal accounts and commercial sites. The sites of the following resources, however, provide focused research articles and other trustworthy information.

The National Center for Complementary and Alternative Medicine (NCCAM), a component of the National Institutes of Health, conducts scientific research on the diverse medical and health-care systems, practices, and products that are not generally considered part of conventional medicine. The organization states that its mission is "to define, through rigorous scientific investigation, the usefulness and safety of complementary and alternative medicine interventions and their roles in improving health and healthcare."

NCCAM has four primary areas of focus: It funds research projects at scientific institutions both in the United States and globally; supports training programs for new researchers and encourages existing researchers to investigate CAM; provides timely, accurate information through its Web site, through social media such as Twitter and Facebook and through its information clearinghouse, fact sheets, and continuing medical education programs; and promotes those CAM therapies proven safe and effective.

PubMed contains a searchable database of published scientific papers on many medical topics, including CAM.

The Web site of the CDC, a U.S. government organization focused on maintaining and improving health, features a comprehensive list of diseases and conditions (communicable, genetic, environmental, and self-inflicted), healthy living, and traveler's health.

WHO, the health authority within the United Nations system, "is responsible for providing leadership on global health matters, shaping the health research agenda, setting norms and standards, articulating evidence-based policy options, providing technical support to countries and monitoring and assessing health trends." The organization's Web site contains informative links on a variety of health topics and publications. Although WHO is focused on conventional medicine, it also provides information on CAM.

While most medical centers in the United States contain public information on conventional medicine, many also provide CAM resources through searchable databases. Medical centers with searchable databases include the Mayo Clinic (http://www.mayo-clinic.com) and the UCLA Medical Center (http://www.uclahealth.org).

Robin L. Wulffson, M.D., FACOG

FURTHER READING

Crawford, Gregory A. *The Medical Library Association Guide to Finding out About Complementary and Alternative Medicine: The Best Print and Electronic Resources.* New York: Neal-Schuman, 2010. A comprehensive resource on CAM, with coverage of both Web-based and print sources.

Freeman, Lyn. *Mosby's Complementary and Alternative Medicine: A Research-Based Approach.* 3d ed. St. Louis, Mo.: Mosby/Elsevier, 2009. Providing a comprehensive overview, this text includes practical, clinically relevant coverage of CAM, with commentary by well-known experts, descriptions of medical advances, case studies, and discussion of the history and philosophy of each discipline.

Health On the Net Foundation. United Nations. http://www.hon.ch.

Hock, Randolph. *The Extreme Searcher's Internet Handbook: A Guide for the Serious Searcher.* 3d ed. Medford, N.J.: CyberAge Books, 2010. A guide to Internet research for librarians, teachers, students, writers, business professionals, and health consumers.

Micozzi, Marc S., ed. *Fundamentals of Complementary and Alternative Medicine.* 4th ed. St. Louis, Mo.: Saunders/Elsevier, 2011. An evidence-based approach that focuses on treatments best supported by clinical trials and scientific studies. Covers the foundations of CAM, traditional Western healing, and traditional healing systems of Asia, Africa, and the Americas.

National Center for Complementary and Alternative Medicine (NCCAM). http://nccam.nih.gov.

Owen, David J. *The Herbal Internet Companion: Herbs and Herbal Medicine Online.* New York: Haworth Information Press, 2002. A guide to herbal products and herbal medicine on the Web.

PubMed. National Center for Biotechnology Information. http://www.ncbi.nlm.nih.gov/pubmed.

World Health Organization. http://www.who.int.

See also: CAM on PubMed; National Center for Complementary and Alternative Medicine; Office of Dietary Supplements; Popular practitioners of CAM; Pseudoscience; Regulation of CAM.

Interstitial cystitis

CATEGORY: Condition

DEFINITION: Treatment of severe and chronic inflammation of the bladder.

PRINCIPAL PROPOSED NATURAL TREATMENTS: None

OTHER PROPOSED NATURAL TREATMENTS: Arginine, dietary changes, glycosaminoglycans, guided imagery, quercetin, transcutaneous electrical stimulation

INTRODUCTION

Interstitial cystitis (IC) is a severe, chronic inflammation of the bladder that is both disruptive and painful. Many more women than men have the condition. Of the 700,000 people with IC at any given time, 90 percent are female.

The symptoms of IC are notoriously variable and can differ from one person to another, or for one person from day to day. People with IC usually have an urgent and frequent need to urinate. They may experience recurring discomfort, tenderness, pressure, or intense pain in the bladder and surrounding pelvic area. This pain often intensifies as the bladder fills and may be exacerbated by sexual intercourse. Certain foods may trigger symptoms; the most commonly mentioned include tomatoes, vinegar, spicy foods, coffee, chocolate, alcohol, and fruits and vegetables.

IC is generally diagnosed after other conditions with similar symptoms, such as bladder infection, herpes, and vaginal infection, have been excluded. The cause of IC is unknown. Although its symptoms resemble a bladder infection, IC does not appear to be caused by bacteria. One theory proposes that IC is caused by an infectious agent that simply has not been detected. A different theory holds that IC is an autoimmune reaction; still another theory is that it is related to allergies. Because it varies so much in symptoms and severity, IC may be not one disease but several.

A variety of treatments are often tried alone or in combination before one is found that works. Oral antihistamines such as hydroxyzine (Atarax) and certirizine (Zyrtec) may provide relief, and the drowsiness they produce often wears off over time. Other medications used for IC include pentosan polysulfate sodium (Elmiron), pyridium, and anti-inflammatory drugs.

Distending the bladder by filling it to capacity with water for two to eight minutes is frequently useful, but although the beneficial effects may persist for months, symptoms usually return eventually. In some cases, medications such as dimethyl sulfoxide and heparin may be introduced into the bladder with a catheter; actual surgical alteration of the bladder is rarely used to treat IC.

OTHER PROPOSED TREATMENTS

There are no well-documented natural treatments for interstitial cystitis, but a few supplements have shown promise.

Quercetin. Quercetin is a bioflavonoid that may have anti-inflammatory properties. A small, double-blind, placebo-controlled trial found that a supplement containing quercetin reduced symptoms of interstitial cystitis.

Arginine. The amino acid arginine helps the body make nitric oxide, a substance that relaxes smooth muscles like those found in the bladder. Based on this mechanism, arginine has been proposed as a treatment for IC.

A three-month double-blind trial of fifty-three persons with interstitial cystitis found only weak indications that arginine might improve symptoms of interstitial cystitis. Several participants dropped out of the study; when this was properly taken into account using a statistical method called ITT analysis, no benefit could be proven.

Glycosaminoglycans. There is some evidence that in interstitial cystitis, the surface layer of the bladder is deficient in protective natural substances called glycosaminoglycans. This in turn might allow the bladder to become inflamed; it might also initiate autoimmune reactions.

Based on these preliminary findings, the use of supplemental glycosaminoglycans in the form of mesoglycan or chondroitin sulfate has been suggested for interstitial cystitis. However, there is no reliable evidence that they really work.

Transcutaneous electrical stimulation. Transcutaneous electrical stimulation is primarily used (with mixed results) in the treatment of muscular pain. It has also been tried for interstitial cystitis, but the evidence that it works is preliminary.

Diet. Although there is no solid scientific evidence that dietary changes can relieve IC, many people find that certain foods increase their symptoms. The most frequently cited offenders are coffee, chocolate, ethanol, carbonated drinks, citrus fruits, and tomatoes. Based on these reports, it may be worthwhile to experiment with one's diet.

Guided imagery. Preliminary evidence suggests that guided imagery may help some women with IC. In one study, listening to a script designed to focus attention on healing the bladder, relaxing the pelvic-floor muscles, and quieting the nerves specifically involved in IC showed some benefit. Without an adequate placebo comparison, though, it is questionable whether these improvements were significant.

EBSCO CAM Review Board

FURTHER READING

Carrico, D. J., K. M. Peters, and A. C. Diokno. "Guided Imagery for Women with Interstitial Cystitis." *Journal of Alternative and Complementary Medicine* 14 (2008): 53-60.

Cartledge, J. J., A. M. Davies, and I. Eardley. "A Randomized Double-Blind Placebo-Controlled Crossover Trial of the Efficacy of L-Arginine in the Treatment of Interstitial Cystitis." *BJU International* 85 (2000): 421-426.

Palylyk-Colwell, E. "Chondroitin Sulfate for Interstitial Cystitis." *Issues in Emerging Health Technologies* 84 (2006): 1-4.

See also: Arginine; Bladder infection; Vaginal infection; Women's health.

Iodine

CATEGORY: Herbs and supplements

RELATED TERMS: Elemental iodine, iodide

DEFINITION: Natural substance of the human body used as a supplement to treat specific health conditions.

PRINCIPAL PROPOSED USE: Nutritional deficiency

OTHER PROPOSED USE: Cyclic mastalgia

OVERVIEW

The thyroid gland, located just above the middle of the collarbone, needs iodine to make thyroid hormone, which maintains normal metabolism in all cells of the body. Principally found in sea water, dietary iodine can be scarce in many inland areas, and deficiencies were common before iodine was added to table salt. Iodine deficiency causes enlargement of the thyroid, a condition known as goiter.

However, if a person is not deficient in iodine, taking extra iodine will not help the thyroid work better, and it might even cause problems. For reasons that are not clear, supplementary iodine might also be helpful for cyclic mastalgia.

REQUIREMENTS AND SOURCES

The official U.S. recommendations (in micrograms) for daily intake of iodine are as follows:

Infants to six months of age (110) and seven to twelve months (130); children one to eight years (90);

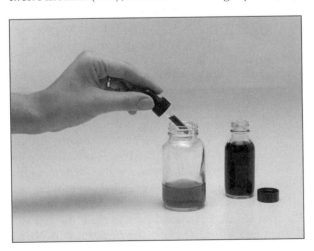

Iodine being dropped into a bottle of water, foreground. Bottle of iodine in the background. (Clive Streeter/Getty Images)

males and females nine to thirteen years (120) and fourteen years and older (150); pregnant women (220); and nursing women (290).

Iodine deficiency is rare in developed countries today because of the use of iodized salt. Seafood and kelp contain very high levels of iodine, as do salty processed foods that use iodized salt. Most iodine is in the form of iodide, but a few studies suggest that a special form of iodine called molecular iodine may be better than iodide.

THERAPEUTIC DOSAGES

A typical therapeutic dosage of iodide or iodine is 200 micrograms daily.

THERAPEUTIC USES

Iodine supplements have been proposed as a treatment for cyclic mastalgia. Cyclic mastalgia is characterized by breast pain and lumpiness that usually cycles in relation to the menstrual period.

SCIENTIFIC EVIDENCE

Three clinical studies provide weak evidence that supplements providing iodine may be helpful in treating cyclic mastalgia. These studies suggest that either iodide or iodine (the pure molecular form) might be useful. In the one double-blind, placebo-controlled trial among this group, a study that enrolled fifty-six individuals, molecular iodine was found superior to placebo in relieving pain and reducing the number of cysts.

Another of these studies compared molecular iodine to iodide. Molecular iodine was no more effective than iodide but was deemed superior because it induced fewer side effects and did not affect the thyroid.

SAFETY ISSUES

When taken at the recommended dosage, iodine and iodide are safe nutritional supplements. However, excessive doses of iodide can actually cause thyroid problems, including both hypothyroidism and hyperthyroidism. There is also a speculative link between excessive iodide intake and thyroid cancer. For these reasons, iodide intake above nutritional recommendations is not advised except under physician supervision.

EBSCO CAM Review Board

FURTHER READING

Ghent, W. R., et al. "Iodine Replacement in Fibrocystic Disease of the Breast." *Canadian Journal of Surgery* 36 (1993): 453-460.

See also: Breast pain, cyclic; Hyperthyroidism.

Ipriflavone

CATEGORY: Herbs and supplements
DEFINITION: Natural plant product used to treat specific health conditions.
PRINCIPAL PROPOSED USE: Osteoporosis
OTHER PROPOSED USE: Bodybuilding

OVERVIEW

Isoflavones are water-soluble chemicals found in many plants. Ipriflavone is a semisynthetic version of an isoflavone found in soy.

Soy isoflavones have effects in the body somewhat similar to those of estrogen. This should be beneficial, but it is possible that soy could also present some of the risks of estrogen. In 1969, a research project was initiated to manufacture a type of isoflavone that would possess the bone-stimulating effects of estrogen without any estrogen-like activity elsewhere in the body. Such a product would help prevent osteoporosis but cause no other health risks.

Ipriflavone was the result. After seven successful years of experiments with animals, human research was started in 1981. Today, ipriflavone is available in more than twenty-two countries and in most drugstores in the United States as a nonprescription dietary supplement. It is an accepted treatment for osteoporosis in Italy, Turkey, and Japan.

According to all but one study, ipriflavone combined with calcium can slow and perhaps slightly reverse bone breakdown. It also seems to help reduce the pain of fractures caused by osteoporosis. However, since it does not appear to have any estrogenic effects anywhere else in the body, it should not increase the risk of breast or uterine cancer. On the other hand, it will not reduce the hot flashes, night sweats, mood changes, or vaginal dryness of menopause, nor will it prevent heart disease. A large study found that ipriflavone might reduce white blood cell count in some individuals.

REQUIREMENTS AND SOURCES

Ipriflavone is not an essential nutrient and is not found in food. It must be taken as a supplement.

THERAPEUTIC DOSAGES

The proper dosage of ipriflavone is 200 milligrams (mg) three times daily, or 300 mg twice daily. A calcium supplement providing 1,000 mg of calcium daily should be taken as well.

THERAPEUTIC USES

Ipriflavone appears to be able to slow down and perhaps slightly reverse osteoporosis. It may be helpful for this purpose in ordinary postmenopausal osteoporosis, as well as in osteoporosis caused by medications. Ipriflavone also seems to ease the pain of fractures caused by osteoporosis. Ipriflavone has also been proposed as a bodybuilding aid, but there is no meaningful evidence that it is helpful for this purpose.

SCIENTIFIC EVIDENCE

Numerous double-blind, placebo-controlled studies involving a total of more than 1,700 participants have examined the effects of ipriflavone on various forms of osteoporosis. Overall, it appears that ipriflavone can slow the progression of osteoporosis and perhaps reverse it to some extent. For example, a two-year, double-blind study followed 198 postmenopausal women who showed evidence of bone loss. At the end of the study, there was a gain in bone density of 1 percent in the ipriflavone group and a loss of 0.7 percent in the placebo group. These numbers may sound small, but they can add up to a lot of bone over time.

However, the largest and longest study of ipriflavone found no benefit. In this three-year trial of 474 postmenopausal women, no differences in the extent of osteoporosis were seen between the ipriflavone and placebo groups. How can this failure be accounted for in view of all the successful trials that came before? Perhaps because the researchers in this study gave women only 500 mg of calcium daily. All other major studies of ipriflavone gave participants 1,000 mg of calcium daily. It is possible that ipriflavone requires the higher dose of calcium in order to work properly.

Ipriflavone, like estrogen, probably works by fighting bone breakdown. However, there is some evidence that it may also increase new bone formation.

Combining ipriflavone with estrogen may enhance antiosteoporosis benefits. However, it is not known for sure whether such combinations increase or reduce the other risks, or benefits, of estrogen.

Ipriflavone may also be helpful for preventing osteoporosis in women who are taking Lupron or corticosteroids, medications that accelerate bone loss. However, the combined use of ipriflavone and drugs that suppress the immune system, such as corticosteroids, presents potential risks. Finally, for reasons that are not clear, ipriflavone appears to be able to reduce pain in osteoporosis-related fractures that have already occurred.

SAFETY ISSUES

About three thousand people have used ipriflavone in clinical studies, and in all but two, no significant adverse effects were seen. However, these trials (a three-year, double-blind trial of almost five hundred women, as well as a small study) found worrisome evidence that ipriflavone can reduce levels of white blood cells called lymphocytes. For this reason, anyone taking ipriflavone for the long term should have periodic measurements taken of white blood cell count.

In addition, ipriflavone should not be used by anyone with immune deficiencies, such as human immunodeficiency virus (HIV), or by those who take drugs that suppress the immune system, except under physician supervision. There are other potential risks. Because ipriflavone is metabolized by the kidneys, individuals with severe kidney disease should have their ipriflavone dosage monitored by a physician. Individuals with ulcers should also avoid ipriflavone.

In addition, although ipriflavone itself does not affect tissues outside of bone, some evidence suggests that if it is combined with estrogen, estrogen's effects on the uterus are increased. This might mean that the risk of uterine cancer would be elevated over taking estrogen alone. It should be possible to overcome this risk by taking progesterone along with estrogen, which is standard medical practice. However, this finding does make one wonder whether ipriflavone-estrogen combinations also raise the risk of breast cancer, an estrogen side effect that has no easy solution. At present, there is no available information on this important subject.

Additionally, ipriflavone may interfere with certain drugs by affecting the way they are processed in the liver. For example, it may raise blood levels of the older asthma drug theophylline. It could also raise levels of caffeine, meaning that if individuals drink coffee while taking ipriflavone, they might stay up longer than they expect. Ipriflavone could also interact with tolbutamide (a drug for diabetes), phenytoin (used for epilepsy), and Coumadin (a blood thinner). Such interactions are potentially dangerous, especially since phenytoin and Coumadin cause osteoporosis, and some people might be tempted to try taking ipriflavone at the same time.

IMPORTANT INTERACTIONS

Individuals who are taking theophylline, tolbutamide, phenytoin (Dilantin), warfarin (Coumadin), or any other drug metabolized in the liver should be aware that ipriflavone might change the levels of that drug in their bodies. For people who are taking estrogen, ipriflavone might help estrogen strengthen their bones even more. However, it might also increase the risk of uterine cancer. Drugs that suppress the immune system, such as corticosteroids, methotrexate, or cyclosporine, should not be used simultaneously with ipriflavone except under medical supervision.

EBSCO CAM Review Board

FURTHER READING

Agnusdei, D., and L. Bufalino. "Efficacy of Ipriflavone in Established Osteoporosis and Long-Term Safety." *Calcified Tissue International* 61 (1997): S23.

Alexandersen, P., et al. "Ipriflavone in the Treatment of Postmenopausal Osteoporosis." *Journal of the American Medical Association* 285 (2001): 1482-1488.

Maugeri, D., et al. "Ipriflavone-Treatment of Senile Osteoporosis." *Archives of Gerontology and Geriatrics* 19 (1994): 253-263.

Moscarini, M., et al. "New Perspectives in the Treatment of Postmenopausal Osteoporosis: Ipriflavone." *Gynecological Endocrinology* 8 (1994): 203-207.

Scali, G., et al. "Analgesic Effect of Ipriflavone Versus Scalcitonin in the Treatment of Osteoporotic Vertebral Pain." *Current Therapeutic Research* 49 (1991): 1004-1010.

See also: Estrogen; Isoflavone; Osteoporosis; Soy; Sports and fitness support: Enhancing performance.

Iridology

CATEGORY: Therapies and techniques
RELATED TERMS: Iris diagnosis, sclerology
DEFINITION: The alternative technique of predicting a person's state of health by examining the iris of his or her eye.
PRINCIPAL PROPOSED USE: Diagnosis

OVERVIEW

Hungarian physician Ignatz von Péczely invented the technique known as iridology in the nineteenth century. After studying the iris, the part of the eye that determines its color, Péczely suggested a direct relationship between the markings in the iris and tissue changes and organ function in the body.

MECHANISM OF ACTION

Iridology assumes that every organ in the human body is connected by nerve impulses to a particular location in the iris. The health of an organ can be predicted by examining patterns in the iris using a magnifying glass and a flashlight, and then using computer analysis of photographs of the eye rather than examining the organ itself to predict a person's health.

USES AND APPLICATIONS

Iridology claims that the patterns, structures, colors, and degrees of lightness or darkness in the iris reveal sites of irritation, injury, degeneration, or disease of specific tissues and organs. Levels of toxicity, and nutritional and chemical imbalances, can be observed. Appropriate action can then be taken to cleanse and strengthen the body.

SCIENTIFIC EVIDENCE

The medical profession recognizes that certain symptoms of nonocular disease (those diseases affecting a part of the body other than the eyes) can be detected by examination of the eye. Iridolgy goes much further by suggesting that the state of a particular organ in the human body, and not only disease symptoms, can be determined by looking at a particular section of the iris. Iridology charts divide the iris into zones and link each zone with different organs of the body.

Many rigorous double-blind tests have found no significance to the claims of iridology, mainly because the fundamental premise of iridology contradicts the medical observation that the iris does not undergo any substantial change during a person's life. Research has indicated that the iris of each person is unique and virtually unchangeable.

In 1979, three prominent iridologists failed a scientific test in which they examined photographs of the irises of 143 people. The practitioners typically identified sick people as healthy and vice versa, with much disagreement among the findings of these practitioners. In the late 1980s, five Dutch iridologists failed to distinguish between thirty-nine people with gall bladder disease and thirty-nine healthy persons. In 2005, a well-known iridologist examined the photographs of the irises of 110 people, 68 of whom had common forms of cancer. He correctly diagnosed only 3 of the 68 people. In still other controlled experiments, iridologists have performed statistically no better than chance in determining the health of a person by examination of the iris.

SAFETY ISSUES

Although iridology is safe, the misinterpretation of the condition of organs by a practitioner of iridology can unnecessarily frighten people, lead them to spend money seeking medical care for nonexistent problems, or create a false sense of security that can defer or delay needed medical care if an actual health problem does exist.

Alvin K. Benson, Ph.D.

FURTHER READING

Barrett, Stephen, and William T. Jarvis, eds. *The Health Robbers: A Close Look at Quackery in America.* Amherst, N.Y.: Prometheus Books, 1993.
Ernst, E. "Iridology: Not Useful and Potentially Harmful." *Archives of Ophthalmology* 118 (2000): 120-121.
Jensen, Bernard. *The Science and Practice of Iridology.* 2 vols. Winona Lake, Ind.: Whitman, 2005.

See also: Bates method; Night vision, impaired.

Iron

CATEGORY: Herbs and supplements
RELATED TERMS: Chelated iron, iron sulfate
DEFINITION: Natural substance of the human body used as a supplement to treat specific health conditions.

PRINCIPAL PROPOSED USES: Iron deficiency, sports performance enhancement

OTHER PROPOSED USES: Attention deficit disorder, enhancing mental function in women, fatigue, human immunodeficiency virus infection support, menorrhagia, reducing side effects of angiotensin-converting enzyme-(ACE)inhibitor, restless legs syndrome, stimulating flow of saliva

OVERVIEW

The element iron is essential to human life. As part of hemoglobin, the oxygen-carrying protein found in red blood cells, iron plays an integral role in furnishing every cell in the body with oxygen. It also functions as a part of myoglobin, which helps muscle cells store oxygen. Without iron, the body could not make adenosine triphosphate (ATP, the body's primary energy source), produce deoxyribonucleic acid (DNA), or carry out many other critical processes.

Iron deficiency can lead to anemia, learning disabilities, impaired immune function, fatigue, and depression. However, individuals should not take iron supplements unless laboratory tests show that they are genuinely deficient in iron.

REQUIREMENTS AND SOURCES

The official U.S. recommendations (in milligrams) for daily intake of iron are as follows:

Infants to six months of age (0.27) and seven to twelve months (11); children one to three years (7) and four to eight years (10); males nine to thirteen years (8) and nineteen years and older (8); females

---

Iron and Mental Function

The element iron is essential to human life. Iron is an integral part of hemoglobin, the oxygen-carrying protein found in red blood cells. Marked iron deficiency causes a reduction in red cell size and in hemoglobin content known as iron-deficiency anemia; this in turn causes fatigue, depression, reduced immunity, impaired mental function, and many other symptoms. Iron-deficiency anemia caused by malnutrition is a common problem in developing countries, especially among children. In the United States, however, deficiency occurs most commonly in menstruating girls and women because of cyclical blood loss.

The famous "iron-poor blood" advertisements of the 1950s and 1960s popularized the notion that a majority of women could benefit from iron supplements. However, this idea still lacks widespread acceptance. According to conventional medical wisdom, iron deficiency does not cause symptoms until it reaches the point of causing anemia. In addition, during the 1980s and 1990s, a theory developed claiming that excess iron can increase the risk of heart disease and strokes. The value of iron supplements for women without iron-deficiency anemia is therefore quite controversial.

The situation has begun to change in recent years. The theory that excess iron is associated with increased heart attack has begun to lose ground, and at the same time, a growing body of evidence suggests that marginal iron deficiency does indeed cause problems.

The human body stores iron in the form of ferritin. Accumulating evidence indicates that nonanemic women with low ferritin levels may feel somewhat tired, and that iron supplementation might increase their energy and physical performance. Thus, the "iron-poor blood" advertisements have been partially vindicated. Furthermore, a study published in 2007 suggests that iron supplements may improve mental function in nonanemic women with low ferritin.

This study evaluated 149 women with varying levels of stored iron, ranging from adequate iron through mild deficiency to true iron-deficiency anemia. All participants were given either iron supplements or placebo for sixteen weeks.

At the beginning of the study, tests of mental function showed a direct relationship between iron status and brain function. On average, participants with anemia performed least well on these tests, while participants with mild iron deficiency performed in the middle and those with adequate iron did the best. By the end of the study, performance improved markedly among those who showed an increase in iron stores. In other words, those who were deficient in iron (whether anemic or not) benefited from iron supplements more than they benefited from placebo. However, those who were not deficient did not show improvement.

One should not take iron supplements unless lab tests show that one is genuinely deficient. However, one should also check measures of iron storage (such as ferritin), because even mild iron deficiency, though too mild to cause anemia, may impair physical and mental function.

Steven Bratman, M.D.

nine to thirteen years (8), fourteen to eighteen years (15), nineteen to fifty years (18), and fifty years and older (9); pregnant women (27); and nursing women (9; 10 milligrams if age eighteen years or younger).

Iron deficiency is the most common nutrient deficiency in the world; worldwide, at least seven hundred million individuals have iron-deficiency anemia. Iron deficiency is widespread in the developing world, and it is prevalent in developed countries as well. Groups at high risk are children, teenage girls, menstruating women (especially those with excessively heavy menstruation, known as menorrhagia), pregnant women, and the elderly.

There are two major forms of iron: heme iron and nonheme iron. Heme iron is bound to the proteins hemoglobin or myoglobin, whereas nonheme iron is an inorganic compound. (In chemistry, "organic" has a very precise meaning that has nothing to do with farming. An organic compound contains carbon atoms. Thus, "inorganic iron" is an iron compound containing no carbon.) Heme iron, obtained from red meats and fish, is easily absorbed by the body. Nonheme iron, usually derived from plants, is less easily absorbed.

Rich sources of heme iron include oysters, meat, poultry, and fish. The main sources of nonheme iron are dried fruits, molasses, whole grains, legumes, leafy green vegetables, nuts, seeds, and kelp. Contrary to popular belief, there is no meaningful evidence that cooking in an iron skillet or pot provides a meaningful amount of iron supplementation.

Iron absorption may be affected by antibiotics in the quinolone (Floxin, Cipro) or tetracycline families, levodopa, methyldopa, carbidopa, penicillamine, thyroid hormone, captopril (and possibly other angiotensin-converting enzyme [ACE] inhibitors), calcium, soy, zinc, copper, manganese, or multivitamin/multimineral tablets. Conversely, iron may also inhibit the absorption of these drugs and supplements. In addition, drugs in the H_2 blocker or proton pump inhibitor families may impair iron absorption.

THERAPEUTIC DOSAGES

The typical short-term therapeutic dosage to correct iron deficiency is 100 to 200 milligrams (mg) daily. Once the body's stores of iron reach normal levels, however, this dose should be reduced to the lowest level that can maintain iron balance.

THERAPEUTIC USES

The most obvious use of iron supplements is to treat iron deficiency. Severe iron deficiency causes anemia, which in turn causes many symptoms. Iron deficiency that is too slight to cause anemia may also impair health. Several, though not all, double-blind trials suggest that mild iron deficiency might impair sports performance. In addition, a double-blind, placebo-controlled study of 144 women with unexplained fatigue who also had low or borderline-low levels of ferritin (a measure of stored iron) found that iron supplement enhanced energy and well-being. Another study found that iron supplements improved mental function in women who were iron-deficient. However, individuals should not take iron just because they feel tired; they should make sure to get tested to see whether they are indeed deficient. With iron, more is definitely not better.

Excessively heavy menstruation (menorrhagia) can certainly cause iron loss, and thereby may warrant iron supplements. Interestingly, a small double-blind trial found evidence that iron supplements might actually help reduce menstrual bleeding in women with menorrhagia who are also iron-deficient.

A study of seventy-one human-immunodeficiency-virus-positive (HIV-positive) children noted a high rate of iron deficiency. One observational study of 296 men with HIV infection linked high intake of iron to a decreased risk of acquired immunodeficiency syndrome (AIDS) six years later.

Individuals taking drugs in the ACE inhibitor family frequently develop a dry cough as a side effect. One study suggests that iron supplementation can alleviate this symptom. However, iron can interfere with ACE inhibitor absorption, so it should be taken at a different time of day.

Pregnant women commonly develop iron deficiency anemia. Iron supplements, however, can be hard on the stomach, thereby aggravating morning sickness. One study found evidence that a fairly low supplemental dose of iron (20 mg daily) is nearly as effective for treating anemia of pregnancy as 40 mg or even 80 mg daily and is less likely to cause gastrointestinal side effects.

Iron has been suggested as a treatment for attention deficit disorder. However, there is only preliminary evidence that it may effective in hyperactive children with low iron levels as indicated by ferritin levels.

Preliminary studies have linked low iron levels to restless legs syndrome. However, a small double-blind study found no benefit when iron supplements were given to healthy people, that is, those who were not iron-deficient. In addition, one study tested whether supplemental iron could increase rate of saliva flow, but it failed to find benefit.

SCIENTIFIC EVIDENCE

Sports performance. A double-blind, placebo-controlled trial of forty-two women without anemia but with evidence of slightly low iron reserves found that iron supplements significantly enhanced sports performance. Participants were put on a daily aerobic training program for the latter four weeks of this six-week trial. At the end of the trial, those receiving iron showed significantly greater gains in speed and endurance, compared with those given placebo. In addition, a double-blind, placebo-controlled study of forty elite athletes without anemia but with mildly low iron stores found that twelve weeks of iron supplementation enhanced aerobic performance.

Benefits with iron supplementation were observed in other double-blind trials also involving mild cases of low iron stores. However, other studies failed to find significant improvements, suggesting that the benefits of iron supplements for nonanemic, iron-deficient athletes are small at most.

Menorrhagia. One small double-blind study found good results using iron supplements to treat heavy menstruation. This study, which was performed in 1964, saw an improvement in 75 percent of the women who took iron, compared to 32.5 percent of those who took placebo. Women who began with higher iron levels did not respond to treatment. This suggests once more that supplementing with iron is a good idea only if an individual is deficient in it.

SAFETY ISSUES

Iron supplements commonly cause gastrointestinal upset, but when they are taken at recommended dosages, serious adverse consequences are unlikely. However, excessive dosages of iron can be toxic, damaging the intestines and liver and possibly resulting in death. Iron poisoning in children is a common problem, so iron supplements should be kept out of the reach of children.

Mildly excessive levels of iron may be unhealthy for another reason: Iron acts as an oxidant (the opposite of an antioxidant), perhaps increasing the risk of cancer and heart disease (although this is controversial). Elevated levels of iron may also play a role in brain injury caused by stroke. In addition, excess iron appears to increase complications of pregnancy, and if breast-fed infants who are not iron-deficient are given iron supplements, the effects may be negative rather than positive.

The simultaneous use of iron supplements and high-dose vitamin C can greatly increase iron absorption, possibly leading to excessive iron levels in the body. One study found that iron does not impair absorption of the drug methotrexate.

IMPORTANT INTERACTIONS

People who are taking antibiotics in the tetracycline or quinolone (Floxin, Cipro) families, levodopa, methyldopa, carbidopa, penicillamine, thyroid hormone, calcium, soy, zinc, copper, or manganese can avoid iron absorption problems by waiting at least two hours following their dose of medication or supplement before taking iron. Individuals who take drugs that reduce stomach acid, such as antacids, H_2 blockers, and proton pump inhibitors, may need extra iron.

Individuals taking iron simultaneously with high doses of vitamin C may be absorbing too much iron. For people taking ACE inhibitors, iron may reduce the coughing side effect; however, to avoid absorption problems, these individuals should wait at least two hours following their dose of medication before taking iron.

EBSCO CAM Review Board

FURTHER READING

Binkoski, A. E., et al. "Iron Supplementation Does Not Affect the Susceptibility of LDL to Oxidative Modification in Women with Low Iron Status." *Journal of Nutrition* 134 (2004): 99-103.

Dewey, K. G., et al. "Iron Supplementation Affects Growth and Morbidity of Breast-Fed Infants: Results of a Randomized Trial in Sweden and Honduras." *Journal of Nutrition* 132 (2002): 3249-3255.

Flink, H., et al. "Effect of Oral Iron Supplementation on Unstimulated Salivary Flow Rate." *Journal of Oral Pathology and Medicine* 35 (2006): 540-547.

Hamilton, S. F., et al. "The Effect of Ingestion of Ferrous Sulfate on the Absorption of Oral Methotrexate in Patients with Rheumatoid Arthritis." *Journal of Rheumatology* 30 (2003): 1948-1950.

Konofal, E., et al. "Effects of Iron Supplementation on Attention Deficit Hyperactivity Disorder in Children." *Pediatric Neurology* 38 (2008): 20-26.

Moriarty-Craige, S. E., et al. "Multivitamin-Mineral Supplementation Is Not as Efficacious as Is Iron Supplementation in Improving Hemoglobin Concentrations in Nonpregnant Anemic Women Living in Mexico." *American Journal of Clinical Nutrition* 80 (2004): 1308-1311.

Murray-Kolb, L. E., and J. L. Beard. "Iron Treatment Normalizes Cognitive Functioning in Young Women." *American Journal of Clinical Nutrition* 85 (2007): 778-787.

Sankaranarayanan, S., et al. "Daily Iron Alone but Not in Combination with Multimicronutrients Increases Plasma Ferritin Concentrations in Indonesian Infants with Inflammation." *Journal of Nutrition* 134 (2004): 1916-1922.

Sharieff, W., et al. "Is Cooking Food in Iron Pots an Appropriate Solution for the Control of Anaemia in Developing Countries? A Randomised Clinical Trial in Benin." *Public Health Nutrition* 9 (September, 2008): 971-977.

Verdon, F., et al. "Iron Supplementation for Unexplained Fatigue in Non-anaemic Women." *British Medical Journal* 326 (2003): 1124.

See also: Attention deficit disorder; Fatigue; HIV support; Iron; Restless legs syndrome; Sports and fitness support: Enhancing performance.

Irritable bowel syndrome

CATEGORY: Condition

RELATED TERM: Spastic colon

DEFINITION: Treatment of a chronic colon condition that occurs without an identifiable medical cause

PRINCIPAL PROPOSED NATURAL TREATMENTS: Flaxseed, peppermint oil, probiotics, traditional Chinese herbal medicine

OTHER PROPOSED NATURAL TREATMENTS: Acupuncture, avoidance of allergenic foods, *Coleus forskohlii*, digestive enzymes (including bromelain and other proteolytic enzymes), fructo-oligosaccharides, glutamine, hypnotherapy, melatonin, relaxation therapy, slippery elm

INTRODUCTION

The term "irritable bowel syndrome" (IBS) is used to describe chronic colon problems that occur in the absence of an identifiable medical cause. Common symptoms include alternating diarrhea and constipation, excess intestinal gas, intestinal cramping, uncomfortable bowel movements, abdominal discomfort following meals, and excessive awareness of the presence of stool in the colon. Despite all these distressing symptoms, in IBS, the intestines appear to be perfectly healthy when they are examined. Thus, the condition belongs to a category of diseases that physicians call "functional." This means that while the function of the bowel seems to have gone awry, no injury or disturbance of its structure can be discovered. (The analogous problem in the stomach is called dyspepsia, and the two conditions frequently overlap.)

Because the cause of IBS is not understood, conventional medical treatment of IBS is highly inadequate. One drug that had shown promise, Zelnorm, was withdrawn from the market for safety issues. Another, Lotronex, was temporarily withdrawn, and then approved again, but only under strict limitations. Other medical treatment approaches for IBS include increased dietary fiber, drugs that reduce bowel spasm, and drugs to address constipation or diarrhea as needed. In addition, various forms of psychotherapy, including hypnosis, have been tried, with some success.

PRINCIPAL PROPOSED NATURAL TREATMENTS

Peppermint. Peppermint oil is widely used for IBS, and the evidence suggests that it is probably useful. A majority of placebo-controlled studies have found peppermint oil to be more effective than placebo. However, most of these studies are small.

Probiotics. Numerous double-blind trials indicate that various probiotics (friendly bacteria) may be helpful for IBS. In a six-week, double-blind, placebo-controlled trial of 274 people with constipation-predominant IBS, in which constipation is a more significant symptom than diarrhea, the use of a probiotic formula containing the bacterium *Bifidobacterium animalis* significantly reduced discomfort and increased stool frequency. In another randomized trial, 266 women with constipation who consumed yogurt containing *B. animalis* and the prebiotic fructo-oligosaccharide twice daily for two weeks experienced significant improvement in their symptoms compared to women consuming regular yogurt as placebo. (Prebiotics are substances that encourage the growth of beneficial bacteria in the colon.)

Another study examined the effects of four weeks of treatment with the bacterium *Lactobacillus plantarum* on intestinal gas in sixty people with IBS. This study found benefits that persisted for an entire year after treatment stopped.

Benefits were seen also in eight other small double-blind trials, using *L. plantarum*, *L. acidophilus*, *L. rhamnosus*, *L. salivarus*, and *Bifidobacterium*, and proprietary probiotic combinations including various strains.

However, there have been a number of negative studies too. Two studies that pooled previous randomized trials on the use of probiotics for IBS came to similar conclusions: Probiotics appear to offer some benefit, most notably for global symptoms and abdominal discomfort. However, these two studies were unable to determine which probiotic species were most effective.

Flaxseed. In a double-blind study, fifty-five people with chronic constipation caused by IBS received either ground flaxseed or psyllium seed (a well-known treatment for constipation) daily for three months. Those taking flaxseed had significantly fewer problems with constipation, abdominal pain, and bloating than those taking psyllium. The flaxseed group had even further improvements in constipation and bloating while continuing their treatment in the three months after the double-blind study ended. The researcher concluded that flaxseed relieved constipation more effectively than psyllium.

Chinese herbal medicine. Chinese herbal medicine is traditionally practiced in a highly individualized way, with herbal formulas tailored to the exact details of each person's case. In a double-blind, placebo-controlled trial, 116 people with IBS were randomly assigned to receive individualized Chinese herbal treatment, a "one-size-fits-all" Chinese herbal formulation, or placebo. Treatment consisted of five capsules three times daily, taken for sixteen weeks. The results showed that both forms of active treatment were superior to placebo, significantly reducing IBS symptoms. However, the individualized treatment was no more effective than the "generic" treatment.

OTHER PROPOSED NATURAL TREATMENTS

One study found evidence that pancreatic digestive enzymes (including proteolytic enzymes plus other enzymes called lipases) might be helpful for reducing the flare-up of IBS symptoms that may follow a fatty meal. Three small studies suggest that the use of the supplement melatonin might reduce symptoms of IBS; it has been suggested that the hormone melatonin may have an effect on the nervous system in the digestive tract.

An herbal combination containing candytuft, matricaria flower, peppermint leaves, caraway, licorice root, and lemon balm has shown some promise for IBS. In one double-blind trial, a combination of lemon balm, spearmint, and coriander showed some promise for reducing symptoms of diarrhea-dominant IBS.

The herbs *Coleus forskohlii* and slippery elm and the supplement glutamine are also sometimes recommended for IBS, but there is no meaningful evidence that they are helpful. One double-blind study failed to find either the herb fumitory or an herbal relative of turmeric helpful for IBS.

The prebiotic supplement fructo-oligosaccharides has been advocated as a treatment for IBS. However, research results are inconsistent at best. For example, a six-week double-blind study of 105 people with mild IBS compared 5 grams (g) of fructo-oligosaccharides (FOS) daily with placebo and returned conflicting results. According to some measures of symptom severity employed by the researchers, the use of FOS led to an improvement in symptoms; however, according to other measures, FOS actually worsened symptoms. Conflicting results, though of a different kind, were also seen in a twelve-week, double-blind, placebo-controlled study of ninety-eight people. Treatment with FOS at a dose of 20 g daily initially worsened symptoms, but over time this negative effect wore off. At no time in the study were clear benefits seen, however. On a positive note, one study did find benefit with a combination prebiotic-probiotic formula.

Food allergies may play a role in IBS, and diets based on identifying and eliminating allergenic foods might offer some benefit. Hypnotherapy has shown some promise for IBS, as has relaxation therapy.

Acupuncture has been proposed as a treatment for IBS. However, study results have failed to show it effective. For example, a thirteen-week study of sixty people with IBS found fake acupuncture just as beneficial as traditional acupuncture. A larger trial of 230 adults with IBS found that acupuncture (six treatments over three weeks) was not associated with

Complementary Approaches to Irritable Bowel Syndrome

Dietary restrictions. Because irritable bowel syndrome (IBS) primarily affects the gastrointestinal (GI) tract, diet is a good place to start treatment. Many people benefit from avoiding certain foods and ingredients, such as caffeine, alcohol, fatty foods, and gas-producing vegetables. For those who find a connection between their symptoms and what they eat, avoiding those foods can be effective.

Fiber. Fiber may improve the colon's function and reduce symptoms, especially in people who tend to be constipated. Scientific research suggests that 20 to 30 grams of fiber per day is optimal. Good sources of fiber include whole grains, fruits, vegetables, and legumes; raw bran; psyllium seeds; and flax seeds.

Peppermint oil. Of the many herbs and supplements that have been recommended for IBS, peppermint oil is one of the few backed by some scientific evidence. The recommended dose is a 0.2-milliliter (ml) capsule three times daily after meals. One should be sure to take the enteric-coated form, so that the capsule will not be broken down in the stomach before it reaches the intestines.

Stress management. Stress management may be able to ease IBS symptoms. Some treatments that may be used to decrease stress include relaxation response (the use of medicine and similar techniques to soothe the response to stress), biofeedback (the use of computers and probes to dampen the physiologic manifestations of stress), and cognitive-behavioral therapy (teaching people to reframe the way they perceive pain and to modify their maladaptive responses).

Exercise. Participating in a regular exercise program can help improve bowel function and other IBS symptoms.

Education. Another important part of treatment is becoming educated about IBS and ways to reduce the symptoms. Joining a support group may also be a good way to learn about the condition and to share one's experiences with others.

Medications. In addition to lifestyle changes, there are a number of medicines that may be helpful in treating the individual symptoms of IBS. In some cases, these medicines may be used in combination. Examples include the following:

- Antispasmodic agents (such as dicyclomine and alverine citrate)
- Antiflatulants (such as simethicone)
- Antibiotics (such as rifaximin)
- Antidiarrheal agents (such as loperamide)
- Low-dose antidepressants
- Probiotics (such as acidophilus)
- Pain relievers (such as acetaminophen)
- Serotonin receptor agonists and antagonists (such as alosetron)

These medicines, though often helpful, are no substitute for a comprehensive lifestyle approach. By finding effective ways to manage stress, exercise regularly, and modify one's diet, a person can attempt to address the complex underlying causes of IBS.

Richard Glickman-Simon, M.D.; reviewed by Brian Randall, M.D.

improved symptoms or severity compared to sham acupuncture.

EBSCO CAM Review Board

FURTHER READING

De Paula, J. A., E. Carmuega, and R. Weill. "Effect of the Ingestion of a Symbiotic Yogurt on the Bowel Habits of Women with Functional Constipation." *Acta Gastroenterologica Latinoamericana* 38 (2008): 16-25.

Ford, A. C., et al. "Effect of Fibre, Antispasmodics, and Peppermint Oil in the Treatment of Irritable Bowel Syndrome." *British Medical Journal* 337 (2008): a2313.

Gawronska, A., et al. "A Randomized Double-Blind Placebo-Controlled Trial of *Lactobacillus* GG for Abdominal Pain Disorders in Children." *Alimentary Pharmacology and Therapeutics* 25 (2007): 177-184.

Lahmann, C., et al. "Functional Relaxation as Complementary Therapy in Irritable Bowel Syndrome." *Journal of Alternative and Complementary Medicine* 16 (2010): 47-52.

Lembo, A. J., et al. "A Treatment Trial of Acupuncture in IBS Patients." *American Journal of Gastroenterology* 104 (2009): 1489-1497.

McFarland, L. V., and S. Dublin. "Meta-analysis of Probiotics for the Treatment of Irritable Bowel Syndrome." *World Journal of Gastroenterology* 14 (2008): 2650-2661.

Merat, S., et al. "The Effect of Enteric-Coated, Delayed-Release Peppermint Oil on Irritable Bowel Syndrome." *Digestive Diseases and Sciences* 55 (2010): 1385-1390.

Saha, L., et al. "A Preliminary Study of Melatonin in Irritable Bowel Syndrome." *Journal of Clinical Gastroenterology* 41 (2007): 29-32.

Wilhelm, S. M., et al. "Effectiveness of Probiotics in the Treatment of Irritable Bowel Syndrome." *Pharmacotherapy* 28 (2008): 496-505.

See also: Constipation; Crohn's disease; Diarrhea; Dyspepsia; Flaxseed; Gas, intestinal; Gastrointestinal health; Parasites, intestinal; Peppermint; Probiotics; Traditional Chinese herbal medicine.

Irritable bowel syndrome: Homeopathic remedies

CATEGORY: Homeopathy

DEFINITION: Homeopathic treatment of the abdominal disorder that includes diarrhea, constipation, intestinal gas, bloating, and cramping.

STUDIED HOMEOPATHIC REMEDIES: Asafoetida; colocynthis; *Lycopodium*

INTRODUCTION

The symptoms of irritable bowel syndrome (IBS) include one or more of the following: alternating diarrhea and constipation, intestinal gas, bloating and cramping, abdominal pain, painful bowel movements, mucous discharge, and undigested food in the stool. Despite all these distressing symptoms, people with IBS have normal intestines, so far as any medical examination can show. Thus, the condition belongs to a category of diseases that physicians call "functional." This term means that while the function of the bowel seems to have gone awry, no injury or disturbance of its structure can be discovered. The cause of IBS remains unknown, although stress is thought to play a role.

SCIENTIFIC EVALUATIONS OF HOMEOPATHIC REMEDIES

One homeopathic remedy, asafoetida, has been evaluated as a potential treatment for IBS. In this fourteen-week double-blind trial, about one hundred people with IBS received asafoetida D3 or placebo. The results indicated that participants taking the homeopathic remedy improved to a greater extent than those taking placebo.

TRADITIONAL HOMEOPATHIC TREATMENTS

Classical homeopathy offers many possible homeopathic treatments for irritable bowel syndrome. These therapies are chosen based on various specific details of the person seeking treatment.

The classic symptom picture for asafoetida, the remedy tested in the foregoing double-blind study, includes constipation alternating with profuse, offensive, watery diarrhea; abdominal distention with much flatulence; and the sensation of a lump in the throat that is relieved by swallowing and belching. Symptoms are worse after eating and while sitting; they also are worse at night and on the left side, but they are relieved by pressure and by motion in the open air.

The remedy colocynthis may be suggested when abdominal pain is described as cutting or cramping, often coming in waves, and relieved by firm pressure or by doubling over. Pain is increased by eating or drinking and by the emotions of anger or indignation. Pain often reaches its peak just before the onset of diarrhea. Homeopathic *Lycopodium* may be recommended when symptoms include bandlike pain around the waist, severe flatulence and bloating, and frequent heartburn.

EBSCO CAM Review Board

FURTHER READING

Diamond, J. A., and W. J. Diamond. "Common Functional Bowel Problems: What Do Homeopathy, Chinese Medicine, and Nutrition Have to Offer?" *Advance for Nurse Practitioners* 15 (2005): 31-34, 72.

Joos, S., et al. "Use of Complementary and Alternative Medicine in Germany: A Survey of Patients with Inflammatory Bowel Disease." *BMC Complementary and Alternative Medicine* 6 (2006): 19.

Koretz, R. L., and M. Rotblatt. "Complementary and Alternative Medicine in Gastroenterology: The Good, the Bad, and the Ugly." *Clinical Gastroenterology and Hepatology* 2 (2004): 957-967.

See also: Crohn's disease; Diarrhea; Gas, internal; Irritable bowel syndrome.

Ishizuka, Sagen

CATEGORY: Biography

IDENTIFICATION: Japanese physician who pioneered the concept of food education and who promoted the macrobiotic diet

BORN: March 6, 1850; Japan
DIED: October 17, 1909; Japan

OVERVIEW

Sagen Ishizuka, a Japanese physician, pioneered the concept of food education (*shokuiku*) and the macrobiotic diet. His theory was based on a few guiding principles, including eating a natural, traditional Japanese diet in which the foods consumed are in season and have a correct balance of potassium, sodium, acid, and alkaline.

Ishizuka posited that a person's health was dependent primarily on proper food intake, and he indicated that a person could couple proper diet with physical exercise and hot baths to eliminate excess salts and minerals in the body to maintain health and overcome illness. His practices were rooted in the idea that the body is a self-regulating organism that, given proper fuel (that is, food), could maintain health and balance. He suggested that proper diet and other natural practices could improve not only physical health but also mental health, leading to happiness and satisfaction.

Ishizuka chose to study in the field of traditional medicine at a young age, a decision that was seemingly guided by his being born into a family of traditional doctors. However, because he came from a modest background with little disposable income, he was apparently self-taught to a large extent. He reportedly taught himself a number of languages (English, French, German, and Dutch), in addition to a variety of scientific disciplines, including chemistry, physics, botany, and anatomy.

Ishizuka joined the Japanese army when he was twenty-four years old and served as a doctor in training. He received a degree as a military pharmacist at the age of thirty-one and, later, the title of military physician. He practiced in the military for about twenty-two years, and retired as a chief military pharmacist.

Ishizuka reportedly developed a distaste for Western medicine after several years at practice and, over time, became a proponent instead of traditional medicine, which he concluded to be more effective. He may have suffered certain ailments as a young man that could be overcome not with conventional Western medicine but with traditional Japanese medicine, including diet variation. Ishizuka would develop a theory that a person's health was dictated by the person's ability to strengthen the body internally by following a balanced regime, which was largely dependent on the person's diet.

After his retirement from the army, Ishizuka opened a free clinic around 1908 and treated patients solely by dictating dietary recommendations. He performed many clinical trials and published two large volumes of his work. It has been written that many of his Japanese supporters referred to him as Dr. Miso Soup and Dr. Brown Rice because of his recommendations for these particular foodstuffs.

Brandy Weidow, M.S.

FURTHER READING

Brown, Simon. *Macrobiotics for Life*. Berkeley, Calif.: North Atlantic Books, 2009.
Kotzch, Ronald E. *Macrobiotics: Yesterday and Today*. New York: Japan Publications, 1985.
"Macrobiotics." In *Complementary and Alternative Medicine Sourcebook*, edited by Amy L. Sutton. Detroit: Omnigraphics, 2010.

See also: Diet-based therapies; Hufeland, Christoph Wilhelm; Macrobiotic diet; Ohsawa, George.

Isoflavones

CATEGORY: Herbs and supplements
RELATED TERMS: Red clover isoflavones, soy isoflavones
DEFINITION: Natural plant product used to treat specific health conditions.
PRINCIPAL PROPOSED USES: High cholesterol, menopausal symptoms
OTHER PROPOSED USES: Aging skin, blood sugar control (prediabetes), cancer prevention, cyclic mastalgia, enhancing mental function, female infertility, osteoporosis, premenstrual syndrome, weight loss

OVERVIEW

Isoflavones are water-soluble chemicals found in many plants. This article focuses on a group of isoflavones that are phytoestrogens, meaning that they cause effects in the body somewhat similar to those of estrogen. The most investigated phytoestrogen isoflavones, genistein and daidzein, are found in both soy products and the herb red clover. Soy additionally contains glycitein, an isoflavone that is more estrogenic than genistein and daidzein but is usually present in relatively low amounts. Red clover also contains two other isoflavones: biochanin (which can be turned into genistein) and formonenetin (which can be turned into daidzein).

Certain cells in the body have estrogen receptors, special sites that allow estrogen to attach. When estrogen attaches to a cell's estrogen receptor, estrogenic effects occur in the cell. Isoflavones also latch onto estrogen receptors, but they produce weaker estrogenic effects. This leads to an interesting two-part action. When there is not enough estrogen in the body, isoflavones can stimulate cells with estrogen receptors and partly make up for the deficit. However, when there is plenty of estrogen, isoflavones may tend to block real estrogen from attaching to estrogen receptors, thereby reducing the net estrogenic effect. This may reduce some of the risks of excess estrogen (for example, breast and uterine cancer), while still providing some of estrogen's benefits (such as preventing osteoporosis).

Isoflavones also appear directly to reduce estrogen levels in the body, perhaps by fooling the body into thinking that it has plenty of estrogen. Isoflavones are widely thought to be the active ingredients in soy products. However, growing evidence suggests that there are other active ingredients, such as proteins, fiber, and phospholipids.

REQUIREMENTS AND SOURCES

Although isoflavones are not essential nutrients, they may help reduce the incidence of several diseases. Thus, isoflavones may be useful for optimum health, even if they are not necessary for life like a classic vitamin.

Roasted soybeans have the highest isoflavone content: about 167 milligrams (mg) for a 3.5-ounce serving. Tempeh (a cake of fermented soybeans) is next, with 60 mg, followed by soy flour with 44 mg. Processed soy products, such as soy protein and soy milk, contain about 20 mg per serving. The same isoflavones found in soy are also contained in certain red clover products.

THERAPEUTIC DOSAGES

When purified isoflavones from red clover or soy are used, the dose generally ranges from about 40 to 80 mg daily. This is considerably higher than the average isoflavone intake in Japan, which is about 28 mg daily. (Postmenopausal Japanese women may consume closer to 50 mg daily.)

There are three major isoflavones found in soy: genistein, daidzein, and glycitein. Each of these isoflavones can occur in two types or states. The first type, predominant in raw soy products, is called an isoflavone glycoside. In an isoflavone glycoside, the isoflavone is attached to a sugarlike substance known as a glycone. The second type, predominant in fermented soy products, is called an isoflavone aglycone. These consist of isoflavones without a glycone attached and are also called free isoflavones. Because isoflavone aglycones are the most pure form of isoflavones, it has been hypothesized (but not proven) that they are more effective than other forms.

THERAPEUTIC USES

Soy products are known to improve cholesterol profile, but isoflavones may not be the active cholesterol-lowering ingredient in soy. Isoflavones may, however, improve other measures linked to cardiovascular risk, such as levels of blood sugar, insulin, and fibrinogen.

According to some but not all studies, soy protein or concentrated isoflavones from soy or red clover may slightly reduce menopausal symptoms, such as hot flashes and vaginal dryness. However, isoflavones have failed to prove effective for the hot flashes that often occur in breast cancer survivors. There is conflicting evidence regarding whether soy or isoflavones may be helpful for preventing osteoporosis, but on balance, the evidence suggests a modest beneficial effect.

One study tested a purified soy isoflavone product (technically, isoflavone aglycones) for treatment of aging skin. In this double-blind trial, twenty-six Japanese women in their late thirties and early forties were given either placebo or 40 mg daily of soy isoflavone aglycones for twelve weeks. Researchers monitored two types of wrinkles near the eye: fine and linear. The results indicated that use of the soy product significantly reduced fine wrinkles compared with placebo. (Effects on linear wrinkles were not significant.) As a secondary measure, researchers also analyzed skin elasticity and found an improvement in the women given the isoflavones, compared with those given placebo. This was much too small a study for its results to be taken as reliable.

A small and poorly reported double-blind, placebo-controlled study provides weak evidence that red clover isoflavones might be helpful for cyclic mastalgia. A combination product containing soy isoflavones, black cohosh, and dong quai has shown some promise for menstrual migraines.

One study found that use of soy isoflavones improved the effectiveness rate of in vitro fertilization (used for female infertility). A double-blind study performed in China found that use of a soy isoflavone supplement improved blood sugar control in healthy postmenopausal women.

In a small double-blind trial, use of soy isoflavones appeared to reduce some symptoms of premenstrual syndrome (PMS). A very small study found hints that soy isoflavones might help reduce buildup of abdominal fat.

Observational studies hint that soy may help prevent breast and uterine cancer in women. If this connection is real and not a statistical accident (observational studies are notorious for falling prey to statistical accidents), the explanation may lie in the estrogen-like action of soy isoflavones. As noted above, isoflavones decrease the action of regular estrogen by blocking estrogen receptor sites and may also reduce levels of circulating estrogen. Since estrogen promotes breast and uterine cancer, these effects could help prevent breast cancer. Soy also appears to lengthen the menstrual cycle by a few days, and this also would be expected to reduce breast cancer risk. However, only a large, long-term intervention trial could actually show that soy or isoflavones reduce breast and uterine cancer risk, and one has not been performed.

Observational studies also hint that soy might help prevent prostate cancer in men. Men have very low levels of circulating estrogen, so the net effect of increased soy consumption might be to increase estrogen-like activity in the body. Since real estrogen is used as a treatment to suppress prostate cancer, perhaps the mild estrogen-like activity of isoflavones has a similar effect. Isoflavones might also decrease testosterone levels and alter ratios of certain forms of estrogen, both of which would be expected to provide benefit. In one double-blind study, men with early prostate cancer were given either isoflavones or placebo, and their PSA levels were monitored. (PSA is a marker for prostate cancer, with higher values generally showing an increased number of cancer cells.)

Isoflavones for Hot Flashes

Some women try herbs or other plant products to help relieve hot flashes, a symptom of perimenopause. These products include soy (a plant in the pea family that contains isoflavones, a type of phytoestrogen) and phytoestrogen-containing herbs.

- *Soy isoflavones.* Soy contains phytoestrogen isoflavones. These are substances from a plant that may act like the estrogen made by the body. There is no clear proof that soy or other sources of phytoestrogens relieve hot flashes, and the risks of taking soy products such as pills and powders are not known. The best sources of soy isoflavones are foods such as tofu, tempeh, soymilk, and soy nuts.
- *Other sources of phytoestrogens.* These include herbs such as black cohosh, wild yam, dong quai, and valerian root. There is not enough evidence that these herbs, or pills or creams containing these herbs, help with hot flashes. Also, not enough is known about the risks of using these products.

The results did show that use of isoflavones (60 mg daily) slightly reduces PSA levels. Whether this meant that soy actually slowed the progression of the cancer or simply lowered PSA directly is not clear from this study alone. However, in another study of apparently healthy men (not known to have prostate cancer), soy isoflavones at a dose of 83 mg per day did not alter PSA levels. Taken together, these two studies provide some direct evidence that soy isoflavones may be helpful for treating or preventing prostate cancer, but the case nonetheless remains highly preliminary.

According to most but not all studies, soy isoflavones do not improve mental function. One study failed to find that soy protein with isoflavones improved general quality of life (health status, depression, and life satisfaction) in postmenopausal women. Soy isoflavones have also failed to prove effective for reducing levels of homocysteine.

SCIENTIFIC EVIDENCE

High cholesterol. Numerous studies have found that soy can reduce blood cholesterol levels and improve the ratio of low-density lipoprotein (LDL, or bad cholesterol) to high-density lipoprotein (HDL, or good cholesterol). Although it was once thought that isoflavones are the ingredients in soy responsible for improving cholesterol profile, on balance, current evidence suggests otherwise. Nonisoflavone constituents of soy, such as proteins, fiber, and phospholipids, may be as important as, or perhaps even more important than, the isoflavones in soy.

It is also possible that the exact types of isoflavones in a particular product made a difference. One study of red clover isoflavones found evidence that biochanin but not formononetin can reduce LDL cholesterol.

Another study found that soy products may at times have an unusual isoflavone profile, containing high levels of the isoflavone glycitein rather than the more usual genistein and daidzein. Glycitein could be inactive regarding cholesterol reduction.

Finally, some evidence hints that soy isoflavones may be effective for reducing cholesterol only when it is converted by intestinal bacteria into a substance called equol. It appears that only about one-third of people have the right intestinal bacteria to make equol.

Menopausal Symptoms. Although study results are not entirely consistent, the balance of the evidence suggests that isoflavones from soy may be helpful for symptoms of menopause, especially hot flashes. Improvements in hot flashes, as well as other symptoms, such as vaginal dryness, have been seen in many studies of soy, mixed soy isoflavones, isoflavone aglycones, or genistein alone. However, the effects have been slight or nonexistent in other studies. At least two studies found that people who are equol producers may experience greater benefits. The herb *Pueraria mirifica*, which also contains a number of isoflavones, has also shown some benefit for menopausal symptoms.

However, several other studies have failed to find benefit with whole soy or concentrated soy isoflavones. Another study failed to find benefit with a mixture of soy isoflavones and black cohosh. Isoflavones from red clover have also shown inconsistent benefit, with the largest and most recent trial failing to find any reduction in hot flash symptoms. Furthermore, in double-blind, placebo-controlled trials, soy or purified isoflavones failed to reduce hot flashes among survivors of breast cancer.

What can one make of this mixed evidence? The problem here is that placebo treatment has a strong effect on menopausal symptoms. In such circumstances, statistical noise can easily drown out the real benefits of a treatment under study. Estrogen is so powerful for hot flashes and other menopausal symptoms that its benefits are almost always clear in studies; it is likely that soy or concentrated isoflavones have a more modest effect, not always seen above the background.

Osteoporosis. Estrogen has a powerfully protective effect on bone. Studies exploring whether isoflavones have the same effect have produced inconsistent results. On balance, it is probably fair to summarize current evidence as indicating that isoflavones (as soy, genistein, mixed isoflavones, or tofu extract) have at least a modestly beneficial effect on bone density.

The best evidence is for genistein taken alone. In a twenty-four-month, double-blind study of 389 postmenopausal women with mild bone loss, use of genistein at a dose of 54 mg daily significantly improved bone density, compared with placebo. (All participants were additionally given calcium and vitamin D.)

However, it is not clear that isoflavones consumed in the diet, even at high concentrations are beneficial. For example, in a placebo-controlled study involving 237 healthy women in the early stages of menopause, the consumption of isoflavone-enriched foods (providing an average of 110 mg isoflavone aglycones daily) for one year had no affect on bone density or metabolism. One small but long-term study suggests that progesterone cream (another treatment proposed for use in preventing or treating osteoporosis) may decrease the bone-sparing effect of soy isoflavones.

Bone is always subject to two influences: bone building and bone breakdown. Estrogen primarily works by reducing the bone breakdown part of the equation, thereby leading to a net result of increased bone growth. Growing evidence suggests that isoflavones act on both sides of this equation, directly stimulating new bone creation, while at the same time slowing bone breakdown. There is mixed evidence that isoflavones are more effective for osteoporosis in people who have the intestinal bacteria to produce equol.

Menstrual migraines. In a twenty-four-week, double-blind study, forty-nine women with menstrual migraines (migraine headaches associated with the menstrual cycle) received either placebo or a combination supplement containing soy isoflavones and extracts of dong quai and black cohosh. Beginning at the twentieth week, use of the herbal supplement resulted in decreased severity and frequency of headaches, compared with placebo. However, it is not clear which of the ingredients in the combination was helpful. The authors of the study apparently considered black cohosh and dong quai as phytoestrogens, but the current consensus is that they do not belong in that category.

SAFETY ISSUES

Studies in animals have found soy isoflavones essentially nontoxic. The long history of the use of soy as food in Asia would also tend to suggest that they are safe. Even though absolute safety cannot be assumed from historical consumption of soy as food, it is reassuring to note that researchers found no evidence of ill effects when they gave healthy postmenopausal women 900 mg of soy isoflavones a day for eighty-four consecutive days. In Japan, the maximum safe intake level of soy isoflavones has been set at a total of 70 to 75 mg daily (food plus supplement sources).

Still, concerns have been raised about estrogenic and other potential side effects of excessive soy isoflavone intake. Overall, the estrogenic effect of soy isoflavones in women seems to be fairly minimal. Nonetheless, it is not zero. According to most but not all studies, use of soy has enough of an estrogen-like effect to slightly alter the menstrual cycle and change levels of sex hormones in young women. Thus, some of the risks of estrogen could, in theory, apply to isoflavones as well.

For example, because estrogen can stimulate breast cancer cells, there are theoretical concerns that isoflavones may not be safe for women who have already had breast cancer. While isoflavones in general should have an antiestrogenic effect by blocking real estrogen, some studies in animals have found evidence that under certain circumstances, soy isoflavones might stimulate breast cancer cells. Studies directly examining the effects of isoflavones on human breast tissue have produced contradictory results. However, on balance, there is no convincing evidence that consuming moderate amounts of soy isoflavones (at levels typical of an Asian diet) increases the risk of breast cancer in healthy women or worsens the prognosis of women with breast cancer. Nevertheless, given the theoretical risk and the absence of large randomized trials investigating the safety of isoflavone supplements, prudence suggests that women who have had

breast cancer, or are at high risk for it, should consult a physician before taking any isoflavone product.

Estrogen also stimulates uterine cells, leading to an increased risk of uterine cancer. Most studies have found that isoflavones do not stimulate uterine cells. However, one fairly large (365 participants) and long-term (five years) study did find uterine stimulation in 3.37 percent of women on isoflavones and 0 percent of those on placebo. This could indicate a slightly increased risk of uterine cancer with high-dose isoflavone use.

Similarly, preliminary studies and reports have raised concerns that intensive use of soy products or isoflavones by pregnant women could exert a hormonal effect that impacts fetuses. Use of soy formula by infants is also of concern along these lines, as an infant subsisting on soy formula has a relatively enormous isoflavone intake; on a per-weight basis, it may exceed the average Asian adult isoflavone intake by a factor of ten.

The drug tamoxifen blocks estrogen and is used to help prevent breast cancer recurrence in women who have had breast cancer. One animal study found that soy isoflavones might remove the benefit of tamoxifen treatment.

One double-blind study of postmenopausal women found the use of red clover isoflavones at a dose of 80 mg daily for ninety days resulted in increased levels of testosterone. The potential significance of this is unclear. In men, isoflavones might decrease testosterone levels, but the effect appears to be slight at most.

Other concerns relate to soy's potential effects involving the thyroid gland. When given to individuals with impaired thyroid function, soy products have been observed to reduce absorption of thyroid medication. In addition, some evidence hints that soy isoflavones may directly inhibit the function of the thyroid gland (though perhaps only in people who are iodine-deficient). To make matters more confusing, studies of healthy humans and animals given soy isoflavones or other soy products have generally found that soy either had no effect on thyroid hormone levels or actually increased levels. In view of soy's complex effects regarding the thyroid, individuals with impaired thyroid function should not take large amounts of soy products except under the supervision of a physician.

Although some experts have expressed fears that soy isoflavones might interfere with the action of oral contraceptives, one study of thirty-six women found reassuring results. Some evidence suggests that the isoflavone genistein might impair immunity. One study in mice found that injected genistein has negative effects on the thymus gland (an organ that is important for immunity) and also causes changes in the prevalence of various white blood cells consistent with impaired immunity. Although the genistein was injected rather than administered orally, the blood levels of genistein that these injections produced were not excessively high; they were comparable to (or even lower than) the amount given children fed soy milk formula. In addition, there are several reports of impaired immune responses in infants fed soy formula. While it is too early to conclude that genistein impairs immunity, these findings are a potential cause for concern.

One observational study raised concerns that soy might impair mental function in adults. However, observational studies are far less reliable than clinical trials. Direct studies designed to test the potential effects of isoflavones on brain function, lasting up to twelve months, have found either no effect or a slightly positive effect on brain function. While this does not rule out a harmful long-term effect on cognition, it is reassuring.

There exists one case report in which soy isoflavone supplements caused migraine headaches in a man who had never experienced migraines before; presumably this was a highly individual reaction, such as an allergy. Similarly, while soy products are sometimes recommend for reducing blood pressure, there is also a well-documented case report in which use of high-dose soy isoflavones caused extreme elevation in blood pressure in a woman participating in a scientific study (of soy isoflavones).

Some researchers have raised concern that genistein may influence the ability of blood to clot properly. A placebo-controlled study involving 104 healthy women, however, found no evidence that the isoflavone genistein had any significant adverse effect on blood clotting.

EBSCO CAM Review Board

FURTHER READING

Brink, E., et al. "Long-Term Consumption of Isoflavone-Enriched Foods Does Not Affect Bone Mineral Density, Bone Metabolism, or Hormonal Status in Early Postmenopausal Women." *American Journal of Clinical Nutrition* 87 (2008): 761-770.

Chandeying, V., and M. Sangthawan. "Efficacy Comparison of *Pueraria mirifica* (PM) Against Conjugated Equine Estrogen (CEE) With/Without Medroxyprogesterone Acetate (MPA) in the Treatment of Climacteric Symptoms in Perimenopausal Women: Phase III Study." *Journal of the Medical Association of Thailand* 90 (2007): 1720-1726.

Jou, H. J., et al. "Effect of Intestinal Production of Equol on Menopausal Symptoms in Women Treated with Soy Isoflavones." *International Journal of Gynaecology and Obstetrics* 102, no. 1 (2008): 44-49.

Khaodhiar, L., et al. "Daidzein-Rich Isoflavone Aglycones Are Potentially Effective in Reducing Hot Flashes in Menopausal Women." *Menopause* 15 (2008): 125-132.

Thorp, A. A., et al. "Soy Food Consumption Does Not Lower LDL Cholesterol in Either Equol or Nonequol Producers." *American Journal of Clinical Nutrition* 88 (2008): 298-304.

Torella, M., et al. "Endometrial Survey During Phytoestrogens Therapy in Postmenopausal Women." *Minerva Ginecologica* 60 (2008): 281-285.

Trifiletti, A., et al. "Haemostatic Effects of Phytoestrogen Genistein in Postmenopausal Women." *Thrombosis Research* 123, no. 2 (2008): 231-235.

See also: Cancer risk reduction; Cholesterol, high; Infertility, female; Menopause; Osteoporosis; Premenstrual syndrome (PMS).

Isoniazid

CATEGORY: Drug interactions
DEFINITION: An antibiotic drug used for the treatment of tuberculosis.
INTERACTIONS: Vitamin B_3, vitamin B_6, vitamin D
TRADE NAMES: Laniazid, Nydrazid

VITAMIN B_6

Effect: Supplementation Likely Helpful

Persons who take isoniazid may develop nerve problems such as tingling or numbness in the arms, hands, legs, and feet. The cause is believed to be the drug's interference with the action of vitamin B_6. The use of isoniazid is one cause of the few occasions in which vitamin B_6 deficiency is seen in the developed world.

To prevent these complications, one should take vitamin B_6 supplements at a dose of 15 to 30 milligrams per day when using isoniazid.

VITAMIN B_3
Effect: Supplementation Possibly Helpful

According to animal studies, isoniazid can interfere with the body's ability to produce vitamin B_3 (niacin) by blocking a key enzyme. This can produce either a subtle or an all-out niacin deficiency (known as pellagra). Taking niacin supplements at standard U.S. Dietary Reference Intake (formerly known as the Recommended Dietary Allowance) doses should help a person get needed niacin.

VITAMIN D
Effect: Supplementation Possibly Helpful

Isoniazid may interfere with the body's ability to use vitamin D. Although it is not clear whether this actually causes symptoms of vitamin D deficiency, it still might be a good idea to take vitamin D supplements at standard U.S. Adequate Intake (AI) dosages.

EBSCO CAM Review Board

FURTHER READING

Ishii, N., and Y. Nishihara. "Pellagra Encephalopathy Among Tuberculous Patients: Its Relation to Isoniazid Therapy." *Journal of Neurology, Neurosurgery, and Psychiatry* 48 (1985): 628-634.

Mandell, G. L., and W. A. Petri. "Antimicrobial Agents: Drugs Used in the Chemotherapy of Tuberculosis, *Mycobacterium avium* Complex Disease, and Leprosy." In *Goodman and Gilman's The Pharmacological Basis of Therapeutics*, edited by Laurence L. Brunton et al. 11th ed. New York: McGraw-Hill Medical, 2011.

See also: Food and Drug Administration; Rifampin; Supplements: Introduction; Vitamin B_3; Vitamin B_6; Vitamin D.

Isotretinoin

CATEGORY: Drug interactions
DEFINITION: A drug related to vitamin A that is used to treat severe acne.

INTERACTIONS: St. John's wort, vitamin A, vitamin E
TRADE NAME: Accutane

VITAMIN A
Effect: Probable Harmful Interaction

Both vitamin A and isotretinoin can cause toxic symptoms if taken in excess. It is presumed that the simultaneous use of vitamin A and isotretinoin would tend to amplify the risk. For this reason, persons using isotretinoin should not take vitamin A at doses higher than the recommended daily allowance. Because most people get enough vitamin A from the diet, it might be preferable to take no vitamin A supplements at all. (Supplements that use beta-carotene to supply vitamin A are probably safe.)

ST. JOHN'S WORT
Effect: Indirect Harmful Interaction

Because isotretinoin can cause birth defects, women who use it are often advised to take oral contraceptives (birth control pills). The herb St. John's wort is thought to interact with birth control pills and reduce their effectiveness, raising the risk of pregnancy. For this reason, people taking Accutane and oral contraceptives should avoid using St. John's wort.

VITAMIN E
Effect: Possible Helpful Interaction

One preliminary study hints that vitamin E might reduce the side effects of isotretinoin.

EBSCO CAM Review Board

FURTHER READING

Murphy, P. A., et al. "Interaction of St. John's Wort with Oral Contraceptives: Effects on the Pharmacokinetics of Norethindrone and Ethinyl Estradiol, Ovarian Activity, and Breakthrough Bleeding." *Contraception* 71 (2005): 402-408.

Pfrunder, A., et al. "Interaction of St. John's Wort with Low-Dose Oral Contraceptive Therapy." *British Journal of Clinical Pharmacology* 56 (2003): 683-690.

See also: Acne; Adolescent and teenage health; Contraceptives, oral; Food and Drug Administration; Herbal medicine; Pregnancy support; St. John's wort; Supplements: Introduction; Vitamin A; Vitamin E; Vitamins and minerals; Women's health.

Ivy leaf

CATEGORY: Herbs and supplements
RELATED TERM: *Hedera helix*
DEFINITION: Natural plant product used to treat specific health conditions.
PRINCIPAL PROPOSED USE: Asthma
OTHER PROPOSED USES: Acute bronchitis, chronic bronchitis, colds and influenza

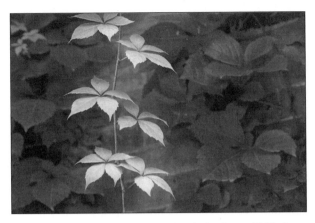

The ivy leaf has a long history of medicinal use. (© Jinfeng Zhang/Dreamstime.com)

OVERVIEW

The climbing ivy that adorns the sides of buildings has a long history of traditional medicinal use. Herbalists used ivy for such disparate conditions as arthritis, bronchitis, dysentery, and whooping cough. Topical applications of the herb were used for skin problems, such as lice, eczema, and sunburn.

THERAPEUTIC DOSAGES

A typical dose of standardized ivy leaf extract is twenty-five drops twice per day in children or fifty or more drops twice per day in adults.

THERAPEUTIC USES

Ivy leaf is one of many herbs used in Europe as an expectorant, a substance said to thin mucus and thereby loosen coughs. (In the United States, the herbal product guaifenesin takes this role in almost all over-the-counter cough formulas.) Germany's Commission E has approved ivy leaf for treatment of mucus in the respiratory passages. On this basis, ivy leaf is often recommended for asthma, acute bronchits, chronic bronchitis, colds and flu, and other respiratory problems. However, there is almost no evidence that ivy leaf (or, indeed, any other expectorant) actually offers meaningful benefits.

Only one double-blind, placebo-controlled study of ivy leaf has been reported. In this study, a total of twenty-four children with asthma received either placebo or ivy leaf extract twice a day for three days. The results showed modest improvement in asthma symptoms as measured by formal testing.

Other studies on ivy leaf compared various forms of the product to each other and thereby do not prove anything about efficacy. One double-blind study found ivy leaf just as effective as the expectorant drug ambroxol for chronic bronchitis; however, because ambroxol itself has not been proven effective, this study proves little.

SAFETY ISSUES

Fairly extensive monitoring indicates that ivy leaf rarely causes any noticeable side effects. Nausea and vomiting are possible with excessive doses, or in very susceptible people. Ivy leaf is not recommended during pregnancy because of its emetine content. Safety in pregnant or nursing women, young children, or people with severe liver or kidney disease has not been established.

EBSCO CAM Review Board

FURTHER READING

Hofmann, D., et al. "Efficacy of Dry Extract of Ivy Leaves in Children with Bronchial Asthma." *Phytomedicine* 10 (2003): 213-220.

Houtmeyers, E., et al. "Effects of Drugs on Mucus Clearance." *European Respiratory Journal* 14 (1999): 452-467.

Ziment, I. "Herbal Antitussives." *Pulmonary Pharmacology and Therapeutics* 15 (2002): 327-333.

See also: Asthma; Bronchitis; Colds and flu.

J

Jensen, Bernard

CATEGORY: Biography

IDENTIFICATION: American chiropractor and nutritionist who promoted a variety of complementary and alternative approaches

BORN: March 25, 1908; Stockton, California

DIED: February 22, 2001; Escondido, California

OVERVIEW

Bernard Jensen was an American iridologist, chiropractor, nutritionist, and entrepreneur, and the author of numerous books and articles on health and healing. He was born in Northern California, where he later attended college to study chiropractic (the profession of his father). It is said that Jensen's health began to deteriorate at a young age, and that he was later diagnosed with bronchiectasis, which is an incurable lung disease. However, he was reportedly mentored by a Seventh Day Adventist physician, who taught him principles rooted in using good nutrition and other natural approaches to manage his health. Using these practices, Jensen reportedly nursed himself back to relatively good health and went on to open a chiropractic practice in California around 1929.

Jensen reportedly relied on a combination of chiropractic and other natural methods to treat his patients. Specifically, he was said to recommend a healthy diet, regular exercise, sufficient rest, management of stress, and maintaining vigor for life that involved providing service and support to fellow human beings. He posited that a combination of such natural steps would serve to maintain or improve a person's health.

Jensen was eventually mentored by a Norwegian homeopath, Victor Rocine, learning the importance of physician-patient interactions and the need for long-term care for the well-being of some persons with chronic illnesses. Based on this idea, he went on to develop multiple nature cure sanitariums in California, where he treated persons with serious illnesses such as cancer, arthritis, weight disorders, and other degenerative diseases. He reportedly treated hundreds of thousands of patients in these sanitariums using natural approaches and gained some notoriety for these efforts.

In addition to his notable work in iridology, which studies the iris of the eye to determine a person's health status, he also supported numerous other methods that fall within the classifications of complementary or alternative medicine, including hydrotherapy, fasting, reflexology, homeopathy, and acupuncture. Jensen reportedly taught his methods to several doctors around the world, and he wrote hundreds of works during his lifetime.

Jensen's teachings and enterprise have been maintained after his death. His daughter-in-law, Ellen Tart-Jensen, continues to apply and teach his practices.

Brandy Weidow, M.S.

FURTHER READING

Jensen, Bernard *Dr. Jensen's Guide to Body Chemistry and Nutrition.* Columbus, Ohio: McGraw-Hill, 2000.

_____. *Dr. Jensen's Juicing Therapy: Nature's Way to Better Health and a Longer Life.* Columbus, Ohio: McGraw-Hill, 2000.

_____. *Dr. Jensen's Nutrition Handbook: A Daily Regimen for Healthy Living.* Columbus, Ohio: McGraw-Hill, 2000.

See also: Chiropractic; Diet-based therapies; Iridology.

Jet lag

CATEGORY: Condition

DEFINITION: Treatment of disruptions to the body's internal clock from air travel across many time zones.

PRINCIPAL PROPOSED NATURAL TREATMENT: Melatonin

OTHER PROPOSED NATURAL TREATMENTS: Natural treatments for insomnia, nicotinamide adenine dinucleotide, tyrosine

INTRODUCTION

The body has an internal clock of sorts that follows the rhythms of night and day. Air travel confuses this clock, causing the phenomenon known as jet lag. Persons who have crossed several time zones during a flight have probably experienced jet lag to some degree. A person may have felt exhausted in the morning and wide awake at night, and between those times may have experienced symptoms such as fatigue, loss of concentration, dizziness, lightheadedness, irritability, nausea, and headache.

Ordinarily, the body clock resets itself within a few days. It is possible to speed up this natural process by deliberately using stimuli to "inform" the body when it should wake up and when it should fall asleep. Common methods involve social activity and outdoor exercise during the daytime, combined with mealtimes appropriate to the new time zone. It is also generally considered important to stay awake upon arrival in the new time zone until night falls. The use of sleeping pills may be helpful at first, so one does not stay awake. In addition, some physicians are experimenting with wakefulness drugs such as modafinil (Provigil) that are used for conditions such as narcolepsy to help travelers stay active and alert on arrival.

PRINCIPAL PROPOSED NATURAL TREATMENTS

Melatonin is a natural hormone that plays a role in the day-night cycle (the circadian rhythm). During

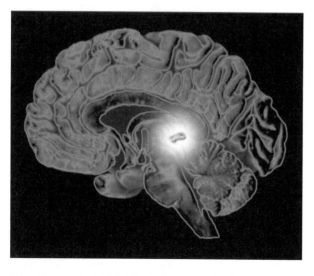

The pineal gland (highlighted) secretes the hormone melatonin. (Pasieka/Getty Images)

daylight, the pineal gland in the brain produces an important neurotransmitter called serotonin, but at night, the pineal gland stops producing serotonin and instead makes melatonin. This melatonin release helps trigger sleep.

The amount of melatonin production varies according to the intensity of light to which a person is exposed; for example, the body produces more melatonin in a completely dark room than in a dimly lit one.

This cyclic pattern of melatonin release helps set the body's biologic clock. Melatonin supplements taken by mouth can be used to reset this clock, an effect that is of potential benefit in jet lag.

According to a review published in 2001, reasonably good evidence indicates that melatonin is indeed effective for this purpose. One of the best supporting studies was a double-blind, placebo-controlled trial that enrolled 320 travelers crossing six to eight time zones. The participants were divided into four groups and given a daily dose of 5 milligrams (mg) of standard melatonin, 5 mg of slow-release melatonin, 0.5 mg of standard melatonin, or placebo. The results of this large study were promising. The group that received 5 mg of standard melatonin slept better, took less time to fall asleep, and felt more energetic and awake during the day than the other three groups.

OTHER PROPOSED NATURAL TREATMENTS

Nicotinamide adenine dinucleotide (NADH) is a chemical that the body manufactures on its own to serve a variety of biologic purposes. In a double-blind, placebo-controlled trial, thirty-five people taking an overnight flight across four time zones were given either 20 mg of NADH or placebo sublingually (under the tongue) on the morning of arrival. Participants were twice given tests of wakefulness and mental function: first at ninety minutes and then at five hours after landing. People given NADH scored significantly better on these tests than those given placebo.

Tyrosine is an amino acid found in meat proteins. A double-blind, placebo-controlled study that enrolled twenty members of the U.S. Marine Corps suggests that tyrosine supplements can improve alertness during periods of sleep deprivation. In this study, the participants were deprived of sleep for a night and then tested frequently for their alertness throughout the following day as they worked. Compared to placebo, 10 to 15 grams (g) of tyrosine given twice daily seemed to provide a "pick-up" for about two hours.

Similar benefits were seen with 2 g of tyrosine daily in a double-blind, placebo-controlled trial of twenty-one military cadets exposed to physical and psychological stress, including sleep deprivation. These findings suggest that tyrosine could be helpful for jet lag.

Besides these supplements, all the natural treatments used for insomnia may be helpful for getting a good night's sleep on the first night of travel.

EBSCO CAM Review Board

FURTHER READING

Deijen, J. B., et al. "Tyrosine Improves Cognitive Performance and Reduces Blood Pressure in Cadets After One Week of a Combat Training Course." *Brain Research Bulletin* 48 (1999): 203-209.

Herxheimer, A., and K. J. Petrie. "Melatonin for Preventing and Treating Jet Lag." *Cochrane Database of Systematic Reviews* (2001): CD001520. Available through *EBSCO DynaMed Systematic Literature Surveillance* at http://www.ebscohost.com/dynamed.

Larzelere, M. M., J. S. Campbell, and M. Robertson. "Complementary and Alternative Medicine Usage for Behavioral Health Indications." *Primary Care* 37 (2010): 213-236.

Neri, D. F., et al. "The Effects of Tyrosine on Cognitive Performance During Extended Wakefulness." *Aviation, Space, and Environmental Medicine* 66 (1995): 313-319.

Rios, E. R., et al. "Melatonin: Pharmacological Aspects and Clinical Trends." *International Journal of Neuroscience* 120 (2010): 583-590.

Suhner, A., et al. "Comparative Study to Determine the Optimal Melatonin Dosage Form for the Alleviation of Jet Lag." *Chronobiology International* 15 (1998): 655-666.

See also: Fatigue; Insomnia; Melatonin.

Juniper berry

CATEGORY: Herbs and supplements
RELATED TERM: *Juniperus communis*
DEFINITION: Natural plant product used to treat specific health conditions.
PRINCIPAL PROPOSED USES: None
OTHER PROPOSED USES: Diuretic, osteoarthritis

OVERVIEW

The Dutch word for juniper is *geniver*, from which came the English word "gin." Juniper, however, is not only good for making martinis. Its berries (actually not berries, but a portion of the cone) were used by the Zuni Indians to assist in childbirth, by British herbalists to treat congestive heart failure and stimulate menstruation, and by American herbalists in the nineteenth century to treat congestive heart failure, gonorrhea, and urinary tract infections.

THERAPEUTIC DOSAGES

Juniper tea can be made by adding 1 cup of boiling water to 1 tablespoon of juniper berries, covering, and allowing the berries to steep for twenty minutes. The usual dosage is 1 cup twice a day. However, juniper is said to work better as a treatment for bladder infections when combined with other herbs. Combination products should be taken according to label instructions.

Bladder infections can go on to become kidney infections. For this reason, individuals should seek medical supervision if their symptoms do not resolve in a few days, or if they develop intense low back pain, fever, chills, or other signs of serious infection.

THERAPEUTIC USES

Contemporary herbalists use juniper primarily as a diuretic (water pill) component of herbal formulas designed to treat bladder infections. A typical combination might include goldenrod, dandelion, uva ursi, parsley, cleavers, and buchu. The volatile oils of juniper reportedly increase the rate of kidney filtration, thereby increasing urine flow and perhaps helping to "wash out" offending bacteria. However, there is no direct scientific evidence that juniper is effective for bladder infections. Only a double-blind placebo-controlled study can prove a treatment effective, and none has been reported with juniper

Recently, gin-soaked raisins have been touted as an arthritis treatment. This is probably just a fad, but some weak evidence suggests that juniper may possess anti-inflammatory properties. In addition, in test-tube studies, certain constituents of juniper have been found to inhibit the herpes virus. However, it is a long way from such studies to the conclusion that juniper is helpful for herpes infections.

SAFETY ISSUES

Although juniper is regarded as safe and is widely used in foods, it is not recommended for use during pregnancy. (Pregnant women should also not drink gin.) Remember, juniper was used historically to stimulate menstruation and childbirth. It has also been shown to cause miscarriages in rats. Persons taking the medication lithium should use herbal diuretics, such as juniper, only under the supervision of a physician, because being dehydrated when taking this medication can be dangerous.

Some texts warn that juniper oil may be a kidney irritant, but there is no real evidence that this is the case. Nonetheless, people with serious kidney disease probably should not take juniper. Safety for young children, nursing women, and those with severe liver disease has also not been established. Individuals who are taking lithium should not use juniper except under the supervision of a physician.

EBSCO CAM Review Board

FURTHER READING

Newall, C., et al. *Herbal Medicines: A Guide for Health-Care Professionals.* London: Pharmaceutical Press, 1996.

Pyevich, D., and M. P. Bogenschutz. "Herbal Diuretics and Lithium Toxicity." *American Journal of Psychiatry* 158 (2001): 1329.

See also: Loop diuretics; Osteoarthritis.

K

Kava

CATEGORY: Herbs and supplements
RELATED TERM: *Piper methysticum*
DEFINITION: Natural plant product used to treat specific health conditions.
PRINCIPAL PROPOSED USE: Anxiety
OTHER PROPOSED USES: Alcohol withdrawal, headaches, insomnia, tension headaches

OVERVIEW

Kava is a member of the pepper family that has long been cultivated by Pacific Islanders for use as a social and ceremonial drink. The first description of kava came to the West from Captain James Cook on his celebrated voyages through the South Seas. Cook reported that on occasions when village elders and chieftains gathered together for significant meetings, they would hold an elaborate kava ceremony. Typically, each participant would drink two or three bowls of chewed kava mixed with coconut milk. Kava was also drunk in less formal social settings as a mild intoxicant.

When they learned about kava's effects, European scientists set to work trying to isolate its active ingredients. However, it was not until 1966 that substances named kavalactones were isolated and found to be effective sedatives. One of the most active of these is dihydrokavain, which has been found to produce a sedative, painkilling, and anticonvulsant effect. Other named kavalactones include kavain, methysticin, and dihydromethysticin.

High doses of kava extracts are thought to cause muscle relaxation and even paralysis (without loss of consciousness) at very high doses. Kava also has local anesthetic properties, producing peculiar numbing sensations when held in the mouth.

The method of action of kava is not fully understood. Conventional tranquilizers in the Valium family interact with special binding sites in the brain called GABA receptors. Early studies of kava suggested that the herb does not affect these receptors. However, more recent studies have found an interaction. The early researchers may have missed the connection because kava appears to affect somewhat unusual parts of the brain. An accumulation of case reports suggests that kava products may rarely cause severe liver injury, and this has led to a banning of kava by many countries.

High doses of kava extracts are thought to cause muscle relaxation and even paralysis (without loss of consciousness) at very high doses. (Inga Spence/ Getty Images)

THERAPEUTIC DOSAGES

A typical dosage of kava when used for treatment of anxiety is 300 milligrams (mg) daily of a product standardized to contain 70 percent kavalactones. A lower dose of 150 mg daily has also been tested but may be less effective. The typical dosage for insomnia is 210 mg of kavalactones one hour before bedtime.

THERAPEUTIC USES

In 1990, Germany's Commission E authorized the use of kava for relieving "states of nervous anxiety, tension, and agitation," based on evidence from several double-blind studies. However, case reports of liver damage later led Germany and other countries to ban the sale of kava.

Like other anxiety-reducing drugs, kava could be useful for insomnia, but most of the supporting evidence for this use remains highly preliminary. One small, double-blind study found that daily use of kava reduced sleep disturbances linked to anxiety. However, a larger study failed to find benefits in people with both insomnia and anxiety.

One animal study suggests that kava may also have value as an aid to alcohol withdrawal. (However, individuals who abuse alcohol are probably at increased risk of harm from kava.) Kava has been additionally proposed as a treatment for tension headaches, but it has not been evaluated for this purpose.

SCIENTIFIC EVIDENCE

Anxiety. There have been a minimum of about one dozen placebo-controlled studies of kava, involving a total of more than seven hundred people. Most found kava helpful for anxiety symptoms.

One of the best of these was a six-month, double-blind study that tested kava's effectiveness in one hundred people with various forms of anxiety. Over the course of the trial, they were evaluated with a list of questions called the Hamilton Anxiety Scale (HAM-A). The HAM-A assigns a total score based on such symptoms as restlessness, nervousness, heart palpitations, stomach discomfort, dizziness, and chest pain. Lower scores indicate reduced anxiety. Participants who were given kava showed significantly improved scores beginning at eight weeks and continuing throughout the duration of the treatment.

This study is notable for the long delay before kava was effective. Previous studies had shown a good response in one week. The reason for this discrepancy is unclear.

Several double-blind, placebo-controlled studies have specifically tested kava for the treatment of the anxiety that often occurs during menopause. In one study, forty women were given either kava plus standard hormone therapy or hormone therapy alone for a period of six months. The results showed that women given kava experienced greater improvement in symptoms than those given hormone therapy alone.

However, not all studies have been positive. One double-blind, placebo-controlled study failed to find kava effective for people with generalized anxiety disorder. Another study failed to find kava more effective than placebo for people with both anxiety and insomnia.

Besides these placebo-controlled studies, one six-month, double-blind study compared kava against two standard anxiety drugs (oxazepam and bromazepam) in 174 people with anxiety symptoms. Improvement in HAM-A scores was about the same in all groups. Another study found kava and the drugs buspirone and opipramol equally effective.

A five-week, double-blind, placebo-controlled trial studied forty people who had been taking standard antianxiety drugs (benzodiazepines) for an average duration of twenty months. Participants were gradually tapered off their medications and switched to kava or placebo. Individuals taking kava showed some improvement in anxiety symptoms. This would appear to indicate that kava can successfully be substituted for benzodiazepine drugs. However, participants who were switched from benzodiazepines to placebo showed little to no increase in anxiety, suggesting that perhaps they did not really need medication after all. Thus, the results of this study are hard to interpret.

This trial involved close medical supervision and very gradual tapering of benzodiazepine dosages. Individuals should not discontinue antianxiety medications without supervision; withdrawal symptoms can be life-threatening.

One study purported to find evidence that kava helps reduce reactions to stressful situations. However, the results mean little because the study lacked a placebo group.

SAFETY ISSUES

Until recently, kava had been considered a safe herb. Animal studies have shown that kava dosages of up to four times the normal amount cause no health problems, and thirteen times the normal dosage causes only mild problems in rats. A study of 4,049 people who took a rather low dose of kava (70 mg of kavalactones daily) for seven weeks found side effects in 1.5 percent of cases. These were mostly mild gastrointestinal complaints and allergic rashes.

A four-week study of 3,029 people given 240 mg of kavalactones daily showed a 2.3 percent incidence of basically the same side effects. One review of the literature concluded that the data support kava's safety in treating anxiety with 280 mg kava lactones daily for four weeks.

However, a growing number of case reports have raised serious concerns about kava's safety. These reports suggest that occasionally even normal doses of kava can cause severe liver injury. Based on these reports, regulatory agencies have taken action in numerous countries banning or restricting sale of kava. However, case reports are notorious for failing to show cause and effect, and some well-regarded experts who have reviewed the literature feel that kava has not been shown to be unsafe. In a report examining twenty-six alleged liver toxicity cases in kava users, consuming the herb at the recommended daily dose (less than 120 mg) and duration (less than three months) was clearly linked with only one case. In all other cases, kava either was not implicated, was taken inappropriately, or was combined with another drug.

At present, it is recommended that individuals who wish to use this herb seek physician supervision to monitor for liver inflammation. People who have liver problems, who drink alcohol excessively, or who take medications that can harm the liver are probably at increased risk of harm by kava.

There are other safety concerns as well. For example, kava should not be used by individuals who have had "acute dystonic reactions." These consist of spasms in the muscles of the neck and movements of the eyes, which are believed to be related to effects on dopamine. They are typically caused by antipsychotic drugs, which affect dopamine. Kava might also trigger such reactions.

At ordinary doses, kava does not appear to produce mental cloudiness. However, high doses cause inebriation and can lead to charges of driving under the influence of drugs.

One study suggests that kava does not amplify the effects of alcohol. However, there is a case report indicating that kava can increase the effects of certain sedative drugs. For this reason, kava probably should not be combined with any drugs that depress mental function. Kava should also not be combined with antipsychotic drugs or drugs used for Parkinson's disease, because of the potential for increased problems with movement.

The German Commission E monograph warns against the use of kava during pregnancy and nursing. Safety in young children and individuals with kidney disease has not been established.

IMPORTANT INTERACTIONS

Individuals who are taking medications for insomnia or anxiety, such as benzodiazepines, should not take kava in addition to them. For people who are using antipsychotic drugs, kava might increase the risk of a particular side effect consisting of sudden abnormal movements, called a dystonic reaction. Kava also might reduce the effectiveness of levodopa, which is taken for Parkinson's disease. In addition, individuals taking medications that can irritate the liver should avoid kava. Numerous medications have this potential, and individuals should consult with a physician to determine whether this concern applies to them.

EBSCO CAM Review Board

FURTHER READING

Anke, J., and I. Ramzan. "Abstract Kava Hepatotoxicity: Are We Any Closer to the Truth?" *Planta Medica* 70 (2004): 193-196.

Cairney, S., et al. "Saccade and Cognitive Impairment Associated with Kava Intoxication." *Human Psychopharmacology* 18 (2003): 525-533.

Geier, F. P., and T. Konstantinowicz. "Kava Treatment in Patients with Anxiety." *Phytotherapy Research* 18 (2004): 297-300.

Jacobs, B. P., et al. "An Internet-Based Randomized, Placebo-Controlled Trial of Kava and Valerian for Anxiety and Insomnia." *Medicine* 84 (2005): 197-207.

Lehrl, S. "Clinical Efficacy of Kava Extract WS 1490 in Sleep Disturbances Associated with Anxiety Disorders." *Journal of Affective Disorders* 78 (2004): 101-110.

Teschke, R., et al. "Kava Hepatotoxicity: A Clinical Survey and Critical Analysis of Twenty-Six Suspected Cases." *European Journal of Gastroenterology and Hepatology* 20 (2008): 1182-1193.

Thompson, R., et al. "Enhanced Cognitive Performance and Cheerful Mood by Standardized Extracts of *Piper methysticum* (Kava-Kava)." *Human Psychopharmacology* 19 (2004): 243-250.

See also: Anxiety; Headache, tension; Insomnia.

Kelp

CATEGORY: Herbs and supplements

RELATED TERM: Kombu

DEFINITION: Natural plant product used to treat specific health conditions.

PRINCIPAL PROPOSED USE: Nutrition

OTHER PROPOSED USES: Cancer prevention, colds and influenza, herpes, high blood pressure, human immunodeficiency virus infection support, weight loss

OVERVIEW

Kelp refers to several species of large, brown algae that can grow to enormous sizes far out in the depths of the ocean. Kelp is a type of seaweed, but not all seaweed is kelp: The term "seaweed" loosely describes any type of vegetation growing in the ocean, including many other types of algae and plants.

Kelp is a regular part of a normal human diet in many parts of the world, such as Japan, Alaska, and Hawaii. It is also incorporated into some vitamin and mineral supplements because of its nutrient value. Kelp is a good source of folic acid (a B vitamin), as well as many other vitamins and minerals–especially

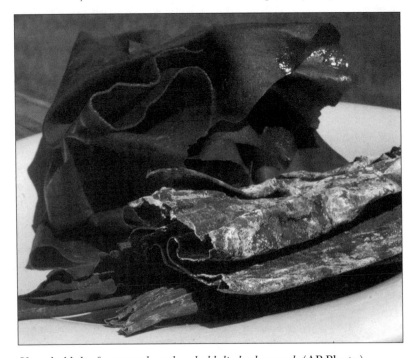

Uncooked kelp, foreground, and soaked kelp, background. (AP Photo)

iodine; but iodine is also a potential source of side effects.

REQUIREMENTS AND SOURCES

Supplements containing kelp can be purchased at most pharmacies and health food stores. Kelp used in food preparation is available at groceries that stock specialties for Asian cooking.

THERAPEUTIC DOSAGES

There is no appropriate therapeutic dosage of kelp, as it is not known whether kelp is truly therapeutic for any conditions. However, because of its high iodine content, it is important not to overdo the use of kelp. The iodine content in seventeen different kelp supplements studied by one group of researchers varied from 45 to 57,000 micrograms (mcg) per tablet or capsule. The recommended daily intake for iodine is 150 mcg per day for people over the age of four, and taking a great deal more than this can cause thyroid problems.

THERAPEUTIC USES

Kelp is used primarily as a nutrient-rich food supplement. The results of highly preliminary test-tube and animal studies have suggested other potential uses for kelp. For example, there is some evidence that elements in kelp might help to prevent infection with several kinds of viruses, including influenza, herpes simplex, and human immunodeficiency virus (HIV). Similarly weak evidence hints that kelp possesses cancer-preventive effects and may lower blood pressure. However, far more research, including double-blind, placebo-controlled studies, would be necessary to know whether kelp is actually helpful for any of these health problems.

Additionally, kelp has been marketed as a weight-loss product, but there are no meaningful scientific studies to indicate that it is effective for this purpose. Another common claim regarding kelp is that, because of its high iodine content, it can help all kinds of thyroid problems. This claim, however, is misleading and even dangerous. It is true that kelp is probably good for people who are deficient in iodine, but iodine deficiency is rare, and taking extra iodine when it is not needed can cause dysfunction of the thyroid.

SAFETY ISSUES

Taking excessive kelp can overload the body with iodine and cause either hypothyroidism or hyperthyroidism, conditions in which the thyroid gland produces either too little or too much thyroid hormone. This potentially dangerous side effect is definitely cause for caution. Individuals whose thyroid gland is already functioning incorrectly should avoid high doses of kelp except on a physician's advice.

Additionally, published reports describe two cases of acne apparently caused or worsened by taking large doses of kelp. This effect is also believed to be due to the large amounts of iodine in the supplement.

Finally, some kelp supplements have been found to contain levels of arsenic high enough to be toxic. Seawater contains highly diluted arsenic, but kelp, like other ocean life, can concentrate arsenic in its tissues, and there are reports of two people with symptoms of arsenic poisoning who had been consuming kelp.

EBSCO CAM Review Board

FURTHER READING

Amster, E., et al. "Case Report: Potential Arsenic Toxicosis Secondary to Herbal Kelp Supplement." *Environmental Health Perspectives* 115 (2007): 606-608.

Clark, C. D., et al. "Effects of Kelp Supplementation on Thyroid Function in Euthyroid Subjects." *Endocrine Practice* 9 (2003): 363-369.

Shan, B. E., et al. "Immunomodulating Activity of Seaweed Extract on Human Lymphocytes In Vitro." *International Journal of Immunopharmacology* 21 (1999): 59-70.

See also: Cancer risk reduction; Colds and flu; Herpes; Hypertension; HIV support.

Kidney stones

CATEGORY: Condition
RELATED TERMS: Bladder stones, calcium oxalate stones, nephrolithiasis, renal calculi, urinary calculi, urolithiasis

DEFINITION: Treatment of crystallized chemicals in the kidneys.
PRINCIPAL PROPOSED NATURAL TREATMENT: Citrate
OTHER PROPOSED NATURAL TREATMENTS: Aloe, goldenrod (and other diuretic herbs, such as buchu, cleavers, dandelion, juniper, parsley, horsetail, and rosemary), fish oil, gamma-linolenic acid, magnesium, pumpkin seeds, rose hips, vitamin B_6
HERBS AND SUPPLEMENTS TO USE ONLY WITH CAUTION: Calcium, grapefruit juice, phosphorus, vitamin C

INTRODUCTION

The sharp and irregular objects known as kidney stones travel down the slender tube (ureter) leading from the kidney to the bladder, and from the bladder to the urethra, following the path by which urine exits the body. Tiny stones may pass unnoticed, but a larger stone can induce some of the worst pain that humans experience.

Most kidney stones are composed of calcium and oxalic acid, substances present in the urine that can crystallize inside the kidneys. Although these chemicals occur in the urine of all humans, natural biochemistry is usually able to prevent them from crystallizing. However, sometimes these protective methods fail and a stone develops. Less commonly, kidney stones may be made from calcium and phosphate, from another substance called struvite (usually the result of an infection) or, rarely, from uric acid or cystine. This article focuses mainly on the calcium oxalate stones.

It is not known why some people develop kidney stones and others do not. However, once a person has a stone, he or she is fairly likely to develop another.

Low fluid intake greatly increases the risk of developing virtually all types of stones. For this reason, persons at risk of developing stones are often advised to increase their fluid intake. However, while there is evidence that fluids in the form of coffee, tea, beer, and wine can decrease risk of kidney stone development, apple juice and grapefruit juice may have the opposite effect.

High intakes of sodium and protein (particularly animal protein) may also increase the risk of calcium oxalate stones, although some studies have found that protein has no such effect. Oxalate-rich foods, such as spinach, rhubarb, and cocoa, may also increase the risk of developing calcium oxalate stones. Indirect evidence suggests that the regular use of cranberry concentrate tablets might also increase the risk of kidney stones. In addition, vitamin D affects calcium levels in the body, and prolonged use of extremely excessive doses of vitamin D has been known to cause kidney stones. High-calcium foods, however, do not seem to increase the risk of calcium oxalate stones.

Conventional treatment for kidney stones varies depending on symptoms and the location and chemical composition of the stones. For those who pass a stone spontaneously, the main treatments are painkillers and fluids. The chemical composition of passed stones can be analyzed to determine their cause. Other stones may be detected earlier, when they are still in the kidney. Treatment depends on their location and symptoms. Those stones that cause problems may be treated with extracorporeal shock-wave lithotripsy, a technique that can break up the stones from outside the body, allowing them to pass more easily. Occasionally, however, surgery may be necessary.

"Silent" stones, or those causing no symptoms, are often treated with preventive measures alone. These methods include increasing fluids, modifying the diet, and taking drugs or supplements to alter the chemistry of the urine.

PRINCIPAL PROPOSED NATURAL TREATMENTS

Citrate. Citrate, or citric acid, is an ordinary component of the human diet, present in high amounts in citrus fruits. Citrate binds with calcium in the urine, thereby reducing the amount of calcium available to form calcium oxalate stones. Citrate also prevents tiny calcium oxalate crystals from growing and massing together into larger stones. Finally, citrate makes the urine less acidic, which inhibits the development of both calcium oxalate and uric acid stones.

One form of citrate supplement, potassium citrate, was approved by the U.S. Food and Drug Administration in 1985 for the prevention of two kinds of kidney stones: calcium stones (including calcium oxalate stones) and uric acid stones. In a three-year double-blind study of fifty-seven people with a history of calcium stones and low urinary citrate levels, those given potassium citrate developed fewer kidney stones than they had previously. In comparison, the group given placebo had no change in their rate of stone formation.

Potassium-magnesium citrate was studied in a three-year trial involving sixty-four participants with a history of calcium oxalate stones. During the study,

new stones formed in only 12.9 percent of those taking the potassium-magnesium citrate supplement, compared to 63.6 percent of those taking placebo. Benefits have been seen in other small studies too.

Citrate is available in the form of calcium citrate. Besides increasing citrate in the urine, this supplement has the advantage of being a readily absorbed form of calcium for those seeking to increase their calcium intake for other health reasons. However, calcium citrate has not been studied as a preventive for kidney stones.

Some physicians have proposed drinking citrus juices as a means of increasing urinary citrate levels. Like potassium citrate, orange juice decreases urinary acidity and raises urinary citrate, but it also raises urinary oxalate, which might tend to work against its beneficial effects. Lemon juice may be preferable, as it has almost five times the citrate of orange juice. A small study found that drinking two liters of lemonade daily doubled urinary citrate in people with decreased urinary citrate. One should avoid regular consumption of grapefruit juice, however: In one large-scale study, women drinking eight ounces of grapefruit juice daily increased their risk of stones by 44 percent.

It was first thought that citrate supplements were helpful against kidney stones only in persons who did not excrete the normal amount of citrate in their urine. Some researchers now suggest that citrate treatment may also be useful for those at risk for stones whose citrate excretion is normal. The proper dosage of citrate depends on the chemical form and should be individualized under medical supervision.

Potassium citrate can irritate the gastrointestinal tract, causing upset stomach or bloating in 9 to 17 percent of people who take it. Potassium-magnesium citrate may potentially cause the same problem, although one study found it to be no more irritating than placebo.

Supplements containing potassium have the potential to raise blood levels of potassium too high, primarily in people with impaired kidneys or those taking a potassium-sparing diuretic such as triamterene. Taking too much citrate can also result in overly alkaline blood, again particularly in people with kidney disease.

Citrate-induced reduction of urinary acidity can lead to decreased blood levels and effectiveness of numerous drugs, including lithium, methotrexate, oral diabetes drugs, aspirin and other salicylates, and

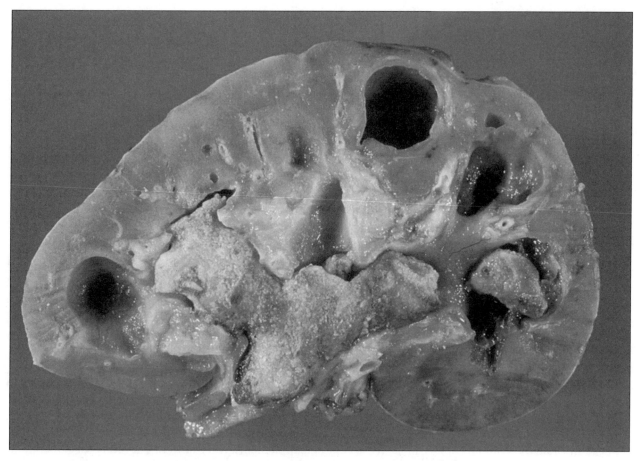

Sectioned kidney showing stone. (Dr. E. Walker/Getty Images)

tetracycline antibiotics. In addition, the urinary antiseptic methenamine is less effective in alkaline urine. Conversely, the blood levels of other drugs could increase, possibly increasing the risk of toxicity. These drugs include stimulants, such as ephedrine and methamphetamine, and the drugs flecainide and mecamylamine.

OTHER PROPOSED NATURAL TREATMENTS

Magnesium, in the form of magnesium oxide or magnesium hydroxide, may help to prevent calcium oxalate stone development. Magnesium inhibits the growth of these stones in the test tube and decreases stone formation in rats. However, human studies on magnesium have shown mixed results. In one two-year open study, 56 persons taking magnesium hydroxide had fewer recurrences of kidney stones than 34 persons not given magnesium. In contrast,

a double-blind (hence, far more reliable) study with 124 people found that magnesium hydroxide was essentially no more effective than placebo.

Two studies performed in Thailand hint that pumpkin seeds might help to prevent kidney stones among children at high risk for developing them. However, this research looked only at chemical changes in the urine suggestive of a possible preventive effect, not at actual reduction of stones. Furthermore, the design of the studies did not reach modern standards.

The herb rose hips might also improve the chemical composition of urine and thereby reduce kidney stone risk. However, rose hips are very high in vitamin C, and vitamin C itself has shown potential risks in people with a tendency toward stones.

Vitamin B_6 might help prevent calcium oxalate stones in certain persons. Deficiencies in this vitamin increase the amount of oxalate in the urine of animals

Symptoms of Kidney Stones

The symptoms that accompany urinary stone disease are dependent on the location of the stone, the size of the stone, how long the stone has been present, whether infection is associated with the stone, and the degree of obstruction to urinary flow caused by the stone. Stones caught in the renal pelvis, prior to entry into the ureter, generally cause an intermittent, sharp pain in the back or side. Stones that pass into the ureter can cause pain in the back as well as points distant from the urinary system (the groin, the lower abdomen, and the testicles and penis in men); this phenomenon is known as referred pain. Occasionally, stones in the lowest portion of the ureters will cause pain only with urination or produce the desire to urinate frequently but only in small amounts.

John F. Ward, M.D., and Prodromos G. Borboroglu, M.D

and humans, and a small uncontrolled study found that supplementation decreased oxalate excretion in people with a history of stones. In addition, a fourteen-year observational study of more than 85,000 women with no history of kidney stones found that women with high intakes of vitamin B_6 developed fewer stones than those with the lowest intake. A large-scale observational study of more than 45,000 men found no link between vitamin B_6 and stones. (Observational studies are notorious for producing misleading results. Only double-blind trials can provide evidence of benefit.) Several supplements, including fish oil, gamma-linolenic acid, glycosaminoglycans, and vitamin A and aloe, are also sometimes recommended for kidney stones, but there is only scant preliminary evidence to suggest that they are helpful.

A variety of herbs are often recommended for kidney stones, on the theory that they increase urine flow, which will help pass kidney stones. These herbs include asparagus, birch leaf, bishop's weed fruit, buchu, cleavers, couch grass, dandelion, goldenrod, juniper, rosemary, horsetail, java, lovage, parsley, petasites, shiny restharrow, and stinging nettle herb and root combinations. However, there is no meaningful evidence that they are effective.

One study claimed to find trigger point injection (a form of treatment somewhat related to acupuncture) helpful for reducing the pain of kidney stones.

However, because the study lacked a placebo group, the results are unreliable.

HERBS AND SUPPLEMENTS TO USE WITH CAUTION

According to some research, the use of vitamin C supplements can slightly raise levels of oxalate in the urine, which could, in turn, increase the risk of kidney stones. However, large-scale observational studies have found that people who consume large amounts of vitamin C have no increased risk or even a decreased risk of kidney stone formation. Nonetheless, it seems that in certain people, high vitamin C intake can lead to a rapid increase in urinary oxalate, and in one case stones developed within a few days. People with a history of kidney stones should probably limit vitamin C supplements to about 100 milligrams daily.

Calcium supplements also present concerns, because they could conceivably increase formation of calcium oxalate or other calcium-based stones. Observational studies and other forms of preliminary evidence do suggest that the use of calcium supplements may slightly increase kidney stone risk. Increased intake of calcium from food, however, does not seem to be associated with increased risk of kidney stones and could even help prevent them. Therefore, persons with a history of kidney stones might be best advised to get their calcium from food rather than from supplements. Alternatively, one study suggests that if calcium supplements are taken with food, no harm results. Furthermore, the use of calcium as calcium citrate may present no increased risk, presumably because the citrate portion of the supplement has activity against kidney stones.

Some evidence hints that excessive consumption of phosphorus in the form of soft drinks might increase kidney stone risk, but study results are contradictory, and if there is an effect, it appears to be small. Also, regular consumption of grapefruit juice may significantly increase the risk of stones.

EBSCO CAM Review Board

FURTHER READING

Allie-Hamdulay, S., and A. L. Rodgers. "Prophylactic and Therapeutic Properties of a Sodium Citrate Preparation in the Management of Calcium Oxalate Urolithiasis." *Urological Research* 33 (2005): 116-124.

Curhan, G. C., et al. "Beverage Use and Risk for Kidney Stones in Women." *Annals of Internal Medicine* 128 (1998): 534-540.

Heller, H. J., et al. "Effect of Dietary Calcium on Stone Forming Propensity." *Journal of Urology* 169 (2003): 470-4.

Kirdpon, S., et al. "Changes in Urinary Compositions Among Children After Consuming Prepared Oral Doses of Aloe (*Aloe vera* Linn.)." *Journal of the Medical Association of Thailand* 89 (2006): 1199-1205.

Rodgers, A. "Effect of Cola Consumption on Urinary Biochemical and Physicochemical Risk Factors Associated with Calcium Oxalate Urolithiasis." *Urological Research* 27 (1999): 77-81.

Sakhaee, K., et al. "Stone Forming Risk of Calcium Citrate Supplementation in Healthy Postmenopausal Women." *Journal of Urology* 172 (2004): 958-961.

Traxer, O., et al. "Effect of Ascorbic Acid Consumption on Urinary Stone Risk Factors." *Journal of Urology* 170 (2003): 397-401.

See also: Calcium; Gallstones; Pain management.

Kombucha tea

CATEGORY: Herbs and supplements
RELATED TERMS: Kargasok tea, Kargasoki mushroom, Kargasoki tea, Kombucha mushroom, Manchurian mushroom
DEFINITION: Natural plant product used to treat specific health conditions.
PRINCIPAL PROPOSED USES: None

OVERVIEW

Just as friends can pass along sourdough starter, a small, round, flat, gray, gelatinous object has become a popular gift among those interested in natural medicine. Individuals insert this object in sweetened black tea and let it ferment for seven days. By the end of the week, it creates a strong-tasting drink and a big, flat, gray, gelatinous object that can be cut up and passed on to friends.

Described variously as Manchurian mushroom, Kombucha tea, or just Kombucha, this tea is said to have been used for centuries to cure a wide variety of illnesses. The earliest known scientific analysis of Kombucha occurred in Germany in the 1930s, and subsequent studies have provided accurate information about this dubious product.

The word "kombucha" literally means "tea made from kombu seaweed." However, what is called Kom-

bucha tea today has no seaweed in it. Furthermore, despite the name "Manchurian mushroom," Kombucha is not a mushroom either. The gelatinous mass is a colony of numerous species of fungi and bacteria living together, and the same microorganisms permeate the tea. The precise composition of any sample of Kombucha depends to a great extent on what was floating around in the kitchen when it was grown.

The microorganisms most commonly found in Kombucha tea include species of *Brettanomyces*, *Zygosaccharomyces*, *Saccharomyces*, *Candida*, *Torula*, *Acetobacter*, and *Pichia*. However, some analyzed specimens have been found to contain completely different organisms, and there is no guarantee that they will be harmless.

THERAPEUTIC DOSAGES

The use of homemade Kombucha tea is not recommended. Commercially produced Kombucha should be safer, but it has no known medicinal effects.

THERAPEUTIC USES

Kombucha tea is widely supposed to have miraculous medicinal properties, ranging from curing cancer to restoring gray hair to its original color. Other reputed effects include normalizing weight, improving blood pressure, increasing energy, decreasing arthritis pain, restoring normal bowel movements, removing wrinkles, curing acne, strengthening bones, improving memory, and generally solving every health problem that exists. However, there is no evidence that Kombucha tea is effective for these or any other uses.

SAFETY ISSUES

In a set of animal studies, researchers prepared a batch of Kombucha and found that it was essentially nontoxic when taken at appropriate doses. However, because Kombucha is a complex and variable mixture of microorganisms, it is not clear that any other batch of the tea would be equally safe. In fact, there are case reports which suggest that Kombucha preparations can cause such problems as nausea, jaundice, shortness of breath, throat tightness, headache, dizziness, liver inflammation, and even unconsciousness. It is not clear whether the cause of these symptoms is an unusual reaction to a generally nontoxic substance or a response to unusual toxins that developed in a particular batch of Kombucha.

In addition, there is one case report of severe lead poisoning caused by regular use of Kombucha brewed in a ceramic pot. When it is brewed or stored in some ceramics, a risk of lead poisoning results because Kombucha tea is acidic. Many ceramic glazes contain a low level of lead that would not make the pottery dangerous for ordinary use, but if an acidic solution like Kombucha is steeped in them for a long time, a dangerous amount of lead may leech into the solution.

There is also one report of Kombucha becoming infected with anthrax and passing along the infection to an individual who rubbed it on his skin to alleviate pain. Apparently, anthrax from nearby cows got into the Kombucha mixture and grew.

EBSCO CAM Review Board

FURTHER READING

Vijayaraghavan, R., et al. "Subacute (Ninety Days) Oral Toxicity Studies of Kombucha Tea." *Biomedical and Environmental Sciences* 13 (2000): 293-299.

See also: Black tea.

Krill oil

CATEGORY: Functional foods
DEFINITION: Natural food product promoted as a dietary supplement for specific health benefits.
PRINCIPAL PROPOSED USES: Dysmenorrhea, high cholesterol, premenstrual syndrome
OTHER PROPOSED USES: Allergies, Alzheimer's disease, angina, ankylosing spondylitis, asthma, attention deficit disorder, bipolar disorder, borderline personality disorder, cancer treatment support, chronic fatigue syndrome, congestive heart failure, Crohn's disease, depression, diabetic neuropathy, eczema prevention, epilepsy, gout, heart disease prevention, human immunodeficiency virus infection, hypertension, kidney stones, liver disease, lupus, macular degeneration, male infertility, migraine headaches, multiple sclerosis, osteoporosis, postpartum depression, pregnancy support, prevention of premature birth, prostate cancer prevention, psoriasis, Raynaud's phenomenon, retinitis pigmentosa, rheumatoid arthritis, schizophrenia, sickle-cell anemia, stroke prevention, surgery support, ulcerative colitis, undesired cancer-related weight loss

OVERVIEW

Krill are tiny, shrimp-like crustaceans that flourish in the Antarctic Ocean and provide food for numerous aquatic animals. Oil made from krill appears on the market as an alternative to fish oil. Like fish oil, krill oil contains the omega-3 fatty acids eicosapentaenoic acid and docosahexaenoic acid. Krill also contains omega-6 fatty acids, an antioxidant in the carotenoid family called astaxanthin, and substances called phospholipids.

SOURCES

Many grains, fruits, vegetables, sea vegetables, and vegetable oils contain significant amounts of essential fatty acids, but krill oil is an especially rich source. Carotenoids are also found in many foods, especially yellow-orange and dark green fruits and vegetables. Carotenoids are not essential nutrients (except insofar as some can be converted to vitamin A), but they might offer some health benefits. Phospholipids are utilized in the body for numerous purposes, but they are not essential nutrients.

THERAPEUTIC DOSAGES

A typical recommended dose of krill oil is 1 to 3 grams (g) daily.

THERAPEUTIC USES

Based on its omega-3 fatty acid content, krill oil would be expected to have many of the same effects as fish oil. A few studies have evaluated krill oil specifically. In one double-blind, placebo-controlled study, 120 people with high cholesterol were given krill oil, fish oil, or placebo. The results for a three-month-period showed that krill oil (taken at a dose ranging from 1 to 3 g daily, depending on body mass and what group the participants were assigned to) improved all aspects of cholesterol profile compared with placebo, and it was more effective than fish oil (taken at the fixed dose of 3 g daily). Krill oil also reduced blood sugar levels. Though these results need to be confirmed by independent trials, they are certainly promising.

Another double-blind study compared krill oil with fish oil for the treatment of symptoms of premenstrual syndrome and dysmenorrhea (menstrual cramps). This study had many problems in design and reporting, but it appeared to show that krill oil was more effective than fish oil for treating both of these conditions. A badly designed study hints that krill oil might be helpful for both osteoarthritis and rheumatoid arthritis.

SAFETY ISSUES

Based on its known constituents, krill oil would be expected to have little to no toxicity. Side effects seen in studies are limited to occasional digestive distress and allergic reactions. The only known potential concerns relate to possible blood-thinning effects: Fish oil is known to decrease blood coagulation, and in one case report it increased the effect of the blood-thinning medication warfarin (Coumadin). People who are at risk of bleeding complications for any reason should consult a physician before taking krill oil. Maximum safe doses in young children, pregnant or nursing women, and people with severe liver disease have not been established.

EBSCO CAM Review Board

FURTHER READING

Buckley, M. S., et al. "Fish Oil Interaction with Warfarin." *Annals of Pharmacotherapy* 38 (2004): 50-52.

Bunea, R., et al. "Evaluation of the Effects of Neptune Krill Oil on the Clinical Course of Hyperlipidemia." *Alternative Medicine Review* 9 (2005): 420-428.

Deutsch, L. "Evaluation of the Effect of Neptune Krill Oil on Chronic Inflammation and Arthritic Symptoms." *Journal of the American College of Nutrition* 26 (2007): 39-48.

Sampalis, F., et al. "Evaluation of the Effects of Neptune Krill Oil on the Management of Premenstrual Syndrome and Dysmenorrhea." *Alternative Medicine Review* 8 (2003): 171-179.

See also: Cholesterol, high; Dysmenorrhea; Fish oil; Functional foods: Introduction; Premenstrual syndrome (PMS).

Kudzu

RELATED TERM: *Pueraria lobata*

CATEGORY: Herbs and supplements

DEFINITION: Natural plant product used to treat specific health conditions.

PRINCIPAL PROPOSED USES: None

OTHER PROPOSED USES: Alcoholism, common cold, menopausal symptoms

OVERVIEW

The herb *Pueraria lobata*, best known as kudzu, is cooked as food in China, and it also is used as an herb in traditional Chinese medicine. However, in the United States, kudzu has become an invasive plant pest. It was deliberately planted early in the twentieth century for use as animal fodder and to control soil erosion. The plant turned out to be incredibly prolific and soon spread throughout the southern United States. Kudzu can grow one foot per day during the summer months and as much as 60 feet each year, giving it the folk name "mile-a-minute vine." It wraps around telephone poles and trees and invades yards and fields.

THERAPEUTIC DOSAGES

The standard dosage of kudzu ranges from 9 to 15 grams daily and is consumed in tea or taken as tablets.

THERAPEUTIC USES

Besides cooking with it, feeding it to animals, and weaving baskets out of its rubbery vines, people have also used kudzo in treating alcoholism. In Chinese folk medicine, a tea brewed from kudzu root is believed to be useful in sobering up people who are intoxicated by alcohol. A 1993 study evaluated the effects of kudzu in a species of hamsters known to drink alcohol to intoxication. Ordinarily, if given a choice, the Syrian golden hamster will prefer alcohol to water, but administration of kudzu reversed that preference.

This animal study, along with another one involving rats, led to widespread speculation that kudzu may be useful in the treatment of alcoholism in humans. However, the results of small reported human trials are conflicting.

In academic Chinese herbology (as opposed to Chinese folk medicine), kudzu has different applications. One classic herbal formula containing kudzu is used for the treatment of colds accompanied by neck pain. However, there is no scientific evidence that it is effective for this condition.

Kudzu contains isoflavones similar to those found in soy. These substances are known to have an estrogen-like effect. On this basis, kudzu has been proposed as a treatment for menopausal symptoms. However, a published double-blind trial failed to find benefit.

SAFETY ISSUES

Based on its extensive food use, kudzu is believed to be reasonably safe. However, safety in young children, pregnant or nursing women, and those with severe kidney or liver disease has not been established.

Reviewed by EBSCO CAM Review Board

FURTHER READING

Lukas, S. E., et al. "An Extract of the Chinese Herbal Root Kudzu Reduces Alcohol Drinking by Heavy Drinkers in a Naturalistic Setting." *Alcoholism, Clinical and Experimental Research* 29 (2005): 756-762.

Shebek, J., and J. P. Rindone. "A Pilot Study Exploring the Effect of Kudzu Root on the Drinking Habits of Patients with Chronic Alcoholism." *Journal of Alternative and Complementary Medicine* 6 (2000): 45-48.

Woo, J., et al. "Comparison of *Pueraria lobata* with Hormone Replacement Therapy in Treating the Adverse Health Consequences of Menopause." *Menopause* 10 (2003): 352-361.

See also: Alcoholism; Colds and flu; Folk medicine; Herbal medicine; Isoflavones; Menopause; Soy; Traditional Chinese herbal medicine; Women's health.